WOMEN'S SEXUAL HEALTH

WOMEN'S
SEXUAL HEALTH

Edited by
Gilly Andrews RGN, ENB A08
Clinical Nurse Specialist in Family Planning,
King's College Hospital;
and Clinic Sister, Menopause and PMS Clinic,
The Lister Hospital, London, UK

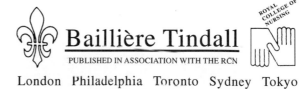

Baillière Tindall
PUBLISHED IN ASSOCIATION WITH THE RCN

London Philadelphia Toronto Sydney Tokyo

BAILLIÈRE TINDALL

An imprint of Harcourt Brace and Company Limited

© 1997 Baillière Tindall
© Harcourt Brace and Company Limited 1998
except Chapter 14, pp 336–364, copyright © Kathy Abernethy

Cover portrait of Susan Lamb, entitled 'Heaven and Earth', © Paula Cox

This book is printed on acid-free paper

A catalogue record for this book is available from the British Library

ISBN 0–7020–1898–8

Produced by Addison Wesley Longman China Limited, Hong Kong
GCC/02

CONTENTS

A colour plate section appears between pages 276–277

CONTRIBUTORS

Kathy Abernethy, RGN, FP Cert, ENB 225, Clinical Nurse Specialist (Menopause), Northwick Park Hospital, Watford Road, Harrow, Middlesex HA1 3UJ

Gilly Andrews, RGN, ENB A08, Clinical Nurse Specialist in Family Planning, King's College Hospital; and Clinic Sister, Menopause and PMS Clinic, The Lister Hospital, London

Gillian Aston, RN, RM, ADM, PGCEA, MA, Lecturer, School of Life, Basic Medical and Health Sciences, Division of Nursing and Midwifery, The Nightingale Institute, King's College, University of London, Cornwall House, 1 Waterloo Road, London SE1 8WA

Gay Curling, RGN, Onc. Cert, Clinical Nurse Specialist, Breast Diagnostic Unit, Royal Marsden NHS Trust, 203 Fulham Road, London SW3 6JJ

Mary Dolman, RGN, BSc, ENB 978, ET, Clinical Nurse Specialist/Continence, East Berkshire Community Health NHS Trust, St Marks Hospital, Maidenhead, Berks SL6 6JU

Suzanne Everett, RGN, RM, ENB 900, AO8 998, ENB 998, Diploma Counselling Skills, Clinical Nurse Specialist in Family Planning, Margaret Pyke Centre and Research Nurse, Margaret Pyke Trust, 73 Charlotte Street, London W1P 1LB

Kati Gray, RGN, RMN, BA (Hons) Registered Psychoanalytic Psychotherapist, Member of the Guild of Psychotherapists, Elizabeth Garrett Anderson Hospital for Women (UCL Hospitals NHS Trust), 144 Euston Road, London NW1 2AP

Marjorie Hickerton, RGN, FETC FP100 and Inst. ENB 985, A08, Cert in Counselling, Course 901 coordinator, Senior Nurse Specialist in Family Planning, Wandsworth, Merton and Sutton Community Trust, 63 Bevill Allen Close, Amen Corner, Tooting SW17

Liz Illman, RGN, ENB 900, AO8, Clinical Nurse Specialist in Family Planning and Women's Health, Nurse Counsellor, TOP Service, Gospel Oak Health Centre, Lismore Circus, London NW5 4QF

Jim Nash, RGN, RMN, BTTA, BSc (Hons), Dip N (Lond), PGCE, Nurse Teacher, Bloomsbury and Islington College of Nursing and Midwifery, Chenies Street, London, W1P 8AN

Sandy Nelson, BEd (Hons) Cantab., Lecturer in Sexual Health, Thames Valley University, Wolfson School of Health Sciences, 32–38 Uxbridge Road, Ealing, London W5 2SU

Vicky Padbury, RGN, ENB 900, A08, 998, Clinical Nurse Specialist in Family Planning, Liaison Family Planning Nurse for Secondary Schools, East Surrey, Contraception Helpline Information Worker, Family Planning Association, 2–12 Pentonville Road, London N1 9FP

Mary Power, SRN, SCM, IVF Coordinator, Lister Hospital, Chelsea Bridge Road, London SW1W 8RH

Imogen Rider, BSc (Hons), RGN, RM, ENB 225, ENB 998, ENB 901, Midwife, Obstetric Hospital, University College Hospital, Huntley Street, London WC1 6AE and Family Planning Nurse, King's College Hospital, London

Jane Selby, RGN, FPA, Cert, FETC, ENB A08, Clinical Nurse Specialist in Family Planning and Psychosexual Nurse Counsellor, Margaret Pyke Centre, 73 Charlotte Street, London W1P 1LB

Jill Steele, SRN, RHV, CMB (part 1), FPA Cert, Formerly Research Nurse, Department of Obstetrics and Gynaecology, UCL Hospitals NHS Trust, 86–96 Chenies Mews, London, WC1E 6HX

Catriona Sutherland, RGN, ENB A08, ENB 998 Practice Nurse and Clinical Nurse Specialist in Family Planning, Paxton Green Group Practice, 1 Alleyn Park, London SE21 8AU and Family Planning Nurse, Brook Advisory Centres, London

Karen Tierney, RGN, BSc, Onc. Cert. Advanced Breast Care Course, Macmillan Breast Care Nurse, St George's Hospital, Blackshaw Road, Tooting, London SW17

ACKNOWLEDGEMENTS

A multi-contributor book of this size inevitably involves a lot of hard work, liaison and research by all concerned, as well as the significant consumption of midnight oil in order to meet editorial deadlines. I am enormously grateful to all the authors for their support, enthusiasm and commitment to the idea of *Women's Sexual Health*. In writing their individual chapters each of them in turn has received support and advice from their partners, families, friends and work colleagues: my thanks are also due to them for their patience and encouragement. Maddy Ward (formerly Nurse Tutor at the Margaret Pyke Centre) and John Studd (consultant gynaecologist at the Chelsea and Westminster Hospital) both merit a particular mention from me for their guidance and wise advice throughout the preparation of this book.

Liz Illman, author of the chapter on promoting a healthy lifestyle, would like to record the help and advice she received from Pat Holder (Community Dietician, Royal Free NHS Trust); Carmel McLaughlin (Primary Care Nurse, Cleveland St Needle Exchange, Camden and Islington Community NHS Trust); Jane Pullin (Senior CNS, Alcohol Advisory Service, Camden and Islington Community NHS Trust); Lyn Szczpura (School Nurse, Severn NHS Trust); and Philippa White (Stop Smoking Programme Coordinator, Worcester and District Health Authority).

Jane Selby wishes to acknowledge groups of nurses, midwives and health visitors who have been leading groups in the study of psychosexual nursing, and without whom her chapter on psychosexual care could not have been written.

The staff at the Margaret Pyke Centre, particularly Ann Eady, have been a source of considerable advice and support to Sue Everett in her chapter on contraception and safe sex, as has Jane Urwin, medical information officer at the Family Planning Association.

Vicky Padbury, writer of the chapter on cervical screening, thanks Dr Joan Austoker of the Cancer Research Campaign, and, for their help in providing slides for the colour section, Peter Greenhouse from Ipswich Hospital and Professor McLean and Sister Carmel Flynn from The Royal Free Hospital, London.

Finally, I should like to thank Sarah James of Baillière Tindall for her unfailing patience, encouragement and sense of humour, ever since our first conversation which sowed the seeds for the project which has now borne fruit with the publication of *Women's Sexual Health*.

Gilly Andrews

INTRODUCTION

Sexual health is an increasingly high profile issue for health professionals, particularly since publication of the Government's *Health of the Nation* document (DOH, 1992). But the term 'sexual health' is used in many different ways: to some it simply means medical and physical problems associated with sexual activity, whilst to others it has broader connotations concerned with self-esteem and mutual fulfilment.

Recognizing these varying usages, this book, *Women's Sexual Health*, attempts to give a holistic and balanced view of women's sexual well-being, and of the inseparability of physical and mental health. It could perhaps have been entitled 'Women's Health' or 'Women's Health Problems' but neither of these alternatives was felt adequately to reflect the breadth of the issues it covers: how a particular illness or problem can influence a woman's sexuality and affect not only herself but also her family, her relationships, her job, her hopes and her fears.

The idea for a book on *Women's Sexual Health* sprang from a realization that there was no single comprehensive text book for nurses covering the whole range of women's health issues, though there are numerous excellent books available on specific subjects. In my roles both as an instructing nurse and as a lecturer on women's health issues, I am frequently asked by nurses of all levels of experience to recommend a suitable broad-based book that is well-researched and based on the requirements of today's nurses: I hope that this book meets their needs.

Women's Sexual Health is written specifically for nurses who are involved or interested in women's health matters, whether in primary care or within a hospital environment, whether pre-registration or undertaking further training. It is hoped that the book will be interesting and informative to other health professionals, and that they will find in it issues of relevance to their own fields of work.

The authors of each chapter have been chosen for their skill, expertise and knowledge of the subject, with the aim of giving the reader a thorough appreciation of the issues involved. All the chapters include suggestions for further reading, a comprehensive resources list for individual research and, where appropriate, suggestions of books suitable for recommendation to clients. Each chapter examines how a woman's sexuality can be affected by a particular disorder, and how you can acknowledge these concerns and incorporate holistic care into your own professional practice.

In order to feel confident in dealing with the broad issues surrounding sexual health and well-being, you should think carefully about three basic areas where you might need further training: your own personal knowledge base, your own values and beliefs, and your own skills, whether of a clinical and technical nature or in the field of counselling and communication. *Women's Sexual Health* should stimulate your thoughts in all these areas.

The book is divided into three sections. Section One, 'Women Today', explores the concept of sexuality within physical, psychological and social dimensions. It discusses the view that women's sexuality is not just about sex and is influenced throughout life by many important factors, such as culture, ethnicity, the environment, sexual orientation and lifestyle.

Section Two, 'Family Planning', discusses many of the issues surrounding female fertility. For centuries women have tried to control their own fertility: a concept difficult to imagine at the beginning of this century but now virtually a reality due to the advances in contraception over the past three decades. Many women, however, still assume that conception will follow immediately after contraception is stopped, and have not considered the possibility of subfertility problems. Others, whether using contraception or not, find unplanned and unwanted pregnancies occurring only too easily. This section explains and explores the options surrounding contraception, subfertility and unplanned pregnancy, and also focuses on sexuality during and after pregnancy.

Section Three, 'Women's Health Issues', concentrates on specific women's health problems. It provides referenced, up-to-date and accessible information, whilst adopting a health-oriented stance where appropriate. Screening programmes for cancer of the breast and cervix are now well established, and women's general health has improved dramatically over this century. However, in spite of these advances, women continue to have health problems that are unique to them as women. This section explains what these disorders are and outlines the treatment options available.

In your position as a nurse, you are perceived by your patients to be more approachable and to have more time available than the doctor to deal with what are often felt to be trivial 'women's problems'. Not only can this pose difficulties with time management, but you may feel uncertain of your knowledge, and be anxious as to how best to help your patients. *Women's Sexual Health* will provide a source of reference, enabling you to give an informed and positive response to their initial enquiries.

Internationally, women are becoming increasingly vocal on a number of issues, including their rights as women, their health, their education, their reproductive rights, poverty and violence. The 1995 United Nations Fourth World Conference on Women, held in Beijing, discussed all these areas of concern, and the World Health Organization (WHO) firmly stated that health security lies at the core of women's physical and mental well-being and should cover their entire lifespan. The WHO Global Commission on Women's Health called for government action to sustain the realization of women's health security by setting 'goals and targets to improve women's health, enhance their education and access to quality care, as well as to assure that women attain the highest possible level of health' (WHO, 1995).

In the UK we are continuing to improve women's health not only by Government initiatives such as *Health of the Nation*, and breast and cervical screening campaigns, but also by providing good quality health promotion, treatment and care within the primary care 'network' at local level. Women are becoming empowered to make free, informed and responsible choices regarding their health, but to do so they need the advocacy and support of the nurses who care for them. Nurses need to foster and build on the trust that their patients place in them: you are a key element in all healthcare teams and are playing a leading role in service provision.

References

Department of Health (1992) *The Health of the Nation.* HMSO, London.

World Health Organization (1995) WHO calls for better women's health security. Press release: WHO/53, Geneva.

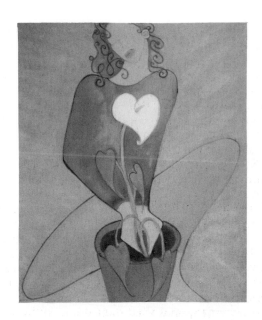

WOMEN TODAY

Women's sexuality
Promoting a healthy lifestyle
Psychosexual and emotional care
Young people and sex
Women with special needs and concerns

1: Women's sexuality
Sandy Nelson

OBJECTIVES

After reading this chapter you will have an understanding of:

♦ the relationship between gender and sexuality

♦ theories of sexuality

♦ female sexual development

♦ bisexual and lesbian sexuality

♦ the relationship between culture, ethnicity, religion and sexuality.

Introduction

The purpose of this chapter is to explore female sexuality. The way we think about sexuality directly influences practice and has implications for the services we provide. It is necessary to understand women's sexuality in holistic terms, otherwise we are likely to be limited in the help we offer.

Nurses are expected to promote sexual health as part of holistic health care. Yet the definition of sexual health implicit in the services provided focuses narrowly on contraception, disease control and the treatment of dysfunction. The World Health Organization provides a much broader definition. It defines sexual health as: 'the integration of the somatic, emotional, intellectual and social aspects of sexual being, in ways that are positively enriching and that enhance personality, communication and love.'

It is essential to think about sexuality in these broader terms, so that the needs of each woman can be reflected in the care provided. However, sexuality is one of the most difficult areas of human experience to define. It is complex, varied and contradictory. It involves desire and excitement,

intimacy and tenderness, risk and danger, love and hate in sometimes confusing combinations. Historically, how we think about sexuality has changed over time, and within our own lives we are likely to think about, experience and express our sexuality in many different ways. The same sexual act can be experienced variously as unique and exciting, or mundane and repetitive, depending on expectations, mood and the circumstances that surround it.

It is the most intimate and private aspect of our lives, yet the Church and State have always been involved in controlling sexuality. Consequently, it is both intensely personal and a matter of public concern. It is learnt through interactions with others in the home, at school and through the media but also meaning is created individually. Hence, although we are influenced by the expectations of others we also experience our own desires, which may differ from theirs.

Moreover, the history of human sexuality has, in many senses, been the history of male sexuality. Women's sexuality has mostly been seen as mysterious and unknown. It is constructed in relation to male sexuality, as basically reactive and responsive. Women, particularly in the last three decades, have challenged this way of seeing female sexuality and have provided important new insights.

There are many competing theories of female sexuality, some of which will be introduced in this chapter. What is of fundamental importance is to question the theories that inform current practices and to be aware of the assumptions made about women's sexuality as these affect sexual health in ways that are both subtle and powerful.

The relationship between gender and sexuality

A discussion of women's sexuality implies that female sexuality is distinct and separate from male sexuality. It seems evident that this is so as most sexual health services are predicated on that understanding. Indeed, it is almost impossible to separate gender and sexuality in our thinking. We think of biological sex and gender interchangeably. Biological sex refers to male or female physical characteristics, whereas gender refers to how we are expected to behave as men and women and has different meanings in different cultures and times. Biological sex itself is sometimes hard to determine, and transsexuals confound all our rigid assumptions about the relationship of gender to biology.

Gender and sexuality are fundamental to our sense of self, and because they are seen as natural, the beliefs and assumptions which are implicit in how we think about them are taken for granted. This has important implications when we consider sexual health care. It is imperative to look critically at both gender and sexuality and become aware of the way they are socially constructed.

How each woman constructs her own understanding of what it means to be a woman and to be sexual will influence her profoundly. Whether or not a woman uses contraception, or is able to negotiate safer sex, will necessarily involve how she thinks about her sexuality and herself as a woman. Apparently simple decisions, such as whether 'to go on the Pill', will be imbued with meaning and will involve conscious and unconscious, rational and irrational elements as well as social and cultural values.

The relationship between gender and sexuality is complex and multifaceted. Consequently, it is possible that someone could see pregnancy as proof that they were a real woman. Indeed, many societies reinforce this view by according status to fecundity. This belief might then affect contraception use because of a conflict between a rational decision that pregnancy should be avoided, and a desire, not necessarily conscious, to get pregnant in order to affirm an insecure sense of gender identity or to attract social approval. This demonstrates how understanding a woman's beliefs about gender and sexuality can help to explain behaviour that may otherwise seem puzzling.

In the West, female sexuality has been constructed in terms of stereotypes of the whore and the Madonna. Women are seen sexually either as voracious and all consuming or pure and chaste. Women who are sexually active are often condemned for their behaviour and labelled as whores. Whilst this attitude has modified considerably it continues to affect women. Despite changes in the law, judges still question women who have been raped about their sexual histories, making their sexual behaviour as much on trial as the activities of the rapist. Young women may worry about their reputations and being called a 'slag' is a potent term of abuse (Holland *et al.*, 1990).

Women suffer the consequences of sexual activity through sanctions against them. In recent history women were placed in psychiatric hospitals because they were unmarried and pregnant. Prostitutes have long been seen as a source of disease and blamed for their work. In the UK, the Contagious Diseases Acts from 1864 until 1883 were directed against women working as prostitutes and the language used was moralistic and condemnatory, whereas the examination of soldiers was abandoned in 1859 as 'repugnant to the feelings of the men' (Davenport-Hines, 1990).

More recently, Cindy Patten (1994) explores how prostitutes were seen by epidemiologists and policymakers as a source of HIV infection to heterosexual men rather than as at risk of infection *from* men. This was despite the probability that female sex workers are more at risk from men because of the greater risk of male to female transmission of HIV infection (Johnson and Johnstone, 1993).

At the other extreme female purity is venerated, and honour and virtue are connected with chastity. In the nineteenth century, sexologists promoted the idea that sexual desire amongst respectable women did not exist (Caplan, 1987). Although these ideas have changed they still have relevance. In the United States there is an increasing trend for young women to pledge that they will remain virgins until they marry and the traditional nuclear family is still revered by many as the ideal.

Of course, women's total experience of sexuality does not fit in with either of these extremes. Actual behaviour and consciously held attitudes and beliefs always lie in uneasy relationship with one another and never more so than in relation to sexuality. However, it can be seen from this how difficult it can be for women to see their sexuality as positive and healthy. Young women, in particular, may feel vulnerable as they attempt to create an identity for themselves as adult, sexual and female amidst the contradictory messages they receive.

Gender-specific expectations are a filter through which sexual encounters are endowed with meaning. For example, men are often expected to separate sex from love whereas women are expected to relate sex to love (Holland *et al.*, 1990). This can lead to very different ways of seeing the same sexual encounter and can cause distressing communication problems as couples struggle to understand one another.

Men are seen as active in sex, as the knowing sexual agent; women as innocent and passive. If being active sexually is defined as male then for women to carry condoms can seem to threaten femininity.

The construction of femininity as passive conflicts with women's ability to negotiate safer sex. This is evident in the research into young women's sexual practices conducted by the Women, Risk and AIDS Project. They provide illuminating examples of how young women know about safer sex and intend to use condoms but undermine themselves because of ideas of appropriate female sexual behaviour. One young woman described her boyfriend telling her that the condom should be blown up before use. She knew that this was wrong but felt unable to tell him because boys are supposed to know about sex whereas women are not. Penetrative sex is still regarded as the definitive sex act. As a result, although young women were aware that their pleasure in sex was not necessarily related to penetration, they continued to define sexual relationships as 'going the whole way' or not (Holland *et al.*, 1990).

Although women are expected to be passive, female sexuality is presented as powerful and dangerous, able to provoke uncontrollable lust in men. Men are not held responsible for their sexual behaviour because of the supposedly overwhelming nature of their sexual urges. Women are held responsible for controlling male sexual behaviour as well as their own. The threat of male sexual violence is used to justify women's need for protection and safety and controls women's ability to freely express their sexuality. Men's frequent sexual irresponsibility is a contemporary problem because of the need to encourage men to use condoms to prevent the transmission of HIV infection.

Women see their bodies and their sexuality presented everywhere in Western society as a commodity. Women's bodies are presented as objects which must fit certain criteria in order to be seen as desirable. As a result, younger and younger women go on diets and become anorexic and older women resort to face lifts and plastic surgery in an attempt to fit the current definition of good looks. There is no place here for the ill or the elderly, and women who have had radical surgery, for example, have to find some way to come to terms with these pressures.

There are many subtle and complex connections between power and sexuality. The possession of money and power can determine the ability and ease of procuring and demanding sexual satisfaction. The lack of power women experience in patriarchal families may be partly responsible for the difficulty women have defining and insisting on their own sexual desires. Rape is an act of power over someone else where sex is used as the means of domination. Perpetrators of sexual abuse are attracted by the vulnerability of their victims. The need to empower women is, therefore, fundamental to sexual well-being.

A woman's sense of ownership of her own body, her understanding of her own sexuality and how she wishes to express it are essential preconditions for good sexual relationships. Gender expectations may create considerable conflict for women and limit their capacity to enjoy a positive female sexuality.

The power of women to define their own sexuality is also crucial in that male definitions of female sexuality have prevailed throughout history. An example of this is the following quotation from the work of Van de Velde, a sexologist who wrote in

1928: 'The wife must be *taught* not only how to behave in coitus, but, above all, how and what to feel in this unique act!' (Caplan, 1987).

More pertinent, perhaps, is the influence the male perspective has had on medical practices. A well-known example of this is the way many gynae-cologists used to insist that hysterectomies were good for women with the rationale that if women no longer needed a womb to bear children it would be better removed. A practice which came from a male perspective was presented as good medicine. Other practices can be seen to have more to do with male desire than female health. In the 1970s on billboards in California Caesareans were marketed for women with the slogan 'Keep your birth canal honeymoon fresh, have a caesar'. The 'marriage' stitch, which was an extra stitch given after birth to women with episiotomies to tighten the vaginal canal for their male partners, was another example. Women have challenged these practices and changes have resulted, but it is a useful reminder of the need to examine gender biases that might underpin current practices.

Theories of sexuality

The predominant view of sexuality is that it is natural and innate, yet what is taken as natural is by no means straightforward and uncontentious. The idea of sexuality as natural has implicit within it specific ideologies. Sexual behaviour is presented from a hierarchical value system with good, healthy, natural sex (heterosexual and for procreation) opposed to bad, unhealthy, unnatural sex (homosexual, depraved and diseased). Homosexuality and diverse forms of sexual expression occur throughout history and in all cultures. In some senses, therefore, they must count as 'natural' behaviour but this is omitted from these theories.

Biologists have studied sexuality as a natural drive which reveals the animal nature of mankind. A basic premise of all their work is that men and women are fundamentally different in their sexual needs and desires because of their genital and reproductive differences. Theories which purport to describe human sexuality have been based on creatures as different from human beings as worms and sparrows! Their arguments fail to convince for many reasons. First, animal sexual behaviour var-

ies so greatly that virtually any theory could be substantiated depending on what view you wished to promote. Secondly, supposedly scientific descriptions of animal behaviour use terms such as 'gang rape' and 'prostitution'. These descriptions are then presented as scientific evidence to support particular ideologies about sexuality.

Even the language used to describe the activity of sperm is gender coded. Thus it is described as thrusting, competitive, actively fighting its way to penetrate the passive, waiting ova.

Observed gender differences in human sexual behaviour are described as having a biological base:

> Because males have an almost infinite number of sperm, while women have a very restricted supply of eggs, it is deduced that men have an evolutionary propulsion towards spreading their seed to ensure diversity and reproductive success, and hence towards promiscuity, while women have an equal interest in reserving energy, an instinct for conservation and hence a leaning towards monogamy.
>
> (Weeks, 1986)

Biological theories have an appealing plausibility until we realize how much sexual behaviour they fail to explain. Sexual behaviour often proves more imaginative and varied than is recognized by these theories. Undoubtedly biology plays a part in human sexuality; reproductive capacities, in particular, are strikingly different for men and women. What is problematic is the attempt to explain all human behaviour on the basis of biology.

Sociologists provide a different framework for understanding sexuality, yet their arguments have similar flaws in that masculinity and femininity are seen in reductive terms, with social roles replacing biology as the essential root of sexual behaviour. Nurture and learned behaviour take over from biological explanations. In their case society rather than biology is seen as the predominant force. These are important influences on sexuality. The problem occurs when the attempt is made to explain all sexuality in these terms.

Psychoanalysis provides a more satisfactory range of theories of sexuality as it takes into account the meaning individuals give to their sexual activities. The role ascribed to the unconscious gives scope for fantasies, irrationality, contradictions and conflicts as the individual struggles to give meaning to psychic development. Neither gender identity nor sexual object choice (the gender of the desired sexual partner) are easily acquired, rather they are somewhat precariously attained through the resolution of developmental conflicts. There are many competing psychoanalytic theories of sexuality but Freud's work remains central (Freud, 1977). He saw human beings as all potentially bisexual, with gender identity and heterosexuality acquired through difficult developmental challenges which the infant negotiates his or her way through. The meaning each of us gives to sexual acts, to body parts and to relationships is far from straightforward and remains tenuous and provisional throughout our lives.

In psychoanalytic theory the roots of what is known as abnormal sexual behaviour are found in the infantile sexuality of all of us. Perverse solutions to developmental crises are available to everyone and heterosexuality is achieved only with difficulty. Within this framework it is possible to explain practices such as fetishism, and it is comprehensible that someone could be born biologically female, identify themselves as male and choose either gender or both as object choices.

However, there is a tension in Freud's work between his understanding of the complexity and fluidity of sexuality and his idea that there is a true adult sexuality. Homosexuality is regarded as a regression, as infantile, in opposition to heterosexuality which is described as 'mature object love'. His arguments were based on reproduction as the biological aim of sexuality. Because sexual acts *can* lead to procreation, it is argued, that is the purpose of sexuality. This is a basic premise of religious and biological views on sexuality upon which moral systems and scientific theories are founded. The problem is that, once again, human sexuality refuses to conform to this. It manifestly fails to explain the continuation of sexual desire after the menopause, when one partner is infertile, when contraception is being used and in homosexual relationships. The belief that sexual expression ought to be solely for procreation may produce guilt, shame or grief in individuals who are sexually active when not procreative, but it cannot explain the presence of sexual desire in these circumstances.

Also, Freud is less convincing about female sexuality, and his theory of penis envy, the claimed superiority of the vaginal orgasm and patriarchal view of women have been thoroughly critiqued by both psychoanalytic and feminist writers. By comparison, the work of Kinsey *et al.* (1953) and Masters and Johnson (1966) was refreshing. They debunked the myth of the superiority of the vaginal over the clitoral orgasm. They also emphasized the similarities of male and female sexual responses. Masters and Johnson were motivated by their beliefs in the equality of the sexes and their wish to promote good, satisfying sex as the foundation of marriage. However, their conclusions were influenced by this ideological position as much as the data. Consequently, although they emphasize similarities, their research shows that women and men have very different numbers of orgasms and their peak ages of sexual interest and activity are totally incompatible. Their work was funded to help marital happiness, yet, ironically, when orgasm is seen as central to sexual satisfaction the partner is relatively unimportant.

> With orgasm defined as the single, universal goal of what they call human sexual response, masturbation wins out every time as the most effective means of achieving it!
>
> (Segal, 1994)

Indeed, Masters and Johnson's work demonstrates that the penis has no great advantage over a hand, tongue or vibrator in bringing about orgasms, in fact, it rather suggests the reverse. If this is the case, and if orgasm is all important as a sexual goal, then heterosexuality has no inherent superiority over homosexuality.

Their work was conducted in a laboratory and they describe neat stages of responses and a linear progression of sexual excitement. Such descriptions are useful but many sexual encounters are experienced in more diverse ways that do not fit into their account.

These limitations to their theory should not detract from the importance of their contribution. Their work broke new ground and it has been used in combination with other approaches to form new sex therapies that are available to the benefit of many individuals and couples.

More recently, Michel Foucault's writing on sexuality has transformed the whole concept of sexuality, bringing about a radical examination of the concealed agendas in scientific, medical, psychological and sociological definitions of sexuality. His work usefully illuminates hidden assumptions, and brings into question how we think about power, diversity and identity in relation to sexuality (Foucault, 1987–88).

Finally, the feminist, gay and lesbian movements have fundamentally challenged traditional views of sexuality. Their campaigns and questions, in conjunction with the availability of birth control and safe terminations of pregnancy, have probably had more impact than anything else on women's sexuality and health. The availability of reliable birth control has profoundly affected the way women experience and think about their sexuality. It is possible, because of contraception, to separate sexuality from reproduction.

The advent of AIDS has also fundamentally affected how we think about sex. As a result of the AIDS epidemic, actual sexual practice has had to be examined more carefully and explicitly than ever before, and it has become even more imperative to understand sexual behaviour in all its complexity.

Female sexual development

The first thing that everyone wants to know about a newborn baby is its biological sex. People are uncomfortable around infants when neither their name nor their attire indicates their gender. We respond differently in both subtle and obvious ways to boy and girl babies. Our behaviour shapes the child's responses into conforming to gender-appropriate behaviours even, at times, when we consciously intend to do otherwise. How we do this and what we regard as acceptable and unacceptable varies in different eras and in different places. It is also the result of our own personal histories, how we feel about our own mothers and fathers, brothers and sisters. Much of what we communicate will be unconscious and irrational and will contain contradictions and conflicts. Each child will actively construct his or her individual meaning as they attempt to make sense of all these messages.

The way in which girls experience their bodies is crucially different from the way boys experience theirs. Boys handle their penises as a matter of course every day; they are visible, external and the changes in them are instantly obvious. For girls, the exploration of their genitals is less frequently a part of their daily experience. This is not to say that their curiosity and satisfaction in playing with their genitals is less than that of boys, but their actual experience is different in significant re-

spects. Many women have never looked at their own vulvas and indeed to do so is far from easy, given that it requires a mirror. Female genitals are often not accurately named. The vulva is referred to as the vagina. In Webster's dictionary, earlier this century, there was no word for female genitals except the vagina.

> One might question how pride in femininity could flourish at a time when our language did not include a word for the part of the female anatomy most richly endowed with sensory nerve endings and with no function other than that of sexual pleasure.
>
> (Golhor Lerner, 1988)

Vague information regarding sexuality and the nature of sexual differences can lead to anxiety, confusion and shame as the environment provides no language to help describe and understand sexual feelings. Gay and lesbian children face a similar challenge as little in the world around them reflects their experiences.

This sense of female bodies as mysterious and unknowable even to women themselves affects the expression of desire.

> The feminine sex organ is mysterious even to woman herself. . . . Woman does not recognise herself in it and this explains in large part why she does not recognise its desires as hers.
>
> (De Beauvoir, 1953)

The infant does not experience her or himself as either gender. There is ample evidence to indicate that both sexes believe that they could become the other sex. For Freud and other psychoanalytic writers this is central to infantile sexuality. The fear of castration for the boy and the castration that has already taken place for the girl, bring about different paths of development for girls and boys. Both sexes identify initially with the mother and the boy has to separate from her and learn to identify with his father, whereas the girl retains her identification with her mother but learns to desire her father. Whether this happens or not and how the crises are resolved by each individual child will provide the basis for their adult sexuality. The strength of this approach is that it accounts for the complexity of gender and sexual identity and demonstrates the role of fantasy and the unconscious.

Anyone who has contact with children knows that they have a rich and vivid fantasy life and that the distinction between reality and fantasy is only slowly and painfully learned. For the young baby there is no clear boundary between itself and the world. It is perhaps because of this that in all cultures the body is the boundary marker and many social and cultural rituals are organized around the body. In particular, the orifices are seen as central. Some anthropologists have suggested that the body is a metaphor for society and that therefore controlling what comes in and what goes out is crucial. Hence sexuality and its regulation is of public concern for any culture.

To the baby its body products are a source of pride and fascination. There is an erotic charge to sucking and defecating which is given up as controls are learned. These emerge again in foreplay and in many adult sexual activities. To the baby, all body parts and both sexes can be vested with sexual excitement. This is part of infantile sexuality and is given up slowly and with difficulty by the growing child. The roots of all 'abnormal' sexual behaviour can be found here. It reveals how sexuality can seek satisfaction in different ways, through any organ of the body and can be attached to any person we desire, regardless of their gender.

Because they have once been a source of intense pleasure and fascination, our body products can become a source of shame and disgust. Unconsciously we remember our earlier curiosity and feel a mixture of excitement and repulsion that can be hard to deal with. Nurses are constantly in touch with body products in a way that can cause discomfort for both them and their patients. Smell is important to sexual desire, and defecation and urination can be part of sexual activities. Yet the intimacy and potentially sexual nature of nursing tasks is not often thought about or spoken about. When sexuality is talked of, the body as a whole, touch, smell and the substances that issue from the body are ignored. Through examining infantile sexuality, it becomes evident that these are important foundations upon which our adult sexuality is formed.

As we mature, controls are developed but these can break down at critical points in our lives. Transitional maturational points (these are times of major social and biological change) are especially vulnerable times. Our infantile sexual conflicts can re-emerge in different ways at these times. This can add to the stresses experienced at puberty, marriage, pregnancy and at the menopause.

All of these transitions can bring up forgotten primitive anxieties that can shock women with their intensity. Ambivalent feelings and pressures to conform to impossibly conflicting expectations can make these times especially sensitive and demanding. Unlike the infant, adolescent and adult women are influenced by social and cultural values as well as by unconscious impulses and fantasies. This can produce feelings of shame and humiliation as adult controls seem less certain and irrational impulses are more demanding. Each woman will experience these transitions in her sexuality in unique ways. Assumptions we make during our work can inhibit patients from communicating distress they feel because they are not experiencing their pregnancy, for instance, as they think they ought to. Descriptions of puberty and the menopause can all too often become prescriptive as well as descriptive. Because of the values associated with good, natural sex it can be difficult to admit deviations from the hierarchy.

Bisexual and lesbian sexuality

From the picture drawn already about sexuality, lesbianism becomes more comprehensible as a choice all women could make. If we are to believe Freud, all of us are initially bisexual. Moreover, sexuality changes for many people throughout their lives.

Given the mutability of sexuality, it is easy to understand that someone can become lesbian after years of heterosexuality. Other women know they are attracted only to women from puberty and occasionally before. Still others have sexual encounters with women, but do not regard themselves as lesbians. Women may, therefore, identify themselves as lesbian, bisexual or heterosexual and the chosen identity may bear little relationship to the actual experiences of sex with other women. The choice of a lesbian or bisexual identity suggests an acceptance by these women of their sexuality. This is important for sexual health as self-esteem and self-acceptance greatly enhance sexual well-being.

Lesbians have become more visible in recent years but throughout history their existence has been ignored. Queen Victoria refused to believe lesbians existed (Ferris, 1993). This, at least, meant that there is no legislation against lesbians but it rendered them invisible. As female sexuality has been seen through male eyes it remains difficult for many men and women to understand how lesbians can have sex without a penis. Again we are confronted by how much sex continues to be defined by penile penetration. Because lesbians are seen as 'other' their differences from 'normal' heterosexuals are understood through frameworks that come from the dominant defining viewpoints. As a result, lesbians are understood in terms of 'butch' and 'femme' in an attempt to make sense of their practices to heterosexuals. Lesbians may indeed take on these roles, sometimes as a deliberate parody of heterosexual relationships and at other times because the women involved feel these roles to be appropriate. Any attempt to fit lesbian sexuality into these categories is made to render their sexuality less threatening. Lesbians are seen as outsiders. They may evoke strong feelings of excitement and danger, forbidden pleasures, disgust and abhorrence. That they may also be caring mothers, loving partners and may work as health care professionals cannot be contained in the usual construction of their sexuality.

Health care services have not taken into account the sexual health needs of lesbians. Services have been organized around contraception, disease control and fertility. Lesbians may require all of these services but there are many of their needs which are not catered for. The success of the Bernhard Clinic which was set up as part of the genito-urinary services in Charing Cross Hospital, London specifically for lesbians has demonstrated how much of an unmet need there was. This illustrates how narrow definitions of sexuality, embodied in the health care services provided, fail to cater not just for lesbians but for any woman whose sexual needs fall outside of the present parameters. Women who are disabled, who are ill, elderly or have learning difficulties similarly have to struggle to be seen as sexual and find services that cater for their sexual health needs.

Culture, ethnicity and religion

One of the fears most frequently expressed by health workers is of giving offence to women whose cultural and/or religious beliefs are different from their own. In order to counter this fear, attempts are made to find out the attitudes to sexuality found in other religions and cultures. This is a fascinating field of study but it is import-

ant that we are careful in how we use this information. Lists of cultural norms are of limited usefulness and can be applied in rigid and potentially racist ways (Montford and Skrine, 1993). Each woman's interpretation of her culture will be unique and the experiences of a second-generation Bengali woman, for instance, will differ from her mother's. There are as many differences within a culture as there are between them.

Also, attitudes and beliefs held publicly may bear little relation to practice. Roman Catholics who practice birth control and who have abortions despite their faith are a good example. This highlights how, for all of us, the beliefs that we hold and the values that we have may not be reflected in our behaviour. This can be a cause of shame and guilt and can be very detrimental to acknowledging our sexual health needs.

The complex relationship between different attitudes and values can also explain conflicting behaviour we observe in patients. For example, in some cultures menstruation is seen as an important regular cleansing for the body and is associated with health (Caplan, 1987). Contraceptives which interfere with menstruation can consequently be rejected as unhealthy because of this. This reminds us once more that it is essential to explore the individual's own understanding of their health and sexuality in order to offer appropriate help.

One danger is that we will overidentify with people who have similar backgrounds to our own, and will assume that their experiences are the same as ours. As a result we fail to notice differences. On the other hand, it is equally possible to regard the experiences of people whose backgrounds differ from our own, as totally foreign and strange. In this case we ignore common experiences. Stereotypes about race and sexuality can bring bizarre fantasies into play that can detrimentally affect health care. It is important to be as aware as we can be of the way these stereotypes can subtly influence us. It is impossible not to be affected by them, but it is crucial to attempt to be as non-judgemental as possible.

Conclusion

Most of us tend to see our own sex life as normal, understandable and natural while the sex life of 'others' may be frightening, bizarre or disgusting.

The danger is that the sex lives of anyone regarded as 'different' are rarely seen in their terms and constantly they face ignorance and prejudice. This affects the elderly, the ill, people with learning difficulties and the disabled, as well as lesbians, prostitutes and cultural and ethnic minorities. The sexuality of all of these people is stereotyped in very different ways, but all of these stereotypes have a destructive effect on potential sexual health.

Nurses are dealing with their own feelings about sexuality whenever they enter the patient's private space. Taking cervical smears, touching, dealing with body products all involve intimacy that can be uncomfortable and disquieting. Yet how patients respond to routine procedures such as cervical smears can provide invaluable information about how they feel about their bodies which can be used by health professionals to promote sexual health.

We fear our own ignorance, feel embarrassed by the inadequate language available to talk about sexuality and worry that we will offend or open up histories of sexual abuse or rape that will overwhelm us. Yet the more we speak and learn the more our confidence grows. There is already a vast improvement from the ignorance prevalent a few generations ago.

How we think about sexuality is constantly changing as new variations on the theme of nature versus nurture emerge. It is possible to think that these debates are irrelevant but in fact they affect health care profoundly. If a young girl of 13 comes in to discuss sexual health, how we think about sexual development will affect our response. Our values will be reflected in how we react if we find out her partner is a woman, 20 years older than her or that she is engaging in anal sex.

If we overemphasize biological differences in the sexual health care we offer we are in danger of ignoring women whose needs are not related to reproduction. On the other hand, if we emphasize similarities between women and men we may fail to cater for gender-specific needs. All aspects need to be reflected in the services we offer.

It may be that the appropriate concern of sexual health is mainly with safety and protection but unless sexuality is seen in much broader terms the care offered will be limited. Sexual health must connect with the experiences of the individual woman if it is to have relevance and meaning for her.

It is vital to remain open to the infinite variations in human sexuality and to acknowledge that sex is always going to be a highly charged and complex issue. To give good sexual health care we need to be curious about how each woman thinks of herself as a woman and a sexual being, and be alive to the fascination, excitement and challenge of sexuality.

Further reading

HOLLAND, J., RAMAZANOGLU, C. and SCOTT, S. (1990) *Women Risk and AIDS Project Papers 1–8*. London: Tufnell Press.

LAWLOR, J. (1991) *Behind the Screens. Nursing, Somology and the Problem of the Body*. Edinburgh: Churchill Livingstone.

LINCOLN, R. (ed.) (1992) *Psychosexual Medicine*. London: Chapman and Hall.

MONTFORD, H. and SKRINE, R. (eds) (1993) *Contraceptive Care*. London: Chapman and Hall.

SAVAGE, J. (1987) *Nurses, Gender and Sexuality*. London: Heinemann Nursing.

VAN OOIJEN, E. and CHARNOCK, A.J. (1993) *Sexuality and Patient Care: A Guide for Nurses and Teachers*. London: Chapman and Hall.

WEEKS, J. (1986) *Sexuality*. London: Routledge.

References

ARCHER, J. and LLOYD, B. (1982) *Sex and Gender*. Harmondsworth: Penguin.

BANCROFT, J. (1989) *Human Sexuality and its Problems*, 2nd edn. Edinburgh: Churchill Livingstone.

BEAUVOIR, DE S. (1953) *The Second Sex*. London: Jonathon Cape.

CAPLAN, P. (ed.) (1987) *The Cultural Construction of Sexuality*. London: Routledge.

COLE, M. and DRYDEN, W. (eds) (1988) *Sex Therapy in Britain*. Milton Keynes: Open University Press.

DAVENPORT-HINES, R. (1990) *Sex, Death and Punishment*. London: Fontana.

FERRIS, P. (1993) *Sex and the British. A Twentieth Century History*. London: Michael Joseph Ltd.

FOUCAULT, M. (1987–88) *The History of Sexuality*, Vols 1, 2 and 3. Harmondsworth: Penguin.

FREUD, S. (1977) *On Sexuality*. Volume 7 of The Pelican Freud Library. Harmondsworth: Penguin.

GOLHOR LERNER, H. (1988) *Women in Therapy*. New York: Harper and Row.

HITE, S. (1993) *The Hite Reports 1972–1993*. London: Bloomsbury.

HOLLAND, J., RAMAZANOGLU, C. and SCOTT, S. (1990) *Women Risk and AIDS Project Papers 1–8*. London: Tufnell Press.

JOHNSON, M. and JOHNSTONE, F. (1993) *HIV Infection in Women*. Edinburgh: Churchill Livingstone.

KITZINGER, S. (1983) *Women's Experience of Sex*. London: Dorling Kindersley.

KINSEY, A.C., POMEROY, W.B., MARTIN, C.E. and GEBHARD, P.H. (1953) *Sexual Behaviour in the Human Female*. Philadelphia and London: W.B. Saunders.

LAWLOR, J. (1991) *Behind the Screens. Nursing, Somology and the Problem of the Body*. Edinburgh: Churchill Livingstone.

LINCOLN, R. (ed.) (1992) *Psychosexual Medicine*. London: Chapman and Hall.

MASTERS, W.H. and JOHNSON, V.E. (1966) *Human Sexual Response*. London: Bantam Books.

MONTFORD, H. and SKRINE, R. (eds) (1993) *Contraceptive Care*. London: Chapman and Hall.

PATTON, C. (1994) *Last Served? Gendering the HIV Pandemic*. London: Taylor and Francis.

SAVAGE, J. (1987) *Nurses, Gender and Sexuality*. London: Heinemann Nursing.

SEGAL, L. (1994) *Straight Sex*. London: Virago Press.

SKRINE, R. (ed.) (1987) *Introduction to Psychosexual Medicine*. Carlisle: Montana Press.

STOLLER, R.J. (1986) *Perversion. The Erotic Form of Hatred*. London: Karnac Books.

TUNNADINE, P. (1992) *Insights into Troubled Sexuality*, revised edn. London: Chapman and Hall.

VANCE, C.S. (1986) *Pleasure and Danger*. London: Pandora Press.

WEEKS, J. (1986) *Sexuality*. London: Routledge.

WELLINGS, K., FIELD, J., JOHNSON, A.M. and WADSWORTH, J. (1994) *Sexual Behaviour in Britain*. London: Penguin.

2: Promoting a healthy lifestyle
Liz Illman ◆

OBJECTIVES

After reading this chapter you will understand:

◆ what is meant by good health

◆ the dimensions of health

◆ the targets of adding life to years and years to life

◆ what is involved in planning, delivery and evaluation of health promotion

◆ how to help clients to make health choices about diet, exercise, smoking, alcohol and other drugs.

Introduction

Before thinking about health promotion, you need first to define 'health'. This is not as easy as it might sound because there is no universally accepted definition of health. Some definitions are as follows:

> Soundness of body: that condition in which its function is duly discharged.
>
> (*Oxford English Dictionary*)

> The state of being bodily and mentally vigorous and free from disease.
>
> (*Collins Dictionary*)

> A process of adaptation. It is not the result of instinct, but of an autonomous yet culturally shaped reaction to socially created reality. It designates the ability to adapt to changing environments, to growing up and to ageing, to healing when damaged, to suffering and to the peaceful expectation of death. Health embraces the future as well, and therefore includes anguish and the inner resources to live with it.
>
> (Illich, 1977)

> A state of complete physical, mental and social well being and not merely the absence of disease and infirmity.
>
> (World Health Organization)

Ewles and Simnett (1992) criticize the above WHO definition for appearing 'to assume that someone somewhere has the ability and the right to define a state of health'.

Health education equally gives us many definitions to do with the enhancement of good health and the prevention of ill-health. Health education is frequently aimed at preventing specific diseases through targeting high-risk groups. The *Health of the Nation* document (DOH, 1992) defines the aim of health education as being 'to ensure that individuals are able to exercise informed choice when seeking the lifestyle they adopt'.

Health promotion is frequently opportunistic and is seen as a major part of the nurse's role in all primary health care settings, particularly since the new funding arrangements for GPs have shifted the focus in medicine from cure to prevention. Health education is seen as an integral part of health promotion.

Your role as a nurse gives you enormous scope for both health education and promotion. However the demands of your job frequently mean that these activities have to take a low priority. Health, as discussed, not only has many definitions but also has different meanings for individual women. For various reasons not all women can achieve the same 'level' of health but in your role as a health carer you should aim holistically to help women feel healthy in all aspects of their lives.

The concepts of health promotion and health education are discussed and explored by Naidoo and Wills (1994) in their book *Health Promotion: Foundations for Practice.*

What does being healthy mean?

Health means different things to different people. Your client may not share your personal or professional ideas about exercise or the benefits of cutting down on red meat or eating more fish. She may regard herself as healthy so long as she feels in control or able to go to work and to cope with everyday routine. She may regard doctors and nurses as people to see only when she is ill.

Scenario

Jenny is 24 and has three children. She and her partner have a two-bedroom flat on a rundown estate. He has been unemployed for two years. Jenny feels constantly tired and stressed. She is overweight and smokes 20 cigarettes a day which, she says, she cannot afford. She knows they are bad for her, but feels unable to do anything about it.

Jenny's story underlines the need for health care practitioners to have a flexible approach to health promotion, which takes account of lifestyle and environmental factors and pressures, which can make it difficult for women like Jenny to change their habits. Jenny needs support with childcare, housing and financial help before she has the strength to tackle the issues such as smoking that are important for her own health.

Figure 2.1 illustrates how the various dimensions of health interact to form an integrated whole, with sexual health overlapping all of these dimensions. Health is influenced by many factors such as the environment, unemployment, nutrition and culture.

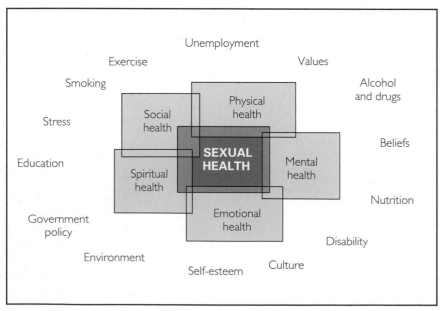

Figure 2.1 *Dimensions of health: a holistic view.*

Health targets

The *Health of the Nation* document (DOH, 1992) sets objectives and targets to 'add life to years and years to life'. These targets are to be met by specific dates and seek reductions in:

♦ cigarette smoking;

♦ average percentage of food energy derived from total fat and saturated fatty acids;

♦ obesity among 16–64 year olds;

♦ mean systolic blood pressure in adults;

♦ alcohol consumption in people drinking more than recommended;

♦ unwanted pregnancies (in under-16s by at least 50% by year 2000); and

♦ sexually transmitted disease and HIV infection.

This might make it sound as if the document has an undue emphasis on 'reductions', but it also stresses the importance of diet and exercise for all; and improving the health of mothers (before, during and after pregnancy) and children. Nurses are expected to play a leading role in implementing these targets and encouraging people to take responsibility for their own well-being.

Health promotion

During the last 20 years there has been much debate over the best ways to promote health. Traditional health education was designed to change the behaviour of the individual towards healthier lifestyles by making people fit the environment. However, this did not make the environment a healthier place to live in; and has resulted in 'victims' being blamed for their own ill-health.

This traditional approach had a further limitation: it was based on the conviction that the expert (usually the doctor) knew best. Ewles and Simnett (1992) point out:

> There is a danger of imposing alien values on a client. Frequently this is an imposition of white, middle-class values on working-class people. For example, a doctor may perceive that the most important thing for a patient is losing weight and lowering blood pressure, but drinking beer in the pub with friends may be far more important to the overweight, middle-aged, unemployed

patient. Who is to say which set of values is right? Whose life is it anyway?

The client-centred approach involves working with clients on their own terms and helping them to make decisions and choices. Clients are valued as equals. The key is self-empowerment evolving from increasing self-awareness and self-esteem. This is in stark contrast to the traditional paternalistic model.

The World Health Organization (1984) defines health promotion as the process of enabling people to increase control over, and to improve their health. The term 'health promotion' is an umbrella term and is used to describe a range of activities which includes health education and prevention.

There are three levels of health education (HE):

♦ *Primary HE* This aims at not only preventing ill-health, but also improving quality of health, and thereby quality of life, through nutrition, contraception and safer sex and accident prevention, for example.

♦ *Secondary HE* This aims to help people with a reversible health problem to adjust their lifestyle, by stopping smoking, changing eating habits and exercising more, for example.

♦ *Tertiary HE* This aims to help people whose ill-health cannot be completely cured to make the most of their lives, for example by rehabilitation training after a stroke, and by minimizing complications arising from diseases such as diabetes, asthma, epilepsy, chronic bronchitis and cancer.

Planning health promotion

You may be able to set up programmes to promote specific aspects of health, for example smoking cessation, to which you invite clients individually or in a group. However, much health promotion is opportunistic – done during a busy clinic or surgery or over the phone. A few minutes may be all that is available – or necessary. Problems that need more time can be identified and followed up at a more convenient time.

Measures you can take to construct a programme for your area could include:

♦ deciding on your aims

♦ setting objectives i.e. goals to be achieved;

♦ deciding which methods/strategies will achieve your objectives;

♦ ensuring support from your manager and colleagues;

♦ contacting the local health promotion department for advice and resources;

♦ talking to local agencies to find out what help they provide and how their referral system works (Can clients self-refer?);

♦ checking that everyone in the programme has the appropriate knowledge and skills;

♦ keeping a list of national and local organizations, helplines and support groups. Ask for their posters and leaflets;

♦ encouraging feedback and building an evaluation strategy into your programme, e.g. through an anonymous questionnaire;

♦ audit helps future planning and to monitor quality standards.

Remember that the best plan can go wrong: the guest speaker fails to turn up; the video breaks down; your client is more concerned about last night's TV programme on breast cancer than her smoking habits. Be flexible and prepared to depart from your plan.

Helping your clients to change

In the formation of your strategy, use the following guidelines:

♦ Develop a partnership with your client in which you use your specialist knowledge, but she remains in control of the choices concerning her health.

♦ Arrange an interpreter/health advocate if necessary.

♦ Decide on the priority. Tackle one thing at a time.

♦ Check your client's knowledge and understanding. She may feel herself to be immune from lifestyle-related disease on account of her age or because of some other factor such as a healthy family history.

♦ Listen carefully and acknowledge her difficul-

ties. Summarizing and reflecting back statements will help to clarify what she wants.

♦ Provide information reinforced with a leaflet, in her own language if possible. Ask her to keep it for reference. If she cannot read, a family member, a friend or health advocate may be able to help.

♦ Repeat key information.

♦ When a client is ready to change, develop an action plan together, encouraging her to use her own ideas.

♦ Set realistic goals.

♦ Emphasize the benefits of healthy changes.

♦ Devise coping strategies.

♦ Monitor her progress at regular intervals.

It is important to acknowledge practical problems that may limit change. Your client may see no need to alter her lifestyle. She may lack the self-esteem and confidence to cope with big changes. She may be unable to change because she lacks control over her life at home or at work, maybe due to lack of money or emotional instability. In addition, you may not have the necessary time she needs in order to help her.

Preconception care and early pregnancy

Preconception care has two aims: (1) to give a baby the best possible start to life by minimizing risks associated with lifestyle, heredity, medical history and maternal age; and (2) to promote the health of the mother.

A woman wishing to conceive, can be given advice concerning the timing of intercourse during the most fertile phase of the menstrual cycle, i.e. 14 days before the expected start of the next period (see also page 208).

In theory, a family planning or well-woman consultation provides an ideal opportunity to discuss plans for having a family, to check your client's general health and to arrange appropriate screening. In practice, however, you may not see your client until she presents for a pregnancy test. A negative result will raise the question as to whether she needs either contraception or preconception counselling. A positive result will enable you either to discuss the issues covered in this section or the possibility of counselling for termination of the pregnancy.

The first four weeks of a pregnancy are the most critical in a baby's development – the time of maximum velocity in cell division, when the heart, brain, spine and other major organs begin to develop. This is why it is so important to give advice to women on diet and health before conception rather than after a client knows she is pregnant, which is almost always after this four-week period. Nevertheless, do not forget that even if your client does not present until she is several weeks pregnant, you can still emphasize that it it is never too late to make healthy lifestyle changes.

In a report for the British Dietetic Association, Doyle (1994) says that women with a high risk of poor pregnancy outcome (Box 2.1) should be targeted for nutrition counselling. Their needs may extend beyond diet and call for a more holistic approach.

Box 2.1 Risk factors for poor pregnancy outcome

♦ Poor obstetric history, e.g. previous low-birthweight baby or previous congenital abnormality

♦ Smoking, heavy drinking or abuse of other drugs

♦ In adolescence

♦ Pre-existing medical conditions, e.g. diabetes, hypertension and malabsorption states

♦ Low socio-economic group and poor housing

♦ Close birth spacing and large families

♦ Very under- or overweight

♦ An inadequate diet, e.g. some vegans with a limited nutritional intake or families with poor cooking facilities

♦ Eating disorders, e.g. anorexia or bulimia.

Preconception and early pregnancy care should include:

♦ A review of medical and family histories

♦ Advice on smoking, alcohol and other drugs

♦ Nutritional advice

♦ Advice on exercise, lifestyle and occupational hazards for both partners.

♦ Information about stopping hormonal contraception and removal of IUD

If a woman becomes pregnant whilst taking hormonal contraception, she should be advised to stop immediately. Reassurance can be given, however, that studies to date have not shown any detectable increased risk of fetal abnormality in babies conceived by women taking hormonal contraceptives (Guillebaud, 1993).

Medical history

A review of general medical history should include disease and long-term medication, such as for diabetes, epilepsy, asthma and mental illness. A client's gynaecological and obstetric history should cover previous pregnancies, miscarriages, abortions, stillbirth and intrauterine death, toxaemia, subfertility, sexually transmitted diseases, hepatitis and HIV status, if known. A check should also be carried out on previous cervical smears, rubella status and sickle cell and thalassaemia trait.

A family history should be taken for both partners, if possible, and screening offered for inherited disorders. Carrier couples may be referred for genetic counselling for conditions such as sickle cell disorders, thalassaemia and Tay–Sachs disease. Screening in specialist centres is also available for conditions such as cystic fibrosis, muscular dystrophy and fragile X syndrome.

Nutrition advice

The importance of a healthy diet for women who are or who want to become pregnant cannot be overemphasized. Women who have an inadequate diet will need advice and supplements and may need to be referred to a dietitian.

Weight control

Women should be advised not to attempt to lose weight if they are actively trying to become pregnant. An obese client should aim to lose weight well in advance of conception in order to let her weight and metabolism stabilize before tackling pregnancy. An underweight woman or one who is over-exercising may have difficulty conceiving. Being underweight also increases the risk of having a small baby. Chronic long-term dieters should try to eat three good meals a day to ensure they are topped up on all the things the baby will need in those all-important first few weeks of gestation (Doyle, 1994).

Folic acid

Supplementation of folic acid can reduce the incidence of neural tube defects (NTD), such as spina bifida. The Department of Health advises women planning pregnancy to take 400 μg folic acid daily, in addition to dietary intake, until the 12th week of pregnancy. If either parent has spina bifida, or if the couple have had a previously affected pregnancy, the woman is advised to take a higher daily supplement of folic acid (5 mg). The DOH (1992) recommended that this daily dose should be reduced to 4 mg if a licensed preparation became available.

Vitamin A

An excessively high intake of vitamin A is associated with birth defects. Pregnant women should be advised to avoid dietary supplements containing vitamin A, or foods known to be high in vitamin A, such as liver or liver products.

Food-related infection

Listeriosis is a bacterial infection common in animals, including cattle, pigs and poultry, that may also affect humans. Maternal infection can result in miscarriage, stillbirth, brain damage or severe illness in a newborn baby.

Foods to avoid in pregnancy include ripened soft cheeses, e.g. Brie, Camembert and blue-veined cheeses. Unpasteurized milk, milk products and pâté may contain high levels of listeria. Cook-chill meals and ready-to-eat poultry should be avoided unless they are thoroughly reheated.

Raw or partially cooked eggs or foods containing raw egg (e.g. mousses and mayonnaise) and undercooked chicken can cause salmonella poisoning and should be avoided in pregnancy.

Exercise, lifestyle and occupational hazards

Advice on exercise is given on page 21. Adequate sleep and relaxation is also important.

Advice should be given for both partners about avoiding occupational hazards, e.g. exposure to chemicals and radiation.

The woman's partner should be encouraged to eat healthily and to cut down or better still stop smoking and reduce alcohol consumption. The mutual support that a partner can give by adopting a similar healthy lifestyle is a positive factor and lays the foundations for bringing up children with a similar approach.

Advise your client about the risk of toxoplasmosis. This is an infection caused by a parasite found in cat's faeces, raw and partially cooked meat and unpasteurized goat's milk and cheese. Exposure in early pregnancy can cause miscarriage and fetal damage, which may lead to mental retardation and blindness. Pregnant women should avoid changing cat litter; but if this is essential, they should wear rubber gloves. They should be especially careful to wash their hands thoroughly after handling animals, cat litter, earth or raw meat; avoid eating rare meat; wash salads thoroughly and wear gloves for gardening.

Women and food

Women play a key role in buying and preparing food and in educating the family about healthy eating. However, dietary preferences of the family at large help to determine what appears on the table. Employment trends and food technology also affect the family menu. Convenience foods appeal to women juggling the conflicting demands of home and outside jobs.

Moreover, a healthy diet can cost more in terms of shopping, preparation and cooking. Local street markets offer cheaper produce which frequently reflects the local variety of ethnic and cultural dietary preferences. If these are not convenient then some women, for example, Afro-Caribbean and Asians, may have to spend more on basic foods which supermarkets classify as 'exotic' if they want to eat their traditional diets.

Self-image also affects the food women buy and eat. Up to 70% of women diet at some time in their lives. Many pursue an elusive ideal figure of the kind promoted by glossy magazines, advertising agencies and the burgeoning dieting industry. Obsessive dieting associated with a distortion of body image can lead to eating disorders.

A good diet

There is an abundance of conflicting advice about diet and what is good or bad to eat. This prompts the question: what is a 'healthy' diet? The most recent recommendations of the Committee on Medical Aspects of Food Policy (COMA) (DOH, 1994) for the UK population include:

♦ Increased consumption of vegetables, fruit, potatoes and bread by 50%. In practice, eat bigger servings rather than more meals.

♦ Replacement of saturated fatty acids with foods containing oils and fats low in saturated fatty acids and rich in monounsaturated fatty acids.

♦ Use reduced fat spreads and dairy products instead of full fat products.

♦ Eat at least two portions of fish, of which one should be an oily fish weekly.

♦ Reduce average salt intake from 9 g to 6 g/day. Do not add salt to food and eat less processed and pre-prepared food.

The HEA (1994) published the *National Food Guide: The Balance of Good Health*, to give the

---

Box 2.2   Body mass index
BMI is calculated by applying the formula:

$$BMI = \frac{Weight\ (kg)}{Height^2\ (m)}$$

BMI grades

Less than 20 = Underweight
20–24.9   = Acceptable
25–29.9   = Overweight (some health risk)
30–40   = Obese (moderate health risk)
Over 40   = Severely obese (high health risk)

---

public a 'consistent and practical message about healthy eating and reduce confusion about what healthy eating means'. The leaflet is based on the Government's Eight Guidelines for a Healthy Diet, for use in schools, workplaces, health centres and supermarkets.

The *Health of the Nation* document (DOH, 1992) sets a target to reduce obesity in 16–64-year-olds by at least 25%. Obesity is defined as a body mass index (BMI) of 30 or over (Box 2.2).

Diet and fertility

What a mother eats before and during pregnancy may influence her child's subsequent health. Research has shown a significant association between retarded growth *in utero*, and increased rates of coronary heart disease, hypertension and non-insulin dependent diabetes later in adult life. Low-birthweight babies or those who are 'small for dates' are at increased risk from these problems in later life. They have been linked to fetal under-nutrition at different stages of gestation (Barker, 1993).

This highlights the need to make all sexually active women aware of what they need to eat. This is particularly important as a woman may not know she is pregnant until she has missed a period, by which time she may be at least four weeks pregnant.

For a couple who want to conceive, the diet should be varied and include adequate quantities of proteins, carbohydrates, fibre, vitamins and minerals from natural sources. Encourage plenty of fresh fruit and vegetables and wholegrain products. 'Fortified' breakfast cereals are a good source of extra vitamins and minerals. Zinc deficiency reduces the sperm count and is believed to be associated with poor pregnancy outcome. Zinc is lost when alcohol intake increases. Calcium is important for adequate mineralization of fetal bone, particularly in the third trimester.

Pregnancy and breastfeeding

During pregnancy and breastfeeding, a good balanced diet is essential. Emphasize the benefits of a healthy, varied diet and the hazards of overeating. Specific points to include are the following:

♦ Appetite is the best guide to energy needs and 'eating for two' during pregnancy is not necessarily a good policy to follow.

♦ Most pregnant women build up a store of 2–4 kg of body fat to support energy requirements for breastfeeding.

♦ Increased quantities of a normal, varied diet will provide all the energy and nutrients most breastfeeding women require for milk production.

♦ Some women need to drink more when breastfeeding, especially as lactation is established.

♦ Calcium requirements during both pregnancy and breastfeeding rise by almost 80% and if there is a deficiency in dietary calcium this will promote demineralization of maternal bone in order to maintain calcium levels in the breast milk. This will increase the risk of osteoporosis in later life (Doyle, 1994).

Adolescence

Teenagers are inclined towards erratic eating habits: missed breakfasts, junk food snacks, irregular meals and (especially girls) crash diets. Yet calorie and nutritional needs are greater in adolescence than at any other time except infancy. Bone mass increases rapidly with the growth spurt, creating great demand for calcium. Pregnant teenagers need extra care but they can be a difficult group to reach: they may not present until late in pregnancy and may disregard nutritional advice.

Adolescents should not be put on reducing diets. These can restrict growth and may precipitate anorexia nervosa which affects about 1% of young women (see also page 82). Bulimia nervosa also affects this age group. Women with eating disorders may need a psychological assessment. An obese or underweight teenager should be referred to a dietitian.

The best way to manage overweight young people is to encourage regular exercise and healthy eating, and to reduce consumption of fatty and sugary foods. This should check weight gain whilst not inhibiting growth. Encouraging them to take part in leisure pursuits (including exercise) will also provide a distraction from eating.

Parents may need education and support in order to encourage their children towards healthier eating. The school nurse may be a good source of help and monitor of progress.

Diet, PMS and the menopause

Eating regular, well-balanced meals throughout the menstrual cycle and avoiding foods containing a lot of salt, sugar and caffeine premenstrually, can help women with premenstrual syndrome (see Chapter 13).

A healthy diet and regular weight bearing exercise will help women prepare for the menopause and guard against osteoporosis.

Helping your client to reduce weight

The following guidelines are useful when helping a client to reduce her weight:

♦ Explore your client's views about her weight. Concern about physical attractiveness and social acceptability may outweigh considerations about health.

♦ Check her BMI – Is she really overweight?

♦ Ask her to keep a diary of what she snacks as well as eats at mealtimes (a bag of crisps in front of the TV, a chocolate bar on the bus), when she eats it and how she feels at the time (hungry, bored or premenstrual?).

♦ Give information on the health risks of being overweight, e.g. for a smoker, diabetic with hypertension, etc.

♦ Explore barriers to losing weight and previous attempts at dieting. Does she prepare food for other people?

♦ Recommend dietary modifications – regular meals (three per day) that are low in fat and sugar. Emphasize the benefits of starchy foods, fruit and vegetables.

♦ Set a realistic target – no more than 6 kg (1 stone) as an initial target. Encourage slow but steady weight loss in preference to a 'crash diet'.

♦ Suggest an increase in exercise. Aim for a permanent change in lifestyle.

♦ Review regularly to give support and set new targets if necessary.

Health and exercise

Exercise has many benefits. These include protection against heart disease and stroke; promotion of psychological well-being; and, to a lesser extent, reduction of anxiety and depression. Researchers, however, have yet to establish if this latter effect is attributable to a biochemically induced response, or to diversion of attention from the source of anxiety.

Most women are aware of these benefits of exercise; what is less well-known is that exercise is also good for the bones. Weight-bearing exercise, such as walking, jogging, dancing and tennis, protects against osteoporosis (see page 345).

The benefits of exercise specific to women do not end there. Pelvic floor exercise helps to promote continence and can increase sexual enjoyment (see page 374). Moderate weight-bearing and non-weight-bearing exercise (e.g. swimming) can improve the course of a pregnancy. Physical activity stimulates metabolism and regular exercise plays a role in preventing weight gain and managing obesity.

Despite all these benefits, women exercise less than men at all ages. You can play an important role by emphasizing the psychological benefits of exercise, and, perhaps, the social aspects of group sessions. Taking exercise can be a good way of encouraging women to make time for and feel good about themselves. Whatever form exercise takes, it must be fun if it is to last.

Recent government research shows that a third of the population is completely sedentary. In March 1996, the Health Education Authority launched the Active For Life campaign to encourage people to lead more active lives, particularly those who do not enjoy taking exercise. The new shift in advice for these people is away from recommending strenuous exercise to 'moderate intensity' exercise. This involves breathing slightly harder; a slightly raised heart rate and feeling warmer, but not out of breath or sweating profusely. Examples include brisk walking, washing the car, dancing, gentle swimming, golf and gardening.

The aim is to build up to 30 minutes of 'moderate intensity' exercise on five or more days a week. This can be split into 10–15 minute bursts. Encourage your client to incorporate exercise into the daily routine by, for example, walking the last couple of bus stops; or climbing the stairs rather than taking the lift. People who are already fit should continue taking more vigorous exercise three times a week, gradually building up the intensity and length of their activity. How vigorous should such activity be? Advise clients that they should be able to continue talking while exercising. Research suggests that three 20 minute sessions per week of vigorous activity provide maximum protection from coronary heart disease and stroke.

Activity and stamina should be built up gradually. Advise clients with medical problems to consult you or the doctor before embarking on a new or more vigorous routine. To reduce the risk of injury, you need to remind your clients to spend about ten minutes 'warming up' and doing some gentle stretching before vigorous exercise. The routine should end with a ten minute 'cool down' period.

The menstrual cycle

There is controversy over whether or not exercise may relieve dysmenorrhoea. According to one theory, exercise triggers the body to produce endorphins, natural opiates that promote a sense of well-being in addition to relieving pain. Anecdotal evidence suggests that moderate exercise can help, perhaps by distracting attention from pain, producing a feeling of warmth and relaxation, and reducing stress. Similarly, exercise may relieve some of the symptoms of PMS.

Yoga and relaxation techniques are recommended for PMS and dysmenorrhoea. Sexual activity and orgasm are also said to help dysmenorrhoea.

Excessive exercise, however, especially in competitive athletes, can lead to irregular periods, anovulatory cycles and amenorrhoea. An inadequate diet or anorexia nervosa can compound such problems, leading to subfertility and the long-term risk of osteoporosis. Periods usually revert to normal and fertility returns to its previous level with an appropriate diet and reduction in exercise.

Pregnancy

Pregnant women should continue to exercise so long as there are no complications (e.g. vaginal bleeding or hypertension). They should consult their midwife if in doubt. Exercise in moderation reduces the risk of miscarriage and premature birth; but women should 'listen' to their bodies and avoid a new, strenuous activity, particularly in the first or third trimesters (Gaskell, 1994).

Beneficial activities include walking, swimming, stationary cycling and yoga. A gradual transition to non-weight-bearing exercises is recommended as the pregnancy progresses and weight increases.

Advise your client to avoid:

♦ Energetic activities, such as jumping, skiing, riding and contact sports

♦ Exercising on an empty stomach (to prevent hypoglycaemia)

♦ Exercising for two hours after a meal

♦ Vigorous physical activity for 6–8 weeks after delivery, or as recommended by their midwife or obstetrician.

Encourage your clients to do postnatal and pelvic floor exercises during this time.

The middle years and beyond

Loss of bone mass is at its greatest in the years immediately after the menopause. Peak bone mass is achieved by the mid-thirties and should be maintained before and after the menopause through diet and weight-bearing exercise such as brisk walking, dancing, cycling, racquet sports and gardening. Swimming helps to protect against heart disease and stroke, but it is non-weight bearing, and does not protect against bone loss. Exercise, apart from maintaining bone density and therefore reducing the risk of osteoporosis, will increase agility and dexterity and help prevent falls and the associated immobilizing fractures.

Exercise should continue after the menopause, with modifications to type and intensity as the years go by. Women disabled by degenerative or neurological disease may need your help to work out appropriate exercise and activities. Walking, golf, bowls, swimming and dancing are all suitable forms of exercise. Many community centres run classes for older people. Have a list of details to hand.

Women and drugs

> The desire to experience some altered state of consciousness seems to be an intrinsic part of the human condition. . . . We are surrounded by drugs . . . the cups of coffee and tea, the glasses of beer, wine and whisky, the cigarettes, the snorts of cocaine, the joints, the tablets of acid, the fixes of heroin and the ubiquitous tranquillisers and sleeping pills . . . . So long as there are drug takers, there will be drug casualties . . . the quest to eliminate drug taking has proved to be the search for a chimera. Drug taking is here to stay and one way or another, we must all learn to live with drugs.
>
> (Gossop, 1993)

It is estimated that twice as many women as men are prescribed tranquillizers; that at least 23% of illegal drug users are women; that increasing numbers of women depend on crack cocaine; and that as many as two-thirds of crack users are women (DAWN, nd, and Westcott, 1994).

The Department of Health's Social Trends survey (DOH, 1995a) reported that in the year ending March 1993, more than 20 000 people attended drug services in Great Britain for the first time, or after an absence of six months or more. Three-quarters were male and over half of both sexes were in their twenties. The main drugs misused were heroin (45%), methadone (15%), and amphetamines (11%). About two in five users reported that they were injecting their main drug. These figures probably reflect only a small proportion of the total.

It is common for female drug users to have a poor self-image and low self-esteem and care should be taken in your dealings with them not to add to these negative feelings. In order to build up an effective therapeutic relationship with such clients it is vitally important that you have a non-judgemental and non-moralistic attitude. When taking a drug history you should use non-judgemental terms such as 'use' rather than 'abuse'. If you have an open and accepting attitude then your clients frequently will respond to your questions accurately rather than give vague responses.

This section discusses the effects of psychoactive drugs, both legal and illegal, therapeutic and recreational, on women. Further information about the physical and psychological effects and legal status of individual drugs are described by the Institute for the Study of Drug Dependence (ISDD, 1994). Alcohol and tobacco are discussed in more detail later. In essence, however, all drugs are used for similar reasons: to feel good, relaxed, happy, to alleviate stress, calm anxiety or to stimulate mind and/or body.

Drugs, the menstrual cycle and fertility

Disruption of the menstrual cycle is common among women using drugs like ecstasy, amphetamines, opiates and anabolic steroids. Their periods may become irregular, and lighter or sometimes heavier; they may experience 'spotting' or even heavy bleeding after taking drugs.

Ecstasy, amphetamines and heroin can suppress appetite. Significant weight loss can result in suppression of ovulation and amenorrhoea. Poor nutrition, a common problem with heavy drug users, and long-term amenorrhoea are risk factors for osteoporosis. Amenorrhoea may lull women into a false sense of security that they will not become pregnant. Consequently they may not use adequate contraception.

Anabolic steroids can affect fertility and sexuality in both sexes. In women, they are associated with menstrual disturbance, increased sex drive, decrease in breast size and irreversible development of virilizing effects. These characteristics may be passed on to a female fetus if the mother is pregnant while taking the drugs. In men, sperm count and sex drive may decrease.

Alcohol and cannabis are sometimes used to 'treat' dysmenorrhoea and premenstrual syndrome, but in some women these drugs may exacerbate PMS symptoms rather than alleviate them.

Drugs, sex and contraception

Ecstasy has been called the 'love drug' and the 'hug drug'. Other drugs reported to promote feelings of closeness and sexual pleasure include cannabis, alkyl nitrites ('poppers'), LSD and amphetamines. However, ecstasy and amphetamines may inhibit orgasm in either sex and reduce the size of a male erection.

Mixing drugs and sex can make it hard to stay in control, and thus to remember to use effective contraception and to practise safer sex. Sharing injecting equipment or having unprotected sex increases the risk of hepatitis, sexually transmitted diseases and HIV.

Drug users may be more inclined to forget to take oral contraception. The combined pill is contraindicated for women with a history of deep vein thrombosis or liver damage, and both are common complications of intravenous drug use. A progestogen injectable or implant are better options: these are highly reliable, non-intercourse-related and may give some protection against sexually transmitted infection. Other possibilities, depending on medical history and sexual lifestyle, include the intrauterine device (IUD), or the levonorgestrel intrauterine system (IUS). The latter may reduce the risk of pelvic infection.

Barrier methods of contraception, if used carefully, are ideal as not only do they provide contraception but also offer protection against sexually transmitted infections. Some women prefer the female condom to the male condom as it gives them more personal control. A diaphragm alone may not be so reliable as rapid weight loss may occur with drug use and a different size diaphragm would then be required (see page 180).

Oral contraceptive users need to know that drug interaction may occur with some antibiotics, antiepileptics, barbiturates, tranquillizers and hypnotics. These drugs can reduce the efficacy of the Pill.

The Pill may also alter the effects of other drugs, including chlordiazepoxide, diazepam, imipramine and amitriptyline. 'Street' drugs mixed with other substances could cause drug interaction. Cocaine, amphetamines and ecstasy can increase blood pressure which, if used frequently or mixed with other drugs, could put oral contraceptive users at greater risk of cardiovascular problems.

Drugs and pregnancy

The lifestyle associated with heavy drug use may put mother and baby at risk through self-neglect and poor nutrition. Drugs also directly affect the baby. The small risk of drug-related malformations is at its greatest in the first trimester.

Many heavy drug users have healthy babies, but heavy drug use (including alcohol and smoking) in pregnancy is associated with miscarriage, premature labour, low birthweight, fetal abnormality and stillbirth. The risk to babies whose mothers take benzodiazepines is believed to be low. However, studies have shown a link between benzodiazepines and cleft palate when they are taken in the first trimester. Babies born to heavy, long-term users of tranquillizers, opiates and barbiturates may show signs of withdrawal.

Women planning a pregnancy or who are already pregnant should be advised to avoid drugs if possible. Those taking prescription medicines should consult their midwife/doctor to discuss whether these need to be continued and if so, the possible risks to a developing fetus. Women who continue using opiates or benzodiazepines should tell their midwife as they may require extra care during pregnancy and labour. Their babies may be at risk from fetal distress and, after birth, from respiratory depression and neonatal drug withdrawal and require extra support from the neonatal care team.

As mentioned earlier, drug users are prone to menstrual irregularities. Women with amenorrhoea may not realize that they are pregnant and may therefore be late in booking antenatal care. Methadone maintenance can improve pregnancy outcome among street drug users. Opiates, barbiturates or tranquillizers should not be withdrawn suddenly. Women wanting to reduce or stop drugs should aim do so slowly during the second trimester, with support and medical supervision. The timing of reduction or withdrawal is important to minimize the risk of miscarriage or premature labour. Inpatient treatment is recommended for barbiturate withdrawal because of the risk of fits.

Tranquillizers and hypnotics

Benzodiazepines are the most commonly prescribed drugs in Britain. Most prescriptions are long-term repeat prescriptions and up to half are issued without consultation or assessment (DAWN, nd). After about two weeks of continuous use, benzodiazepines may become ineffective as sleeping tablets; after four months they are ineffective against anxiety (ISDD, 1994).

Coming off tranquillizers (Box 2.3)

Many women come off tranquillizers without medical or drug agency support whilst others need help from a community drugs team (CDT) or a residential unit. Women with young children often fear they will be taken into care. Very few residential units accommodate children and there are even fewer mother and baby units.

Ideally, women coming off tranquillizers should have access to medical help and counselling. During this time they may be vulnerable to a re-emergence of the problems which led to them taking drugs in the first place. These may be compounded by additional new difficulties.

Box 2.3 Coming off tranquillizers
The Mental Health Foundation booklet, *Helping you Cope* (1994), contains this advice for women coming off tranquillizers:

♦ Talk to your doctor, nurse or street agency about why you want to stop and your expectations of withdrawal.

♦ Ensure you have support. Family, friends and women who have shared the experience may be of special help.

♦ Find out about your local specialist services. You may benefit from counselling, psychotherapy or self-help groups.

♦ Don't stop suddenly – this will cause more severe withdrawal symptoms which may encourage you to start again.

♦ Reduce tranquillizer intake gradually at your own pace. The withdrawal period should never be less than 6–8 weeks. The timetable needs to be flexible to allow for any withdrawal symptoms which may appear.

♦ Keeping a diary can help you to monitor progress and achievements.

♦ Don't go back. If you are finding it too difficult, you are probably cutting down too fast. Try taking smaller steps. You may need to ask for a different strength of tablet to tailor the dosage.

♦ Try not to be too disheartened if you don't manage to withdraw completely at the first or even second attempt. You have already started to take control of life and you can always try again.

Sources of help

When working with clients who use drugs, you will find it useful to compile a list of local services. These could include:

♦ Street agencies

♦ Community drop-in services

♦ Drug dependency units (DDU)

♦ Community drug teams (CDT)

♦ Needle/syringe exchange schemes.

These services are able to provide a wide range of help, including counselling and psychiatric services, advice on safer sex (see page 173), and safer injecting techniques and disposal of equipment, and also outreach group work. Some agencies work with GPs to provide primary health care and a prescribing programme.

Ask these services for their leaflets, posters or information packs so that you can offer up-to-date information to your clients. If possible, arrange to visit them so you can see how they operate.

In the field of drug education it is now recognized that it is more realistic to encourage clients to minimize harm, particularly with clients who have no desire to change their behaviour.

Women and smoking

About 11 million people in Britain have stopped smoking in the last 15 years; more than half the remaining 12.5 million cigarette smokers are reported to want to do so. QUIT (personal communication, 1994) estimates that 1000 people a day give up the habit. It is crucial to focus on women to maintain this trend and to discourage young people from starting to smoke. In 1972, 52% of men and 41% of women smoked. This sexual divide has steadily narrowed, with 28% of women, and 29% of men smoking in 1992 (OPCS, 1994a).

Women are less likely to give up smoking than men and not just because of self-image and fear of gaining weight. Research suggests that women are more likely to smoke under emotional pressure, while men prefer to do so in more relaxed circumstances. Women are also said to rely more on cigarettes to cope with anger and frustration. Research also shows that quitting smoking depends on the interaction of at least three crucial factors: perception of stress, self-confidence and dependence on cigarettes.

Not only do women feel less confident and more dependent on cigarettes than men, but they see themselves as being more under stress – which in turn boosts their sense of dependence on cigarettes (Jacobson, 1986). Moreover, younger women are more likely to start smoking. In England in 1990, about a quarter of girls were regular smokers by the age of 15 (OPCS, 1991). The *Health of the Nation* document (DOH, 1992) set a target to reduce smoking among 11–15-year-olds by a third to below 6% by the end of 1994. The 1993 OPCS Survey showed that 9% of 11–15-year old boys and 10% of girls of the same age were regular smokers (OPCS, 1994b). These figures have not changed significantly.

Most smokers know that the habit is potentially life-threatening, but still continue to smoke. Anti-smoking propaganda has been particularly ineffective among women, so it is important to look at why women smoke within the context of their lifestyle and the barriers which prevent them giving up (Westcott, 1994).

Why do women smoke?

Many women, typically those with a low income and poor housing, see smoking as 'a necessary luxury' to help them cope with bringing up their families (Graham, 1987). Their smoking may be encouraged further by the idea that cigarettes suppress appetite and relieve stress. Women may feel that they are unable to change their lifestyle and smoking in the short term is seen as the 'least of a woman's problems'.

Most smokers start the habit in their teens, or even younger, after exposure to cigarette advertising and promotion. ASH (1994) claims that women are a key target for tobacco companies, with some 'feminine' brands marketed with special emphasis on 'lightness of taste, luxury length and slimness'. This marketing strategy has become more pronounced as tobacco sales to men have fallen.

In Britain, cigarette smoking has been shown to be more prevalent in the white population than in any other groups (Figure 2.2). Although cigarette smoking is rare amongst Asian women, chewing 'pan' (a blend of pan leaf, betel nut and lime to which tobacco is often added) is a social custom. It is chewed for many different reasons. After a meal it is often used to aid digestion and to freshen

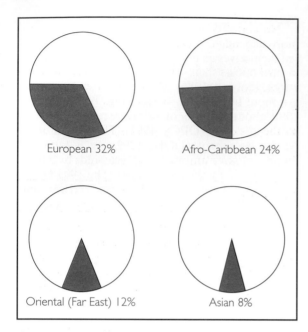

European 32%   Afro-Caribbean 24%

Oriental (Far East) 12%   Asian 8%

Figure 2.2 *Percentage of female smokers by ethnic group in the UK (Waterson, 1989).*

the breath. Like tobacco, the betel nut is said to have a mild stimulant effect. Chewing pan is associated with oral cancer.

Tomorrow's smokers

The tobacco industry needs to recruit 300 smokers a day to replace those lost to smoking-related diseases. The young are a prime target for recruitment. Smoking is still associated with being grown up and staying slim. Sports sponsorship enables cigarette companies to associate smoking with healthy, glamorous and life-enhancing activities. Seeing adults smoking along with tobacco advertising and promotion encourages young people to experiment, which can lead to lifelong addiction. Parents, teachers, music and sport celebrities all act as role models.

Friends who smoke can also create peer pressure to conform. Further pressures can result from low self-esteem, problem behaviour and poor school performance. Teenagers are particularly susceptible to the addictive nature of nicotine. They soon experience cravings, become irritable and suffer sleep disturbances (Bellow and Ramsay, 1991).

Parental smoking is the most important factor influencing young girls' smoking habits. Children from households where one parent smokes are twice as likely to become regular smokers as those from non-smoking homes. Nine per cent of children who have ever smoked had their first cigarette in the company of a parent (White, 1994a).

Smoking and fertility

Smoking can cause fertility problems in both sexes, but quitting appears to restore fertility to that of non-smokers. Women who smoke during pregnancy may condemn their unborn daughters to lower fertility and an earlier menopause; their unborn sons to an increased chance of sperm abnormalities; and, possibly, successive generations to reduced fertility (White, 1994b).

The Health Education Authority (HEA, 1993b) says that women smokers have a twofold increase in risk of ectopic pregnancy, and a 27% increased risk of miscarriage. Premature labour and stillbirth are also more common among smokers, while the risk of perinatal mortality increases by a third. Smokers are twice as likely to have low-birthweight babies, on average 200 g lighter. Some women may see this as an advantage, making labour easier, but it is important to point out that there is an increased risk of mortality and morbidity in infancy and early childhood in low-birthweight babies.

Smoking is also associated with abnormal menstrual patterns; premature ageing, including skin wrinkling; earlier menopause, by 2–3 years; and an increased risk of osteoporosis.

Smoking and cervical cancer were first linked in the late 1970s (see Chapter 11). The estimated degree of increased risk varies from study to study, but there seems to be a twofold risk in the increase of cervical cancer, and up to a 12-fold increase in CIN III in smokers. Several studies have found high concentrations of cigarette smoke components, including nicotine and cotinine, in cervical mucus. These concentrations were higher than those found in the blood levels of the subjects (Szarewski, 1994).

Cigarette chemicals may affect the immune mechanisms of the cervix, reducing the number of Langerhans' cells (immune cells) in women with CIN. Other types of immune cell can be similarly affected. These same immune cells have been found to be reduced in number in women smokers. Thus, smoking may be a co-factor in causing cervical cancer (Szarewski, 1994).

Passive smoking

The problem of passive smoking used to be dismissed as mythical, but recent research suggests that it can cause cancer. The hazards were highlighted by the death of the entertainer Roy Castle, a non-smoker, who spent much of his early working life in smoky nightclubs.

Non-smokers inhale both 'mainstream' smoke inhaled/exhaled by the smoker; and 'sidestream' smoke from the burning end of a cigarette. Only 15% of smoke is inhaled by the smoker. The average passive smoker is estimated to smoke the equivalent of one or two cigarettes a week. Recent research has shown that there is an increased risk of death from lung cancer (10–30%) in non-smokers as a result of passive smoking over long periods. Most at risk from passive smoking are babies and children, especially those with asthma and allergies, who have more hospital visits and inpatient stays for chest and ENT problems. Cot deaths are more common in families where parents smoke (HEA, 1991a, 1993b).

Helping smokers to quit

Nurses in hospital or primary care settings are ideally placed to encourage women to stop and help them design their quit programme. In reality many nurses themselves are smokers despite being well aware of all the risks to their personal health. They smoke for similar reasons as their clients, e.g. stress, pleasure, etc. Some people might question whether nurses who smoke are in a position to encourage others to give up when they still smoke themselves. Nurses who are smokers should address their own personal issues first, but should continue to advise, support and encourage their clients to give up smoking.

Why do women want to quit?

Women want to stop smoking for a variety of reasons. These may include:

- ◆ Social pressure
- ◆ To increase self-respect
- ◆ To feel in control
- ◆ To improve health
- ◆ To save money
- ◆ To set an example to children
- ◆ To smell fresher.

Scenario

 Karen, aged 24, tried to stop several times. She finally succeeded when her five-year-old asked her not to kiss him good night because she smelt so horrible. Karen said: 'I felt really bad and very guilty.'

In case you need to remind your client of the link between smoking and health, a number of the diseases associated with smoking are listed in Box 2.4.

Box 2.4 Smoking-related diseases (US DHHS, 1989; HEA, 1993)
A definite link has been made between smoking and a number of diseases:

Cardiovascular diseases
(Women on the pill who smoke increase their risk times 10.)

- ◆ Coronary heart disease
- ◆ Cerebrovascular disease
- ◆ Atherosclerotic peripheral vascular disease

Diseases of the respiratory system

- ◆ Chronic bronchitis and emphysema

Cancer

- ◆ Lung, mouth, nose, throat, oesophagus, stomach, bladder, kidney, pancreas, cervix, leukaemia

Other diseases

- ◆ Osteoporosis, tobacco amblyopia (a cause of blindness), cataracts, peptic ulcers, complications of diabetes and premature death.

What stops women quitting?

Knowing the risks of smoking does not necessarily help. Women often fail to stop because of the following factors:

◆ Withdrawal symptoms

◆ Possible weight gain

◆ Fear of losing control

◆ Anticipation of increased stress

◆ Enjoyment of smoking

◆ Lack of support

◆ Lack of confidence and low self-esteem.

Some comments frequently made by clients and some possible replies are listed in Box 2.5.

Box 2.5 Frequently heard comments and some suggested replies

'What if I can't do it? I'll feel such a failure.'
'Stopping for good may take more than one attempt. Try to set a realistic target – if you don't succeed you can always try again.'

'I've been harming my body for years. What's the point of stopping now?'
'Research shows that it is never too late to stop. The risks of heart disease and lung cancer begin to go down as soon as you stop smoking.'

'I didn't stop in my last pregnancy and everything was OK.'
'You were lucky. Smoking during pregnancy makes you more likely to have a baby with health problems. Miscarriage is more common and you're twice as likely to have a premature baby and the chances of having a stillbirth or losing your baby soon after birth increase by a third.'

'I've got no will power.'
'A good quit programme can help by giving you the support you need.'

'I never smoke in the same room as the children.'
'That's better than smoking while they are around, but unfortunately it won't necessarily stop them from following your example. Research shows that children of a parent who smokes are twice as likely to become regular smokers themselves.'

Recruiting women to a quit programme

A variety of approaches can be used to recruit women to a quit programme:

◆ Advertising in waiting room, practice/clinic leaflet

◆ Family planning/well-woman clinics

◆ Antenatal clinics

◆ Child health checks

◆ Referral from another health professional

◆ Routine checks for blood pressure, asthma, diabetes, etc.

Women who are pregnant, on the Pill or have young children – especially those with asthma and diabetes – should be prime targets.

Assessing the needs of women who want to quit

During the initial assessment of your client, you will need to evaluate:

◆ her motivation to give up – clarifying her reasons;

◆ any factors influencing smoking behaviour, e.g. family circumstances, parental and peer group pressure;

◆ her knowledge about smoking and health; and

◆ any anxieties about quitting. Any previous attempts?

Taking a smoking history and asking her to keep a smoking diary for a week will give you and your client valuable insight into her smoking habits and nicotine dependence. Remember to check if it is a typical week, and not one which is particularly stressful or relaxed. You cannot change her lifestyle or remove the stresses, but listening and acknowledging her difficulties may help her to feel valued. The quit rate increases with help on a one-to-one basis or in an all-female group (Austoker *et al.*, 1994; Rieder *et al.*, 1994).

You will need to ask your client the following questions:

◆ When does she smoke – when stressed, working, relaxing, bored, drinking coffee or alcohol, etc.?

◆ Which people and places does she associate with smoking?

♦ What time does she smoke the first cigarette of the day?

♦ What is the longest she goes without a cigarette?

♦ How many does she smoke daily?

♦ How long she has been smoking?

When compiling her smoking diary, your client should record:

♦ The date

♦ The time of every cigarette

♦ The reason for having a cigarette, e.g. the situation, with whom, how she is feeling, etc.

Designing a quit programme

There is wealth of information and material available; depending on time and resources, you can either devise a tailor-made programme for the individual or invite her to join a group with its own programme. This may include guest speakers, videos and role play in addition to sharing experiences and giving mutual support. A successful group may go on to create an independent support group. Support from other people is recognized as a major factor in quitting. You must ensure you have sufficient professional support to help your clients complete your programme. There is evidence that the accumulative effect of smoking cessation information and additional counselling has beneficial effects. Make the most of every opportunity to reinforce the message.

Since people smoke for different reasons, there is no right or wrong way to quit. Be creative. If you have a good idea, try it! You might like to base your quit programme on the advice to clients outlined in Box 2.6.

Box 2.6 A quit programme: advice to clients

♦ Write down your reason(s) for quitting. Keep the list handy.

♦ Choose your day: Over the weekend? On holiday or at the start of a working week? This will depend on what sort of smoker you are. Do you smoke more when you are relaxed or when you are busy and/or stressed?

♦ Make a date and stick to it: It may help to tell your family and friends. Ask them to respect your decision.

♦ Try giving up with a friend, colleague or partner for mutual support.

♦ Review your plan the day before Quit Day.

♦ Remove temptation: Dispose of cigarettes, lighters and ashtrays.

♦ Stop completely: Cutting down rarely helps. You may try to phase out the habit by gradually cutting down, only to find that as you smoke less, each cigarette becomes more satisfying. It is really important not to have even one puff.

♦ Reschedule your routine: You may need to avoid pubs/places/people you associate with smoking. Certain times or routines – a cup of coffee or a phone call – may trigger craving.

♦ Keep busy: Try to think about something other than smoking. If you need something in your mouth, try sugar-free gum or a raw carrot. Fiddling with beads or a pen may help to keep your hands busy.

♦ Be positive: Think of all the good you are doing to your body – and the people you live and work with. Look at the benefits chart (Table 2.1) for encouragement as to the long-term gains in quitting.

♦ Think money: Calculate your savings on a day-by-day, week-by-week basis. Plan how you can spend it – on a special treat or a holiday. Twenty cigarettes a day costs over £900 a year.

♦ Congratulate yourself: Plan a reward for the end of the first day, first week, etc.

♦ Practise relaxation: Simple techniques of slow, deep breathing can help to deal with cravings. 'Smoke fresh air' to relieve tension.

♦ Make your goal to get through TODAY without smoking.

Table 2.1 *Cessation of smoking: the benefits chart*	
GENERAL	Ex-smokers spend less time off work, and are healthier
IMMEDIATE	Within 8 hours of quitting, nicotine and carbon monoxide levels in the blood halve
	Senses of smell and taste improve within a few weeks
	Shortness of breath and cough improve
	Fertility increases
	Better chance of a healthy pregnancy and baby
1–2 YEARS	Extra risk of heart attack halves
3 YEARS	Risk of heart attack is similar to that of a life-long non-smoker
10 YEARS	Lung cancer risk falls to about half
15 YEARS	Risk of smoking-related diseases reduced to little more than that of a life-long non-smoker

Source: The Health Benefits of Smoking Cessation. A report of the Surgeon General 1990 (US Department of Health and Human Services).

Withdrawal effects: symptoms of recovery

About one in three smokers withdraw with little or no symptoms, but many experience severe symptoms, often classified as either physical or psychological. In practice, it may be difficult to disentangle one from the other.

Explaining why these symptoms occur may help your client combat unpleasant effects. Tell her that they are a positive sign that her body is recovering from the effects of tobacco. Vitamin C speeds up elimination of nicotine from the body. Exercise helps to relieve tension and irritability.

Withdrawal effects include the following:

♦ *Appetite* This may increase temporarily, which is often a discouraging factor – particularly for women.

♦ *Cough* Reactivation of the cilia, slowing down of mucus production and increased viscosity of the sputum may make coughing more difficult for a few weeks.

♦ *Constipation* This may result from the reliance of the bowel on the laxative action of tobacco.

♦ *Dizziness* This may be due to improved blood supply to the brain as carboxy-haemoglobin is eliminated and the red blood cells carry a greater concentration of oxygen.

♦ *Mouth ulcers and sore tongue* These may be due to changes in the bacterial flora.

♦ *Sleep disturbances* These may include insomnia and nocturnal tobacco craving. Insomnia may be related to a temporary fall in electro-cortical activity when smoking stops. This period may be followed by difficulty in concentrating and staying awake during the day.

♦ *Tingling sensations* These may occur with improved circulation. Elimination of nicotine from the body restores normal arterial tone, lowering the heart rate and blood pressure.

Nicotine replacement therapy

The Imperial Cancer Research Fund (ICRF) reported that smokers almost doubled their chances of quitting by using nicotine replacement therapies (NRT) in conjunction with a quit programme (Silagy *et al.*, 1994).

Transdermal patches and chewing-gum can be bought at pharmacies. They cannot be prescribed on the NHS, but a private prescription may work out cheaper as it avoids paying VAT. There is some variation in the price of different preparations, but generally the 10–12 week weaning period costs no more than 20 cigarettes a day.

Data sheets warn that smokers should stop completely when using NRT. Patches should not be worn during pregnancy, breastfeeding or by patients with cardiovascular problems. However, the risks of NRT need to be offset against the risks of continued smoking.

Patches are available in three strengths, released over 16 or 24 hours. Research has shown little difference in the efficacy of the 16- and 24-hour patches. Women craving nicotine on waking may find the 24-hour patch better, though it is more likely to cause sleep disturbances and dreaming. The 16-hour patch is worn during 'waking' hours. Patches can cause itching and erythema, and should be applied to non-hairy areas such as the upper arm or thigh.

Nicotine gum comes in two strengths and should be chewed until the taste becomes strong, then placed between the gum and cheek. It should be re-chewed when the taste fades. The process is repeated for about 30 minutes to release the rest of the nicotine. Gum can be chewed when the urge to smoke is felt, usually about ten pieces

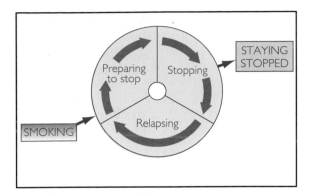

Figure 2.3 *Preparing to stop smoking. Source:*
Stopping Smoking Made Easier, *HEA, 1992. The
diagram is like a revolving door. Many smokers
go round several times before leaving it. This is
encouraging. The person trying to stop should
keep on trying and eventually will succeed.*

a day, for a period of three months. Intake should
be reduced gradually.

A nicotine nasal spray is now available on prescription.

Other aids to giving up smoking include
hypnotherapy, acupuncture, relaxation therapy
and counselling. This may be carried out either
on a one-to-one or group basis. Helplines are also
available.

Helping relapsers (Figure 2.3)

Many smokers go round the cycle several times
before quitting for good. This is not necessarily a
bad thing as they can learn from the experience.
You can help your clients by exploring what happened last time and finding a more effective strategy for the future. Feelings of failure and guilt are
common and may put them off trying again. You
may also feel demoralized when clients fail to reach
their goal and wonder if you are giving them the
right advice. It is worth remembering that a realistic success rate is only 5–10% (White, 1994).

Your continuing support and non-blaming,
non-judgemental approach may spur clients on to
have another go. You can suggest:

◆ Checking on the reasons for quitting. Does she
  really want to stop? Is she committed?

◆ If withdrawal symptoms were a severe problem,
  try nicotine replacement.

◆ Seeking more support – maybe by joining a
  group.

◆ Working out the best time to have another go
  at quitting.

◆ Having a break until she is ready to try again.

Women and alcohol

Alcohol, the most popular drug in Western society, is associated with good times: celebrations,
weddings, social occasions and family gatherings
– when many young people experience their first
drink. It is also a means of 'drowning our
sorrows'.

Until recently, problem drinking was predominantly associated with men, but the move to sexual equality is believed to have encouraged women
to drink more. Alcohol advertising and promotion
is frequently directed at women and young people,
with companies promoting images of women who
drink as glamorous, successful and generally more
attractive. Promoting concern among teenagers
about alcohol misuse is hard when advertising
equates adult success and attractiveness with
drinking. In reality, women often drink excessively
because they are lonely, unhappy and lacking confidence and support.

Total UK alcohol consumption almost doubled between World War II and 1979. This is attributed, in no small part, to the fall in the cost of
alcohol in relation to rising income: drinking became cheaper in real terms. Today, more women
are in paid employment, with more disposable
income. Social and cultural influences are also
significant (Ritson, 1990). Alcohol Concern's data
for 1992 suggest that the proportion of men drinking at risky or dangerous levels had been constant
since 1986. In contrast, the proportion of women
drinking at such levels had risen 'without
remission' since 1984.

Concealment of women's drinking misled researchers about the true scale of problem drinking.
Changing social attitudes towards women are believed to have encouraged more accurate research
which suggests that (Breeze, 1985; HEA, 1991b;
Alcohol Concern, 1994):

◆ in England, 89% of girls and boys have had their
  first 'proper' drink by the age of 13;

♦ in 1992, 27% of men and 11% of women in the UK exceeded 'safe drinking' units;

♦ 9% of men and 4% of women in the UK are 'problem' drinkers;

♦ of all age groups, 18–24-year-olds drink the most. Women most at risk from alcohol misuse are under 25, single and career orientated. They account for 45% of heavy drinkers.

Young people are heavily influenced by their parents' attitude and use of alcohol. In a multi-racial study on 9–15-year-olds, Afro-Caribbean and white children (71% and 65% respectively) were most likely to have tried alcohol. Only 19% of Asian children were reported to have done so. For a significant proportion of 15–16-year-olds drinking is an established habit rather than an occasional treat (HEA, 1991b).

More women are beginning to seek help with alcohol-related problems. Research in the 1980s suggested that women were more likely than men to acknowledge their problems, but less likely to attribute them to alcohol. (Anecdotal evidence in the 1990s suggests that this sexual divide is narrowing.) Social taboos still make it generally unacceptable for women to be drunk. Thus, women at risk

---

Box 2.7 Warning signs of harmful drinking

♦ Needing alcohol close at hand

♦ Making drink the number one priority

♦ Drinking faster than others in social situations

♦ Having to increase the amount or type of drink to maintain the effect, i.e. developing a tolerance to alcohol

♦ Feeling angry/irritated when others talk about your drinking

♦ Feeling tired/lethargic, sick

♦ Having hangovers, 'the shakes' or sweats

♦ Sleep problems

♦ Disruption of relationships and friendships

♦ Drink-related accidents or injuries

♦ Difficulty maintaining normal routine at home and work.

Some problem drinkers may show only one of these signs; others may show several.

---

are more inclined to consult people not specifically associated with alcohol abuse (Thom, 1986). GPs and primary care nurses fall within this category, are readily accessible and there is no stigma attached to consulting them. This gives them the opportunity to reach many women with alcohol problems who might otherwise be neglected.

Why do women drink?

Women drink alcohol for many reasons, including:

♦ to socialize;

♦ to boost confidence;

♦ to relax and to promote sleep;

♦ to cope with work, domestic and financial pressure;

♦ to 'treat' sexual problems;

♦ to relieve stress, boredom and loneliness;

♦ to help cope with major life events (e.g. bereavement, job loss, abuse); and

♦ to switch off.

Anxiety, depression, shame, guilt, grief, can all trigger and be exacerbated by drinking. Depression in women may be more marked premenstrually, postnatally and at the menopause. Drink can cause a vicious circle in which depression triggers drinking which, in turn, results in low self-esteem and lack of confidence which, in turn, aggravates depression.

Women play a central role in the family, often putting others' needs before their own. Women in general and problem drinkers in particular often feel guilty about taking time for themselves. In addition, they may wrongly perceive themselves to be 'bad mothers' or 'bad partners'. They need to learn how to meet their own needs (Plant, 1993). Another potential problem – 'the empty nest syndrome' – may develop when children leave home, and can be a trigger in increasing alcohol intake.

Less well-known is the susceptibility of lesbian women: a third are reported to have alcohol problems. A survey conducted among isolated young lesbians found the figure to be almost 70%. US research suggests that lesbians are vulnerable because they socialize in gay bars, and feel the need to 'hide away from the world' and 'escape their feelings about being different' (Lesbian Information Service, 1992).

Women with a history of sexual or physical or emotional abuse, or of problem drinkers in the family, are also at increased risk.

Women and the effects of alcohol

Women are more vulnerable to the effects of alcohol than men as they have a higher proportion of fat to water. This results in higher blood alcohol concentrations after drinking the same quantity of alcohol.

Drinking the same amount of alcohol at different phases of the menstrual cycle is reported to produce varying blood alcohol levels. The peak is said to occur during ovulation and premenstrually. Oral contraception slows down metabolism of alcohol, meaning that it takes longer for blood alcohol levels to revert to zero. (Alcohol is normally metabolized at the rate of a unit per hour.) A woman on oral contraception may be more likely than a non-pill-taker to be over the legal driving limit the morning after an evening of drinking. Even small amounts of alcohol (1–2 units) can impair judgement, especially in young people. The message should be do not drink anything if you are going to drive.

Alcohol is a central nervous system depressant and potentiates the action of sedative drugs. The combination of alcohol with tranquillizers, antidepressants and narcotics is potentially dangerous and sometimes lethal. Prolonged heavy use of alcohol causes increased metabolism of some drugs, including antiepileptics, hypoglycaemic agents and metronidazole.

Fatty deposits in the liver from heavy alcohol exposure will resolve if drinking stops and the liver is given a rest. Failing that, alcohol-induced hepatitis may follow. Prolonged heavy drinking leads to scarring and cirrhosis and possibly to cancer. Women, on average, develop cirrhosis within 13 years, nine years earlier than men (Plant, 1993; Webb, 1988).

Alcohol, sex and contraception

Drink-related sexual problems are associated with loss of libido, dyspareunia and vaginismus. Affected women may resort to alcohol to 'treat' themselves, reinforcing the popular myth that it enhances sexual pleasure. They may even perceive it to be an aphrodisiac, perhaps because of its disinhibiting effect. But as Shakespeare observed: 'It provokes the desire, but takes away the performance'. It is not only performance that may be lost as the disinhibiting effect of alcohol discourages effective contraception and safer sex. A Scottish survey found that young adults who frequently combined alcohol and sexual activity were seven times more likely to engage in risky sex than other young people, increasing the risk of unwanted pregnancy, HIV and other sexually transmitted infections (Bagnall et al., 1990).

Alcohol and the menstrual cycle

Women who drink heavily are susceptible to menstrual disturbances and reduced fertility, whilst heavy drinking men may experience temporary impotence after a drinking binge. Five units a day can reduce sperm counts.

PMS is more common in women with alcohol-related problems. Many sufferers are reported to 'self-medicate' with alcohol in the hope of relieving symptoms. Alcohol can trigger hot flushes at the menopause, and heavy consumption is a risk factor for osteoporosis, especially in smokers. Excess drinking puts osteoporotic women at increased risk of falls and fractures.

Alcohol and pregnancy

Alcohol freely crosses the placenta, so the concentration of alcohol in the developing baby will be the same as that in the mother. A baby's liver is less efficient at eliminating alcohol.

The Royal Colleges of General Practitioners, Physicians and Psychiatrists have jointly recommended that a pregnant woman should not drink more than one or two units of alcohol more than once or twice a week. The US Surgeon General was more cautious, ruling that there is 'no threshold' which is safe for all women. He recommended that women should not drink at all during pregnancy, nor when trying to conceive.

In practice, it is not always possible to give preconception advice as so many pregnancies are unplanned, leaving women unaware that they are pregnant until several weeks after conception. Thus, all sexually active women should be aware of the effect of alcohol on the fetus.

Maternal alcohol consumption may:

♦ increase the risk of spontaneous abortion;

♦ retard intrauterine growth (small babies); or

♦ cause damage to the developing fetus ranging from minor problems to full-blown fetal alcohol syndrome.

Breastfed babies may also be affected by alcohol passing into the breast milk in small quantities, disturbing their feeding, sleeping and bowel habits. Breastfeeding mothers should follow the same advice as given in pregnancy.

Alcohol and breast cancer

Recent research has focused on a possible relationship between moderate alcohol consumption and development of breast cancer. However, Plant (1993) says that while there is enough consistency in the data to suggest an association, there is little evidence to prove a causal relationship.

Sensible drinking

There has been a move away from the previously accepted, weekly, sensible drinking levels of 14 units for women and 21 units for men. The Department of Health's *Sensible Drinking* report, published in December 1995, recognizes the variability in individual responses to alcohol; and suggests a daily benchmark of between two and three units for women and between three and four units for men. Consistently drinking more carries an increasing health risk.

The report says that one or two units a day can provide some protection against coronary heart disease in postmenopausal women and men aged 40 and over. This effect may be negated by other predisposing factors such as smoking.

It is important to emphasize the risks of intoxication and binge drinking, to which young people are especially vulnerable. You may need to explain the importance of avoiding alcohol for 48 hours after heavy drinking.

How can you help?

Nurses working in primary care and women's health are in an excellent position to identify and help women at risk of developing a drink problem. Nurses are often thought of as more approachable and as having more time than doctors. But what about the nurses themselves? Many feel that they lack the skills to handle the complex underlying causes of alcohol problems particularly if they drink heavily themselves. Before helping others, nurses will need to think about the reasons they themselves drink and try to sort out their personal situation first. Developing counselling skills helps to build up confidence and expertise to open up the subject, encouraging clients to discuss their drinking habits in an open and honest way. In addition many local alcohol services or health promotion units now offer training/education sessions in alcohol awareness.

A client may present with anxiety, depression, general malaise or a fractured wrist, and may not recognize or admit that her problem is alcohol-related. Regular visits to the surgery with such problems may indicate a serious underlying problem she has not yet voiced.

Taking a drink history

Asking about alcohol consumption in a routine health check can encourage discussion without causing offence. Questions must be open and non-judgemental. A client may ask if she is drinking too much. An effective response may be to ask how drink is affecting her life (Box 2.7). Keeping a drink diary for a week or two may help her to establish if she is at risk. A diary can also pinpoint situations when she feels vulnerable and in need of a drink. Emphasize that for the diary to be useful, it must be a true record. Tell your client that she does not have to show it to anyone unless she wishes, which should encourage honesty.

Check that she understands about units of alcohol and the different strengths of alcoholic drink. A pub measure of spirits in England and Wales (25 ml) contains one unit; a drink poured at home may contain much more. She may not know, for example, that extra strong lager contains almost three times as much alcohol as ordinary lager. A 440 ml can of extra strong lager contains four units. For more information see *That's the Limit. A Guide to Sensible Drinking* (Health Education Board for Scotland, 1994).

The diary should record:

♦ Date and time of each drink

♦ Type and amount of drink (in units)

♦ Where and who with

♦ The circumstances – how does she feel before and after drinking?

♦ Cost.

Avoid pressurizing your client to stop drinking: women who drink heavily use alcohol as a coping mechanism. Physically dependent drinkers should not stop suddenly or without medical supervision.

Use the initial assessment to find out what your client wants to do. You can help her to explore her options: to continue drinking at current levels, to cut down or to stop. Many women can cut down successfully, but a dependent heavy drinker will probably need to stop completely, and may recognize that abstinence is her only hope.

Self-assessment and acceptance that alcohol is – or could be – a problem marks a major step

forward. Your client may need further information, referral to a GP or specialist alcohol service, and support from a social worker or health visitor. Encourage her to play an active role in planning her own recovery by, for example, suggesting that she books her own appointments.

What else can you do?

Compile a list of local agencies and visit them if possible. Ask if they provide women-only services, drop-in or crêche facilities (usually few and far between). Self-help and support groups for people with drink problems are often dominated by men which some women find intimidating.

Find out about residential/day-care facilities and their referral systems. Can a client self-refer for counselling or advice to the community psychiatric team? Can she have detoxification at home through a community alcohol team? There may be a need for this if residential accommodation is unavailable and if a woman has a young family.

Stress

Stress is a normal part of everyday life. Short-term stress can have a positive effect, making us take stock of difficult situations, or alerting us to potential threats or hazards. In contrast, long-term, unresolved stress is potentially destructive. The so-called stress response, which prepares the body for 'flight or fight', helps with short-term emergencies, for example, attack by man or animal. Long-term stress in modern life can result in a state of over-alertness and prolonged worry which prevents the body from winding down. Coping with a job or unemployment while trying to bring up a family can cause prolonged stress. The breakdown of the traditional extended family has compounded stress in family life by leaving women unsupported.

Stress in women is variable. A source of stimulus for one person may reduce another to a state of nervous exhaustion. Stress in women may be caused by all sorts of factors:

♦ Raising a family – young children, teenagers, single parenting, a low income, poor housing

♦ Employment/unemployment problems

♦ Ill-health

Box 2.8 The following tips may be useful when discussing how to moderate alcohol consumption with a client:

♦ Set yourself a limit for the day/week/or a special occasion e.g. a party.

♦ Enjoy the taste. Make it last. Take smaller sips and put the glass down in between.

♦ Avoid rounds and kitties. Don't feel obliged to keep up with other people.

♦ Dilute spirits with low calorie mixers to make a long drink.

♦ Pace your drinks with non-alchoholic 'spacers'.

♦ Eat a meal before or while drinking.

♦ Avoid cocktails and 'strong' lagers. They contain several units of alcohol.

♦ Find other ways to relax and unwind. Take a walk, have a long bath, try a new hobby or evening class and make friends outside your drinking circle.

♦ Give yourself a treat with the money you've saved.

♦ Caring for an elderly or sick relative

♦ Racism

♦ Sexism

♦ Living in a violent relationship.

Many of the chapters in this book deal with potentially stressful issues, such as infertility, pregnancy, abortion, abnormal smears, PMS, rape and urinary incontinence. Stress associated with issues like these may be exacerbated by lack of information and understanding and by fixed, inaccurate ideas of the 'My mother told me' variety.

Developing counselling skills may help you to help many of your clients. However, some women may need to be referred for more specialist counselling than you can offer – for example, a woman who has been raped.

Health care professionals themselves are not immune from stress and may need support. Personal problems may be exacerbated by professional ones in a health service increasingly beset by job insecurity, heavy workloads, lack of resources and insufficient management support.

There is a dearth of research about the reasons why nurses themselves smoke and drink, and the extent to which they do so to alleviate stress in their professional or personal life. This seems ironic in a profession that is dedicated to health care.

The RCN Counselling and Advisory Service offers free professional counselling to members on a range of issues which may be either personal or work related (see Resources, page 39).

Grace Owen, the author and General Secretary for the National Association for Staff Support (NASS), emphasizes that before trying to help others, health care professionals need to look at their own lives; to recognize their own signs of stress; and to be aware of situations which they find stressful.

They should ask themselves questions like:

♦ How much support do I have from my peers?

♦ Are my working conditions satisfactory?

♦ Do my colleagues and I have opportunities for debriefing?

♦ Am I in the right job?

♦ Am I a valued member of staff?

♦ Do I have the freedom to express my feelings and ideas?

Dealing with stress

Grace Owen also emphasizes the importance of empowerment in the workplace as a means of personal growth and development. This can help to build up confidence, self-esteem and a sense of professional identity which may have an insulating effect against stress.

As outlined in Box 2.9, there are many different responses to stress – many of these are negative but if stress is sensitively dealt with there can be a positive outcome.

Box 2.9   Responses to stress

Negative responses

♦ Drinking

♦ Smoking

♦ Tranquillizer and illegal drug use

♦ 'Comfort eating'

♦ Feeling moody

♦ Relationship problems – lowered libido and sexual functioning.

Positive responses

♦ Making time for yourself

♦ Developing a new interest

♦ Taking regular exercise: going for a long walk, yoga

♦ Learning to be more assertive

♦ Identifying problems and talking about them

♦ Making lifestyle and career changes

♦ Joining a self-help group

♦ Having counselling

♦ Complementary therapies – relaxation and visualization, massage, aromatherapy, reflexology, acupuncture, Alexander technique, shiatsu and therapeutic touch and hypnotherapy.

Relaxation techniques can be effective, easy to teach, and used in many different situations: either alone or in groups; or with an audio cassette. A simple routine which you can recommend is outlined in Box 2.10.

Box 2.10 A simple relaxation routine

♦ Sit right back in a chair and uncross your legs. Rest your hands in your lap.

♦ Put your feet flat on the floor.

♦ Close your eyes and breathe easily and normally.

♦ Tense and relax the main groups of muscles starting with the toes and ending with the face. Notice the difference in the sensations.

♦ When you feel ready, open your eyes. You should feel renewed and refreshed.

Conclusion

Nurses in community and hospital settings can play a key role in health education and health promotion by encouraging women to take care of themselves and their families. Try to empower your client to make her own decision about health and lifestyle, but respect her final decision, even if it runs contrary to your own view. Her upbringing, culture, values and social and financial circumstances will influence her personal response to health promotion.

It is beyond the scope of this chapter to present a fully comprehensive view of health promotion, but we hope that it will stimulate further exploration and learning and will have given you many useful ideas that you can adapt to suit your own clinical practice and local needs.

Resources

Health promotion

Health Education Authority
Hamilton House, Mabledon Place, London WC1H 9TX
Tel. 0171 383 3833
Health Promotion Information Centre
Tel. 0171 413 1995
Provides a wide range of services and resources.

Health Education Board for Scotland
Woodburn House, Canaan Lane, Edinburgh E10 4SG
Tel. 0131 447 8044

Health Promotion Agency for Northern Ireland
18 Ormeau Avenue, Belfast BT2 8HF
Tel. 01232 311611

Health Promotion Wales
Ffynnonlas, Tyglas Avenue, Llanishen, Cardiff CF4 5DZ
Tel. 01222 752222

Healthwise
27 Mortimer Street, London W1N 7RJ
Tel. 0171 636 7866
A Family Planning Association bookshop carrying an extensive range of books on all aspects of women's health. A mail order service is available.

Women's Health
52 Featherstone Street, London EC1Y 8RT
Tel. 0171 251 6580
Provides a wide range of information and leaflets. Send a stamp-addressed envelope for a publications list.

Courses

Universities, colleges of nurse education, the Royal College of Nursing and local health promotion units run courses and workshops, some of which lead to a degree/diploma/certificate or ENB award in:

♦ Health Education and Promotion

♦ Health Studies

♦ Women's Health Screening

♦ Communication and Counselling Skills

♦ Teaching and Facilitating

♦ Smoking Cessation. Drug and Alcohol Awareness

♦ Management Studies

♦ Stress Management.

The RCN and ENB provide course information.

ENB Careers
PO Box 2EN, London W1A 2EN
Tel. 0171 391 6200/6205
Provide information on ENB approved courses.

Institute of Advanced Nursing Education of the Royal College of Nursing
20 Cavendish Square, London W1M 0AB
Tel. 0171 872 0840 or 0171 409 3333

Preconception care and early pregnancy

Maternity Alliance
15 Brittania St, London WC1X 9JN
Tel. 0171 837 1263
Publishes books, reports and leaflets for parents-to-be and professionals on preconception advice, pregnancy and the first year of life.

Video: *'From Chance to Choice'. A multi-ethnic approach to community genetics: the role of the primary health care team.* Costs £30. Available from: Unit of Clinical Genetics and Fetal Medicine. Institute of Child Health, 30 Guilford St, London WC1N 1EH
Tel: 0171 242 9789 ext 2610

Health and exercise

British Sports Association for the Disabled (BSAD)
Solcast House, 13–27 Brunswick Place, London N1 6DX
Tel. 0171 490 4919

The Sports Council
16 Upper Woburn Place, London WC1H 0QP
Tel. 0171 388 1277
Publishes a wide range of materials for the public and professionals. It also publishes jointly with the Health Education Authority.

Women and drugs

ADFAM National
5th Floor, Epworth House, 25 City Road, London EC1Y 1AA
Tel. 0171 638 3700
A charity for families and friends of drug users. It runs a national helpline offering information and support. The office is open between 10 am and 5 pm.

Council for Involuntary Tranquilliser Addiction (CITA)
Cavendish House, Brighton Road, Waterloo, Liverpool L22 5NG
Helpline: 0151 949 0102
Provides support for people withdrawing from tranquillizers.

Drugs and Alcohol Women's Network (DAWN)
c/o GLAAS, 30–31 Great Sutton Street, London EC1V 0DX
Tel. 0171 253 6221
For information and advice about drug and alcohol problems.

Drugs in Schools Helpline
Tel. 0345 366666 (calls charged at local rate)

Institute for the Study of Drug Dependence (ISDD)
Waterbridge House, 32–36 Loman Street, London SE1 0EE
Tel. 0171 928 1211
This is a library and information service on non-medical use of drugs.

MIND (The National Association for Mental Health)
Granta House, 15–19 Broadway, London E15 4BQ
Tel. 0181 519 2122; Information line: 0181 522 1728

National Drugs Helpline
Tel. 0800 77 66 00
For 24 hour advice, counselling and information about local agencies. Advice in other languages is available on request.

Northern Ireland Council for Voluntary Action
127 Ormeau Road, Belfast BT7 1SH
Tel. 01232 321224

Release
Tel. 0171 729 9904
A national drugs advice line operating from 10 am to 6 pm Monday to Friday. For the emergency 24-hour helpline, including legal advice, telephone 0171 603 8654.

Scottish Drugs Forum
5 Oswald Street, Glasgow G1 4QR
Tel. 0141 221 1175

Standing Conference on Drug Abuse (SCODA)
Waterbridge House, 32–36 Loman Street, London SE1 0EE
National coordinating body for organizations concerned with drug abuse and counselling. A directory of drug services nationally is available entitled *Drug Problems: Where to Get Help.*

Welsh Office Drugs Unit
Welsh Office, Cathays Park, Cardiff CF1 3NQ
Tel. 01222 825111

Women and smoking

Action on Smoking and Health (ASH)
109 Gloucester Place, London W1H 3PH
Tel. 0171 935 3519
(Also ASH Scotland, Wales and Northern Ireland).

HEA Local Smoking Action Unit
University of the West of England, Oldbury Court Road, Fishponds, Bristol BS16 2JP
Tel. 0117 976 2173

Provides resources and support for smoking prevention specialists and agencies.

Quitline
Tel. 0800 0022 00
Offers help and advice to smokers trying to stop. Ex-smokers can also ring for encouragement. A *Quitpack* and a *Break Free Pack* (for young people) is available from QUIT, Victory House, 170 Tottenham Court Road, London W1P 0HA.

RCN Nurses Against Smoking Group
20 Cavendish Square, London W1M 0AB
Run campaigns to promote smoke-free living. There is a pack available.

Women and alcohol

Alcoholics Anonymous (AA)
General Services Office, PO Box 1, Stonebow House, York YO1 2NJ
Tel. 01904 644026

Al-Anon and **Alateen** (for young people)
61 Great Dover Street, London SE1 4YF
24-hour helpline 0171 403 0888
Support family and friends of problem drinkers through group meetings.

Alcohol Concern
Waterbridge House, 32–36 Loman Street, London SE1 0EE
Tel. 0171 928 7377
Publishes research (including regular bulletins) and provides information and resources for professionals and the public.

Aquarius – Managing Drink
The White House, 111 New St, Birmingham B24 4EU. A teaching pack for nurses.

Drugs and Alcohol Women's Network (DAWN)
Address as for GLAAS (below). Publishes leaflets and research.

Greater London Alcohol Advisory Service (GLAAS)
30–31 Great Sutton Street, London EC1V 0DX
Tel. 0171 253 6221

Stress

National Association for Staff Support (NASS)
9 Caradon Close, Woking, Surrey GU21 3DU
Tel. 01483 771599
A charitable association providing a networking and resource service for professionals who want to promote good staff support practices. Membership costs £20.00.

NURSELINE
8–10 Crown Hill, Croydon, Surrey CR0 1RZ
Helpline: 0181 681 4030
An independent *signpost* advisory and information service provided by the Royal College of Nursing for all nurses and midwives. It is designed to point nurses towards help for matters of personal anxiety and work-related stress.

Royal College of Nursing Counselling and Advisory Service
8–10 Crown Hill, Croydon, Surrey CR0 1RZ
Tel. 0345 697064
Offers free professional counselling to members. The service is a member of the British Association for Counselling and offers short-term counselling on a range of issues which may be either personal or work related.

References and further reading

ACQUIRE (1994) Alcohol Concern's Quarterly Information and Research Bulletin. no. 7.

ALCOHOL CONCERN (1994) Alcohol Concern's Quarterly Information and Research Bulletin. *Acquire* no. 7.

ASH Scotland (1994) *Action On Smoking and Health*, leaflet.

AUSTOKER, J., SANDERS, D. and FOWLER, G. (1994) Smoking and cancer: smoking cessation. *British Medical Journal* **308**: 1478–82.

BAGNALL, G., PLANT, M.A. and WARWICK, W. (1990) Alcohol, drugs and AIDS-related risks: results from a prospective study. *AIDS Care* **2**: 309–17.

BARKER, J.P. (1993) Fetal nutrition and cardiovascular disease in adult life. *Lancet* **341**: 938–41.

BELLOW, B. and RAMSAY, I. (1991) Towards a smoke free generation. London: HEA and DOH.

BETTER LIVING BETTER LIFE (1993) A primary healthcare resource on lifestyle interventions for coronary heart disease and stroke prevention. Oxon: Knowledge Hse (multi author).

BREEZE, E. (1985) *Women and Drinking*. Office of Population Censuses and Surveys. London: HMSO.

CAMBERWELL COUNCIL ON ALCOHOLISM (1980) *Women and Alcohol*. London: Tavistock.

CURTIS, H., HOOLAGHAN, J. and JEWITT, C. (eds) (1995) *Sexual Health Promotion in General Practice*. Oxford: Radcliffe Medical Press.

DAWN (nd) *Women and Drinking*, booklet. London: DAWN (no date of pub.– approx. 1990).

DOH (1991) *While You Are Pregnant: Safe Eating and How to Avoid Infection from Food and Animals*. London: HMSO.

DOH (1992) *Folic Acid and the Prevention of Neural Tube Defects*. Report from an Expert Advisory Group. London: HMSO.

DOH (Department of Health) (1992) *The Health of the Nation. A Strategy for Health*. London: HMSO.

DOH (1994) *Committee on Medical Aspects of Food Policy. Report of the Cardiovascular Review Group*. London: HMSO.

DOH (1995a) *Social Trends*, 25. London: HMSO.

DOH (1995b) *Sensible Drinking*. Report of an Interdepartmental Working Group. London: DOH.

DOH (1956) *Sensible Drinking*. Report of an Interdepartmental Working Group. London: DOH.

DOYLE, W. (1994) *Teach Yourself Healthy Eating*. London: Hodder & Stoughton.

EWLES, L. and SIMNETT, I. (1992) *Promoting Health. A Practical Guide*. London: Scutari Press.

GASKELL, J. (1994) No pause for pregnancy. *Practice Nurse* 1–14 March: 207–10.

GOODWIN, K. (1993) *Planning a Pregnancy*, booklet. London: FPA.

GOSSOP, M. (1993) *Living With Drugs*, 3rd edn. Aldershot: Ashgate.

GRAHAM, H. (1987) Women's smoking and family health. *Social Science and Medicine*, **25**: 47–56.

GUILLEBAUD, J. (1993) *Contraception: Your Questions Answered*, 2nd edn. Edinburgh: Churchill Livingstone.

HEA (Health Education Authority) (1991a) *Passive Smoking. Questions and Answers*. London: HEA.

HEA (1991b) *Factfile: Young People and Drink*. Drinkwise Campaign. London: HEA.

HEA (1993a) *Every Woman's Health*. Information and resources for group discussion. London: HEA.

HEA (1993b) *Smoking and Pregnancy: Guidance for all Health Professionals Supporting Pregnant Women who Want to Stop Smoking*. London: HEA.

HEA (1996) *Promoting Physical Activity in Primary Health Care: Guidance for the Primary Health Care Team*. London: HEA.

HEA, DEPARTMENT OF HEALTH, THE MINISTRY OF AGRICULTURE, FISHERIES AND FOOD (1994) *The National Food Guide: The Balance of Good Health*. London: HEA.

HMSO (1988) *Fourth report of the Independent Scientific Committee on Smoking and Health*. London: HMSO.

ILLICH, I. (1977) *Limits to Medicine – Medical Nemesis: the Exploration of Health*. London: Pelican Books.

ISDD (Institute for the Study of Drug Dependence) (1993) *Druglink Factsheets 4 and 5*. London: ISDD.

ISDD (1994) *Drug Abuse Briefing*, 5th edn. London: ISDD.

ISDD (1995) *Drugs Pregnancy and Childcare. A Guide for Professionals*. London: ISDD.

JACOBSON, B. (1986) *Beating The Ladykillers: Women and Smoking*. London: Pluto Press.

LESBIAN INFORMATION SERVICE (1992) *Lesbians and Alcohol: A Resource List*. London: Alcohol Concern.

McCONVILLE, B. (1991) *Women under the Influence: Alcohol and its Impact*. London: Grafton.

McPHERSON, A. (ed.) (1993) *Women's Problems in General Practice*, 3rd edn. Oxford: Oxford University Press.

MARKHAM, U. (1990) *Women Under Pressure. A Practical Guide for Today's Woman*. Shaftesbury: Element Books.

MENTAL HEALTH FOUNDATION (1994) *Helping You Cope. A Guide to Starting and Stopping Tranquillisers and Sleeping Tablets*. London: Mental Health Foundation.

NAIDOO, J. and WILLS, J. (1994) *Health Promotion. Foundations for Practice*. London: Baillière Tindall.

NATIONAL OSTEOPOROSIS SOCIETY (1992) *Exercise and Physiotherapy in the Prevention of Osteoporosis*. London: National Osteoporosis Society.

OPCS (Office of Population Censuses and Surveys) (1991) *Survey of Smoking among Secondary Schoolchildren in 1990*. London: HMSO.

OPCS (1992/1994) *General Household Survey*. London: HMSO.

OPCS (1994a) *General Household Survey 1992*. London: HMSO.

OPCS (1994b) *Survey of Smoking Among Secondary Schoolchildren in 1993*. London: HMSO.

PLANT, M. (1993) Drink problems. In McPherson, A. (ed.) *Women's Problems in General Practice*. Oxford: Oxford University Press.

RIEDER, A., SCHOBERBERGER, R. and KUNZE, M. (1994) First experiences in women's smoking cessation in Austria. International Congress on Smoking Cessation held in Glasgow.

RITSON, B. (ed.) (1990) *Alcohol and Health. A Handbook for Nurses, Midwives and Health Visitors*. London: The Medical Council on Alcoholism.

ROYAL COLLEGE OF PHYSICIANS (1991) *Medical Aspects of Exercise*. London: RCP.

RUTHERFORD, D. (1988) *A Lot of Bottle*. London: Institute of Alcohol Studies.

SILAGY, C., MANT, D., FOWLER, G. and LODGE, M. (1994) Meta-analysis on efficacy of nicotine replacement therapies in smoking cessation. *Lancet* **343**: 139–42.

SIMNET, I. (1995) *Managing Health Promotion: Developing Healthy Organizations and Communities*. Chichester: John Wiley & Sons.

SZAREWSKI, A. (1994) *A Woman's Guide to the Cervical Smear Test*. London: Optima.

THOM, B. (1986) Sex differences in help-seeking for alcohol problems. 1. Barriers to help-seeking. *British Journal of Addiction* **81**: 777–88.

THOMAS, B. (ed.) (1994) *Manual of Dietetic Practice*, 2nd edn. London: Blackwell Scientific.

TREVELYAN, J. and BOOTH, B. (1994) *Complementary Medicine for Nurses, Midwives and Health Visitors*. London: Macmillan.

US DHHS (Department of Health and Human Services) (1990) *The Health Benefits of Smoking Cessation: A Report of the Surgeon General*. Atlanta: Public Health Service Centers for Disease Control.

WATERSON, E.J. and MURRAY-LYON, I.M. (1989) Alcohol, smoking and pregnancy: some observations on ethnic minorities in the United Kingdom. *British Journal of Addiction* **84**: 323–25.

WEBB, I. (1988) *Breaking the Habit. Guide to Alcohol Education*. London: Thames Television.

WEBB, I. (1992) *A Woman's Guide to Alcohol*. London: Alcohol Concern.

WELLS, R. with TSCHUDIN, V. (eds) (1994) *Wells' Supportive Therapies in Health Care*. London: Baillière Tindall.

WESTCOTT, P. (1994) *Women's Health. Nursing Times* special publication, pp. 60–62.

WHITE, P. (1994a) Tackle tomorrow's smokers today. *Practice Nurse* 1–14 March: 193–96.

WHITE, P. (1994b) World talks about quitting. *Practice Nurse*, 15–31 May: 523–25.

WILSON, M. (1989) *Living with a Drinker: How to Change Things*. London: Pandora.

WORLD HEALTH ORGANIZATION (1984) Health promotion: a WHO discussion document on the concepts and principles. Reprinted in: *Journal of the Institute of Health Education*, **23**(1) 1985.

3: Psychosexual and emotional care

Jane Selby

OBJECTIVES

After reading this chapter you will understand:

♦ that it is appropriate for nurses to enquire about a woman's sexual life as part of holistic care

♦ how to observe, listen to, reflect and respond to a woman's sexual anxieties

♦ that psychosexual nursing skills are not about having to find a solution

♦ that grief and bereavement affect people in a variety of ways

♦ the different stages of grief

♦ that there are other types of loss apart from death

♦ how to make appropriate referrals either for psychosexual or for emotional problems.

Psychosexual nursing

This section describes how the sexuality of patients can be addressed as part of normal clinical practice. Psychosexual nursing should be accepted and practised wherever and whenever the opportunity presents, whether you are in training or a qualified nurse, midwife or health visitor. A move can then be made away from pathology and this will allow you and your patient the opportunity to talk more freely about feelings associated with sexuality and life events.

Most women whom you meet professionally do not have deep-seated psychological causes for their worries and anxieties. Women may use any consultation with you to ask about sexual matters, sexual development and anxieties. They see you as not being personally involved with their life, and welcome the opportunity of a consultation with a concerned and sensitive nurse. The aim of this chapter is to encourage you to use and increase the skills that you already possess but which often lie dormant and unrecognized. Sometimes it may take just as much courage for you to overcome your inhibitions with patients as it does for them to be brave and raise sexual matters with you.

Nurses are human beings, and you share the same gifts, faults and failures as your patients. You have emotional experiences and personal events which can be drawn upon when talking to women, but you should remember that these belong to you alone and must never be personalized in a consultation. There is an additional problem that we like some patients and some patients like us more than others, i.e. we feel we 'work well' and relate with them, but we may have negative attitudes towards others. It is often felt that nurses should not react in this way, but all human beings have these prejudicial emotions. The recognition and sharing of these emotions with patients and colleagues can be revealing and is often enough to relieve anxiety. In itself, this can be a significant help to the patient. Sexuality is still seen to be private even with today's more liberal attitudes and thinking. Therefore the patient's behaviour can be noted and her wishes respected.

When patients make enquiries to you about sexual matters, you 'hear' but are often fearful of the outcome and fail to respond appropriately because you think 'I might be seen to be prying' or 'I might get out of my depth' and go on to think 'I don't know how to solve the problem'. In psychosexual nursing the most important thing to learn is that you do not have to solve the patient's problems. It is the patient who has to do that, with your help.

A knowledge of emotional development must be attained to acknowledge sexual maturation. This can be done by looking at everyday behaviour around you, reading novels and magazines, watching television as well as by professional study. Then practise your new learning by observing, and studying how you relate to each patient and how the patient behaves towards you. You will then be able to notice when normal steps in sexual growth seem to have been missed out, or events have happened that cause or leave damage and trauma, which appear to affect a woman's sexual health. An enquiry can then be made and interpreted with her. We all learn from our patients and John Bowlby (1986) dedicates his book on *Loss, Sadness and Depression* to 'My patients who have worked hard to educate me'.

Psychosexual nursing is often painful and frightening for both you and your patient. The temptation is not to stay with uncomfortable emotions but to go down the safer route of pathology and clinical illness: the familiar route where the patient may feel more comfortable and you feel more skilled.

It is your responsibility to listen, understand and share these ordinary everyday fears and worries, and enable your patient to explore her problems with you and then lead her to an understanding of them. You will then discover that you have skills, often hidden and not used, that allow you to make a move forward in offering psychosexual care. This can give satisfaction not only to your patient but also to yourself.

Scenarios are included throughout this chapter as examples to illustrate how problems can be presented to you, and to show that the presenting problem may well cover deep unspoken sexual anxieties. Recognition of this fact alongside sensitive questioning can mean that a small amount of help from you may be all that is needed to prevent minor anxieties becoming major psychosexual problems.

Presentation of sexual anxieties

Sexual anxieties are presented in a variety of ways and you need the knowledge and skills to be alert to these in order to communicate effectively. Nurses who work in women's health have a valuable opportunity to ask about sexuality as part of their holistic care. Alas, such enquiries do not always take place, and if they do they may well come from the patient herself rather than from the nurse.

The overt presentation

Anxiety may be openly presented by your client in various forms:

◆ A client may just ask you a direct question about sexuality or sexual life. This usually comes as a surprise and you may feel taken aback initially, sometimes even bordering on panic, for instance during a consultation when sexual abuse is revealed.

◆ The patient may feel she wants to 'test you out'. In spite of feeling you have been asking relevant questions in your consultation which might have allowed her to voice an anxiety, nothing has actually been revealed. It is only when she feels she can trust you and your attitude, that she can say something.

◆ Sometimes the patient waits to the very end of the consultation until she asks the question. It may be that she has had to screw up her courage to raise her anxiety. This can create a reciprocal anxiety for you because time is running out and other patients are waiting. It then becomes difficult to deal with the problem satisfactorily. You should endeavour to talk about sexuality issues early in the clinical consultation.

Tears represent a variety of emotions (Box 3.1). Some people cry easily and will then apologize afterwards. Others remain dry-eyed even whilst telling harrowing stories when you feel they should be crying. Absence of tears does not necessarily indicate a lack of feeling. You need to recognize and interpret with the patient the feelings that lie behind the need to cry.

Box 3.1 Types of tears

♦ *Happy tears* of excitement and joy are perhaps the easiest to cope with. They may represent relief from anxiety as well as joy, e.g. childbirth, or on hearing that a breast lump is not malignant.

♦ *Tears of anger* that 'come in bucketfuls' may be a result of a feeling of frustration with a problem at home, or perhaps with medical care; a treatment may not be working or an old complaint may be recurring; in women's health, cystitis and vaginal discharge are common causes for anger as these not only affect general health but are also closely tied up with sexual life. The anger is not only with the initial complaint, but also with themselves and their partner.

♦ *Tears of sadness* that well out of the eyes and roll down the cheeks, despite the woman's attempts to control them, may make the nurse feel she has provoked sadness by an innocent enquiry. Loss is often the clue in such a situation. It may not be a recent event; the emotional pain may have been controlled not just for days or weeks but sometimes many years, e.g. the termination of an earlier pregnancy.

♦ *Sobbing tears* where the whole body seems to be involved can occur in acute stress situations, e.g. divorce. The woman has felt perhaps for some considerable time that she must stay in control and when she meets you, who appear empathetic, it is then that she breaks down.

Scenario

Sandra, a young woman of 23, married for just two months, had come to see the nurse in the surgery. She was the last patient of a late clinic. When she was called in she shot through the door, sat down and burst into tears. The nurse held her hand and waited – not easy for the time-pressed nurse. Sandra blurted out that 'she didn't love her husband and nearly didn't marry him, but felt too frightened to say no'. The nurse felt taken aback. Sandra then said she thought she might be pregnant. Her husband wanted a baby and they had not used contraception, but she didn't want a baby yet. The nurse thought he sounded most uncaring. The pregnancy test was indeed positive and Sandra revealed that her husband was in the waiting room. The nurse went to fetch him, and found a young man who appeared very concerned and quite different from her assumptions. She left them to talk together. The husband walked out as the nurse returned, and Sandra appeared calmer and said she wasn't going to have a termination. She and her husband then went in to see the doctor and on returning to the waiting room she flung her arms round the nurse saying 'thank you'.

For Sandra, the emotional upheaval of marriage and a quick pregnancy was just like receiving an electric shock: frightening and overwhelming. The nurse shared these emotions, she waited and used the skill of touch, a professional privilege, to 'stay' with Sandra throughout this encounter. The way Sandra said goodbye to the nurse was important, as she showed relief and grateful appreciation of her help and concern.

The covert presentation

Hidden and often unspoken anxieties will require all your skills of observation and listening, if you are to uncover the real problem.

Nurses are well trained in clinical observation, which is one of the early skills learnt in basic training, but psychosexual nursing observations are about the patient's feelings and emotional life; these require very perceptive antennae. Nurses sometimes feel that it is unprofessional and not part of the job to pry into women's sexual lives.

This can be overcome and it should be the responsibility of the sensitive nurse to offer an opening for any patient to talk about her sexual health during a consultation.

The setting and first observations

This could be the surgery, the clinic, the outpatient department, the ward, the waiting room and even the corridor. The way she walks into the room and greets you can be an important clue. Who accompanies her? A child, children, her boyfriend, partner, husband or friend? How does she behave with them? What does she bring with her? Does she bring lots of bags – this may be only the shopping, but note how she organizes the bags; she may need support even from them. If she comes on her own, does she seem to be in control but not very confident? Could this be hiding some painful emotional feelings?

Appearance

Is she dressed appropriately for her age group? Does she dress up or down? Observe her make-up and appearance of her nails; if they are bitten it will often indicate anxiety. Hair, particularly for the young is an excellent curtain to hide behind. If you see someone regularly, note any changes from one visit to the next. You do not always have to verbalize your thoughts to the patient but appearances indicate mood and emotional changes as well as life changes. It may be useful to make a comment and acknowledge these changes at a later consultation.

Smell

This can be unpleasant and embarrassing both for the patient and for you. Is it the smell of a dirty body, unwashed or dirty clothes? Is it the smell of urine? If so, you could raise a question about her continence as she may suffer from stress incontinence which she has never felt able to discuss before. As all continence advisers will tell us, it is a common problem which affects all age groups and once the question has been raised and incontinence acknowledged, help is often gratefully received (see Chapter 15).

Alcohol on the breath may well be a sign of a problem, especially if the time of day appears to

be inappropriate. Alcohol and drugs are widely used to help both short-term anxieties and long-term emotional problems, but they also can cause havoc with people's sexual lives.

Scenario

 Sally was a professional woman aged 36 and held a responsible administrative job. She appeared tired and overweight. She had come for a repeat pill prescription. The nurse noticed a smell of alcohol on her breath although it was mid-morning. Sally said that although she and her partner both worked for the same organization they hardly ever saw each other. On enquiry from the nurse, she also admitted there was hardly any sexual life. She was worried about her recent increase of weight and admitted that her eating habits were erratic as she was always home late and her partner was even later. She was a non-smoker which then led to the nurse enquiring about her drinking habits. She had to entertain at lunchtime – often with wine– and had a drink again when she got home in the evening. On discussing this she was shocked to realize that over the last six months she had started with one glass of wine in the evening but now quite frequently finished the bottle by herself. Her health and sexual life were in jeopardy, and the small clue to this unhappiness was the faint whiff of alcohol mid-morning that the nurse had noticed and sensitively enquired about.

Facial expressions

The eyes often give the clue – sad, flashing, defiant, or unable to look at you. Look at the face as you talk to your patient and obtain information from her. Note any change in facial expressions – all the emotions can be expressed, ranging from excitement to sadness. The nose that wrinkles, as in a family planning consultation, where the nurse learnt from the young girl that they were using condoms as she had a new boyfriend. She knew that the nurse was expecting to hear that they were practising safer sex, but the nurse noted the nose twitch and the brief downward look. On commenting 'You don't look very happy about that' she learnt the true story where the condom was not always used and a gamble was consequently taking place for both HIV and contraception. One small sign gave the observant nurse the opportunity to discuss other methods of contraception and the importance of safer sex.

Common sexual anxieties and problems

Women come to you to seek and receive professional help, information and advice, often with the added pressure of asking you to find a solution for them. In psychosexual nursing the patient has to find the solution for herself, but you can help her. Women frequently present with problems that seem irrelevant and this can confuse both of you. It is up to you to try to sift out and clarify what is relevant to your nursing role. The importance of identifying the real anxiety becomes your primary task, whether it is physical, emotional or a combination of both.

The feelings that adversely affect a woman's sexuality are summarized in Box 3.2.

The encounter can be uncomfortable for both of you and patience may be required as usually nothing significant will be revealed if the woman is feeling hassled. Silence may hide the distress of a woman struggling with her inner feelings which she feels are unspeakable. Try not to be afraid of this silence, bear with it and more often than not you will be rewarded with a response.

Many events and changes in women's lives only cause temporary sexual anxieties and not long-lasting problems. They are certainly more likely to be temporary if they are discussed early on rather than later or not at all.

Sexual anxieties and problems are often classified as being *primary* or *secondary*. Primary problems have been present since the start of sexual activity whereas secondary problems develop after a period of satisfactory sexual function. Common forms of sexual anxiety and dysfunction are listed in Table 3.1.

Loss of libido

Loss of libido is defined as a loss of interest and desire to feel a sexual person. It is sometimes referred to as 'feeling frigid'. This is a common

Box 3.2 Feelings that adversely affect a woman's sexuality

Misunderstanding about sex
♦ Ignorance about sex
♦ Not knowing what to expect
♦ How to behave
♦ Expectations too high.

Bad feelings about sex
♦ Fear of being caught
♦ Fear of making too much noise and being overheard
♦ Fear of being interrupted
♦ Fear of failing to perform 'normally'
♦ Fear of being undignified or incontinent
♦ Guilty, believing that sexual intercourse or sexual acts are wrong
♦ Disgust that sex is dirty and messy.

Problems in the relationship
♦ Feeling angry, even rage and violence
♦ Feeling resentful and bitter
♦ Feeling contempt for a partner
♦ Feeling insecure
♦ Fear of being physically hurt
♦ Fear of partner leaving
♦ Fear of the future.

Bad feelings from women
♦ Depression
♦ Worthlessness
♦ Low self-esteem
♦ Unattractive
♦ Unhappy with her body image.

Circumstances which cause lack of sexual feelings
♦ Too tired
♦ Worried
♦ Preoccupied with other things
♦ Babies and children of all ages
♦ Lack of warmth and comfort
♦ Losses and bereavement
♦ No privacy.

Table 3.1 *Sexual anxiety and dysfunction*	
DYSFUNCTION	**CAUSE**
Loss of libido	Emotional
Dyspareunia	Physical and emotional
Vaginismus	Physical and emotional
Dry vagina	Physical and emotional
Orgasmic dysfunction	Emotional

complaint and many women have a feeling of failure both for themselves and their partners.

Primary lack of sexual libido may be the result of difficulty during early sexual maturation, e.g. child sexual abuse or rape.

Secondary lack of libido presents more frequently and is likely to be associated with either present life events or a past emotional or physical event. Women may also feel generally depressed with their current situation. Such situations could include:

◆ Difficulties in a relationship with poor communication between the couple

◆ Infertility problems

◆ Pregnancy, birth and postnatal problems

◆ Redundancy, job failure or career changes

◆ Retirement and ageing

◆ Bereavement

◆ Losses, e.g. leaving home, selling and moving house

◆ Anxieties over medical problems and ill-health

◆ Gynaecological problems including cervical cell changes and the effects of colposcopy.

It is usually the anger, frustration and resentment at the above situations which leads to a withdrawal of feelings to have a sexual relationship.

Scenario

Carol came to the surgery to have a cut finger dressed. She was well-known to the nurse and asked if she remembered telling her last time that 'she felt nothing when making love'. The nurse did not remember the remark but she did this time!

Carol was now six months postnatal after her third child and commented 'I never felt like this after the other two'. The nurse offered to examine Carol and noticed that the episiotomy had healed well with no pain but Carol then said her vagina felt 'numb'. The nurse felt baffled, just as Carol felt, so suggested she should return for some counselling. It was then that Carol said very angrily that would be impossible as she was having to move across the country because of her husband's job. The nurse recognized and identified with her this feeling of anger, which led on to Carol saying she did not want to leave this happy neighbourhood and all her friends, but had to move as the house was now sold. The discussion that followed made her realize she was also angry with her husband, leaving her no desire to make love as well as having a 'numb' vagina.

The nurse's skill during this encounter was to work with the angry feelings of Carol which were only revealed when the nurse examined her. A relatively minor complaint may cover and disguise a far larger problem and may only be revealed when the woman has found a sympathetic listener.

Dyspareunia

Dyspareunia is pain during or after sexual intercourse. This can occur for pathological reasons and a cause should always be investigated first, e.g. infection. Dyspareunia can also be an expression of emotional pain where there is muscle tension. If digital vaginal examination shows there is no evidence or expression of pain from the woman, then further enquiries may reveal the true anxiety. Factors leading to dyspareunia can include:

◆ Parental influence

◆ Past sexual experiences

◆ Termination of pregnancy

◆ Childbirth

◆ Previous gynaecological disease

◆ Fear of cancer

◆ Ill-health

◆ Feeling inadequate as a sexual partner.

Scenario

 Diane, a 22-year-old, came to the nurse complaining of pain on intercourse for the last nine months. She was in a loving relationship but now 'dreaded' having intercourse. The nurse asked when they last had sex and was told that it was over a month ago and it had been very infrequent since she had a colposcopy nine months previously. The nurse wondered if that had been the problem, as Diane described the experience of colposcopy as 'quite a shock as it was so painful'. The nurse shared this experience with her and explained the necessity for colposcopy treatment. Diane described the pain as 'being outside and very sore as he entered'. She was examined by the doctor who identified some slight soreness of the fourchette and prescribed salt baths and a short treatment of oestrogen cream to aid healing. The nurse then went on to discuss with Diane her fear of sex and of her boyfriend hurting her and why she had waited so long to discuss this. An appointment was made to return in two weeks to see the nurse. When she returned the pain had gone and Diane described having sexual intercourse as 'great again'.

Here the problem was identified by the patient but she needed both prescriptive help and emotional help from the nurse. To make a brief follow-up appointment to share the outcome is always a good idea as it will encourage you in future consultations with patients with similar problems. If the problem had not been resolved then more skilled psychosexual counselling and help should be made available.

Vaginismus

Vaginismus occurs when there is an involuntary spasm of the muscle surrounding the lower third of the vagina, making penetration difficult or impossible. It is often described as 'a blockage' and experienced as pain, representing an unconscious expression about a woman's vagina.

Primary vaginismus indicates there has been no penetration of the vagina by the woman herself or the penis. Non-consummation is no penetration of the vagina in a sexual partnership. The sexual response of the woman in all other ways may be normal, she can be orgasmic and makes use of other sexual expressions to satisfy her sexual needs, e.g. masturbation and oral sex. This can leave her partner feeling impotent and he may also have erectile problems. Presentation is often after some years in a partnership when there is a wish to start a family, or in starting a new relationship where a previous relationship has not been consummated. A lot of courage may have been required for a woman to present with this failure in her sexual relationship. Specialist psychosexual counselling should always be offered and an appropriate referral made if you meet this problem.

Secondary vaginismus may take place after sexual or emotional trauma, including sexual abuse and gynaecological examinations. Other causes include:

♦ Infertility investigations and the demands of treatments

♦ Discharges and vaginal infections – the vagina is felt to be dirty

♦ Fantasies of thinking the vagina is too small or the penis will damage the inside

♦ Ante- and postnatal anxieties

♦ After hysterectomy or bladder surgery

♦ Anxiety about contraception.

You will need to explore the feelings surrounding vaginismus and the anxiety it poses for the individual women. It can be helpful for her to explore or re-explore her vagina with your help as described on page 51.

Dry vagina

If the natural vaginal secretions are impaired for any reason then penetration by the penis can be uncomfortable and painful. The emotional reasons stated under dyspareunia will also cause a feeling of dryness. Sexual stimulation may be unsatisfactory and foreplay may be either too slow or too quick and the woman not sufficiently sexually aroused. For the peri- and post-menopausal

woman the physical complaint of the vagina becoming dry and tight is due to a fall in oestrogen
levels and can be treated by local or systemic
oestrogen. Water-based jellies and lubricants are
an alternative treatment for some women. There
may also be other changes going on in their lives
which will require emotional care and support.

Orgasmic dysfunction

Orgasmic dysfunction means difficulty in having
an orgasm despite a normal sexual responsiveness, and only becomes a problem when the
woman regards it as such. Orgasm can occur
through stimulation by a partner or from self-
masturbation and is a unique experience which
makes it difficult to define and where a loss of
control will take place. As Joan Coombs writes
in her chapter on 'Problems with orgasm' (Skrine,
1989): 'Arousal and orgasm have something to
do with forgetting the outside world'.

Women sometimes enquire what is an orgasm
or how can they become orgasmic? You cannot
make them orgasmic, but you can listen to the
contributory factors that may be expressed:

♦ She has high expectations aroused by the media,
but in real life orgasm seems ordinary

♦ Orgasm does not happen as frequently as she
wishes

♦ She never has vaginal orgasm but comes before
or after penetration

♦ They do not 'come together'

♦ Their sexual technique is poor or inadequate

♦ She has a real fear of losing control and 'letting
go'

♦ She feels she is abnormal and simulates orgasm
to protect her self-esteem

Postnatal lack of orgasm is common, and is
hardly surprising with the many changes that have
taken place: tiredness, breastfeeding, physical discomfort, as well as the birth itself which may not
have been as she wished. Anorgasmia is a disappointment and the woman may feel she is failing
her partner.

Scenario

*Pat had recently registered at the surgery, so was
unknown to the nurse. She called
Pat in to her room where she sat
very upright with her hands clasped,
her face quite expressionless apart
from the occasional wry smile. The
nurse felt uncomfortable but asked
how she could help. Pat said 'I want help with my
sex life'. Pat then told her she was 39 years old and
had a previous relationship of eight years, but she
now had a new boyfriend and she had never had
an orgasm. She then sat back and waited. The
nurse wondered where to start. She asked some
questions but all Pat replied was 'I don't know'. The
nurse felt quite irritated by this behaviour and felt
that her enquiries and the negative responses were
getting nowhere. She suggested she should make
an appointment to see the counsellor in the
surgery which was accepted by Pat. The nurse,
reflecting on the encounter later on, realized that
this degree of control by Pat and denial of any
feelings was going to make it very difficult for her
to become orgasmic. Perhaps deep down there
was some hidden pain which never allowed her to
'let go'.*

Defence mechanisms for nurses and patients

When working in the field of women's sexual
health, both nurses and patients put up barriers.
These act as a means of defence against working
with emotional feelings and any pain involved in
the consultation. These barriers protect you and
your patient from discomfort. It is often difficult
at the time of the consultation to identify what is
happening and why the encounter may not be
going too well, but a clue can often be found in the
ebb and flow of communication which takes place
during the consultation. The interest that you and
your patient show in each other can range from
boredom to being over anxious. It is therefore
important that you, the nurse, recognize these
defences and how they affect verbal and non-
verbal communication. They should be treated
with respect and not dismissed as a sign of failure.
This then allows you to make changes in your

nursing practice, to accept and work with defensive as well as positive feelings.

You arrive at work with the same variety of emotions as patients have when they come to see you. Sometimes you feel well and on top form, and other days you arrive feeling strained and stressed. You may have left children ill, the child-minder has arrived late, there are financial anxieties, a row with your partner, bereavement or any other event which upsets the routine. Your training in your professional role enables you to continue to work with people when you feel like this, but such training is aimed at giving information, advice and using well-practised skills and techniques to give treatment. Talking about sexual health is different as this is about exploring and discovering reality with your patient. The demands that come from your patient may be overwhelming for you, and you can experience a feeling of helplessness and uselessness and not wanting to be involved. Then what do you do? Frequently you may try to make things better by talking too much or asking lots of closed questions, desperately hoping to find a solution. The responses often reveal irrelevant information and you and your patient may feel you are getting nowhere. A referral may be made which can be equally unhelpful and the moment for helping your patient is lost and her anxiety is not explored. The patient feels let down, and often dissatisfied. It is these defences that you may use that you need to recognize in your day-to-day work with your patients.

Reassurance

How often do you read the word 'reassured' in medical notes? What does it mean? What has been offered to the patient? Reassurance implies that the patient requires comfort, and therefore there is some worry, anxiety or even anger. The facts behind this anxiety may be unknown or felt too awful to communicate. Inevitably this can increase anxiety and not allay it. Physiological and pathological questions can be answered by clinical knowledge, but with sexuality, where the emotional pain and anxieties are often hidden, 'reassurance' is easier to record. If you see this in your patient's notes, refer back to the initial consultation and make another enquiry. The problem

may not be so acute but often it has not been fully resolved or understood by the patient.

Lack of time

Lack of time is another major defence that nurses tend to use. Even a brief amount of time if carefully planned can be used effectively for your patient. It is the quality of time given and not the quantity that is important (Balint and Norell, 1973). The excuse of 'lack of time' is frequently used to avoid listening and hearing the spoken or unspoken cry for help from your patient. Of course it is not only nurses who have this excuse; patients may often use the same defence – pleading that they are in a hurry rather than verbalize a problem. They may also appear to want to have a social chat, rather than asking for your professional help. You should remember that your patients are often busy as well and may have waited to see you and to use the consultation time for 'social chat' may be an 'avoiding technique' for you both. The disciplined use of time by using appropriate and professional remarks at the introduction as well as during the consultation and at its conclusion can be very effective. It is easy to find an excuse not to have time for your patient when you have a waiting room full of people, or are working on a busy ward.

You may feel that talking about sexuality will take even more time. Why does it feel like that? It seems easier for nurses to ask women about their last menstrual period or when their bowels were open, details which are just as intimate for the patient concerned, than to ask about their sexual life. Because sexual maturation has so often not been recognized as an integral part of health care, then 'lack of time' will continue to be used as an excuse not to discuss the matter. When you are able to routinely include sexuality in your care, it is seen to be time well spent for both you and your patient, and offers a high quality of care. The importance of being punctual and keeping to the boundaries is as important for your patient as it is for you. The sharing of limited time becomes disciplined and the offer to continue the discussion later will always be appropriate. You may be disappointed if your patient fails to return, but it may not necessarily be for negative reasons; your patient could have had time to think, reflect and feel positive about her initial consultation with you.

Lack of confidence

Sexuality is frequently not raised as an issue because you fear you will be 'out of your depth', 'make the situation worse' or you feel that you 'cannot offer a solution'. This lack of confidence makes you think and feel that only 'experts' talk about sexuality. This is not true as women choose the place and 'the face' where they feel comfortable and able to discuss everyday emotions about their sexuality and feelings. They will not usually talk about sexual dysfunction and rarely about sexual deviation, but will often wish to share the emotional feelings surrounding sexuality. During a vaginal examination, how often do you hear colleagues say 'just relax'. Try to do the same when discussing sexuality with a patient – relax and be yourself, and realize there is no need to feel out of depth or to produce a solution. Women generally respond very positively when they meet a nurse who is uninhibited, sensitive and flexible in approach. It is rewarding to try.

Lack of privacy

Lack of privacy can act as another excuse not to open or even respond to a question about sexual health. Sexuality is a private area and Dr Margaret Gill comments in her chapter 'Defences in the patient': 'The private parts are not so called for nothing' (Skrine, 1989). There are degrees of privacy for everyone, depending on our upbringing and circumstances. As nurses we perform daily tasks which are very intimate, such as: washing a patient, cleaning the incontinent, passing a catheter, dressing a surgical wound such as a mastectomy or colostomy, vaginal examination, passing a speculum and treatment of sexually transmitted diseases. The midwife has similar tasks: examination and delivery of a baby followed by postnatal care of the perineum and breasts. Sometimes these tasks are performed with only curtains as a barrier but the patient may still choose such a moment to confide in you. This can sometimes be identified as 'a moment of truth' when she is enabled to talk about her inner feelings, where intimacy and touch by you are the releasing factors. Some women do not feel the need to wait and find privacy; they can accost nurses in the corridor, the waiting room or even in the supermarket. It is usually only *your* feelings of embarrassment and intrusion that get in the way. It is the woman's choice when to talk about an anxiety and acknowledgement of this is always appropriate, but it must be your professional judgement that decides about future consultations. Your offer of finding privacy may be brushed aside with a comment such as 'I just wanted to ask you now', and once again the moment may be lost for the patient.

Finding a solution

The need to find a solution for your patient's anxieties could mean that you start advising on techniques in sexual nursing for which you have not been trained. he works of Masters and Johnson (1970) and their techniques (a behaviourist therapy) are frequently quoted and offered by nurses to their patients because it is seen to be constructive and therefore better than nothing. This is not good practice, as all recognized therapies require training, practice and supervision before they are offered to patients. The important factor which enables you to move forward in psychosexual nursing is to realize that you do not need to find a solution for your patient and the anxiety should always belong to the patient and not to you. Be available to listen, share and reflect on what you hear but remember your role is to facilitate your patient finding her own solution.

Referral

It is well-recognized that some doctors use the prescription pad as a defence mechanism when they are running late or do not know the answer to a patient's problems. This excuse is not generally available to nurses, so instead of prescribing nurses may suggest to the patient that they should see the doctor to ask their discomforting questions. Some doctors have training in psychosexual skills just as some nurses are trained, but many have no more skills than nurses and their perception and experience of patients are the same. Again, you should ask yourself 'Why did the patient choose me?' Do you have skills you fail or choose not to recognize? Do you fear that colleagues will mark you out as 'the nurse who always deals with sex problems'?

You may feel the need for additional training to increase your skills. In psychosexual nursing it is always worth trying 'to stay' with the woman rather than referring her, but be aware of the defences from you both that may hinder or stop your work. It is never easy, often painful but immensely satisfying and rewarding for both you and your patient.

Approaches to vaginal examination

Throughout women's lives the vaginal examination is one of the most frequent and intimate examinations given by the medical and nursing profession. It should never become routine but as will be discussed here, should be observed and thoughtful each time it is undertaken. Vaginal examination is a skill for all nurses and midwives to learn, practise and revise when necessary and it can then become a basis for psychosexual nursing. It has been well-documented that a vaginal examination can often offer 'the moment of truth' for women who have troubled sexuality (Tunnadine, 1970, 1992).

In medical practice, vaginal examination is usually done to exclude pelvic pathology or to assess progress during labour. In nursing it is possible to use a vaginal examination as an extension of your psychosexual nursing skills. In such cases it becomes therapeutic and can help both you and your patient towards a better understanding of a problem and for some women the revealing of a hidden difficulty. The examination does not necessarily have to be a bimanual examination but can be a digital examination or the passing of a speculum or only the examination of the external genitalia. You may become aware of a degree of vaginismus. Nurses and midwives may need to involve the doctor in order to make a clinical diagnosis and if a woman requests a doctor then her wish must be respected. More often than not women are only too pleased to have continuity of care from the nurse to whom they initially revealed their anxiety.

Occasionally women will ask for a vaginal examination when it is not appropriate. Some reasons for this are listed in Box 3.3. Clearly, a valid indication for a vaginal examination should be established before the procedure is started.

> **Box 3.3** Some reasons why women come for examination where it may not be appropriate
>
> ♦ Some women want to be examined to be told they are normal.
>
> ♦ Some women feel they *should* be examined. Are they missing out? What have they lost? Perhaps the loss of never having had sexual intercourse?
>
> ♦ They receive a request to have a cervical smear. Compliance seems to be important for them although there is no clinical indication for a smear as no vaginal intercourse has ever taken place.

Observations

It is relevant to notice the woman's reaction to the suggestion of a vaginal examination and the defences she may put up to avoid it such as:

♦ Menstruation at repeated visits

♦ 'I haven't washed'

♦ 'I'm in a hurry today'

♦ Arriving late for an appointment

♦ Keeping her pants on as she gets on the couch.

All of these can be observed and an appropriate comment made which can allow the woman to voice an anxiety. It is not always possible to predict how a woman will react to a vaginal examination. Women who you think of as likely to be difficult to examine may lie back, appear relaxed and 'behave' perfectly.

Scenario

Maria was complaining to the nurse of soreness and feeling dry during intercourse. The nurse noted a history of recent thrush and genital warts which had been treated and Maria had been given the 'all-clear'. During the discussion Maria said quite angrily 'He gave it to me'. The nurse offered to look again but Maria was reluctant and said 'I've been examined so much'. The nurse encouraged her to have another examination and the vulva and vagina showed no indication of soreness or

dryness. The nurse wondered 'what was going on here' and remembered the anger in Maria's answers. She enquired how Maria felt about her partner and learnt that she was very angry with him for 'infecting her' as she said. A short discussion followed where they felt it could be the emotional anger with him which was making intercourse uncomfortable and Maria acknowledged that the nurse's examination did not hurt. The anger and fury (soreness and dryness) really got in the way of her sexual life and the nurse was able to make this interpretation with Maria.

On the other hand, it may only be when an examination is attempted on an outwardly relaxed woman that you realize she may have difficulties. There is no guarantee that if examinations have been done previously with no problems that the woman's behaviour will be 'perfect' on a subsequent examination. All nurses, whether they are observing, chaperoning or performing examinations, must be alert and observe any distress signs at each particular occasion.

There is acceptable and unacceptable behaviour during an examination. A very detached, uncaring attitude from your patient where there appears to be no modesty, may indicate that she really does not value her sexuality or her vagina. She almost 'throws it away' and can make you feel uncomfortable at the lack of some degree of modesty. Too much modesty, on the other hand, may be indicated by vaginismus, abductor spasms, moving up the couch as you approach, the lifting of buttocks and arching the back off the couch, as well as a verbal expectation of pain. All these reactions arouse different feelings in you, which may include sympathy, impatience, annoyance and occasionally anger. If you are sensitive and have gained insight and understanding then you can share and enquire about these feelings with her rather than being tempted to ask a barrage of questions and ignore your patient's verbal and non-verbal signs. The examination can then have a positive outcome for your patient. Her attitude at the time may indeed also be a clue to the way she affects her partner, or vice versa, and more may be gained if this issue is discussed during the examination rather than waiting until later.

Preparation for examinations

Your patients should be adequately prepared for an examination by a clear explanation of the procedure as well as by discussing any fears and anxieties they may have. There are many myths, even nowadays, about vaginal examinations and it is relevant to discuss the women's attitude to menstruation and her experience of sexual intercourse. Never make an assumption that your patient is or has been sexually active but ask 'Have you ever had sexual intercourse?' If the reply is 'no' then the reason for coming for an examination can be discussed. Vaginal examination in a woman who is sexually active and sexually mature is usually achieved with few problems.

Preparation can also include:

♦ showing the woman a speculum if she wishes, and explaining that it is smaller than a penis;

♦ using a hand mirror to look at the genitalia or the cervix when the speculum is in position;

♦ allowing the woman to insert the speculum herself.

The flexibility of your approach is the secret of success. Sadly, insensitive examinations all too frequently take place, leaving women with anxieties about vaginal examination that are never forgotten. This is similar to an experience of violent intercourse and the mental and physical pain will always be remembered.

During the examination

Women must be asked to lie in a comfortable and correct position. The dorsal position is the most common, with the shoulders off the pillow and easy access to a light. It is also easier for you to observe the non-verbal communication of your patient. Some gynaecologists use the left lateral position and in some instances this position is necessary for clinical reasons. It is helpful to insert a finger before insertion of the speculum so that the size of the introitus can be assessed and the position of the cervix identified before taking a cervical smear.

At this point it may be useful to assess the woman's attitude towards her vagina by asking a few careful questions (Box 3.4). You may suggest that it is quite acceptable and normal for a woman to explore her vagina and that she can try it now or in private at home if she wishes. She might need a simple anatomy lesson first and is often grateful for this as she feels she should know more about herself but is frightened to reveal her own ignorance. A simple diagram can be helpful as well as describing the best position to feel inside, e.g. by putting one foot on a chair or by squatting on her heels and inserting one or two fingers into the vagina in a downward direction towards the floor.

Box 3.4 Questions you could use that may reveal the women's attitude towards her vagina

◆ *'Do you use tampons with an applicator?'* The use of these indicates that she feels able to insert something into her vagina and feels no blockage. However, there is a cardboard tube and therefore no need to actually feel inside the vagina.

◆ *'Do you use tampons without an applicator?'* With these there will be finger contact with the introitus and vagina. Some women will say they have tried without success and 'it hurt'. If they want to try again a simple explanation, usually of the direction to push the tampon is all that is required.

◆ *'Have you ever felt inside your vagina?'* The answer may be 'no' and implies that the woman may think that part of her is private and not your business, or she may feel unsure of your reaction if she says 'yes'. She may think she should not feel inside or you may think her 'dirty'.

There is no right or wrong way for self-examination but you should aim to make it acceptable and achievable for your patient. Sadly for some, self-examination remains abhorrent despite referral and skilled help.

During a vaginal examination you can talk to the woman and ask her to perform simple tasks to help you. Perhaps you could ask her to:

◆ put her hands underneath her buttocks to tilt her pelvis if the cervix is difficult to visualize;

◆ contract and relax the vaginal muscles and introitus;

◆ bear down to aid removal of the speculum;

◆ cough to expose the cervix.

If a woman complains of dyspareunia, this must always be explored by asking:

1 At what stage of intercourse does she feel the pain (e.g. penetration or at other times during sexual intercourse)?
2 Can she describe the pain?

Clinical problems

Pathology must be excluded and this will require examination by a doctor. If tests and investigations are necessary, these in themselves often give rise to further anxiety. If there is no clinical reason for dyspareunia it is helpful to find out what might be getting in the way.

Women often express hidden feelings by asking questions or making comments:

◆ 'How big is the vagina?'

◆ 'My vagina seems too small' (or too big).

◆ 'My vagina is dry.'

◆ 'My partner seems to be very big.'

◆ 'It starts to sting and hurt as he goes in.'

◆ 'It always seems so messy.'

◆ 'I don't like using contraception.'

◆ 'I wish he would use a condom.'

◆ 'I never seem to "come".'

◆ 'I often think of other things when *he* makes love.'

Vaginal fantasies

Many women have fantasies about their vagina, which can get in the way both of sexual intercourse and vaginal examination. These fantasies are not controlled by factual knowledge and although she may know her anatomy theoretically, intellectually she feels that *her* vagina is different.

Women may ask questions which can offer a clue to these fantasies, such as 'Where does it go to?' 'Is it really very small?' or 'Are the walls rigid?' She may describe her vagina as dark, dirty, disgusting, messy or red and raw – all bad feelings. The good feelings of the vagina like 'velvet', 'soft and comfortable' or 'soft and crinkly' and 'it feels surprisingly familiar just like the inside of the mouth' are also sometimes expressed.

Perhaps a woman thinks her vagina is remote and does not belong to her, so how does she give or offer it to anyone else? She may feel she needs to be given permission to use her vagina. Does marriage give permission? Sometimes being a virgin before marriage is important for religious or cultural reasons. Others may have tried to have sexual intercourse before marriage and failed, but hope that when they get married everything will be different. Sadly, this is often not the case. The woman feels a failure and finds it difficult to seek help. You may be tempted to 'take over' and can give inappropriate instructions in a desperate attempt to improve the situation. Logical thought and explanations are really not effective against illogical, inexpressible fears and fantasies of the vagina or of an examination. You should seek to refer these women to a skilled psychosexual counsellor for help.

Psychosexual referrals

The reason for referral to a psychosexual counsellor must be established between you and your patient before referral is made and the woman must be willing to see someone else. She should be encouraged to make her own appointment as this gives her some control and then she is more likely to keep this appointment. Waiting lists for psychosexual counselling are often long, and in some cases this is due to women who are unwilling or not yet ready for counselling. Some women may have previously sought advice or had counselling, often over a period of years, and it is important to find out why this was not satisfactory before making another referral. Some women 'do the rounds', which is not necessarily their fault as previous referrals for help may have been inappropriate. When women become desperate for help they may self-refer to an agency or therapist, often at great expense to themselves. In vain, women try to seek help from various people; some of these will be skilled but others may be unskilled and offer dubious therapy, with a poor outcome.

Psychosexual help within the National Health Service is very patchy and there will often be long waiting lists. Some GPs, family planning and hospital doctors have undertaken seminar training, a psychodynamic approach under the Institute of Psychosexual Medicine, but the counselling offered is not intended to be an extended therapy. Such sessions are held in GP surgeries, family planning clinics and in some hospitals. Nurses may also have the opportunity to work alongside doctors as independent psychosexual nurse counsellors in some areas.

Counsellors or social workers in primary care, community or hospital clinics may only offer general counselling and do not necessarily work with their patient's sexuality, although some community psychiatric nurses may offer sexual counselling. Before referring any woman it is important that you establish how the counsellor works and that they are capable of working with sexual anxieties.

Some women are unfortunately referred to busy gynaecological departments, where staff change frequently and clinical problems are examined and discussed, but rarely the emotional anxieties associated with the complaint. In hospital, with the high turnover of inpatients and busy outpatient departments, you may observe and hear of sexual anxieties, but these will usually have a low priority over other more pressing problems.

Although you wish to make a referral you may feel restricted because of a lack of knowledge and contacts in your district. Where troubled sexuality is identified, communication must be made between professionals. Where you know of no counselling facilities, you can alert the GP, district nurse, health visitor, or community midwife by letter or by a personal telephone call rather than leaving the problem and hoping that someone else will 'pick up the pieces'! Nurse specialists with counselling skills play a very important role, particularly the breast counsellor, continence adviser, stoma adviser, infertility counsellor and family planning nurse specialists. The conditions presented to these advisers can have an impact on all aspects of sexuality.

Outside the NHS there are many counsellors with a wide variety of training and experience. Again, before referring it is important to check what they offer as many may only give general counselling and do not necessarily work with sexual anxieties. Find out how they work and whether they would be suitable for a particular woman's problem. There will be fees to pay so it is important that you have up-to-date information.

Relate (formerly Marriage Guidance Council)

have trained psychosexual counsellors offering a behaviourist therapy. All clients are assessed before being accepted for a course of therapy and it is normal practice to be seen as a couple. They also have marital and reconciliation counselling where they will see single people. Some Relate offices are able to offer an assessment in a crisis situation. Donations or fees are required for their services.

To summarize it is helpful to keep a list of counsellors, agencies and services available for appropriate help in your locality. Use the checklist in Box 3.5 to obtain relevant information.

Box 3.5 Questions to ask of counsellors, agencies and services

1 Who is available?
2 Where are they?
3 When do they work – days and times?
4 How long is the waiting list?
5 What sort of therapy or treatment do they offer?
6 What type of training have the counsellors received?
7 Do they offer short- or long-term therapy?
8 How do you refer a woman?
9 Do they make an assessment first and then decide to offer therapy?
10 What payment is required, or is it free?

Finally, if it is possible, arrange to meet those offering the service, and see where they work. Then you can give first-hand information to your patient and be sure that you are sending her to the right place. With the difficulty of finding skilled help, it is even more necessary nowadays for you to know what is available and if it is appropriate for the individual woman or couple.

Training in psychosexual nursing

In order to be effective, training in psychosexual nursing has to be tailored to your role as a nurse. The skills learned must be relevant and possible to use in your day-to-day clinical practice. Expectations that training will give you answers and make you an expert must be dispelled. A knowledge of emotional development and an understanding of sexual maturation (see Chapter 1) is important, just as the knowledge of anatomy and physiology is essential for clinical nursing. Skill is needed to communicate effectively with all women about

sexual matters whether they are well or unwell, and you will need continuing opportunities where the individual nurse/patient relationships can be studied to assess and develop these skills. There is very little training in psychosexual nursing around the country, so it is a bonus when sexual care is well integrated into pre- and post-registration courses. Training is expensive and nurses often have to find the finances themselves. Sadly nurses who wish to gain psychosexual skills have to 'fight' to be heard by their managers and educators. Holistic care is difficult to measure and unfortunately 'value for money' is frequently measured in terms of quantity of patients and not quality of care.

It is necessary to recognize that in psychosexual nursing your role is not the same as either the doctor, the social worker or the counsellor. But like doctors, you have the privilege and ability to touch, examine and treat women intimately. Female patients perceive you to be a 'carer' and will trust and confide in you. This can provide you with the opportunity to make positive use of your professional role to share women's fantasies, fears and joys. The encounters with women who have sexual anxieties are often brief with little opportunity for follow-up. This brief encounter can be just as important to the patient as a longer consultation.

Reasons for psychosexual training

There are many reasons why you might want to have further training in psychosexual skills, ranging from a genuine desire to help to 'collecting another certificate'. These reasons could include the following:

◆ Women are asking you questions about their sexuality and sexual health. You feel inadequate and feel you require further skills.

◆ You want to know about psychosexual problems and how best to help.

◆ You have been on lots of training days and none of them have answered your needs, so you continue searching.

◆ You have your own personal problems and difficulties which are unresolved. In this case, personal therapy would be more appropriate before undertaking psychosexual training.

Choosing suitable training

Training needs to be at a convenient location as travelling is both time-consuming and expensive and requires a positive commitment. Questions that you should consider include:

♦ What training is on offer?

♦ What work do they require of you?

♦ How much time do you have available?

♦ What approach does the course have?

♦ Who will be the tutors – what are their skills and experience?

♦ How long is the course?

♦ Is further training offered if required?

♦ Is there a recognized qualification?

Post-registration courses

Post-registration courses offer an ideal opportunity to extend skills in psychosexual training, particularly for those who work in women's health. Your own individual life experiences have increased as well as your nursing skills and you have started to recognize any difficulties you may have in discussing patients' sexuality.

You are also beginning to expand your own role, taking on more responsibilities and specializing with growing confidence, often training other nurses and setting standards for a pattern of care. Sexuality must be integrated throughout a post-registration course from the beginning if it is to be of value, and not offered as a 'one-off' or 'token' lecture at the end of a course. The discussion of sexuality and the opportunities to practise communication skills can take place and clinical encounters from your daily work can be reflected on during the course. You should be encouraged to get away from thinking there is a right and wrong way to work with sexuality and not to make assumptions because you feel uncomfortable discussing feelings. You may then feel able to offer help without a fear of saying the wrong thing.

The English National Board have courses on psychosexual counselling for nurses (ENB 985). The future of these courses is uncertain and of the few that are currently running their methods of training vary.

Counselling and communication courses

There are numerous courses offered by a variety of organizations and agencies. Some are specialized, such as abortion or bereavement counselling, but many are more general and only offer basic counselling skills. Some nurses feel very disappointed with the outcome of the course they attended, thus emphasizing the need to find out beforehand what the course offers and that it will be helpful and relevant for your psychosexual work.

Courses on sexuality

Courses on sexuality are often multi-disciplinary and offer a theoretical knowledge, with the expectation that you will be prepared to discuss your own anxieties about sexuality during training. With such a course you will need to think carefully about whether you are able to share your private feelings and experiences and whether it will be relevant to your patient care. Role play and problem-solving exercises are often offered as the method of study, and your day-to-day work may not be explored. Some courses may require you to undergo personal therapy yourself before or during training.

Seminar training

Seminars are an experiential training, when a group of nurses meet together with a leader and present clinical encounters from their daily work. The aim of such seminars is to increase skills by honest discussion and reflection where counselling is seen as an integral part of clinical care. The focus of the work is on the interaction between the nurse and the patient and the feelings invoked, offering participants the opportunity to listen, think and discuss not only their own work with patients' sexual anxieties but also those of others in the group. The training is similar to a pattern of training developed by the Institute of Psychosexual Medicine. For seminar training to be effective nurses must be working in clinical practice, so that changes they make in their practice can be self-assessed and evaluated within the group. It is therefore not suitable for short training but it has been recognized that six seminars at monthly intervals does allow new thinking and some exploration and discovery of skills with patients (English National Board Course A08 for Advanced Family Planning Nurses). A more permanent change can take place after 20–30 seminars of two hours each held weekly or fortnightly.

A 'taster' of a short course of seminars is better than nothing, and allows those who are interested the opportunity to extend their skills with further seminars.

Workshops

Workshops can be very valuable as you will participate in group work, and they may take place over one or more days. Some nurses find it threatening to participate in a group, particularly when there is a fear of having to put their own feelings about sexuality forward. The skill of the facilitator is paramount in establishing an atmosphere where feelings about sexuality can be discussed freely, and the focus must be on the patients, the nurses' clinical practice and the relationship between them. Many sensitive nurses feel they work in total isolation with their patients' sexuality, as colleagues do not always take this subject seriously and seem unsupportive when concerns are raised. Signs of amusement and laughter will often cover other people's embarrassment. In a workshop you are given the chance to meet other nurses who are committed to an holistic approach and this allows you to acknowledge skills and feelings that you may have hidden from your colleagues.

Lectures

Lectures are generally 'one-off' events where listen, take notes and there are no demand get involved. Lectures usually represent a threatening form of education. Theoretical kn ledge and information is given and you may some insight into sexual problems and anxie by listening to new ideas and different commu cation skills. You may then come away fired wit enthusiasm to try them in your own clinical practice. Often, unfortunately it is easier to revert to old ways of practice and fail to address your patients' sexual care. On the other hand, the information learnt may be very positive and inspire you to seek further training.

Support groups

In support groups nurses can meet for discussion of cases and for mutual support. Unfortunately, there is often no aim or structure to these groups or even a designated facilitator. The tendency is then for the group to become a 'social' group of professionals where training and therefore learning is minimal.

The need for further training is an individual matter, but an enormous amount of job satisfaction can be gained when you can offer your patients a more holistic approach by integrating the theory of sexuality with increased counselling skills.

Conclusions

All women go through life with sexual feelings, fears and fantasies which may persist into old age and can include sexual experience of masturbation, heterosexuality or homosexuality. Many changes take place during their sexual maturation, both physical and emotional. For some women their sexual lives are fulfilled and they feel happy, supported and loved, whilst others feel their lives are in a turmoil and they feel depressed, angry, confused and lonely.

It is important for all nurses to realize that you can help by developing your observing and listening skills when you meet women in your everyday clinical practice where their sexuality, sexual health care and sexual lives can be nursed with the same respect and equality as the other care that you offer and give.

HumatroPen™3

s
cl
sta
bere

Lilly

reaction and will not be known until the event itself. The feeling of being out of control is strong and can be frightening. We can read about the effects of bereavement and the processes of mourning that take place in preparation for ourselves, and to help us to work with our patients, but it is often bewildering and puzzling how individual people react to loss, and it may be very different from the behaviour expected both of ourselves and our patients. The actual process of grief is little understood and there is no right or wrong way to grieve. It does not mean that people are coping when they do not show their grief like everyone else. Patients need to be allowed to feel and behave as they are – individuals.

The study of grieving and loss is crucial for all nurses, as there is a profound effect on the psychosocial and psychosexual lives of those concerned. Nurses not only meet loss that is current, but also loss from the past, where grieving, for whatever reason, has not taken place. Where this has not been expressed, emotional trauma can remain hidden, leaving damage for the patient you are seeing as well as for partners, husbands, family and friends. An illustration of this sometimes occurs when a midwife takes an obstetric history from a pregnant woman. Routine questions about previous pregnancies are asked but the midwife may not stop to ask how the woman is feeling now about a previous termination of pregnancy, miscarriage, stillbirth or death of a child. All these questions may provoke memories of a loss that has not been resolved and can then cause emotional anxiety. The midwife can observe the response of the woman, which may be obvious, such as welling tears or she may appear quite dismissive of the loss. This is often a clue that the grief is hidden and there is still unexplored psychological pain. If the midwife can then share the woman's feeling of dismissal and of not wanting to talk about past events, then the woman may feel able to say something like 'I feel so silly and anyhow it was a long time ago'. Work can then start to allow some resolution of her loss before the birth of the next baby. Many of us, whether nurses, midwives or health visitors, underestimate our skills and the very fact that the loss has been raised, acknowledged and discussed is frequently enough for self-healing to take place. If the emotional pain is too great then referral to a bereavement counsellor or an organization such as Cruse may be an appropriate solution (see Resources, page 64).

The period of mourning should normally be completed within two years. This does not mean forgetting, but a fading of feelings which allows emotional healing to take place, and the opportunity to start to build a new, separate life. The grief process describes the common reactions and feelings which are normal and appropriate. Most people who experience bereavement are not ill themselves, and if they are treated as being unwell they may retreat into helplessness, i.e. withdrawing from what is going on around them, to get away from the pain, rather than allowing themselves to experience the necessary stages of emotional pain to stop grieving. Grief has been studied in depth by Colin Murray Parkes and his book *Bereavement* (Parkes, 1986) is a highly informative and useful book for all health professionals.

It is important for you as a nurse to relate the identified stages of grief and feelings to your everyday clinical practice, with the knowledge that anyone you meet may be experiencing loss in a variety of forms. This may not necessarily be the death of a loved person, but could also be the loss of a job, divorce, financial loss or burglary, as well as loss experienced through surgery and illness. Loss not only involves the patient you meet but their family as well; whether in hospital, general practice, the community or the home, they all may need your support and care.

When you are nursing a child or adult with a chronic illness you will have noticed how much has to be sacrificed by the carers, the family and the patient. There are many losses, one of which can be a sexual life for the carers as well as for the adult patient. You can sometimes wonder in these circumstances who is the 'real' patient. Is it the carer or the sufferer? It is also important to recognize that all those who are involved have their own emotional needs that may require your help at different times.

In Western culture, bereavement is still seen as private and not to be publicly displayed. In other cultures, particularly Asian, there is often a set period of mourning with open tears and acceptance of rituals and behaviour which helps all those involved to come to terms with their loss.

The stages of grief

Shock

This phase usually lasts for a short while. It will be particularly pronounced when death is sudden and unexpected, leaving a state of confusion where reactions will vary, from feeling completely numb or apathetic to being overreactive. As Lily Pincus in *Death and the Family* says, 'for physical shock, rest and warmth are the recognized methods of treatment' (Pincus, 1974). The same treatment applies equally to emotional shock and it should be remembered that to 'keep going' is not necessarily a good cure for emotional pain. The need for tender loving care will be important particularly when the main feeling is of being left alone and abandoned. The return of the bereaved to the family home, after leaving hospital following a death where perhaps only a short time previously everything had been normal, gives rise to feelings of disbelief, which can rapidly turn to extreme distress bordering on hysteria. Feelings of being out of control, not able to cope, fear, the inability to relax and restlessness are all common. Sleep patterns are disturbed and it could be you who might encourage the bereaved to take medication at this stage.

Nowadays people live much more in isolation, with relations and family often living far away and neighbours and friends out at work during the day. In fact neighbours may only be known by sight and not by name. Thus the feeling of loneliness can be intensified.

When the death has been expected, and some preparation for mourning has already started, the immediate reaction may be one of relief rather than shock. This reaction will vary with the individual situation and the temperament of the bereaved, but it does not mean to say the emotions will be any less intense.

During this stage of grief arrangements have to be made, the funeral organized and the bereaved will be supported by relatives and friends. It is important for you to remember, whatever your work setting, that many other people will be mourners and may be grieving as well as the immediate relatives. This is particularly relevant for those in a close community.

Nurses must also mourn. Where nursing care has been given, often over a long period of time,

either on a one-to-one basis or with a team approach, nurses can become very close to both the dying and their relatives, so it is only to be expected that they should experience a similar reaction. In hospital the turnover in bed occupancy is so rapid that there may be no time for adjustment to a new patient in a bed where a death has recently occurred. The bed is remade and clean and it becomes hard to remember the recent death and nurses might even have a feeling of guilt that this can happen so quickly. Time should be made on a ward or in general practice for discussion of individual deaths and acknowledgements of the feelings that other nurses and professional colleagues have. Other patients may also need support; they have watched the comings and goings and wonder what has happened. They know when a death has taken place and their enquiries must be answered truthfully. Even though other patients' deaths may not be imminent, there is always the individual knowledge that they will die at some time in the future. This can be frightening. The death of someone else will often evoke painful memories of a previous experience of death.

In home nursing, the contact between the nurse and patient is much more intense. The acceptance of care comes from the patient and those living in the home, and a close relationship often develops. Even then the role of the nurse has to be nonintrusive, especially at the time of dying. Nevertheless, for the nurse to be present and available is usually seen to be important to the family; to be on call in the event of change in the patient's condition is reassuring for everyone. The nurse who is unable to be present at the end may have feelings of 'letting the family down' and of leaving the task incomplete both for her and the relatives. Contact with the bereaved is much more likely to continue after a home death, particularly where the nurse may be known and seen in the neighbourhood. This is often a real benefit in the healing process for both the nurse and those who are bereaved.

Searching

After the initial shock response, relatives and friends leave and a feeling of isolation takes over. The bereaved may start looking for the lost person, with the inability to accept this loss. Pining is a noticeable wish for the lost person. The adult may see this as irrational behaviour, but that does not mean they are out of control. Their behaviour may be restless and tense with lots of repetitive talking and recalling past events. The bereaved may give vivid descriptions of 'seeing' the dead person or feeling their presence. This is a common phenomenon and can be a comfort to them and is not necessarily upsetting. These symptoms will decrease as the reality of the loss is accepted.

Some people may experience feelings which are new to them of anger and aggression, even over trivial events. Nurses may be aware of hostile feelings often directed towards them and other medical staff as the bereaved feel the need to express blame. Depression, not necessarily pathological, and despair are common; these may not be prolonged but have acute phases and then disappear. The feeling of guilt about what might have been said or not said, or regrets that they should have done something can leave a feeling of unfinished business. For the bereaved, there is sometimes a loss of interest in their personal appearance as there is no one to make an effort for and no one to compliment them.

Concentration, whether at home or at work is always difficult. Many women have jobs, either full or part time, and usually only a brief leave of absence is given or taken. It may be therapeutic to return to work as the activity keeps them occupied, but it can also leave feelings of not being able to cope and being less efficient, resulting in a lack of confidence.

The home becomes difficult to organize and the family may feel neglected, especially if there are young children, who may find it difficult to understand why routines are upset and they are not receiving the same attention as before. Children need just as much support and understanding during a bereavement as adults. The mother can then feel guilty as she is not able to be the provider and organizer for her children whilst she is trying to cope with her own grief.

Possessions may become very important. Sometimes there is the temptation to get rid of everything too early but it is important to allow some time before making final decisions as regrets are then less, and specific possessions will remain as reminders of happy times. Other people get rid of nothing or may leave a room untouched. The possessions then seem to remain a 'living' memorial. Memories and recollections are particularly painful throughout this time but happier memories will replace them as the pain starts to fade. When death was sudden and there was no time for farewell, the bereaved may feel that they never had a chance to say 'goodbye' which makes the task of mourning even harder, and longer.

Acceptance and adaptation

During this phase the emotional pain of bereavement lessens and acceptance of the loss becomes a reality. Changes take place and a new identity is established with the environment where the deceased lived or the loss took place. Relationships which may have suffered within the family may need to be renewed, even if the idea seems totally alien to other members of the family. It then starts to become possible to reinvest emotional feelings in new relationships. Family affairs have to be reorganized and where the bereaved has never dealt with financial matters these have to be understood and new skills learnt.

If the wife and mother becomes the provider, family administrator and planner she is often surprised at how well she can cope. Support and encouragement will continue, but it is important to stop grieving otherwise the new identity will not develop. Colin Murray Parkes (1986) describes 'turning points; that is events associated with a major revision of their feelings, attitude and behaviour'. He goes on to point out that 'the timing of such turning points is important'. They can be an anniversary, a holiday or a memorial service and should not go unnoticed by those around. It is at such 'turning points' that problems can be discussed and arrangements for the future made which will continue to allow further adaptation to the new situation.

Pathological grief

The signs that all is not well are when physical symptoms persist with no pathology; there may be excessive guilt or anger; an anxiety state with uncontrollable tears and depression. Maybe the grieving is being avoided or the problem as in chronic grief is how and when to stop this process. You need to be able to identify that there is a problem and offer suitable support and perhaps onward referral, which can then lead to an acceptance of the bereavement.

Other types of loss

Other types of loss take place throughout life and are more frequent and cover a wide range of issues (Box 3.6). The feelings of grief are exactly the same. Some losses pass quickly, fade equally quickly and leave little or no trauma. But for others, because it is not necessarily a death of a person, it is difficult to understand why the feelings of grief should be there at all. Nurses feel the same and wonder why a loss which appears remote or happened a long time ago should have

---

Box 3.6 Losses which can affect women's sexual health

Most of these losses take place in a normal lifecycle and many of them are mentioned elsewhere in this book but it was felt important to group them together in this section on bereavement. You will encounter many different types of loss in your daily clinical work:

♦ Loss of parental control; children rejecting parents, teenage trauma, truancy from school, running away from home, drugs, alcohol and eating disorders

♦ Children leaving home for school, college, university, a new job or to live with a partner

♦ Loss of virginity – particularly traumatic following sexual abuse and rape

♦ Loss of confidence and self-esteem

♦ Getting engaged and married

♦ Loss of husband or partner through separation, divorce or death. Partners separated by work

♦ Loss of parents and close relatives

♦ Never having had the opportunity to have children

♦ Pregnancy; unable to have a normal delivery; unable to breastfeed

♦ Loss of employment, redundancy, financial loss, early retirement as well as retirement at the standard age

♦ Buying and selling a house; moving neighbourhood, moving to a new country

♦ Menopause with loss of periods and loss of fertility

♦ Death of a pet

♦ Burglary.

Physical loss

♦ Medical illness which can be short or long term, acute or chronic or progressive and incurable, e.g. diabetes, asthma, stroke

♦ Changes in personality; memory loss, senility

♦ Loss of function in any part of the body by accident or illness

♦ Paraplegia

♦ Incontinence of bladder and rectum

♦ Infertility.

Surgical loss

♦ Loss of limb

♦ Hysterectomy, vulvectomy

♦ Mastectomy

♦ Miscarriage, ectopic pregnancy, stillbirth

♦ Termination of pregnancy

a bearing on the current situation. Even if we are told of a 'loss event' the interpretation of this may be difficult, and we fail to 'hear' the patient's emotional pain and continue to concentrate on the physical symptoms. The temptation to ignore a recent loss is common as you may feel the event is 'too close' and be afraid of upsetting the patient and provoking sadness and tears. Women themselves have the same fear that 'I should be getting over it now' and will often apologize for crying.

You may also find that your own personal experiences of loss and bereavement may not have been adequately resolved and consequently get in the way of working with your patients over their own experiences of loss.

The positive message for you as a nurse involved in women's health is that you must be open and willing to listen to the psychosocial events that surround women's lives and then make enquiries. You will gain information on loss whilst taking a medical history, in conversation with a patient during a consultation, from a concerned professional colleague with or without referral and even from the 'grapevine'. You must aim to acknowledge this loss, to pause and then allow the patient to share her feelings with you. It need only be very brief but it is important to resist the temptation to ignore or pass over the loss. You need to observe how the woman responds to your acknowledgement of her loss. It may be so painful that it is dismissed with 'I'm alright'. Experience tells you they are seldom 'alright'. You can then ask a pertinent question, such as 'Tell me what you mean by alright?' This allows the patient to hear that you are listening and empathetic. Then her true feelings may be revealed, which you can identify and share with her as being a normal reaction to her loss. This is often a relief and a revelation, especially where the loss has been hidden. At this stage of talking about loss you are not offering counselling and therapy, but acting as a concerned nurse alongside the woman. It will be your observations and clinical experience that will determine with the women the need for more time and counselling in the future.

As we have seen already, the value to the patient of being allowed to recognize her feelings over the loss is often therapy itself. When working in women's health we should constantly remember that we are not only caring for a woman's physical needs, but also her psychosexual and psychosocial well-being. Remember that the loss can be exciting and pleasurable, such as loss of virginity, and therefore not always one of trauma and sadness.

Summary of help you can offer the bereaved

1 Your help should be an enabling process where you endeavour to help the bereaved cope for themselves. You should avoid telling them what to do.
2 A consultation with you can be very short or more prolonged, just as in the grieving process itself.
3 One of the crucial skills you require is to be able to listen to really painful events and information without becoming emotionally swamped yourself.
4 Let your genuine concern and care show, but be able to stand back and think about your responses.
5 Allow the bereaved to express how they are feeling in the 'here and now'; listen and hear what they want to share with you. When the subject is too painful it is only too easy to try and change the subject which can then allow both of you to run away from the pain. Try to stay with the current situation.
6 If you are asking questions, make them open ended. 'How are you feeling now?' elicits a fuller reply than 'Are you feeling a bit better now?', when the answer is often 'Yes', even if they are not! Questions that start with 'how', 'what', 'when' and 'why' will give your patient more time to express herself fully.
7 Encourage women to be patient and not to expect too much of themselves too quickly.
8 Encourage the family to talk about their individual feelings. Communication in families is often poor and remote, but distress if shared can be a positive benefit.
9 The friends and family you meet will also want to know how they can help. They can be encouraged to just listen, even if it may be repetitive!
10 The bereaved must have the true facts about the death which may relieve their individual feelings of guilt and blame. This is especially

important in accidents and in instances of sudden death.

11 Allow them to understand that the reactions and feelings they have are 'normal' and experienced by others in similar situations.

Difficulties you might experience when offering help

1 You may feel so helpless yourself that you imagine you will be of no use. Patients are your educators and you can learn by listening to them. If you have experienced a loss or bereavement yourself and you feel you have come to terms with it, you will have much to offer to others. Never be tempted to personalize from your own experiences.

2 You may be tempted to avoid talking about emotions and painful events because you want to try and make patients feel better. Do not try to change the subject to make it more comfortable for you and run away from the pain that the woman is feeling.

3 Empathize rather than sympathize. You must avoid saying 'I know how you must be feeling'. You may like to think you know, but everyone's grief pattern is different and individual to them. It is important not to belittle or devalue their feelings and not to make assumptions.

4 Avoid the temptation to tell patients how they should be feeling now and how they will feel in the future and what they should do.

5 Try not to feel sorry for the patient. This can then lead to a feeling of pity or even contempt, which will stop your care for the bereaved. This should not be confused with the sadness that is appropriate when dealing with your patient's loss.

Conclusion

Bereavement and grief are commonplace and cover many types of loss apart from death. If you as a nurse can acknowledge your patient's sadness and participate in helping her through the grief process then the care you can offer your patients will be truly holistic.

Resources

Psychosexual nursing and counselling

British Association of Sexual and Marital Therapy
PO Box 62, Sheffield S10 3TL

British Association of Counselling
1 Regents Place, Rugby, Warwickshire CV21 2PV
Tel. 01788 578328

Institute of Psychiatry
De Crespigny Park, London SE5
Tel. 0171 703 5411

Institute of Psychosexual Medicine
11 Chandos Street, London WM1 9DE
Tel. 0171 580 0631

Relate Central Office
Herbert Grey College, Little Church Street, Rugby CV21 3AP
Tel. 01788 573241

Sexual Dysfunction Clinic
St Georges Hospital, Blackshaw Road, Tooting, London SW19

Tavistock Institute
120 Belsize Lane, London NW3 5BA

Training

There are numerous courses on counselling at all levels and these can be found at local Colleges of Further Education, Colleges of Nursing, and Universities.

English National Board for Nursing, Midwifery and Health Visiting
Victory House, 170 Tottenham Court Road, London W1P 0HA
Tel. 0171 388 3131

Scottish National Board for Nursing Midwifery and Health Visiting
22 Queens Street, Edinburgh EH2 1JX
Tel. 0131 2267371

Welsh National Board for Nursing Midwifery and Health Visiting
Floor 13, Pearl Assurance House, Greyfriars Road, Cardiff CF1 3RT
Tel. 01222 395535

Enquiries for psychosexual nurse training, seminars or workshops can be made to:
Mrs Doreen Clifford, 15 Ferrymore, Ham, Richmond, Surrey TW10 7SD
Mrs Jane Selby, 28B York Gardens, Clifton, Bristol, BS8 4LN

Bereavement

Child Bereavement Trust
1 Millside Riversdale, Bourne End, Bucks, SL8 6EB
Tel. 016285 21908

Child Death Helpline
(Great Ormond St and Camden Social Services)
Evening helpline (7 pm – 10 pm) 0171 829 8685

Compassionate Friends
53 North Street, Bristol BS3 1EN
Tel. 0117 953 9639 (Helpline) or 0117 966 5202 (Head office)

Cruse Bereavement Care
126 Sheen Road, Richmond, Surrey TW9 1UR
Tel. 0181 940 48180 or Bereavement line 0181 332 7227

Foundation for the Study of Infant Deaths
14 Halkin Street, London SW1X 7DP
Tel. 0171 235 0965 (Cot death helpline) or 0171 235 1721

Hospice Information Service
St Christopher's Hospice, 51–59 Lawrie Park Road, Sydenham SE26 6DZ
Tel. 0181 778 9252

Miscarriage Association
c/o Clayton Hospital, Northgate, Wakefield, WF1 3JS
Tel. 01924 200799

National Council for the Divorced and Separated
13 High Street, Little Shelford, Cambridge CB2 5ES
Tel. 01533 708880

Road Peace
PO Box 2579, London NW10 3PW
Tel. 0181 964 1021
Support for those bereaved by road accidents.

SAMM (Support After Murder and Manslaughter)
Cranmer House, 39 Brixton Road, London SW9 6DZ
Tel. 0171 735 3838

SANDS (Stillbirth and Neonatal Death Society)
28 Portland Place, London W1N 4DE
Tel. 0171 436 7940 (Office) or 0171 436 5881 (Helpline)
Will put in touch with other bereaved parents. Variety of booklets available.

SATFA (Support Around Termination for Abnormality)
73–75 Charlotte Street, London W1P 1LB
Tel. 0171 631 0280 (Office) or 0171 631 0285

Video

When Our Baby Died. A video for use by health care professionals for parents. Available from Professional Care Productions, 1 Millside Riversdale, Bourne End, Bucks SL8 5EB.

References and further reading

Psychosexual nursing and counselling

BALINT, E. and NORELL, J.S. (1973) *Six Minutes for the Patient*. London: Tavistock.
BALINT, M. (1957) *The Doctor, His Patient and the Illness*. London: Pitman.
BANCROFT, J. (1989) *Human Sexuality and its Problems*, 2nd edn. Edinburgh: Churchill Livingstone.
BERNE, E. (1985) *Games People Play*. Harmondsworth: Penguin.
BRECHER, R. and E. (eds) (1967) *An Analysis of Human Sexual Response*. London: Panther.
BURNARD, P. (1992) *Counselling. A Guide to Practise in Nursing*. London: Butterworth-Heinemann.
CASEMENT, P. (1985) *On Learning from the Patient*. London: Tavistock.
DAINOW, S. and BAILEY, C. (1988) *Developing Skills with People*. Chichester: Wiley.
DOYLE, C. (1994) *Child Sexual Abuse. A Guide for Health Professionals*. London: Chapman and Hall.
ENDACOTT, J. (1989) Coping with psychosexual problems. *Nursing Standard* 3(42): 29–31.
HASLETT, S. and JENNINGS, M. (1992) *Hysterectomy and Vaginal Repair*, 3rd edn. Beaconsfield, Bucks: Beaconsfield.
HILTON, P. (1988) Urinary incontinence during sexual intercourse. *British Journal of Obstetrics and Gynaecology* **95**: 377–81.
JENKINS, D. (1986) *Listening to Gynaecological Problems*. Berlin: Springer-Verlag.

LINCOLN, R. (ed.) (1992) *Psychosexual Medicine. A Study of Underlying Themes*. London: Chapman and Hall.

MASTERS, W.H. and JOHNSON, V.E. (1970) *Human Sexual Inadequacy*. Edinburgh: Churchill Livingstone.

MONTFORD, H. and SKRINE, R. (eds) (1993) *Contraceptive Care. Meeting Individual Needs*. London: Chapman and Hall.

MUNRO, E., MANTHEI, R. and SMALL, J. (1988) *Counselling: A Skills Approach*. London: Routledge.

NURSE, G. (1980) *Counselling and the Nurse*. Aylesbury: H.M.&M.

ORBACH, SUSIE (1994) *What's Really Going on Here*. London: Virago.

RANDALL, E. (1992) *Preparation for Psychosexual Nursing*. Report on a Survey of the ENB Course 985, Lewisham Hospital. London: The Centre for Inner City Studies, Goldsmiths College.

SAVAGE, J. (1988) *Nurses, Gender and Sexuality*. London: Heinemann Medical.

SELBY, J. (1990) Psychosexual nursing. *Practice Nurse* June, 99–101.

SKRINE, R. (ed.) (1989) *Introduction to Psychosexual Medicine*. London: Chapman and Hall.

SKYNNER, R. and CLEESE, J. (1984) *Families and How to Survive Them*. London: Methuen.

TUNNADINE, P. (1970) *Contraception and Sexual Life*. London: Tavistock (out of print).

TUNNADINE, P. (1992) *Insights into Troubled Sexuality. A Case Profile Anthology*, revised edn. London: Chapman and Hall.

TUNNADINE, P. *Sense and Nonsense about Sex*. Family Doctor series, London: BMA (out of print).

VALINS, L. (1992) *When a Woman's Body says No to Sex*. Harmondsworth: Penguin.

WAKELEY, G. (1991) *Sexual Abuse and the Primary Care Doctor*. London: Chapman and Hall.

WRIGHT, H. (1989) *Groupwork Perspectives and Practice*. London: Scutari Press.

Bereavement

BOWLBY, J. (1986) *Loss, Sadness and Depression*, volume 3. London: Pelican.

HILL, S. (1977) *In the Spring Time of the Year*. Harmondsworth: Penguin.

HILL, S. (1990) *The Family*. Harmondsworth: Penguin.

KUBLER-ROSS, E. (1970) *On Death and Dying*. London: Routledge.

LIVELY, P. (1977) *The Road to Lichfield*. Harmondsworth: Penguin.

LIVELY, P. (1990) *Passing On*. Harmondsworth: Penguin.

MANDER, R. (1994) *Loss and Bereavement in Child Bearing*. Oxford: Blackwell Scientific.

NEUBERGER, J. (1994) *Caring for Dying People of Different Faiths*, 2nd edn. St Louis: C.V. Mosby.

PARKES, C.M. (1986) *Bereavement*, 2nd edn. Harmondsworth: Penguin.

PINCUS, L. (1974) *Death and the Family*. London: Faber & Faber.

STEWART, A. and DENT, A. (1994) *At a Loss: Bereavement Care when a Baby Dies*. London: Baillière Tindall.

THOMAS, J. (1993) *Supporting Parents when a Baby Dies Before or Soon After Birth*, 2nd edn (published privately). Available from: The Child Bereavement Trust, 1 Millside Riversdale, Bourne End, Bucks SL8 5EB.

THOMAS, J. and KOHNER, N. (1993) *Grief After the Death of Your Baby*. Bourne End: Child Bereavement Trust.

WHITAKER, A. (ed.) (1984) *All in the End is Harvest*. London: Cruse.

WORDERN, J.W. (1991) *Grief Counselling and Grief Therapy*, 2nd edn. London: Routledge.

4: Young people and sex
Catriona Sutherland ◆

OBJECTIVES

After reading this chapter you will understand:

◆ how the law affects young people with regard to contraception, abortion and other related issues

◆ the confusion surrounding sex education in schools

◆ that young people have many needs when seeking advice but that their greatest anxiety is that confidentiality will be broken

◆ the extra problems that peer group pressure can exert, with particular regard to eating disorders.

Introduction

Young people have their own special needs both as a generic group and as individuals. These needs – particularly in the areas of sex education, contraception, advice and counselling – can only be met with special services that are accessible and relevant to them.

This chapter is intended to help you to extend your knowledge and skills in relation to the needs of young women. The particular skills needed include sensitivity, the ability to listen, respect for others, being non-judgemental and well-informed.

The term 'young woman' is generally used throughout, in preference to girl, teenager, child or adolescent.

Legal issues affecting under-16s

Age of majority

The Family Law Reform Act 1969, in England and Wales, reduced the age of majority from 21 to 18.

This means that young people of 18 and above can vote and marry without the consent of their parents.

Section 8 of this Act puts the age of medical majority at 16. Therefore young people, once 16, can consent to their own surgical, medical or dental treatment without reference to their parents. This means that a young woman of 16 can consent to use any method of contraception or to have an abortion.

Contraceptive advice and treatment to under-16s

Contraceptive advice and treatment to under-16s is lawful. In 1974 the Department of Health and Social Security issued a Memorandum of Guidance (DHSS, 1974) which stated that a doctor was: 'not acting unlawfully provided he acts in good faith in protecting the girl from the harmful effects of intercourse'.

In 1980 the DHSS issued a revised Memorandum which stressed the hope that the doctor: 'will always seek to persuade the child to involve the parent or guardian'. The wording of the revised

Memorandum made it quite clear that it would be the normal procedure to obtain parental consent, and to do anything else would be exceptional. There was considerable concern about the interpretation of this advice and the understanding of what was to be thought 'exceptional'. A resolution to this confusion took many years.

Then in 1980 Mrs Victoria Gillick sought an assurance from her local Area Health Authority (AHA) that her daughters under 16 years would not be given contraceptive advice or treatment without her consent. This assurance could not be given. In 1982 Mrs Gillick looked for a High Court ruling against her AHA and the DHSS. This ruling went against her and in 1984 she went to the Appeal Court.

As a result of the Gillick case, there was a ruling from the House of Lords in 1985. This ruling was felt, once and for all, to have clarified that the giving of contraceptive advice to under-16s was not unlawful. Following the House of Lords ruling, in 1986 the DHSS issued a Health Circular specifying that when giving contraceptive advice and/or treatment to under-16s certain guidelines should be used. The guidelines stated that contraceptive advice could be given, without the knowledge of parents, provided the doctor was satisfied:

(i)   that the girl, regardless of age, will understand the doctors' advice;
(ii) that they cannot persuade her to inform or to allow him/her to inform the parents that she is seeking contraceptive advice;
(iii) that she is very likely to begin or to continue having sexual intercourse with or without contraceptive treatment;
(iv) that unless she receives contraceptive advice or treatment her physical or mental health or both are likely to suffer;
(v)   that her best interests require him/her to give contraceptive advice, treatment or both without parental consent.

What this means is that young people under 16 are legally able to consent, on their own behalf, to any surgical, medical or dental procedure provided, in the doctor's opinion, they are capable of understanding the nature and possible consequences of the procedure.

It is important for persons under 16 seeking contraceptive advice to be aware that the doctor is legally obliged to discuss the value of parental support. However, it does not have to go any further than a discussion and the doctor must respect the young person's confidentiality.

The publicity and discussion generated while the Gillick case was running greatly affected the accessibility and availability of contraceptive advice to under-16s. Many young women still mistakenly believe that if they ask for advice the doctor will insist that their parents are informed. It is vital that health care workers continue to stress this point to all those seeking advice who are under 16 years old. The Department of Health's *Health of the Nation* document (DOH, 1992) has as one of its targets 'to reduce the number of conceptions among the under 16's by at least 50%' by the year 2000. If we are to have any chance of achieving this target then we must make certain that young women have correct contraceptive advice freely available when they need it.

Obviously it would be best for a young woman to have the support of her parents at this significant stage in her life. But her own wishes are more important. Establishing a trusting relationship with the doctor or nurse will do more to promote health than the refusal to see the young woman without involving her parents. Not all young women have caring families and many have very difficult family relationships. Some are abused; some want to protect their parents; some are desperate for their own independence; some just want to make some very mature decisions with privacy.

♦ 'If I have to tell my dad would chuck me out. That's what he did with my older sister.'

♦ 'If you tell my mum she will try to stop me from seeing my boyfriend. But it won't make any difference and I may have to leave home.'

♦ 'I can't tell my parents. They are having terrible fights at the moment and my dad is threatening to leave. If I told them it would only make things worse and my dad would blame my mum.'

Consent to treatment

Consent to treatment can be implied, spoken or written

(DOH, 1990).

Implied consent is mainly a non-verbal communication that the patient consents to undergo an examination or treatment. She may roll up her sleeve to have her blood pressure taken; she may remove the relevant clothing, voluntarily, and lie on the couch to have a cervical smear taken. This is a valid form of consent, but there can still be problems. There may be a misunderstanding between the patient and the nurse about what the nurse is proposing to do. She may not be aware of the intention of the nurse.

Spoken, or *verbal*, *consent* is what most nurses rely on in their day-to-day work. For example, you may simply ask 'Have you come for your smear test?' and receive the reply 'yes'.

Care needs to be taken that assumptions are not being made that the procedure is understood. This may be particularly true of young people. The nurse needs to ensure that the young woman understands the purpose of the procedure, what has and has not been done. The limits of the procedure need to be explained and understood. For example, a routine blood test for anaemia will not tell the patient her blood group or if she has HIV; a cervical smear test is not taken to detect a vaginal infection and does not routinely include a pelvic examination.

When asking for consent for a procedure an open question, rather than a closed one, will usually elicit a more useful response. For example, even though the nurse suspects that the woman has booked for a cervical smear, the open question 'What can I do for you today?' may get the response 'You know that I have come for my smear'. However, it may get 'I don't know, I received a letter telling me to come' or 'I was told I couldn't have any more pills until I had been to see you', and neither of these replies could be construed as giving consent to any procedure.

The age of consent

It is an offence for any male aged over 14 to have intercourse with a girl aged under 16. It is not the girl who is acting illegally. It is an absolute offence for a male aged over 14 to have unlawful sexual intercourse with a girl aged under 13.

It is no longer a legal requirement to report the knowledge of an act of unlawful intercourse. This duty was removed in 1967.

Abortion

A young woman under 16 can consent to a termination of pregnancy even if her parents have refused consent. The circumstances surrounding this would generally be considered most exceptional. Equally, a termination of pregnancy cannot be carried out against an under-16s' wishes, even if her parents have consented. Young women in such circumstances inevitably need considerable support and counselling in helping them reach a decision (see also page 145).

Homosexuality

In England and Wales the Sexual Offences Act 1967 legalized homosexual acts between men provided that: they both consent, it takes place in private and they are both aged over 21. The 1994 Criminal Justice Act included a clause lowering the age of homosexual consent to 18. This is still out of line with the age of 16 years for heterosexual consent.

The only law relating to female homosexuality is that of indecent assault. Lesbian acts are therefore legal, provided both women consent and are aged 16 or over.

The Children Act 1989

The Children Act 1989 brings together for the first time the public and private law relating to children. The most important principal of The Children Act is that the welfare of the child is of paramount consideration. Parents have new rights and responsibilities under the Act. However, children under 16, whether or not they are 'in care', can give or refuse their own consent to medical treatment depending on their capacity to understand the nature of the treatment.

Sex education

Sex education is not just about sex. It is about knowledge, information and understanding. It is about feelings and relationships. It is about empowering young people to make safe decisions regarding their sexual health. It is about being responsible. It is about life.

What is sex education for?

Sex education is about acquiring accurate information. It is about learning how to make safe decisions. It is about having a high self-esteem. It is about being assertive. It is about knowing how to say 'no' or 'yes'. It is about being enabled to make important personal choices.

There is evidence that those people who are better informed and have a higher self-regard will make better choices about their sexual health. Conversely, poor information about sexual matters helps to confirm feelings of guilt, which may be damaging to relationships. Massey (1990) suggests that ignorance is likely to perpetuate prejudice in such matters as sexism, homosexuality and unplanned pregnancy.

Where do young people get their sex education?

Most young people acquire their knowledge of sex from their parents and families, from their friends, from the media and from their schools.

Parents

Ideally sex education should be part of the whole learning process. It should not be a formal topic to be tackled when a child reaches a particular age, but accepted as a part of everyday life. Questions should be answered and information given by parents within the family context. The depth of the questions and the complexity of the information to be given grows as the child matures and develops.

A number of surveys over the last ten years have come up with similar findings. Allen (1987) found that most parents believe that their children should have adequate sex education, as do the young people themselves. Although parents feel that, ideally, this information should come from them – a survey by the Schools Health Education Unit (1994) supports this – they often feel ill-equipped to provide the information and education, and consider that school is the best

place for this to be given in a carefully planned setting.

Parents may feel that they are not the right people to provide sex education for a number of reasons. It could be that they feel embarrassed and consider that they are ill-equipped and ill-informed for answering questions about sex and sexuality. The majority of parents also felt their own sex education was poor or non-existent.

What most parents would like is a partnership with the schools. Parents have clear views on the topics they wish the schools to cover, which include basic bodily changes, pregnancy, contraception and AIDS. A significant number of parents believe that the schools should have the sole responsibility for covering sex education.

♦ 'I can't talk to my daughter about that, it's much too embarrassing.'

♦ 'Where can I find out what I should tell them? My mother never told me anything and I don't know how much to tell at what age.'

♦ 'They find out what they need to know when the time comes.'

Friends

Every young person receives some sex education from their friends and many young people will ask their friends for advice even though they are aware that these friends themselves may be, for the most part, ill-informed. At its best the advice is informative, helpful, supportive and safe, but at its worst it can be a mish-mash of rumour and hearsay. Such bad advice can help to perpetuate the myths and misconceptions that surround sex and is not always helpful, and may indeed be harmful.

♦ 'My friend says that you always start your pills seven days after your period.'

♦ 'My boyfriend says that I can't get pregnant if he does not come inside me.'

♦ 'I didn't know about the morning after pill, but my friend knew what to do and where to go.'

♦ 'My boyfriend says I can't ask him to wear a condom, it would mean that I didn't trust him.'

♦ 'My friend knew where to go for a pregnancy test.'

The media

Parents are often worried about the influence of pornographic videos and magazines. In books, newspapers and magazines there are constant references, both in words and pictures to sex and sexuality. These references reinforce and perpetuate stereotypical behaviour and prejudices. Some magazines run useful 'agony aunt' pages, which often give straightforward and factual advice about situations that young women often feel too embarrassed to ask their friends and parents about. The worries may be about periods, masturbation, physical changes, sexual feelings or how to handle difficult sexual situations and how to say 'no'. As long as the information is correct then these columns have a useful function.

Schools

It is generally accepted that sex education should be part of a programme of 'personal, health and social education', and while at the present time it is not compulsory, most schools have some sort of policy and have incorporated this in the curriculum.

What actually happens in individual schools varies enormously. At one end of the scale, a school may not have a policy, and may only be compelled to formulate one and consider formal sex education in response to a crisis, for example when a pupil becomes pregnant. At the other end of the scale, a school may have an excellent policy, and a well-planned and executed programme that is being regularly evaluated and altered in response to any local or topical needs (Box 4.1).

In the majority of schools it is the teachers who carry out sex education; usually it is the responsibility of an interested biology teacher. This may be why there is often a purely biological emphasis to sex education, paying little attention to aspects that concern sexuality and relationships. Sex education and related topics are not part of the teacher training programme and consequently many teachers feel ill-equipped to tackle the subject.

Some schools ask a professional from outside to come in and 'do' sex education. However, they may be given totally unrealistic targets of what to cover in the time available. It has been known for a professional to be asked to go in and speak to thirty-five 14-year-olds for a total of 40 minutes

Box 4.1 Sex education
Some comments from young people on their experience of sex education:

♦ 'I can talk to my mum about anything. I can't remember being sat down and told the facts of life, or anything like that. We would just discuss new topics when they came up. I never felt that any big deal was being made of it.'

♦ 'When we had our sex education the teacher seemed really embarrassed. I think we all knew more than him.'

♦ 'It was really stupid when we did our sex education. The boys all sat in a group and said ignorant, macho things. They made it impossible for us girls to join in and ask questions. All it did was show themselves up.'

♦ 'It was brilliant the way they did sex education in our school. They had someone in from outside. She came several times. We would break up into small groups, where we would work on all sorts of topics. You feel more comfortable in a little group, you can say all sorts of things and not feel stupid.'

♦ 'They do your sex education much too late. It should have to start while you are in junior school.'

♦ 'Sex education classes never tell you what you really want to know.'

♦ 'One thing we did in sex education was how to recognize difficult situations. Then we worked on how to be assertive. We did work on how to say "no" to things we didn't like. It was really helpful and I think it taught the boys something.'

and to cover menstruation, contraception, pregnancy, drug abuse, HIV and AIDS in this time.

Some teachers are very proprietorial about the teaching of sex education and are unwilling to share this subject with health professionals. However, other schools have an excellent relationship with such professionals, who may be school nurses, family planning nurses or sex education outreach workers.

Some local authorities employ sex education outreach workers, who can help with the development of a sex education policy, programme development and teacher training. The outreach worker is there to support the teachers, not to take the work away from them. In one area, a youth worker reported, 75% of the pupils said they would prefer to have an outside speaker, rather than a teacher from the school. Over recent years there has been an increase in the number of outreach workers as local authorities, hospital trusts and other agencies realize that they need to go out to where the young people are to give advice rather than wait for them to go to their doctor or a clinic when it is often too late. The outreach workers also work with young men. Hopefully these initiatives will help reduce the pregnancy rate in the under-16s as outlined in the *Health of the Nation* document.

Additionally the outreach worker may be reaching young people out of school, through youth clubs, young mothers' groups, tuition centres, the probation services and young people with special needs, which may include the young homeless.

Whatever the policy and however much schools feel that they have 'dealt with' sex education, there are still huge gaps in many young people's knowledge (Box 4.2). This can be demonstrated by a 'teenage' pregnancy rate in the UK of 69 per 1000. This compares with a rate of 9.2 per 1000 in the Netherlands – the lowest teenage pregnancy rate of any developed country. For many years the Dutch have had a very effective sex education

programme which has led to a well-informed population. There is no National Curriculum in schools, but sex education is compulsory, and starts at a much earlier age than in the United Kingdom.

Francis (1994) found that there appear to be three main differences between the UK and the Netherlands concerning the provision of sex education:

1. The Dutch have a much more accepting attitude to teenage sexuality and the need for contraception.
2. Young people are given more consistent messages from the government, the media and the schools about contraception: 'pill scare' stories are rare.
3. Young people know they can trust their doctor and are given the same degree of confidentiality as adults.

None of this leads to sexual activity starting at an earlier age. In fact, the emphasis is one of individual choice and personal responsibility for safer sexual behaviour. One outcome of this has been the 'double Dutch' method of contraception, i.e. the use of the Pill and condoms as protection against pregnancy and also infection.

Additionally young men are specifically targeted for sex education in the Netherlands as it was considered that in the past their needs had been overlooked and sex education was mainly for young women. This is in contrast to the experience of many young men in the UK.

♦ 'All I got on sex education in school was a 30 minute film on having a baby. And I'm gay.'

Legislation and official guidance concerning sex education

In 1986 the report of Her Majesty's Inspectorate supported the teaching of sex education. The HMI report states:

> the importance of sexual relationships in all our lives is such that sex education is a crucial part of preparing children for their lives now and in the future as adults and parents.

The report suggested that the topics covered should include: under-16s; homosexuality and abortion.

Box 4.2 Some statistics about young people and sex

♦ In 1992/93 45% of under-16s who visited Brook Advisory Centres came for emergency birth control or a pregnancy test.

♦ Forty to fifty per cent of 14, 15 and 16-year-olds use no birth control at first intercourse.

♦ Twenty per cent of 16–19-year-olds have unprotected sex the first time.

♦ Teenage (age 15–19) pregnancy rates per 1000 (1990):
England and Wales 68.6
Netherlands 9.2

♦ UK (except Northern Ireland) age of consent 16: 50% of young people have had first sexual experience by this age.

♦ Netherlands age of consent 12: average age of first sexual experience is 17.5 years.

The 1986 Education Act gave school governors the power to decide if sex education would be taught in their own school. If sex education was to be part of the curriculum, the governing body had to formulate a policy. Such a policy should be made in consultation with the headteacher and take into account the needs and beliefs of the local community. The local authority then has the obligation to see that the school curriculum is one which:

(a) promotes the spiritual, moral, cultural, mental and physical development of pupils at the school and of society; and

(b) prepares such pupils for the opportunities, responsibilities and experiences of adult life.

Section 28 of the Local Government Act 1988 amended Section 2 of the Local Government Act 1986 and prohibited local authorities from promoting homosexuality by teaching or publishing material. However, the Department of the Environment advised that Section 28 only applied to the local authorities themselves and not to schools. This is because school governors have been given the responsibility for decisions on sex education in their own schools.

By 1993 legislation ensured that all maintained schools should provide sex education (including education about HIV and AIDS and other sexually transmitted diseases) to all registered pupils. These schools should all have an up-to-date written policy available to all parents. Any sex education should be given: 'in such a manner as to encourage young people to have regard to moral considerations and the value of family life.'

Parents of a pupil can withdraw their child from all or part of the sex education programme.

The National Curriculum

Health education, of which sex education may be a part, is named as one of five cross-curricular themes in the National Curriculum. None of these themes is compulsory, unlike the ten core subjects which are. Sex education is only compulsory when it forms part of the science core subject.

The health education theme in the National Curriculum is broken down into nine components:

♦ Substance abuse and misuse

♦ Sex education

♦ Family life education

♦ Safety

♦ Health-related exercise

♦ Nutrition

♦ Personal hygiene

♦ Environmental aspects of health education

♦ Psychological aspects of health education.

Guidance is given over appropriate topics and areas of study at key stages. The key stages relate to age groups (Box 4.3).

Box 4.3 Examples of guidance on sex education for pupils at key stages 2, 3 and 4

Key stage 2 (age 7–11)
Pupils should 'begin to know about and have some understanding of the physical, emotional and social changes which take place at puberty.'

Key stage 3 (age 11–14)
Pupils should 'understand that organisms (including HIV) can be transmitted in many ways, in some cases sexually; be aware of the range of sexual attitudes and behaviours in society.'

Key stage 4 (age 14–16)
Pupils should 'consider the advantages and disadvantages of various methods of family planning in terms of personal preference and social implications; recognize and be able to discuss sensitive and controversial issues such as conception, birth, HIV/AIDS, child rearing, abortion and technological developments which involve consideration of attitudes, values, beliefs and morality; be aware of the need for preventive health care and what this involves; be aware of partnership, marriage and divorce and the impact of loss, separation and bereavement; be able to discuss issues such as sexual harassment in terms of their effect on individuals.'

Over the years stories and rumours about the provision of sex education have abounded. Sensational stories often appear in the popular press about inappropriate information being given to children who were too young to understand. This information is frequently reported as being of a near pornographic nature. The truth is usually that a responsible teacher or health professional was answering direct and explicit questions by pupils as accurately as possible.

In 1994 the Department For Education published a circular making changes to sex education provision (DFE, 1994). The effects of these changes are that:

1 all maintained schools must provide sex education to all registered pupils;
2 teaching on AIDS, HIV, sexually transmitted diseases and aspects of human sexual behaviour is only allowed when included in biological aspects of human sexual behaviour of the National Science Curriculum;
3 parents are allowed to withdraw their children from sex education, when not part of the National Curriculum.

In addition, the circular stated that it would be inappropriate for teachers to give contraceptive advice to under-16s without parental knowledge or consent.

This last point inevitably places some teachers in a difficult position. They are trusted by their pupils to keep secret any confidences, and yet are prohibited by the Department For Education from giving advice and help to their pupils when it is requested. It is likely that teachers, if they want to, will be able to get around this prohibition by employing a hair-splitting interpretation of the guidance. For example, they can talk in general terms about contraception and advice agencies, without appearing to be giving specific direction to a particular pupil.

Teachers are not allowed to promise confidentiality but neither are they legally obliged to reveal anything. However they may be under strong pressure to reveal that they have given advice or that they have been given confidential information. Some schools are now moving towards a 'whole school health policy' which would make it difficult for parents to remove their children from these classes.

Confidentiality

Many young people (particularly those under 16) are reluctant to seek medical help or contraceptive advice as they fear that a consultation will not be confidential and will be mentioned to others.

The Shorter Oxford English Dictionary defines confidential as: 'Spoken or written confidence; enjoying another's confidence; entrusted with secrets.'

The duty of confidentiality in medicine goes back to the fifth century BC and Hippocrates. The Hippocratic Oath states:

> whatever, in connection with any professional practice or not, I see or hear in the life of men which ought not to be spoken abroad, I will not divulge as reckoning that all such should be kept secret.

The United Kingdom Central Council (UKCC) gives guidance to nurses through the Code of Professional Conduct (UKCC, 1992), Clause 10 of which states:

> protect all confidential information concerning patients and clients obtained in the course of professional practice and make disclosures only with consent, where requested by order of a court or where you can justify disclosure in the wider public interest.

The nurse's duty to protect patient confidentiality does not have the same authority as the law (Medical Defence Union, 1992). This means that for a nurse the duty of confidentiality is an ethical one, rather than a legal one.

A patient should be able to speak with total freedom to their doctor or to any other health care professional. This freedom can only come from the trust that the patient has in that particular professional to respect their confidentiality.

A patient may be afraid that personal and private information will be revealed to other people. This anxiety is particularly prevalent in young people. If they fear that their trust will not be respected then they may not ask for medical help or else may not pass on information that is relevant to their medical care. Consequently this may mean that a young woman may not be truthful about her age, she may not reveal that she is taking some specific medication (e.g. for epilepsy), she may not seek advice for a vaginal discharge.

Scenario

 Rebecca, aged 18, came to see the nurse at the clinic several times. The first time she came she said that she had had two epileptic fits, which had been extensively investigated and no

cause found. She was put on drug therapy that she didn't take. At the clinic she was prescribed a higher dose contraceptive pill to counter the effects of the antiepileptic. After she had had several repeat visits to the clinic she told the nurse that the fits had been caused by the drug Ecstasy. She didn't want her GP to know, so she pretended to continue taking the medication.

The doctors' statutory body, the General Medical Council, states:

> patients are entitled to expect that the information about themselves or others which a doctor learns during the course of a medical consultation, investigation, or treatment, will remain confidential.

A person under 16 should expect the same duty of confidentiality as any other person.

A doctor may refuse to give advice or treatment to a person under 16 years if he believes that the young person cannot understand what the advice or treatment may involve. Even if a young person is considered too immature to give valid consent, the consultation should still remain confidential. The fear of betrayal of trust is greater than the reality. Most doctors will respect the confidentiality of those asking for contraceptive advice. However, the suspicion remains that a few doctors, because of their personal beliefs, would breach confidentiality with someone under 16 years. The difficulty for the young person lies in the ability to distinguish between those they feel they can and cannot trust. The consequences of a breach of confidentiality may be devastating to a young person.

♦ 'When I was 16 I went to my doctor for a pregnancy test. The doctor told my mum I was pregnant. Before I could say or do anything I had had an abortion. I had a bad time for a couple of years after that; I went a bit wild. I behaved very badly and took a lot of serious risks. It may have been the right decision, but it wasn't my decision. I can't talk to my mum now.'

The British Medical Association, General Medical Services Committee, Health Education Authority, Brook Advisory Centres, Family Planning Association and Royal College of General Practitioners issued a joint guidance note for doctors in 1993 (BMA *et al.*, 1993). The note spells out clearly that disregarding confidentiality, except in the most exceptional circumstances, is a serious breach of professional ethics. The fear of such a breach is a serious anxiety to many young women, although, there is, in fact, very little evidence that these breaches are made. It has usually happened to 'a friend of a friend'!

♦ 'I can't go and see my doctor about going on the pill. He is a very good friend of my parents and would be bound to tell my mum.'

♦ 'My friend went to the doctor for the pill. He said she had to tell her mum first.'

♦ 'I went to make an appointment at my doctor's for family planning. The receptionist said that I was too young.'

The only way to counter such anxieties is for health professionals to repeat, again and again, that all consultations are confidential, whatever is said in them. However, young people's trust will be greatly tested by the prominent debate and strong guidance from the Department for Education and Science about the role of teachers in the field of sex education. As mentioned earlier, from May 1994 a teacher has not been allowed to give advice on contraception or other sexual matters to a young person under 16, without informing the parents. Whether or not this matter is considered solely politically motivated and so subject to change according to party whim, remains to be seen. This guidance is likely to limit further those professional adults from whom young people can ask for advice, in confidence. Some young people have a complex and troubled family life and a respected teacher may be the only adult in whom they can confide.

Needs and attitudes of young people

Young people have a good idea of the kind of help and advice that they want. The majority know that there is birth control and have a reasonable knowledge of the different methods of contraception. However, many, especially young men, do not know where clinics are or where to go for help. Young people are clear about what they need and would like from a family planning clinic or youth session, which should be confidential, accessible, relevant, professional, non-judgemental and sensitive. These criteria, although relevant to all medical consultations at any age, are particularly pertinent for young people.

Confidential

A survey by Platt *et al.* (1992) demonstrates that this is considered to be one of the most important issues for young people. Though confident in many ways, they still doubt the total confidentiality of the clinics or consultations with their GP. Young people fear that the doctor will write or speak to their parents or that they will be forced to speak to their parents themselves.

Accessible

The timing of the session is important. A lunchtime session may be helpful, but not if pupils are unable to leave school premises. After-school sessions are popular, but not so useful in rural areas, where a young person may miss the only bus to take them home if they stay behind. In urban areas after-school, early evening and Saturday morning sessions are convenient, as these are often held at times when their absence from home can easily be explained:

♦ 'My mum thinks that I'm out shopping with my friend.'

♦ 'They think that I've gone to visit my Nan; I'll go on to see her when I leave here.'

♦ 'My mum thinks that I have stayed on at an after-school club.'

For some young people the precise location of a clinic may be important. Some may have the confidence to walk in, off the street, into a clearly signposted youth advice session or family planning clinic, and are not worried about anyone seeing them, whilst others would prefer the relative anonymity of a health centre, where they may be going to see other health care professionals, such as the dentist or chiropodist.

Some prefer to see their doctor in a group practice, where they may also be going for advice about their acne or ingrowing toenail. Finding appropriate premises may be difficult. In a rural area an attempt was made to set up a youth advice session after school using premises within a secondary school, but the school governors were unhappy about the possibility of being seen to condone under-age sex. Fortunately, premises were found in a youth club next to the school. Currently, in London, a Sixth Form College is starting a session on college premises that is to be run by family planning staff who are experienced in working with young people. Hopefully other schools will show similar initiatives with new schemes.

Relevant

Young people want any service that is offered, whether by their own doctor or a clinic, to be relevant to their needs. They do not want to be just given condoms and told 'not to do it'. Young people want to discuss and have advice on a wide range of topics including:

♦ Contraception

♦ Pregnancy

♦ Abortion

♦ HIV/AIDS

♦ Sexuality

♦ Incest

♦ Sexual abuse

♦ Genetic disorders

♦ Menstruation

♦ STDs

♦ Weight

♦ General health issues.

They also want and need the freedom to discuss relationships. These relationships may be with girlfriends, boyfriends, or parents and family. Their parents may be having their own relationship difficulties which they may want to talk about or there may be anxieties about drugs or alcohol, with their schooling or where they are living.

Professional

Young people want help from people who are professional, up to date, well-informed, and who understand the needs of the local community, e.g. having the clinic open at a time and in a place that is accessible to a young woman who may be closely chaperoned by parents or relatives, or ensuring that all staff are trained and informed of the cultural impact on sexual behaviour and contraceptive choice that comes from different ethnic groups.

They want help from those who have total integrity as far as confidentiality and legal issues are concerned. In short, they want help from someone they can trust to have their best interests as a priority.

Non-judgemental

At the heart of training in youth advice and family planning is the strong belief that any involvement with young people should be non-directive and non-judgemental. You should not make assumptions and moral judgements. No one knows why a young person has come to a clinic until that person says the words. Even then, why they say they have come may not be the reason why they have really come. You need to remember that you are there to help young people to make their own decisions and to learn to take responsibility for their own actions. Young people want to feel good about having come to ask for help. They do not want to feel put down or intimidated; to be made to feel guilty or bad. It needs to be acknowledged that the young person has made a big step in coming to ask for help, often a very difficult decision to take. For many it will be the first mature decision that they have made and they want to be listened to and they do not want to be talked down to or patronized.

Sensitive

Young people can find it very difficult to ask for what they want, or indeed what they think they want. This difficulty may be caused by embarrassment or come from ignorance. For example, a young woman may ask you for a pregnancy test, when what she really needs is emergency contraception, and vice versa. It is essential that you use appropriate language, language that is clearly understood by both parties, and, as far as possible,

reflects the young woman's level of knowledge. The language used must not increase her possible anxiety, particularly during the first visit.

All this has to be achieved while not appearing to be patronizing, but friendly and approachable.

Young people will not come to clinics and ask for help if their needs are not met, or if they do come once they will not return and will certainly not encourage their friends to attend if they did not feel welcome. They are also less likely to persist with their chosen method of contraception or to use it correctly if they felt uncomfortable during the consultation (Hutchinson, 1993; Williams, 1994).

♦ 'I didn't like the clinic I went to. I felt stupid when I didn't understand what they were on about.'

♦ 'I thought I was going to be lectured to and made to feel small. But it wasn't like that at all.'

♦ 'They explained everything to me, then let me decide.'

♦ 'It was really embarrassing having to explain what had happened. But I understand that it was necessary. I went away feeling much better.'

♦ 'They treated me like an adult, not like a silly kid.'

♦ 'I really trust the clinic. There's a counsellor to talk to if you have other problems. I would tell any of my friends to go there.'

♦ 'My mum took me to the doctor's. They did talk to her, but they made it clear that any decisions were mine. That was brilliant.'

Service provision

In order to meet the *Health of the Nation* targets of reducing teenage pregnancies (DOH, 1992), many GP surgeries and family planning clinics are setting up specially designated young people's clinics. If you are involved in setting up a session or clinic for young women in your locality it is important to research fully the needs of young people in your area. You will need to arrange:

♦ staff who understand and are sympathetic to young people's needs;

♦ an informal atmosphere and convenient location;

♦ an appropriate time of day, possibly after school;

♦ provision for 'drop-in' (no appointment) sessions;

♦ publicity emphasizing that the service is totally confidential; and

♦ provision of a professional, comprehensive service.

While this is what should be available to women of any age group, it is particularly important that it is provided for young women because they tend to be more vulnerable and may lack the verbal skills or initiative to seek advice further afield. If they are too frightened to go to a clinic, or if they go and their expectations are not met, or if they are treated insensitively and do not return, then they may be 'lost' for years at a time of need.

Sex and sexual needs and anxieties

Sexuality is thinking about it. Sex is doing it. Sexuality is the interest in sexual activity. This interest develops during the adolescent years, and sexual feelings usually develop earlier in girls than in boys. Along with this interest a range of needs and anxieties emerge.

The sexual needs and anxieties that young women have can be many and varied and stem from a variety of sources:

♦ Some come from the way in which a young woman has been brought up, from her family life and in particular from the way her mother has influenced her view of herself as a female (see Chapter 1).

♦ Some come from the pressures and influences of friends and peers.

♦ Some come from the pressures and influences of society, much of it through the media, which frequently gives conflicting, confusing and complex messages about the role, status and value of young women in society.

The anxieties may be to do with physical changes, with relationships, with sexual relationships, and with sex itself.

The change of body shape at puberty may cause many fears and anxieties and young women need to find a way of accepting their alteration in body image. The transformation from child's body to womanly body appears effortless for some, but for others it turns into a long, hard and awkward process. Breasts and hips may seem to be too big or too small and there may be too much or too little body hair. Greasy skin, spots and acne can be a considerable problem giving rise to a loss of confidence.

Periods usually start at 12–13 years, but they may start as early 9 or as late as 16 or 17 and you need to be able to reassure young women that this is normal. Everyone feels that their own experience of puberty is unique. How a young woman views her periods is very much influenced by how her mother has prepared her for them. So ideas about pain, bad blood, the 'curse' and smell are negative. There can be difficulties and anxieties regarding different types of sanitary protection. There may be practical problems with privacy at school, particularly if she starts her periods while still at junior school. For some young women (and their mothers) there may be fears about attempting to use tampons. You may find that you are in a position to offer sensible and constructive advice, e.g. practising with the smallest tampon, perhaps using a lubricant; practising with different types of tampons, with and without an applicator; and giving reassurance that the tampon cannot get lost. Some young women have problems with period pains and premenstrual syndrome and need to be given help with both these problems.

Some young women are very shy, and lack the maturity and social skills to make relationships. Some are fearful of rejection with friends of either sex. Often, a young woman may be ambivalent about her sexuality – unsure whether or not she is a lesbian. It may be difficult to determine the difference between a 'crush' and real sexual feelings.

The majority of sexual anxieties and needs are to do with sex itself. How a young woman feels about sex is influenced by her family, her friends and by society. How she feels may also be determined by what sexual experiences she has already had. These experiences may include rape, sexual abuse, incest and sexual harassment. Any of these experiences may be in the background of a young woman coming for help for the first time.

There may be particular reasons why a young woman wants a sexual relationship at this time. It may be a mature, planned decision about a deepening and loving relationship. It may be an act of defiance, intended to shock. It may reflect a need for someone to love her. It may be the only way for her to leave her family or home.

Some young women have a lack of knowledge about what sex really is. There are anxieties about vaginal penetration; this can be to do with the size they think their vagina is and the size they think their boyfriend's penis is. They may have been influenced by having had problems using tampons.

♦ 'My mother said that she was very small inside. She said everything was always very difficult. When I was born she had to have a 'Caesar'. She says that I am just like her. I'm really worried that my boyfriend won't be able to get inside me.'

♦ 'The third time I went out with my boyfriend he told me that his penis was 8 inches long. We hadn't talked about having sex at that time. I want to have sex with him, but I'm frightened it'll hurt. Why did he have to tell me about his size?'

There is ignorance about what an orgasm is and how to achieve one. This is hardly surprising, considering that most young women's early sexual experiences are at the hands of equally inexperienced young men and usually only last for a few minutes! It can take trust, experience and a reasonably relaxed location to make sex fulfilling, requirements that may not be met whilst waiting for parents to return home at any minute or on the back seat of a car.

If penetration is difficult for any reason there is the fear of being labelled 'frigid'. This is a term that is usually used by men to describe women, totally disregarding any ineptness or lack of sensitivity that they might have.

Most of the anxieties young women have about sex are to do with communication and with being able to negotiate with a boyfriend about what feels right for her. This may be saying 'no' to a sexual relationship at this particular stage or with this particular person. It may be to do with saying 'yes', but needing to be able to discuss issues of contraception and safer sex first. Mutual respect can be shown by not using these topics as an issue or a weapon, but demonstrating the need to discuss them as a partnership.

Some of the problems surrounding sex are compounded by not having a common language and by using words that are not clearly understood by all concerned. 'Making love' may only mean kissing to one person, whilst to another it means mutual masturbation, and to a third, penetrative vaginal sex. 'Oral sex' may be just kissing, or merely talking about sex. If a clearly understood vocabulary is used then issues of contraception, safer sex and sexual relationships can be negotiated.

No assumptions should ever be made about anyone's level of knowledge. Terms like 'contraception', 'birth control' and 'family planning' may not be understood.

♦ 'I don't want to go to a family planning clinic yet. I'm not thinking of planning a pregnancy and family for a number of years.'

A young woman may come asking for help because she thinks she may need contraception or perhaps emergency birth control. But she may be quite unsure as to whether or not she has had penetrative sex. Sensitive questioning is needed to assess the present risks and help her make decisions for the future.

Perhaps the main area of anxiety for young women is pregnancy. You should remember that young people are individuals and studies show that there is no simple model of sexual behaviour that will enable health professionals to target those at risk of unplanned pregnancy (Woodward, 1995). Teenage pregnancy is a complex problem and you should try to acknowledge and recognize young people's individuality in your dealings with them.

Sometimes a young woman will choose to become pregnant, or at least make no effort to stop becoming pregnant. This may be for a variety of reasons:

♦ She may see it as a way of demonstrating her independence.

♦ She may feel that she is showing devotion to her boyfriend.

♦ She may be desperate for someone of her own to love.

♦ She may have nothing better to do: no status, no expectations.

♦ She may be worried about infertility, not because she wants a baby now, but because she wants to be sure that she can when she wants to.

Somctimes a young woman will deliberately become pregnant and then have an abortion, just to demonstrate her fertility. You may find that this is more likely to occur in some cultures than others.

For most, though, the main anxiety is to prevent pregnancy at this time in their life, although for a few it is because they never, ever want a pregnancy.

♦ 'I'm really worried about becoming pregnant. I take my pills very carefully. I never forget them. And I don't let my boyfriend come inside me. What else can I do?'

♦ 'It would be an absolute disaster if I got pregnant for the next two years. I must use the best, safest birth control. But there mustn't be any side-effects.'

There may be anxieties about being examined, and about having a smear test. Some young women believe that if they go to a clinic or to their GP and ask about contraception, then they have to be examined at that visit and that it is a prerequisite for using any contraception. Yet many of these young women are virgins. A few think the examination is some kind of punishment for their sexuality and a procedure that has to be endured. If you can pick up this anxiety and explain the situation the relief expressed can be enormous. Someone showing extreme anxiety about being examined, or always coming up with an excuse for postponement, needs to be considered carefully. It is an opportunity to reveal underlying psychosexual problems or difficulties (see also page 51).

The same anxieties apply to the smear test. Though, when discussing the smear test, you can use it is an opportunity to talk about a wide range of health-related issues, including menstruation, sexually transmitted diseases, AIDS, smoking, diet, as well as any relevant family history. For many young women this will be the first time that they have had an opportunity to take responsibility for their own health, and make their own decisions.

Your own attitudes at this initial consultation may have an enormous impact on how the young woman views her future sexuality and it is vitally important that you appear relaxed and comfortable whilst discussing sex so that she can pick up these positive feelings from you. Hopefully, if she

feels confident and comfortable then she will encourage her friends to visit you for similar advice. Her first examination and/or smear should be carried out in a non-rushed, private situation and the procedure fully explained. Many women dread vaginal examination later in life as their first experience of this was uncomfortable, intrusive, insensitive and rushed.

Some young women are prescribed the oral contraceptive pill for dysmenorrhoea or menorrhagia, or to 'regulate' their periods, and they have anxieties about being examined. An examination and smear on a virgin is not necessary, as long as there is no concern about any underlying pathology.

Peer group pressure

Peer group pressure can vary enormously and cover a range from subtle, almost subliminal messages through to heavyweight pressure that might almost be called bullying.

Most young people want to fit into a group. They value the opinions and style of their friends and want to be accepted and valued by the group. This may lead them to be pressurized into behaving in certain ways, to conform to group standards. On one level this pressure may be no more than to wear certain clothes or to have a particular hairstyle, but on another level there may be pressure to become involved in dangerous and/or illegal activities.

Smoking

Peer group pressure to smoke is common amongst teenagers. It is not unusual to find that a group of friends will be either all smokers or all non-smokers; boys being more influenced by their peers than girls and girls being more influenced by parental smoking. Some young women see smoking as a way of controlling or reducing their weight (Camp *et al.*, 1993). In fact, some research has shown that smokers have a significantly higher body mass (Townsend *et al.*, 1991). This may be explained by smokers drinking more alcohol, taking less exercise and having a less organized diet. A survey in 1992/3 by the Office of Population Censuses and Surveys into the smoking habits of 11–15-year-olds suggests that 9% of boys and 10%

of girls in that age group smoked regularly (OPCS, 1994).

Dieting

Many young women feel that they have to conform to an ideal body shape. They may try to achieve this through 'dieting', disorganized eating, smoking or by increasing the exercise that they take.

Alcohol

The peak age for experimenting with alcohol is 13–15 years. By 13 years 90% of young people have had some alcohol. Family influences are strong here with young people who see family views as strict and repressive being likely to drink more (see also page 31).

One of the dangers of excessive drinking is the greater likelihood of unprotected and/or unplanned sex. In these circumstances not only is there a high risk of pregnancy but also of infection. There may have been no thought of rational, careful consideration before intercourse.

Drugs

The same is also true for drugs. The vast majority of 15- and 16-year-olds will have been offered drugs. Solvent abuse is also dangerous, but cheap, and appears to be more common with boys than girls. There is no accurate information on how many have taken drugs, though this will range from those who have tried something just once, to those who are more regular users. Young people think they are knowledgeable about drugs: the types, availability, effect and cost. Drugs are very much part of current youth culture and they may be used much more than alcohol.

♦ 'The bars at the clubs don't make any money these days. That's because almost everyone is taking drugs.'

A new programme aimed at reducing the demand for drugs among schoolchildren is planned for implementation in all primary and secondary schools. In some areas there are exciting initiatives to try and combat the problem such as a 'drug' bus that tours with information. A drugs prevention programme is running very successfully in Amsterdam's primary schools, with plans for it to be set up in other Dutch cities. It is hoped that the scheme will have the same level of success as the Dutch sex education programme.

With drugs, as with alcohol, there are known health risks. As a result of the loss of inhibition, there are the risks of unplanned, unprotected or even unwanted sex. As a health professional you could offer advice about drug safety (Box 4.4).

Box 4.4 Advice to give young people about drug safety

This should better be described as 'how to minimize the risk'. These are some suggestions:

♦ If taking Ecstasy don't drink any alcohol, but do drink plenty of water otherwise heat exhaustion can follow.

♦ Make use of needle exchange programmes and don't share 'works'.

♦ Don't take hallucinogenic drugs when you're alone, and if in a group have one person not tripping.

♦ Don't do cocktails of drugs, in the same way you don't mix drinks.

♦ Remember, if on drugs your judgement will be affected and you may put yourself in an unsafe situation personally, sexually (with unplanned, unprotected or even unwanted sex) or both.

Sex

There is pressure to be sexually active, or to appear to be sexually active. A young person can be made to feel immature, unattractive and boring if they do not become sexually active. Unfortunately there is often little planning in their early sexual encounters. The younger a person is when they have their first sexual intercourse, the less likely they are to use any contraception.

There can also be pressure and influence about the kind of contraception that they can or cannot use.

♦ 'You mustn't use the pill, it makes you fat.'

♦ 'You can never have a coil if you have never had a baby.'

◆ 'My friend says I must change my pill. She says that her pill is much better because it costs more than mine.'

◆ 'We didn't use a condom because I was told that you only get pregnant if you have an orgasm. I've never had an orgasm.'

◆ 'He says he can't use a condom because they are all too small for real men.'

A practice nurse relates:

> We have a young woman in the practice who was pregnant, with twins, when she was still 17. She has great influence with a group of other young women, and a number of them became pregnant too. Now that she has had the babies and has chosen to use reliable contraception, we are hoping that her friends can be encouraged to make similar choices.

Bullying

Woolfson (1989) suggests that with girls bullying is likely to be verbal, while with boys it tends to be physical. There is no accurate information on the nature and extent of bullying, but estimates suggest that 10–25% of pupils are directly affected, either as victims or as bullies themselves (Friend, 1992). Schools are being encouraged to develop policies to combat bullying and to encourage pupils and parents to come forward if there is a problem.

Society's expectations

Apart from the peer group pressure to be at the best school, in the best class and to achieve the best results, pupils also feel the pressure of society's expectations, even in the most supportive and unpressurized family or school. Some pupils will become physically ill in the build-up to exams. There is often an enormous pressure on them to achieve; some parents have very unrealistic or inflexible expectations of their children's potential. They want their children to do well academically, perform well at sport, have additional skills and interests, and to have a good group of friends.

There is pressure from both parents and schools for young people not to smoke or drink, not to become involved in drug taking or solvent abuse, and yet young people often feel that they have far greater knowledge in these areas than their parents. Parents want there to be no question about their child's sexual orientation and many would ideally want their child's relationships to be non-sexual. All these pressures may come from parents who smoke and drink themselves, who may take 'recreational' drugs, who are not always honest, and who may have adulterous relationships. It is no wonder that their children are experiencing very conflicting and confusing messages. As so often with young people, it is a case of 'do what I say, not what I do'.

◆ 'I really wanted to talk to my parents about my boyfriend, but I can't. My Dad's having an affair with another woman, and my Mum's in a terrible state.'

Your role as a health care professional is to listen. The young person needs to trust that you are there for her, to support her, to be non-judgemental and to value her concerns. If this is all forthcoming then you can help her.

Young lesbians

Young women are not generally seen as sexual beings in their own right. They are often perceived to need a man to be sexual, and that if they are lesbians they are only infatuated with another girl and they can be 'cured' by a real man. As with gay young men, young lesbians have problems with coming out. Many lack any support from family and friends, and have experienced great personal difficulty. Section 28 of the 1988 Local Government Act (see page 72) has made it difficult, if not impossible, for information to be widely available to young lesbian, gay and bisexual people. There has not, to date, been a successful prosecution but self-censoring by local authorities is widespread. Many young lesbians find it difficult to come out until they leave home. Most find information about advice groups, social groups, etc. from any of the various 'listings' publications.

Eating disorders

Anorexia nervosa and bulimia nervosa are the eating disorders most likely to be encountered in young people.

Anorexia nervosa

Anorexia is a serious illness affecting perhaps as many as 1% of secondary schoolchildren (Crisp *et al.*, 1976). As many as 10% of these pupils may die as a result of the illness. This means there could be as many as 10 000 schoolgirl anorexics in the UK. The Eating Disorders Association suggests that approximately 1 in 500 women between the ages of 15 and 25, or around 6000 people a year in Britain require treatment. In addition, some research suggests that 1 in 50 of university students is affected with an eating disorder. This number rises to 1 in 14 of students at dancing and modelling schools, where the 'ideal' body shape is seen as being ultra slim (Slade, 1984).

The typical anorexic is a female in her mid- to late teens, although the disease can manifest itself at an earlier as well as at a much later age. Males form only 10% of anorexics. The majority of anorexics appear to start 'slimming' because they believe, rightly or wrongly, that they are overweight. However, unlike the average 'dieter' who gives up after a time, the anorexic persists until there is an abnormal weight loss. The longer they persist the more abnormal their thinking and reactions become (Bruch, 1978). Bruch describes anorexia as 'the relentless pursuit of excessive thinness'.

Many anorexics in order to achieve their 'ideal' body weight resort to the use of laxatives so that they lose another pound or two. Once weight has been lost, young women will frequently also have amenorrhoea as the body attempts to conserve energy for the basic activities of life.

There appears to be a genetic predisposition that gives anorexics a specific personality; they are likely to be perfectionists with obsessive compulsions, who are very determined. This type of personality means that when they encounter difficulties they respond by starving themselves. The difficulties may be anything from a chance remark about their weight, exam pressure, family problems, to sexual abuse. The response is to take control in the only way they know. Anorexia is not just about food, it is about doing something perfectly.

Anorexics make an abnormal response to what others might consider a normal but upsetting situation. For example, a young woman turned down by ballet school might decide that if she loses weight then the school will offer her a place after all. A young woman may be anxious about how she will do in her exams, losing weight may be something that she can do very well. A young woman's father may die; so she loses weight to stay a little girl and not grow up. For some it may be a way of avoiding some of the problems of adolescence, particularly those to do with developing sexuality, adolescence being a time of uncertainty and self-consciousness (Palmer, 1989).

Anorexia may be the response of some young women to the profound changes in their lives. It may be a demonstration that they are self-sufficient, independent and have no needs.

Common signs and symptoms of anorexia nervosa are listed in Box 4.5.

Box 4.5 Signs and symptoms of anorexia

♦ **Abnormal desire to be thin**

♦ **Abnormal weight loss – and covering up this weight loss with baggy clothes**

♦ **Distorted body image (thinking of herself as fat), even when obviously underweight**

♦ **Obsession with food, calories and cooking, but denial of dieting**

♦ **Obsession with exercising, sometimes for hours at a time**

♦ **Low self-esteem and lack of confidence**

♦ **Isolation from friends**

♦ **Use of laxatives/vomiting**

♦ **Amenorrhoea**

♦ **Lanugo (an excess of fine body hair)**

♦ **Feeling cold.**

Bulimia

Bulimia is characterized by overeating followed by self-induced vomiting. The amount of food consumed in a bingeing session can be enormous. In addition, excessive exercise and the taking of laxatives and diuretics are used to keep weight down.

The condition usually starts between the ages of 15 and 24 years. It is thought that about 3% of women will be affected at some stage in their lives, but because of the secretive nature of the condition this has to be a conservative estimate. As with anorexia, bulimia may be the response to stressful life events. However, where anorexics 'choose' to starve themselves, bulimics need to show that they are coping and capable, and so keep their chaotic eating a secret (Lawrence and Dana, 1990).

Signs and symptoms of bulimia are listed in Box 4.6.

Box 4.6 Signs and symptoms of bulimia

◆ Irregular periods

◆ Fear of fatness

◆ Binge eating, often huge amounts of food, most commonly in secret

◆ Normal weight

◆ Regular self-induced vomiting

◆ Possible use of large doses of laxatives and/or diuretics

◆ Tooth decay.

Causes

There are various theories as to the origins of the two conditions anorexia and bulimia. These theories include:

◆ Pressures of society

◆ Family pressures, in which the meal becomes the arena for family problems

◆ Child sexual abuse

◆ Depression

◆ Stress, particularly a reaction to some distressing event

◆ Biological changes, as a way of controlling and avoiding physical, bodily changes

◆ Genetic predisposition

◆ Needs, which may be in conflict to upbringing.

Whatever the causes, it is now recognized that more is needed than force-feeding the young woman until her weight is 'normal'. Treatment may consist of behavioural, psychodynamic or family therapy, living in a therapeutic community, self-help groups, or any combination of these. Therapy is seen as the only way of trying to resolve the underlying problems that manifest themselves as an eating disorder. Whatever the methods used, two elements are necessary to achieve a satisfactory outcome. The first is the woman having a

desire to change. The second is the woman having an understanding of the trigger for her disordered eating habit, e.g. a disturbed family relationship (Abraham and Llewellyn-Jones, 1992).

Treatment and prognosis

Unfortunately, there are few specialist eating disorders units in this country; they are mainly located in psychiatric units or hospitals. The prognosis appears to be related to the length of time the disorder has been present; the earlier the condition is recognized and treatment started, the better the outcome.

The majority will recover, but it may take many years. How good the recovery is may be variable: a good outcome being measured by the maintenance of a normal weight and regular menstruation. The young woman with anorexia may be easier to identify because of her extreme weight loss, but the young woman with bulimia may more readily come and ask for help.

A school nurse reports:

◆ 'If a pupil has anorexia then it is her friends who will come and tell you and ask you to do something. If the pupil has bulimia, then she is very likely to come and ask for help herself'.

The consequences of untreated or inadequately treated anorexia or bulimia can be very serious, the effects being broadly grouped depending on whether there is starvation, vomiting or laxative abuse (Box 4.7).

One mother says of her daughter: 'She eats too little to live, but too much to die.' Your role when encountering young women with eating disorders is to be sensitive to the clues that might indicate that there is an eating problem. These clues may be:

◆ Wearing an inappropriate amount of baggy clothing

◆ Anxiety about menstruation

◆ Delayed onset of menstruation

◆ Excessive thinness

◆ Unexplained weight loss

◆ Fainting or dizziness.

When you have identified someone at risk of an eating disorder good health promotion may be all

Box 4.7 Potential damage to health from eating disorders

Anorexia

♦ Severe constipation

♦ Osteoporosis

♦ Muscle wasting

♦ Severe electrolyte imbalance

♦ Death.

Bulimia

♦ Mouth ulcers

♦ Tooth decay and gum disease

♦ Stomach and bowel disorders

♦ Hair loss

♦ Hypokalaemia causing cardiac arrhythmias

♦ Muscle weakness

♦ Kidney damage.

that is necessary. Having calculated the young woman's body mass index (BMI) (see page 19), which should be between 19 and 24.9, you can then advise her of a healthy eating programme. You should be able to discuss the risks to her health of chaotic eating and be able to discover some of her anxieties and her level of understanding of her situation. With this information you should be able to determine if the young woman needs to be referred on for expert professional treatment.

Conclusion

Government strategies have meant that the health situation regarding young people is constantly changing. The targets set by the *Health of the Nation* document (DOH, 1992) for reducing the teenage pregnancy rate seemed unrealistic at first but success is slowly being achieved with local initiatives to improve sex education and greater publicity about the availability of sexual health information. Young people need to know where they can seek sexual health advice preferably before embarking on a sexual relationship, but sex for young people is often unplanned and impulsive so adequate information about emergency contraception also needs to be available.

Having read this chapter you will appreciate many of the difficulties young people experience whilst growing up. Young women will seek your professional help and advice which should be confidential and given in a professional, supportive and non-judgemental manner. If you appear relaxed and comfortable when dealing with young people then they will pick up positive messages from you and encourage their friends to attend. Not only do young people learn from you but you can also learn from them about their needs so that the service you offer can be improved for others. After all, sex and sexuality are human pleasures and you should be able to enjoy your sexual health work with young people.

Resources

Anti Bullying Campaign
10 Borough High Street, London SE1 9QQ
Tel. 0171 378 1446

Brook Advisory Centres
153a East Street, London SE17 2SD
Tel. 0171 701 5171. 24-Hour helpline 0171 617 8000

Childline
Tel. 0800 1111

Children's Legal Centre
University of Essex, Wivenhoe Park, Colchester, Essex CO4 3SQ
Tel. 01206 873820

National Drugs Helpline
Tel. 0800 77 6600

Eating Disorders Association
Sackville Place, 44 Magdalen Street, Norwich, Norfolk NR3 1JE
Tel. 01603 621414

Family Planning Association
2–12 Pentonville Road, London N1 9FP
Tel. 0171 837 5432 (Switchboard)
0171 837 4044 (General helpline)

Further reading

BURNINGHAM, S. (1994) *Young People Under Stress: a Parent's Guide*. London: Virago Press.

LLEWELLYN-JONES, D. and ABRAHAM, S. (1992) *Everygirl*, 2nd edn. Oxford: Oxford University Press.

MCPHERSON, A. and MACFARLANE, A. (1989) *I'm A Health Freak Too!* Oxford: Oxford University Press.

NOONAN, E. (1993) *Counselling Young People*. London: Routledge.

References

ABRAHAM, S. and LLEWELLYN-JONES, D. (1992) *Eating Disorders: The Facts*, 3rd edn. Oxford: Oxford University Press.

ALLEN, I. (1987) *Education in Sex and Personal Relationships*. London: Policy Studies Institute.

BMA *et al.* (British Medical Association, General Medical Services Committee, Health Education Authority, Brook Advisory Centres, Family Planning Association and Royal College of General Practitioners) (1993) *Confidentiality and People Under 16: A Joint Guidance Note*. London.

BROOK ADVISORY CENTRES, *Annual Report* 1992–1993.

BRUCH, H. (1978) *The Golden Cage: The Enigma of Anorexia Nervosa*. London: Open Books.

CAMP, D.E., KLESGES, R.C. and REYLEN, G. (1993) The relationship between body concerns and adolescent smoking. *Health Psychology* **12:** 29.

CRIMINAL JUSTICE ACT (1994) London: HMSO.

CRISP, A.H., PALMER, R.L. and KALUCY, R.S. (1976) How common is anorexia nervosa? A prevalence study. *British Journal of Psychiatry* **128:** 549–54.

DFE (Department for Education) (1994) *Education Act 1993: Sex Education in Schools*. Circular number 5/94. London: DFE.

DHSS (Department of Health and Social Security) (1974) *Family Planning Service Memorandum of Guidance*: issued with circular HSC(IS) 32; May.

DOH (Department of Health) (1990) *A Guide to Consent for Treatment*, HC (90). London: DOH.

DOH (1992) *The Health of the Nation: A Strategy for Health*. London: HMSO.

FPA (Family Planning Association) (1994) *Young People's Attitudes Towards Sex Education*. London: FPA.

FRANCIS, C. (1994) Sex education for teenagers in Holland. *Nursing Standard* **15:** 27.

FRIEND, B. (1992) Blighted childhood. *Nursing Times* **88:** 18.

HMI (Her Majesty's Inspectorate) (1986) *Health Education from 5 to 16 (Curriculum Matters)*. London: HMSO.

HUTCHINSON, F. (1993) Contraceptive needs of young people. *British Journal of Sexual Medicine* 10.

LAWRENCE, M. and DANA, M. (1990) *Fighting Food: Coping with Eating Disorders*. London: Penguin.

LOCAL GOVERNMENT ACT (1988) London: HMSO.

MASSEY, D. (1990) School sex education: knitting without a pattern? *Health Education Journal* **49:** 134.

MEDICAL DEFENCE UNION (1992) *Confidentiality*. London: MDU.

OPCS (Office of Population, Censuses and Surveys) (1994) *Smoking Among Secondary Schoolchildren*. London: HMSO.

PALMER, R.L. (1989) *Anorexia Nervosa: a Guide for Sufferers and their Families*, 2nd edn. Harmondsworth: Penguin.

PLATT, M.J., BATCHELOR, L. and TAYLOR, R. (1992) *Young People and Sexual Health: a Survey of Views, Behaviours and Needs*. Report, Macclesfield Health Authority.

SCHOOLS HEALTH EDUCATION UNIT, UNIVERSITY OF EXETER (1994) *Young People in 1993*. Exeter: HEU.

SLADE, R. (1984) *The Anorexia Nervosa Handbook*. London: Harper & Row.

TOWNSEND, J., WILKES, H., WILKES, A. and JANIS, M. (1991) Adolescent smokers seen in general practice: health, lifestyle, physical measurements, and response to anti-smoking advice. *British Medical Journal* **303:** 949.

UKCC (1992) *Code of Professional Conduct for the Nurse, Midwife and Health Visitor*. London: UKCC.

WILLIAMS, E. (1994) Contraceptive compliance among young people. *British Journal of Sexual Medicine* May/June: 12.

WOODWARD, V. (1995) Why do teenagers fall into the pregnancy trap? *Modern Midwife* August: 15–18.

WOOLFSON, R. (1989) Bullying at school: part 1 – the nature and extent of the problem. *Health at School* **4:** 152.

5: Women with special needs and concerns

Marjorie Hickerton

OBJECTIVES

After reading this chapter you will understand:

♦ how the domiciliary family planning service works and who can benefit from such a service

♦ the importance of sensitivity in dealing with people with learning disabilities

♦ the impact of sexual abuse and rape on women

♦ how different cultures and religions influence female sexuality.

Introduction

The title of this chapter 'Women with special needs and concerns' could cover a wide range of women with very different needs, concerns and problems and easily become a complete book in its own right. It is not within the scope of this chapter to cover the subject in such depth but it is hoped that by concentrating on a few specific areas you will be able to understand and be aware of the sexual health and contraceptive needs of different groups of people in society. Women with special needs are often confused, their problems are complex and you will need time, patience and the ability to enlist the help of counsellors, social workers and others in order to help them.

Domiciliary family planning

Domiciliary family planning is a specialized service visiting women at home to give advice on contraception and sexual health. The service has also been described as: 'preventative community services which should bridge the gap between medical and social services' (Christopher, 1980). This is in line with the *Health of the Nation* document (DOH, 1992), which states that 'family planning services should be appropriate, accessible and comprehensive to meet the needs of those who use or may wish to use them' (Box 5.1).

The provision of domiciliary family planning was established in the late 1950s, when pilot studies were set up in Newcastle, York and Southampton. The aim of the service was to establish and maintain contact with those women who were in need of the service and defined as 'hard to reach' and could not or would not go to family planning clinics.

In 1972, the Secretary of State recommended that the service should be available within the National Health Service and about this time 140–150 domiciliary family planning services were started up throughout the country (Leathard,

1985). These services were mostly situated in the larger cities and in their surrounding areas.

The domiciliary service can be run by nurses with a doctor, or by nurses alone. If it is run solely by nurses, then clients who are unable to attend clinics can be taken to a clinic to be seen by a doctor. This is necessary for clients who choose prescribable methods of contraception for the first time, i.e. the Pill or injection, and for insertion of intrauterine devices. It is hoped that with the general move forward with nurse prescribing that suitably qualified nurses will be able to take over this role in the future.

Staff working in the domiciliary service need considerable experience in all aspects of sexual health and in working within the community. Courses such as the advanced family planning training (ENB AO8), are desirable, thus enabling the nurse to carry out the tasks required, especially if working alone. Close liaison between social services and the domiciliary service may be required in order to provide access to additional support.

> **Box 5.1** Domiciliary services available
> All the following services can be carried out in a domiciliary capacity:
> - ♦ Information and advice on all methods of contraception
> - ♦ Abortion counselling and referral
> - ♦ HIV and AIDS counselling and referral
> - ♦ Cervical screening/breast awareness
> - ♦ Menopause counselling and referral
> - ♦ Post-termination counselling
> - ♦ Preconceptual advice
> - ♦ Pregnancy testing
> - ♦ Pre-menstrual syndrome counselling and advice
> - ♦ Psychosexual counselling
> - ♦ Referral to genito-urinary medicine clinics
> - ♦ Sterilization/vasectomy counselling and referral.

Scenario

Mary, a 15-year-old single girl, was referred to the service having just had her first baby. Her pregnancy was unplanned. She said that as she had not got pregnant after her first experience of unprotected sexual intercourse she was sure she was infertile. Her partner was the same age as her and they both seemed immature for their age.

They eventually married but were divorced within three years, leaving Mary with a second child. Both children were boys and they would have posed a handful to raise even for a more mature couple with no additional problems. The boys seemed beyond parental control by the time the first was 5 years old. The eldest boy had spent short periods of time in care and on one occasion had even set the house on fire.

The boys refused to go to school and their teacher told Mary that when they were there they behaved so badly that it was not acceptable to put them with the other children. There were constant complaints from neighbours about their behaviour and Mary and her family became more and more

isolated. She existed between periods of deep depression, sometimes bordering on suicide, and periods of just managing to cope. Mary herself had spent part of her own childhood in children's homes and desperately did not want the same to happen to her own children.

Originally Mary was on the combined oral contraceptive pill but was an unreliable pill-taker and required emergency contraception on a number of occasions. This failed on one occasion and Mary had a termination. It was about this time that Mary's husband left her. After the termination she needed regular counselling and support. It was decided that a more reliable method of contraception requiring easy compliance was necessary and from the choices offered Mary chose the injectable method.

This proved successful and she remained with this method for the next six years. During this time her eldest child had to be placed in care and was eventually fostered. She regularly called the GP to her remaining son and neglected her own health. She smoked heavily and had a very poor diet. Regular check-ups were given and Mary also received advice on a more healthy lifestyle. After a routine cervical smear test Mary required a colposcopy. She became very anxious and failed to attend numerous colposcopy appointments so eventually the domiciliary family planning nurse accompanied her to the clinic. Mary felt guilty and over-anxious that the necessity for a colposcopy might have been due to her number of sexual partners and was eventually referred for psychosexual counselling.

Her problems resolved after a number of sessions, and her lifestyle and self-esteem improved. Last year she met a new partner who has accepted her and her child and she is pregnant again. This time it is a planned pregnancy and she hopes for a more stable future.

Many of the women seen by the domiciliary service have low-self-esteem, poor education and limited skills. This can lead to a lack of finances and poor housing which in turn compounds the problem. Under these circumstances contraception becomes a very low priority and this in turn leads to even more hardship. If help and advice are given at an early stage then many of the pitfalls that clients experience could be avoided.

Referral system

Clients are referred to the domiciliary service from many sources. Any health care worker who recognizes a woman in need may refer, having first obtained permission from the client. Referrals can be made verbally by telephone or on the appropriate written form. It is the intention of the service that each new client is seen either by a doctor or a nurse within 48 hours of professional contact.

Reasons for referral are often complex and multifactorial, reflecting the crises and difficulties experienced by this client group. Major contributory factors are socio-economic limitations, e.g. a single mother with several young children, lack of motivation by the client and suspicion or fear of conventional facilities. Referrals are also made because of learning disabilities, mental illness, religious or cultural restrictions.

Staff working in domiciliary family planning need to have considerable training in all aspects of health care and a wide variety of experience is required as, on most occasions, nurses will make decisions on their own. Detailed protocols should be in place to give health care professionals guidance and support. The Royal College of Nursing has also produced guidelines for Domiciliary Family Planning Services and this document assumes familiarity with, and an acceptance of, the RCN Nursing Standards of Care for Family Planning Nurses (1989) and the RCN *Family Planning Manual for Nurses* (RCN, 1991b).

There have been those who complain that the domiciliary service is expensive, even though it is, in fact, only marginally more expensive than a visit to the doctor. Success of the domiciliary service, however, cannot be measured by cost alone. Because the women catered for are often poorly motivated and, by nature, intermittent contraceptive users, unplanned pregnancies will still occur, adding to the already difficult situation these women are in, but these pregnancies will be more widely spaced than they would be without the domiciliary service. The benefits to the client in allowing her to take control of her sexuality and lifestyle cannot be measured in terms of cost or client satisfaction.

The service is needed more than ever today in our multicultural society. Many clients come from countries where sex education and contraception are either forbidden or non-existent. They find attending clinics or GP centres intimidating and feel isolated and insecure in strange and often very formal surroundings. They feel more confident having a home visit with their families around them. Family planning services are inexpensive in terms of total NHS expenditure. For every £1 spent on family planning there is a saving of £11 to the taxpayer (McGuire and Hughes, 1995).

Many people involved in domiciliary family planning believe that it is a much underfunded service. Its value and potential need to be recognized by health care workers and especially by GPs, some of whom are completely unaware of the services available and how their patients could benefit. It can cost £1000 per week to keep a child in care, depending on the child's needs. This is money that could easily be directed at expanding the domiciliary service and preventing unplanned pregnancies in those women who find it difficult to attend the usual clinics.

More information about local domiciliary family planning services can be obtained from the District/Trust Health services, the FHSA or from local telephone directories.

Women with learning disabilities

When defining learning disability it was once thought that intelligence was the 'gold standard'. However, intelligence cannot be defined in a precise way; it is made up of a number of components, including cognition, language, motor skills and social abilities (Sims and Owens, 1993). In the past, and in ICD-10 (a WHO classification of mental and behavioural disorders), an IQ score of 70 or below has been regarded as indicative of a learning disability, but the definition is by no means as simple as this.

A survey at one mental hospital showed that of the people admitted, more than half had IQs above 70, a quarter recorded scores above 80, and 7% had scores between 90 and 100. There are, most certainly, genetically and environmentally caused medical disorders which may have a profound effect on physical and mental development. Such conditions include Down's syndrome (a chromosomal abnormality), tuberose sclerosis (a single gene error), cytomegalovirus (due to infection) and fetal alcohol syndrome (resulting from pre-natal environment). A good account of these and many other disorders may be found in Craft and Craft (1985).

People with learning disabilities have the same rights as other individuals within the community and are encouraged to live as independent a life as possible. Recently there have been moves towards greater care at local levels, away from large institutions and into small residential units within the community. Here there are greater opportunities for education and training and many have found worthwhile jobs whilst living in supervised housing. The majority are unaffected by physical handicap and generally have no problems with sexual functioning.

Attitudes towards people with learning disabilities have gradually changed as the general public have become more aware of the needs of this group. There is a growing acceptance that they are as entitled as the rest of the population to lead as normal a life as is possible. However, this requires understanding on the issues relating to their sexuality. Problems can arise if these issues are not dealt with sensitively. An individual's sexuality is intimately connected with her mental health and disruption of one can have a serious effect on the other.

Scenario

Terrie, aged 21 years, suffers from Smith–Lemli–Opitz syndrome, a hereditary syndrome transmitted as an autosomal recessive trait and characterized by microcephaly, mental retardation, hypotonia, a short nose with anteverted nostrils and syndactyly of the second and third toes. She is slim, blonde, of average height and attractive. Her verbal capacity and understanding are limited and her facial movements are minimally distorted. At times she becomes aggressive and will then throw anything within her reach at anyone present at the time.

Terrie lived in residential care but went home to see her parents on a regular basis. She attended a day centre for people with learning difficulties and the staff became aware and concerned that she was becoming sexually active. Terrie had not considered the possible outcomes of sexual intercourse and was not using any form of contraception. A domiciliary family planning nurse was asked to visit the day centre to discuss the matter with her.

On the first contact Terrie was very withdrawn and non-committal and the nurse used this session to assess her level of understanding and the language she used to refer to her own sexuality. Terrie had a limited understanding but recognized her sexual feelings. On the second visit her boyfriend, who also attended the day centre, was present with her. He had a greater understanding of sexual matters and in his presence Terrie was much more communicative.

They discussed with the nurse their relationship and their hopes and plans for the future. They both stated that they wanted a home and a family but realized they would need support to achieve this. The couple set up home together, and with supervision they managed to cope. Terrie was advised on methods of contraception but it soon became obvious that she was unreliable with any method that involved self-compliance.

Terrie eventually became pregnant and when the baby was born the care that was given was limited. Eventually both parents and their baby moved into residential care where greater supervision was available. The baby, a little girl, appeared to be quite normal and the couple were loving and caring parents. Terrie realized that she could not cope with another child and requested a reliable method of contraception that required minimal compliance on behalf of either partner. After discussion of all the methods Terrie eventually chose to have the contraceptive injection.

Terrie and her partner manage, with considerable help, to bring up one child but have realized that more children would put considerable stress on their relationship. Their understanding of sexual matters, contraception and sexuality has increased dramatically since Terrie was referred to the domiciliary service and the involvement of her partner at the outset was of considerable help to her.

It would appear that the old-fashioned argument concerning people with a mental handicap still often applies, 'if we don't talk about it, we won't put ideas into their heads and they will not show any interest in sex'. This is nonsense as all humans have sexual needs and drives and although these may vary from individual to individual they still exist and need to be acknowledged by health professionals.

No human being is asexual. Sexual education and health education are vitally important but should not take place in isolation and should include discussion about relationships and social interactions. Many of these young people will not have the ability to select the appropriate reading materials for themselves or possess the capacity to absorb and interpret their meanings. Most young people learn a significant amount about their sexuality from peer group discussion but this invariably is not the case with young people with learning disabilities.

Schools that cater for children up to the age of 16 years with learning disabilities are increasingly featuring sex education in the curriculum and many have discussion groups about matters surrounding adolescent sexuality at which parents are encouraged to attend. Anxieties can be shared and parents realize that many of the issues they worry about are common problems which can be discussed together, e.g. 'My son aged 14 regularly gets an erection in class, this upsets some of the other pupils who look at him and want to touch him'.

Another common problem is that of masturbation by females, particularly when this is done in public. It is important to acknowledge and recog-

nize the sexual pleasure that is obtained but young women should be told that this is best done in private. Contraceptive advice should always be accompanied by advice and counselling in sexual behaviour and personal relationships. There is a fear amongst those who are not used to dealing with people with learning disabilities, that by educating these young people in matters of sex and sexuality they may be encouraged to explore further with each other.

Parents in general find it difficult to talk to their children about sexuality and this is even more so with young people with learning disabilities who are often more sheltered as their parents or guardians believe that sexual activity is not an option for them. It is unfortunately the case that the carers have become used to making all the decisions for those in their care. Although this is completely understandable it may leave the individual with the disability less likely to think for his or herself and they may then lack the confidence to make decisions for themselves.

Carers of the disabled should be helped and guided by other health care professionals, e.g. the mental handicap and social workers to provide the maximum support in this delicate area of learning. Those working with clients with learning difficulties need to be sensitive when teaching sexual awareness. It is important to be constantly aware of how vulnerable these groups are to the possibility of exploitation and abuse, both mental and physical, without being able to take any action for themselves.

Scenario

Jane, aged 35 years, with a history of mental illness was visited by a family *planning nurse. She could not read or write and had two children by previous partners. Both children had been taken into care. The nurse noticed on the first visit that Jane was very withdrawn and that her present partner never left her alone. Her partner was a few years older than her and was physically disabled with no use of his left arm.*

After a few visits Jane managed to speak to the nurse on her own. She then told her that her partner beat her and never gave her any money.

She was never allowed out on her own and was kept locked in the flat most of the time. This was reported to the appropriate authority and action was taken. Jane's partner was asked to leave the flat and was bound over by the local Magistrate's Court.

Obviously a great deal will depend upon the severity of the disability. Those with severe problems, who are unable to take any meaningful part in society, will need full-time residential care. Others have a good quality of life living at home and receiving day care. Some are able to work and to take part in the community with limited assistance and supervision but all have their sexual wants and needs and these must be addressed by the carers in society.

Concern also needs to be shown for the families of the disabled; their lives can be taken over completely by the person with the disability.

Scenario

The Brown family had a daughter with a severe learning disability. There were two older teenage boys in the family but virtually all the parents' attention was focused on the daughter. The boys naturally felt excluded and eventually both got into trouble and dropped out of school. The family never had a holiday and the whole week's timetable was organized around the activities of the daughter. They refused respite care and other offers of assistance to the obvious detriment of the other members of the family.

Clients with learning disabilities need care and time to help them live as normal a life as possible. Nurses are frequently in a unique position to assess patients' sexual needs and problems due to their close relationship with patients and their families. Many have been rehabilitated very successfully into the community and manage to cope well with day-to-day life events and have been able to develop close relationships, both sexual and platonic. Marriages between people with a learning disability are increasingly common and these are often stable and successful. Genetic counselling may be appropriate in some instances.

Violence against women

Child abuse

Child abuse can be verbal, emotional, physical or sexual. Verbal and emotional abuse can occur when a parent or parents continually fail to show their child love or affection. They may shout at the child, call it names or even threaten or taunt the child about sending it away or leaving it on its own. This causes the child to lose self-confidence and self-esteem and become nervous and withdrawn. Verbal and emotional abuse, although leaving no physical scars, causes psychological damage and can have far-reaching effects.

Sexual misuse or exploitation of children includes three distinct activities: sexual abuse, child prostitution and child pornography. Child sexual abuse, including incest, has ceased to be a taboo subject and is increasingly discussed by the media. Naturally though it still continues to arouse a sense of moral and legal outrage. The actual incidence of child sexual abuse is very difficult to measure as the vast majority of cases go unreported, making it one of the most under-reported forms of crime. Fear, embarrassment and concern about the response of medical, social and legal agencies lead to this lack of reporting, although the number has increased dramatically during the past decade, possibly due to increased surveillance by the social services and better community awareness programmes.

Child sexual abuse occurs mainly within the family by a relative, but can also occur outside the family by someone known to the child (or family) or by a complete stranger. Both boys and girls are abused, and frequently it is the eldest children who are more often affected. Within a family it is more common for just one of the children to be abused and the others left alone. Young children are most at risk, partly due to the fact that they are more vulnerable and cannot seek help. Coitus is rare with younger children, but exhibitionism, fondling and masturbation are common.

Much of the abuse is by the child's parents and is more common where a cohabitant is involved who is not related to the child but is living in the home. Younger parents are more likely to abuse their children than older parents. Sexual abuse is more commonly perpetrated by men, whilst suffocation and Munchausen's syndrome by proxy abuse are usually perpetrated by women. It is common for both parents to be involved in cases of physical abuse or neglect.

The abusing parents do not generally have an identified mental illness though many have personality traits predisposing to violent behaviour or inappropriate sexual behaviour. Men who have poor self-esteem may have considerable anxieties about their own identity and capacity. Sexual activities with children may seem easier, with less resistance to overcome, and less chance of rejection and repetition of earlier humiliation (Bentovim, 1992). Daughters who are victims of incest often suspect that although their mothers know what is going on they are too embarrassed or horrified to broach the topic with them (Cohen *et al.*, 1987).

Abuse and incest occurs in all ranks of society (Renvoize, 1982) but is more likely to be reported in those families who are socially deprived. Abuse is thought to be 20 times more likely if one of the parents has been abused themselves as a child.

Health professionals should be aware of the variety of ways in which children are abused, whether emotionally, physically or sexually, and be aware of the 'risk factors' that make a particular family more vulnerable to abuse than another (Box 5.2).

Box 5.2 Vulnerable families

◆ Disturbed family background

◆ Chaotic relationships

◆ A succession of stepfathers

◆ Previous incest or sexual deviance in the family

◆ A new male member of the household with a record of sexual abuse

◆ When the perpetrator is under the influence of alcohol

◆ Where there is, or has been, sexual rejection

◆ Paedophile sexual orientation in relation to sex rings and pornography.

Children who have been abused may have a variety of symptoms (Box 5.3). Health professionals are often the first professionals, along with teachers, who have the ability and opportunity to make accurate observations of a child they think

may be abused. These observations and the action taken will determine whether the child will ultimately receive the treatment and protection required or whether the cycle of abuse will continue.

Box 5.3 Symptoms and signs of child abuse

Physical symptoms

◆ Trauma

◆ Infection

◆ Perineal soreness

◆ Vaginal discharge

◆ Anal pain or bleeding.

Emotional effects

◆ Loss of concentration

◆ Enuresis

◆ Encopresis (loss of bowel control)

◆ Anorexia

◆ Truancy

◆ Disturbed behaviour from early childhood

◆ Changes in behaviour, e.g. withdrawn or aggressive, or developing obsessive behavioural patterns, e.g. worry about cleanliness

◆ Severely self-destructive behaviour.

Child sexual abuse is neither a rarity or a fantasy. Children who are abused may not realize that they are being abused and may think the experience is a normal part of family life. It is only when they are older and find themselves in different circumstances that they realize they have been abused. This can cause severe emotional, interpersonal and sexual problems in later life.

Scenario

Ann, a 49-year-old single woman, came to the menopause clinic to discuss her symptoms. The nurse learned that she had not had a cervical smear for some years and discussed with Ann the need for this investigation.

While she was being examined Ann began to cry and on gentle questioning told the nurse about her early life.

Ann had been born abroad where she had lived with her parents and three elder brothers on a farm in a remote part of the country. From the age of 10 she had been regularly sexually abused by her father, her brothers and her uncles. Her mother was also abused regularly by the males in the family. It was only when she left home to obtain work that she realized what she had undergone was not a normal part of growing up.

Ann eventually came to this country and over the years she had a succession of male friends but she always terminated the relationships when they became intimate. She said that although she had a successful career her life was lonely and unhappy. She had always wanted to marry and have children and she had neither.

She went on to explain how angry and bitter she felt about her family and how she had not seen or kept in contact with them since she left home. She said it was the first time in her life that she was able to unburden herself of the secret. Ann was given support and counselling for some considerable time in order to help her come to terms with her childhood abuse.

Abuse of women

As with children there is no typically abused adult. Violence and sexual abuse happens to all types of people whether they are children, young people or adults. They can be male or female, although women are consistently more likely than men to be the targets of physical, sexual and emotional abuse. They can come from any family background, any social class or any culture. They can be highly intelligent or with a learning disability, be able bodied or disabled.

Sexual abuse entails all types of sexual activity, often with escalating intrusiveness. Women may be exposed to indecent acts, pornography, photography or external contact in the form of fondling, touching or masturbation. Penetrative sex can be vaginal, anal or oral.

It is very difficult, if not impossible, to assess how often sexual abuse occurs as studies both in the UK and other countries have shown that the vast majority of cases go unreported and of those that are reported only a small percentage ever get to court. Koss (1985) found in the USA that only 5–8% of women who had been sexually assaulted

actually reported the crime. The reasons for this reluctance to report are numerous and include self-blame, fear of reprisal and lack of confidence that justice will be done. Due to an increased awareness of abuse and more open discussion there are now greater numbers of people seeking help.

The effects of violence and sexual abuse of an individual are far reaching both in the short term and with the longer term sequelae. Violence can have a debilitating affect on a woman's health and all her future relationships whether sexual or not. Violence against women will frequently leave a 'legacy of pain' to future generations.

Research has shown that many separated or divorced women gave abuse by their spouse as one of the main reasons for leaving them (McLeod and Cadieux, 1980; Ellis and Ryan, 1987). For some, separation was seen as the solution to marital problems, including psychological, emotional and physical abuse. However such a solution to the problem of spouse/partner abuse appears to have variable effects. Some women who were beaten before separation from their partners found that if they returned the beating ceased whilst others who had not experienced violence before separation reported that they were beaten on their return.

Female economic dependence is associated with a higher rate of severe violence within the relationship (Kalmuss and Strauss, 1982) and women are more likely to sever the relationship if they were working outside the home.

Abuse and violence against women in their own homes is a social problem and is remarkably similar across international samples. The attitude of the police and their response to domestic and sexual abuse is vital, and a number of police forces throughout the UK now have special sections that deal with such problems where the staff involved are given additional training.

Rape

Rape is committed when a man has sexual intercourse with a woman either knowing that she does not consent or being reckless as to whether she consents or not. Consent must be genuine and not obtained through violence, threats, fraud and coercion. It can also be termed rape if intercourse occurs with a woman who is unconscious or asleep; when the rapist impersonates the woman's partner;

or where the woman is not in a position to consent on the grounds of being mentally deficient, too young or drunk.

The slightest penetration of the penis into the outer labia or vagina is sufficient to be termed rape and there is no requirement for the hymen to be broken (in the case of a virgin) nor for there to be any ejaculation of semen. An indecent assault is an assault or battery accompanied by circumstances of indecency. What 'circumstances of indecency' means has never been clearly defined but seems to refer to any overtly sexual conduct which could include kissing.

Perception in society as to what constitutes rape has varied over the years and is constantly changing even in the present day. There have been recent changes in the law and it is now possible for a man to rape his wife. Sexual assault and rape can affect any woman, irrespective of age, class and background. A high percentage of rape cases show that the rape is committed by a person who is known to the victim, and the most common place for this to happen is the victim's home. She may be attacked by more than one assailant and the sexual assault will frequently involve other acts, forcing the victim to take part in sexual activity and degrading practices against her will. One third of all rapists have a sexual dysfunction.

When rape victims first divulge what has happened to them they need gentle handling and considerable support to help them over their immediate problems. Your own reaction is vital and you should encourage the woman to talk and validate the trauma she is experiencing. Victims of rape and assault need to feel in control and they must not be pushed for details which are not immediately relevant.

Women who have been victims of rape and sexual assault may attend the Accident and Emergency Department, their GP's surgery or family planning clinic with a variety of complaints. This can be either immediately after the assault or it may be some considerable time later (see page 124). They may request emergency contraception, a cervical smear, or a referral to the GUM clinic (Box 5.4). It is useful to observe patients carefully when they attend under such circumstances and watch the way they sit, undress and get on the couch. You should listen carefully to any remarks they make during the examination and note if they become tense or anxious. Some may refer to sexual inter-course as being a dirty activity and others may be obsessive about cleanliness and personal hygiene.

Box 5.4 Acute problems encountered with rape victims

♦ Fear of internal damage

♦ Pregnancy

♦ Sexually transmitted infection.

The woman may require considerable support from you not only in the short term but also in the future. Rape can have long-term effects not only for the woman involved, but also with her partner and their relationship. The victims of rape may suffer any or all of the problems listed in Box 5.5.

Box 5.5 Long-term problems suffered by rape victims

♦ Rape trauma syndrome

♦ Guilt and self-blame ('why me?' and 'was it my fault?')

♦ Sleep disorders

♦ Phobias

♦ Panic attacks

♦ Inability to concentrate and work

♦ Sexual problems

♦ Change in lifestyle.

The services of a victim support team may be required and counselling and psychotherapy may help. With time and good care victims can slowly begin to reorganize their lives.

Most victims of rape feel dirty and their first instinct is to wash themselves and their clothing after the assault. This is something that should be strongly discouraged as important forensic evidence will be destroyed. Victims often need time to consider the implications of reporting rape or sexual assault to the police. If they report the attack, they need not necessarily have to go to court, but the information that they give to the police could be helpful when there have been instances of unsolved rape cases. Many police forces now have a 'rape suite' where the victim may be taken for forensic examination.

Police response to rape and domestic violence

is crucial. The victim needs to feel believed and trusted and does not want to be made to feel any more uncomfortable than she already is. The police response will also encourage other victims to come forward and perhaps help in reducing the incidence of such abuse.

Nursing issues in dealing with abused women

In your nursing practice you should learn to recognize the factors that increase the risk of violence towards women and know the cues that could signal abuse. You could incorporate, and enlarge upon, the following questions during your consultation with a woman who you suspect is being abused:

♦ Do you feel safe in your current relationship?

♦ Do you feel your partner controls your behaviour too much?

♦ Have you ever been sexually or physically abused, recently or as a child?

♦ Can you tell me what happened?

You should then be prepared and able to intervene in a sensitive and empowering way. Careful documentation is essential and the woman should be made aware of the various options for assistance that are available to her, including social service support, women's shelters, rape crisis helplines and support groups (see Resources, page 106). She should also be encouraged to seek the help and support of friends, relatives and neighbours where appropriate, although women are often reluctant to involve others initially.

Your initial reaction is vitally important when a client of any age first tells you that she has been sexually abused. A non-threatening, accepting and understanding attitude will reduce her sense of abnormality and encourage her to talk. Too often nurses do not know what to say in such a situation and might be tempted to 'gloss over' or ignore what they are being told. Referral to a psychologist or counsellor may be necessary as these women can take considerable time to come to terms with their abuse. It is important that your client does not feel that you are deserting her if you do decide to refer her for counselling.

It will have taken her a considerable amount of courage to disclose the information to you and she must not feel that she is being 'passed around'.

Continuing nursing education on violence is essential if you are to become better equipped to provide the intervention and effective help that women need in order to survive. Additionally you could establish contacts and links with local community agencies who support abused women and their families and exchange thoughts and ideas in order to provide greater continuity of care for your patients.

Nurses need to know how to empower women to avoid denial, reduce guilt feelings and acknowledge and recognize their past experiences, and then encourage them to move forward and take control of their own lives in the future.

Cultural and religious aspects of sexuality

What do we mean by culture? Culture can be summarized by saying that it describes patterns of learned human behaviour by which ideas and images can be transferred from one generation to another. This transfer is not through biological means. The same newborn child will grow up with a different set of cultural characteristics if it is reared in different cultural groups.

Today, in the UK, you will meet in your everyday work an increasing number of clients from different ethnic and cultural backgrounds. Each of these different cultures look upon sex and female sexuality in different ways and a variety of cross-cultural views co-exist at any one time. Religious beliefs will also affect these attitudes, especially in the case of Asians where religion is an integral part of their lives. It is more than a doctrine or a set of beliefs and governs their way of life, attitudes and culture.

The aim of this section is to point out some of the many pitfalls that may arise by not concerning yourself with the religious and cultural aspects of the client's ethnic group and imposing, however unintentionally, your own religious and cultural beliefs. It would not be correct to assume that all members of the cultural groups mentioned will believe the same things. Many clients will have been born in this country and because of the interaction between them and other cultural groups their attitudes towards sexual matters will have changed.

Women from other cultures, particularly from the Indian subcontinent and the West Indies, tend to have larger families than those who are born in Britain (Cartwright, 1976). This does not necessarily mean that they are opposed to contraception but the advice they require needs to be culturally sensitive to their beliefs. Immigrant families are generally found in cities and they frequently live in poor, overcrowded conditions. However, because of the support system of their extended family, less use is made of social services.

English will not be the first language for many immigrant women, so communication with them may present a problem. You might think that your client has understood what you have been talking about because she has nodded and said 'Yes', but frequently she may be too embarrassed to admit her difficulty. Pamphlets in different languages should always be available, but if not, then you should give her the English language version and encourage her, as best as you can, to get someone to translate this accurately for her.

Interpreters are a considerable help in such situations and can range from a colleague in your clinical practice, a friend or relative of your client to a complete stranger to you both from an outside interpreting agency. Many interpreters are excellent and translate very accurately what you say, but it can be difficult working through a third party as some interpreters may unintentionally distort the questions you ask, and the information they give back to you from your client, and give you their own personal views.

In some areas where there is a significant number of women from another culture it has been considered worthwhile, in an attempt to overcome the language problems, to make an audio or video tape in different languages containing information about health care and contraception that women can listen to and watch whilst waiting to be seen.

It is not possible to discuss fully the special needs of all cultures and religions, but if you come across significant numbers of women from different groups in your clinical practice you should try to acquire some additional understanding of their needs. Often your patients are your best educators!

Hinduism

Hinduism is one of the oldest religions and is widely practised in India, East Africa and the West Indies. Hindu society is patriarchal and the role of the woman is subservient. Sex education is almost totally lacking and girls are expected to be virgins when they marry. Most marriages are arranged and the dowry and caste systems still exist. Men and women do not meet socially and are generally separated from puberty.

In Hindu culture there is a strict code of sexual morality to protect families and the community. Pre-marital and extramarital sex are strictly forbidden. Great shame follows the discovery of illicit liaisons and this may affect the whole family. Parents remain responsible for their children all their lives and the children are expected to obey and care for their parents when they are old.

Marriage is considered to be not just between two people but between two families. It has to be decided whether a family is suitable and whether the son or daughter will be well treated. For the people arranging the marriage love and romance are the last things on their mind (Kapadia, 1966) and the individual's need for personal happiness is not recognized. It is quite common for families to marry off their sons first and use the dowry obtained to pay for the marriage of their daughters.

It is still frowned upon if a Hindu person does not want to marry, although some will delay marriage if they are, for example, in the middle of their education. The eldest son will usually remain with his parents after marriage and has specific religious duties within the family, especially concerning the ritual cremation of his parents after their death. A wife's first allegiance is to her husband and her in-laws and her own family takes second place. A Hindu father without a son is considered to be unlucky, and giving birth to a son will enhance a woman's status within the community.

Scenario

 Two students, aged 19 years, one Hindu and the other a Sikh came to a family planning clinic. The girl requested a pregnancy test. During the initial counselling they were asked what they intended to do if the outcome

of the test was positive. They said that termination of the pregnancy was their only choice. Although they said they were very much in love there was no way that they could marry each other as they were from differing religions. Were they to marry both would be cut off entirely from their respective families for life.

The pregnancy test proved positive. Both were upset and needed time to come to terms with the result. A further counselling session was arranged and they went away to consider all their options. When they returned to the clinic for their appointment they requested a termination of pregnancy. This was arranged and they were seen for counselling on three further occasions in an effort for them to accept their situation.

During these sessions they talked about their future. Their parents lived in London and the Midlands and they both lived in rented accommodation away from their parental homes. The situation they found themselves in caused them deep distress. They decided that they would not tell their parents what had happened but would use a reliable method of contraception. The methods available were explained to them and they chose to use the combined oral contraceptive pill.

The situation described in the scenario here is not an isolated incident and over the years all health professionals have met couples with similar problems. In our multi-racial society such problems are becoming increasingly common.

Contraception for Hindus

In the UK there is a wide range of attitudes among Hindu women about contraception. These vary from the traditionalists who would never consider any form of birth control to the more liberal women who have been born and educated in this country and realize that the social and economic differences in Western life force them to reconsider their traditional customs.

The choice of contraception may exclude all methods that require insertion, as this is taboo in some Asian cultures. Hindu women believe that only the left hand should be used to touch their genital area and this practice would make the diaphragm difficult to use. Another reason why such means of contraception are not chosen by women of Asian cultures is that they find internal examinations shocking and humiliating and may not wish to use a method that requires one. Hindu women will only have been touched by their husbands and will be reluctant to be examined by a male doctor.

When menstruating, Hindu women cannot attend prayers and cannot carry out certain household duties, particularly preparing food and cooking. As the IUD may cause longer periods this method of contraception may not be chosen. The most popular method of contraception in Hindu communities is still the condom but the Pill is becoming acceptable to the younger woman. Many Hindus are vegetarian and it is worth remembering this when teaching clients how to take the Pill, as absorption may be affected due to a high-fibre diet.

General knowledge of contraception is minimal in immigrant Hindu women as there is little sex education in schools. The subject is very private and many women do not even discuss the matter with their husbands. When discussing contraception and sexual issues with Hindu women you should remember these points and approach the subject with sensitivity.

Hinduism is the most complex religious group to describe because the customs and beliefs vary widely, both regionally and from class to class. Hindus form the smallest group of Asian migrants to Britain and those that settle are mostly from agricultural and trading groups of quite high social status.

Islam

Islam is the religion of Muslims: a world religion that is widespread and not just confined to the Indian subcontinent. Nearly all the Muslims in Britain are from Pakistan or from Bangladesh.

Islam means 'complete submission to God' and Muslims have five codes of behaviour; these are sometimes called the five 'pillars' of Islam:

♦ There is only one God

♦ Prayers five times a day

♦ Giving money to charity

Box 5.6   Hindu naming system (from Oueresh, B., GP Hounslow, London)
Hindus have a first or personal name, a middle or complementary name, and subcaste name, which in Britain is used as a surname.
    The husband's subcaste name is adopted by the wife on marriage and is used by the children.
    Both first and middle or complementary names should be used together, sometimes they are written as one word: for example, Arimadevi.
    In Gujarati families the middle name is usually the father's first name, to distinguish between different families called Patel or Shah, or other common subcaste names.

Example

	First name (personal) (male and female different)	*Middle or complementary name* (male and female different)	*Subcaste name*
Female	Arima	Devi	Patel
Male	Naresh	Lal	Chopra

♦ Fasting from dawn to dusk during the month of Ramadam

♦ Performance of pilgrimage, especially to Mecca.

In Muslim society the roles of men and women are made clear by Islamic Law and the Holy Koran. Men are responsible for all matters outside the home and for supporting the families. Women are responsible for rearing and educating children, looking after the family and running the home. Muslim boys must be circumcised before puberty. This procedure is sometimes done in Britain by a Jewish rabbi. Elsewhere it may be done by the family doctor. Circumcision for boys is legal in the UK but the circumcision of girls is illegal (see page 105).

    Beliefs about women's roles and responsibilities influence Muslim parents' decisions about the education and upbringing of their daughters in Britain. It is almost impossible for a Muslim girl to participate fully in the life of her British peers and yet remain a good Muslim.

    Although there are no statements on contraception in the Holy Koran, many conservative Muslims feel that contraception interferes with God's design. The women are considered responsible for producing children and infertility can have serious implications for a couple, leading to eventual rejection and divorce. Conservative Muslim men may be most reluctant to attend fertility clinics with their wives and will feel humiliated and angry at any suggestion that they might be responsible in some way.

Scenario

Jameela, a Muslim aged 24 years had been married for three years. She regularly came to see the nurse at her GP practice in tears as her husband suffered from an erectile dysfunction. It was an arranged marriage; her husband had been born in Britain and she was born in India. Her command of the English language was limited.

Her extended family constantly wanted to know why she was not pregnant and this naturally placed her in a very difficult situation. She had not used any form of contraception as a baby was expected by both the bride and groom's family within the first year. She had undergone basic fertility investigations and her hormone levels and ovarian function appeared to be within normal limits.

After a number of counselling sessions the nurse remained unable to convince Jameela that her husband should also attend, despite the advice and information on the subject she gave Jameela to give to her husband. He refused to attend and on one occasion asked his wife to collect pills for his problem which of course the nurse was unable to supply.

Jameela told the nurse that he would not admit to any family member that the fertility problem could be his. She felt unable to talk to his family about the problem so they all blamed her for not producing a child. She was desperate and said that if she did not become pregnant soon her husband would divorce her and she would be sent back to India to her parents. This would cause her own family considerable shame and embarrassment as there would be no place for her in Muslim society without a husband and children.

Eventually Jameela managed to persuade her husband to attend the doctor to have his problem investigated. Follow-up psychosexual counselling sessions were arranged for both of them to attend.

In Muslim society marriage is compulsory for both men and women and it is now illegal for a man to have more than one wife. Muslims often marry first cousins so genetic counselling may be necessary. Neither men nor women expose their bodies, and a woman should also cover two-thirds of her head.

A Muslim woman is always under the guardianship of a man; this may be her father, her husband, or her sons if she is a widow. This is considered very important in matters concerning the outside world. Within the family, decision making is shared by both men and women. There is a rigid formal code of behaviour between the sexes.

Contraception for Muslim women

Confidentiality is very important for Muslims and sex is very private and rarely discussed. The woman's attitude towards sex is very reserved as the beauty of a woman is considered to be her sexual naivety. Muslim women are forbidden to fast during Ramadan and are not allowed to visit the mosque when menstruating. Therefore any method of contraception that prolongs menstruation or may cause breakthrough bleeding is unacceptable. The diaphragm may also be unacceptable as Muslim women dislike touching their genitals and may only use their left hand for this. Muslim women often refuse to have a vaginal examination within ten days of their period and prefer intrauterine devices to be fitted when they are not menstruating. Conservative Muslim women do not have intercourse for 40 days after a baby is born.

Sikhs

Most of the Sikhs in Britain come from the Punjab, though there are a few that come to this country from East Africa. Sikhism is a relatively new religion, having developed as a reformist movement of Hinduism in the sixteenth century. The founder, Guru Nanak, was opposed to the various excesses of his time such as idolatry, strife between Hindus and Muslims and the evils of the caste system.

At the end of the seventeenth century the tenth and last Guru, Guru Gobind Singh, wished to strike a final blow to the caste system among his followers. He instituted the Sikh naming system in which the last (subcaste) name was dropped and

---

Box 5.7 Muslim naming system

Muslims from different parts of the world have different naming systems.

In those from the Indian subcontinent or of Asian origin from East Africa there are traditionally no names shared by the whole family; and wives and children do not adopt the husband's name.

Muslim men have two or more names, one being a personal name and the other often with a religious connection, such as Mohammed or Ali.

In Britain, families usually use a clan name such as Chaudry or Khan as the surname.

Example

	Names	Record as:
Husband	Mohammed Habib Rahman	(Mohammed) Habib RAHMAN
Wife	Jameela Khatoon	Jameela Khatoon, wife of Mohammed RAHMAN
Son	Shafiur Mia	Shafiur Mia, son of Mohammed RAHMAN
Daughter	Shameema Bibi	Shameema Bibi, daughter of Mohammed RAHMAN

Box 5.8 Sikh naming system
The Sikh naming system is based on the Hindu system. In rural India the subcaste names have been abandoned, but in Britain they may be readopted and used as a surname.

If the subcaste name is not used, Singh may be used as a surname.

All Sikh men have the complementary (or middle) name of Singh (meaning lion) and all Sikh women the complementary middle name of Kaur (meaning princess).

The Sikh first name is used by family and friends, whereas for polite use, as in the outpatients department or surgery, the first and complementary names are used, followed by the subcaste name if used.

The subcaste name is adopted by the wife on marriage and is used by the children.

Some families simply use Singh as the surname for all male members and Kaur as the surname for all female members of the family.

Example

	First name (personal) (male and female usually same)	Middle or complementary name (religious)	Subcaste name
Female	Jaswinder	(all women) Kaur	Gill
Male	Armarjit	(all men) Singh	Bamra

the first (personal) name was used, with a religious second (or complementary) name: Singh (male) and Kaur (female) (Box 5.8).

Sikhs believe in one God and, unlike Hindus, do not worship different manifestations of God. There are very few practical regulations concerning the everyday or religious activities of Sikhs. Every Sikh makes his own relationship with God and worships in his own way. Sikhism emphasizes the practical rather than the theoretical.

The five signs of Sikhism

Sikhs have five signs by which Sikh men and women could be identified and united. These are known as the five Ks and each has a symbolic meaning. The turban traditionally worn by Sikh men has become an important visible symbol of Sikhism.

♦ Kesh – uncut hair

♦ Kangha – a comb

♦ Kara – a steel bangle

♦ Kirpan – a symbolic dagger

♦ Kaccha – special undershorts.

Sikh women are highly respected and have a great influence in important domestic and community matters. Both men and women take part in all important religious ceremonies. Women are educated equally with the men and have considerable freedom and authority although, as among Hindus and Muslims, there is a system of etiquette which influences the behaviour of the sexes in public.

It is important for a Sikh couple to have a son. In rural societies a large family with several sons ensures family prosperity and survival and is regarded as a blessing. Many Sikhs will therefore decide to continue having children until they have at least one son.

Western culture seems to have influenced Sikhs more than the previous two religious groups discussed, Hindus and Muslims. Women are allowed to work outside the home and the cultural environment. This inevitably leads to many Sikh women exercising greater influence over family affairs such as the decision to regulate family size.

Infertility is again a very important factor and, as with Hindus and Muslims, men will look upon this as the fault of the woman and they will regard any suggestion that they could be the cause as a personal affront. In some families failure to produce sons may be regarded as a reason for rejecting a wife.

Asian family life and differing attitudes among Asian women

Asian society has a community-centred organization. The extended family is still the norm and may consist of unmarried sisters, brothers with their wives and families all living under the same roof.

All social events are centred around the family and relatives and any problem encountered will affect the whole family. Although this close network has become more dispersed with families who have settled in Britain, the psychological factors that bind families together remain very strong.

Parenting is not, as was believed some years ago a natural instinct; it is an acquired skill. One of the virtues of the extended family system as seen in Asian families, lies in the parenting skills which the elder members impart to young parents (Laungani, 1989).

The Asian child has several close attachments apart from its mother and father. Whilst growing up the child acquires several role models amongst whom are its grandparents and other elders, uncles and aunts who all play an important part in the child's upbringing. Research has shown that this, combined with the close family network, produces a low incidence of child abuse.

Asian mothers rely on the experience of their elders, who have had children of their own, to learn parenting skills. All elders within Asian families are accorded special status and are very much concerned with the moral and spiritual development of the child. Children are seen as a gift from God. Asian parents foster in their children values which emphasize obedience to parental wishes and respect of their elders and teachers.

Research undertaken in Leicester and London on the Asian community has reported that Sikh and Hindu women are much more authoritative and outgoing than their Muslim counterparts (Leicester Council, 1986). Muslim women, particularly those in the Bangladeshi community consider making decisions on contraception impossible without the approval of their partners. Muslim women prefer the pill whilst their men had a tendency to use condoms.

Sikh women, however, take more responsibility in choosing methods of contraception without encountering opposition from their husbands. Some Hindu women prefer intrauterine devices while the Sikhs are equally happy with pills, IUDs and condoms. Sterilization is accepted on a small scale by all three religious groups.

Afro-Caribbean

Under slavery, Afro-Caribbean women were encouraged to produce children but were forbidden to marry. The women, their children and the fathers of the children were the property and responsibility of the slave owner. Thus the father's place was never secure as he was not the source of provision and protection for the mother and her children. Marriage among Afro-Caribbeans nowadays is considered to be a very serious matter. A man must be able to support his wife, thus marriage in this community tends to occur later in a couple's life.

In some Afro-Caribbean cultures pre-marital sex is accepted. It is important for the woman to prove her fertility to her partner and illegitimacy does not carry the same stigma as it does in Western society (Henriques, 1956; Hiro, 1971). Sexual activity and sexual pleasure is more acceptable in Afro-Caribbean cultures.

Recent studies have shown that the Afro-Caribbeans have a genetic predisposition to hypertension. This is possibly due to increased salt intake or to hypersensitivity to salt. Therefore African and Afro-Caribbean women may be more susceptible to pill hypertension than other ethnic groups.

The Afro-Caribbean community have 87% slow acetylator status. Acetylator status is the rate at which the body inactivates a drug. A client who is of low acetylator status is likely to retain a drug longer, giving increased beneficial effects but also more prolonged side-effects. If an Afro-Caribbean client complains that she cannot tolerate the Pill, a low acetylator status should be taken into account, and a lower dose pill suggested. Acetylator status applies to all drugs.

The IUD is usually preferred by Afro-Caribbean clients. Most like to have normal periods and do not like menstruation to be suppressed. For those clients who suffer from sickle cell anaemia it has been shown that the injectable 'Depo-Provera' lessens the number of sickle crises. Depo-Provera has a stabilizing effect on the cell membrane in sickle cell disease which is a positive health feature.

Rastafarians

Rastafarians can be found in many parts of the world and are easily recognized by both their colourful dress and their hairstyle. They believe in Ras Tafari as a god who is also regarded as a Black Messiah. They see Ethiopia as their promised land.

Contraception is unacceptable to many Rastafarians and is seen as an attempt of white-dominated society to control black fertility. The rhythm method is the only acceptable method of birth control.

Jews

Jewish religion and culture are inextricably entwined. Judaism is based on the belief in one universal God and the religious precepts followed are simply to worship one God, to carry out the ten commandments and to practise charity and tolerance towards one's fellow human beings.

The family is of great importance in Jewish life. In Britain today there is a wide spectrum of observance among Jews from 'reform' and 'liberal' to the ultra orthodox communities whose daily lives are guided by the code of laws contained in the five books of Moses, the 'Torah'. There are strict Sabbath laws which must be observed from 4 pm on Friday to 4 pm on Saturday. There are also a number of feast days.

Judaism is a male-centred religion. Orthodox Jewish women will dress with modesty but are unlikely to make a special request to see a female doctor. Any form of fertility control is opposed by orthodox Jewish religion because it negates the command to 'be fruitful and multiply'. Jewish belief is that the life-giving potential of semen is sacred and any form of contraception which prevents sperm and ova from meeting, or which destroys or wastes sperm is not allowed. Thus the use of barrier methods, spermicides and coitus interruptus are forbidden by the 'Halacha' (the body of the Jewish law). On the same principal, female sterilization is more acceptable than male, since it does not damage the sperm. According to other Jewish authorities, the use of the diaphragm is more acceptable because the sperm is deposited in the vagina and not wasted.

If pregnancy is considered harmful to the health of the woman then contraception may be used. In this case, the use of barrier methods and the use of oral contraception in the form of the Pill are acceptable. Although the latter prevents the sperm from meeting the ova, it does not interfere with the natural act of intercourse and does not directly destroy the male sperm. The use of the IUD is permitted, with reservations based on the mechanism of action of the IUD. If it prevents fertilization it may be acceptable, but if fertilization can occur and the IUD acts by preventing implantation then it may be considered an abortifacient and thus is unacceptable.

Ambivalence about birth control among Jews stems from a tension between the prescription of the marital duty to procreate and the desire to provide adequate sexual companionship. Responsible parenthood is often seen as a more important issue for Jewish families than which method of contraception to choose. Marriages are usually 'arranged' and marrying anyone outside the Jewish religion is forbidden, as is extra-marital sex (Thompson, 1993).

During menstruation women are considered 'unclean' and are forbidden inside the synagogue. Sexual intercourse is also forbidden at this time. This unclean state continues until seven days after menstruation when the 'Mikvah' (the ritual bath) takes place. In consequence, the IUD, which might cause longer menstruation is not desirable.

Circumcision is performed on baby boys on the first opportunity eight days after birth. This is a Bible-based practice and is seen as a covenant with the Torah and God. Circumcision is very widely practised and causes much soul searching for out-married couples, i.e. Jew and non-Jew, as it is seen as a continuity of covenant with being Jewish.

In very orthodox circles the sexes are segregated from an early age, around 7 or 8 years, especially in educational establishments. In the home this is not so pronounced but at any social event outside the home, segregation would take place. For orthodox Jews the dietary laws are strict, and only 'kosher' food is acceptable. Milk and meat are not eaten at the same meal. Meat must be killed according to kosher ritual and is acceptable only from animals which chew the cud and have a cloven hoof, or from poultry. Pig and rabbit meat are forbidden.

Abortion is generally forbidden, but would be allowed in circumstances where the mother's health is at risk or where congenital diseases are detected in the early stage of pregnancy. Ashkenazy Jews are the main ethnic group at risk from Tay–Sachs disease. One in 25 people in this group is a Tay–Sachs disease carrier as opposed to 1 in 250 of the non-Jewish population. Tay–Sachs disease is an incurable neurodegenerative disorder caused by the deficiency of an enzyme called hexosaminidase A (Hex A), which results in the accumulation of a harmful substance in the brain. It causes early death due to progressive mental retardation and motor weakness. As there is no cure for Tay–Sachs disease, treatment focuses on the management of the various complications and on ensuring that the child is as comfortable as possible. Death usually occurs by the age of 4 years.

Chinese

In recent years, in common with many Western countries, Britain has seen a significant increase in the number of Chinese and Vietnamese people who choose to live away from their own native country. Many of them are refugees and will have left behind members of their family and consequently feel isolated and alone. They tend to gather together in this country in small areas in an urban environment.

Almost all Chinese are Buddhists. Buddhism arose in the sixth century BC in the area of the Himalayan Kingdom of Nepal. It took its name from the title 'Buddha' (the Enlightened) given to its founder. Buddhists believe in reincarnation, and so accept responsibility for the ways in which they exercise their freedom in life, since the consequences of their actions may be seen in subsequent lives. It is therefore important that the individual behaves properly. Because there is no 'God' there is no actual worship, but the act of 'Puja' (to respect) is the Buddhist way of acknowledgement of an ideal. There are about 20 000 Buddhists in Britain. Most are native converts.

Infanticide and abortion have been practised in China for thousands of years. The dowry system is still practised and up until the recent interventions in birth control unwanted female children were disposed of. At present in China no marriage is allowed before the age of 24. The laws relating to childbirth and the number of children allowed to a married couple are changing regularly. Currently a couple are only permitted one child and are given State payments and grants if they manage this. A second pregnancy frequently ends in an abortion and grants being withdrawn.

The most common method of contraception used is the IUD. In China the devices are fitted without threads so they are not easily removed.

However, women will occasionally have the device removed and will then pretend that it fell out unnoticed. If they have been seen to be using contraception and become pregnant due to a 'method failure' they are sometimes allowed to keep the second child. Male sterilization is one of the main forms of contraception and China has the highest number of vasectomies in the world.

Scenario

Suzy, a Chinese woman aged 31 years, was living *in Britain whilst studying for a PhD and came to a family planning clinic for advice. Her husband and daughter were still living in China and she had recently visited them. The method of contraception they used was the condom. She now found that she was pregnant and visited the clinic to arrange for a termination.*

During the counselling session she went on to explain that only one child was allowed to each couple in China. There was a possibility that she would have continued with the pregnancy if she could settle in this country but as her husband had a senior position in the Chinese government, his career and hers would suffer as a consequence.

The termination was arranged and at a further counselling session she wanted to know the sex of the fetus. The counsellor was unable to give her this information. Suzy told the counsellor that the sex would not have influenced her decision regarding a termination but that both she and her husband would have liked a son.

She was advised on the methods of contraception available to her in this country and she chose the IUD. She was very much against using any hormonal method as she thought it was 'not natural'.

Vietnamese

In Vietnamese culture large families are traditionally a great source of pride. The size of the family is not in any way related to social status. Vietnamese women reject any argument that it is better to have small families. The appeal of family planning for them is that it enables them to space their children rather than limit their numbers.

Family planning is available in Vietnam on a limited scale and family planning campaigns are carried out by the State. Trained health workers visit towns and villages to give information and advice about contraception. Where available, the most commonly used methods are the Pill, the coil and the condom. Contraception is not freely discussed between the sexes in Vietnam. When family planning talks are arranged the audience will be either all male or all female. In your clinical practice, to avoid embarrassment it may be easier to discuss matters concerning contraception separately with the husband and wife.

If it is necessary to use an interpreter they should be of the same sex as the person you wish to speak to. Vietnamese are often vague about their reproductive anatomy and embarrassed to discuss it. The coil and the Pill are acceptable to some women, although the latter needs careful and adequate explanation as to how it should be used. The diaphragm is not generally available in Vietnam and some women in Britain are initially embarrassed at the idea of inserting and removing it. Their reluctance, coupled with the language barrier, sometimes discourages the doctor or nurse suggesting it as a possible alternative.

In recent years all forms of religious practice have been discouraged by the Vietnamese State. Because of this, some Vietnamese people feel threatened by questions about their religious beliefs and give the response they feel the most diplomatic in the circumstances. Although Vietnam has no official religion, Buddhism, Taoism and Confucianism are the three philosophical traditions that have played a significant part in the development of Vietnamese culture. Roman Catholicism was introduced by the French to Vietnam and although the Catholic population of Vietnam is small, a significant number of Vietnamese in Britain are practising Catholics.

Catholics

The Catholic Church sees itself as the one, true, universal and apostolic Church of Christ. It teaches that there are two specific ways of fulfilling the vocation of love:

1 through marriage characterized by permanence, fidelity and openness to life, or

2 through virginity or celibacy.

Any alternative is viewed as an abuse of human sexuality whether intentional or through immaturity or ignorance.

Many Catholics are faced with tension as they feel caught between the conservative position of the central Church and the current Pope on population issues and the various moves to reform and modernize Catholic doctrine. Recent trends have been in the direction of encouraging responsible parental decision in procreation.

Controversy and discontent with the Church's teaching is now a reality and debate surrounding the above issues will not go away. With today's more liberal outlook attitudes towards pre-marital sex and divorce are being challenged on all sides and restrictions regarding contraception are widely disregarded. All the Catholic Church's teaching on contraception refers to contraception *within* marriage so the question of contraception outside marriage does not arise.

Catholicism, however, is not opposed to family planning in its literal sense but demands self-control or abstinence to achieve this. The rhythm method or safe period is the only method of contraception that is acceptable. Catholic couples can be referred to a suitable agency to learn more about this method (see page 208).

Catholic couples tend to have larger families than other couples as abortion and sterilization are opposed. According to both American and British fertility studies (Woolf, 1972; Cartwright, 1976) in reality all methods of birth control are used and abortion itself is resorted to when a woman feels she cannot face another pregnancy. Some Catholic women, when they feel they have had the number of children they can cope with, will request sterilization.

Catholics in Eire, who wish to practice a method of contraception not accepted by the Church, will travel miles outside their local area to seek family planning advice. Many of their family doctors are now beginning to prescribe the Pill for 'menstrual irregularities' rather than as a method of contraception. Despite the prohibitions on pre-marital sex, pregnancy before marriage frequently occurs. About 4000 Irish women travel to Britain each year to have abortions, and others to have their baby so that their families will not discover the pregnancy.

Some priests are now leaving the decision on

the use of birth control methods other than those advocated by the Catholic Church to the conscience of the woman or couple concerned.

Nursing issues affecting culture and religion

The above is not a definitive list of cultures and religions. It does, however, include the main cultures and religious groups to which a significant number of your clients will belong. Not all the individuals coming from these cultures will still conform and many, particularly if they have been born and brought up in Britain, will be far more Westernized than others. Practices relating to sex, marriage and the family frequently cause conflict between generations with those (usually the old) who wish to preserve traditions and those (usually the young) who wish to adapt and change. The more diverse the population becomes the more attitudes and practices will change.

In your clinical practice you should be aware that culture and religion can have a powerful influence on the way a woman feels about her sexuality and you should try to assess these at your initial consultations. It is also important for you to be aware of your own religious and cultural beliefs about sexuality and not let these influence you in your care of your client if they are in opposition. You should be able to demonstrate an accepting, non-judgemental attitude towards all your clients regardless of their ethnic background in order to provide the professional nursing care they need.

Female genital mutilation

Female genital mutilation is widely practised and an acceptable norm in many African ethnic groups and in some parts of the Middle East and South-East Asia. Some practise it with a belief that it is a religious requirement for Muslims. However, the Holy Koran does not include a single mention of circumcision of girls although it refers to many issues pertaining to women such as pregnancy, childbirth, breastfeeding, divorce and menstruation. Female genital mutilation is practised by Christians, Muslims and non-believers alike.

The incidence of female genital mutilation or 'female circumcision' was fairly rare in Britain until the 1970s when an increasing number of immigrants and refugees began to arrive from parts of the world where it is practised. There can be no doubt that female genital mutilation is an extreme form of physical assault on a defenceless child, which has a life-long effect on the victim. Such mutilation of a child's genitalia, for no good medical reason, is a violation of the child's human rights and is, in effect, 'child abuse'.

In Britain it is estimated that 10 000 female children are at risk (Hedley and Dorkenoo, 1992). In 1985 the British government passed a Bill which made 'female circumcision' illegal in Britain. Consequently some immigrant families take their daughters out of the UK to their home country for a 'holiday' to have this procedure carried out. A girl who is not circumcised can have difficulty finding a husband.

The simplest form of genital mutilation is called *circumcision* and involves cutting off the hood of the clitoris. *Excision* is the amputation of the clitoris with or without removal of the labia minora. *Infibulation* involves the removal of the clitoris, the labia minora and much of the labia majora. The sides of the vulva are then sewn together, leaving only a tiny opening at the perineum for the passage of urine and menstrual blood.

The 'operation' is usually carried out under poor aseptic conditions that are likely to be unhygienic, and the infection rate is high. Ninety-five per cent of female genital mutilation is performed on girls between 1 day old and 16 years, i.e. before they become too vocal and able to understand the long-term implications. The more wealthy parents tend to use trained surgeons.

A woman who has undergone female genital mutilation as a child may not present until she is pregnant (childbirth and female genital mutilation is discussed on page 125). Others may present earlier with problems of non-consummation, infertility, dysmenorrhoea, recurrent urinary tract and vaginal infections and psychosexual problems. The initial consultation provides an ideal opportunity for giving information and for sensitive counselling. Sometimes a de-infibulation procedure may be decided upon after such counselling and support.

All health visitors, family planning nurses, midwives and school nurses need to be aware of this practice as they will occasionally come across women and children from other cultures who have undergone female genital mutilation. Those who come into contact with families who have cultural or racial links with countries where this practice is endemic should use their skills to advise parents of the health risks involved. Such clients require an approach that is culturally sensitive and non-judgemental.

Conclusion

This chapter has highlighted some of the situations where health professionals might find they need extra resources to enable them to help women in different circumstances. The domiciliary family planning service, where it is available, can successfully cope with many of these requirements. People with learning disabilities are encouraged to become more independent and are being cared for in the community – they need the skills of caring professionals to help them cope with their sexuality.

Women within violent relationships need sensitivity in helping them come to terms with what has happened to them and recover. Over the past few decades the UK has become a more homogeneous mix, with people from many ethnic backgrounds, cultures and religions living together in relatively small communities.

Women with special needs are more vulnerable; not only do they need special care for their own individual situations but they may also have problems with many of the issues that are discussed elsewhere in this book, e.g. unplanned pregnancy, subfertility, psychosexual problems and premenstrual syndrome to name but a few. Many changes are taking place within the health service and it is important that women with special needs should receive the more individual care that they require.

Resources

Buddhist Hospice Trust
PO Box 51, Herne Bay, Kent CT6 6T
Tel. 01580 891650

Catholic Marriage Advisory Council
Natural Family Planning Service, Clitherow House, 1 Blythe House, Blythe Road, London W14 0NW
Tel. 0171 371 1341

Childline
Freepost 1111, London N1 0BR
Tel. 0800 1111 (freephone)
Telephone counselling service for young people who have been sexually abused.

Equal Opportunities Commission
Overseas House, Quay Street, Manchester 3
Tel. 0161 833 9244

Hindu Centre (London)
39 Grafton Terrace, London NW5
Tel. 0171 485 8200

Islamic Cultural Centre
London Central Mosque, 146 Park Road, London NW8
Tel. 0171 724 3362

National Children's Bureau
8 Wakley Street, London EC1V 7QE
Tel. 0171 843 6000
Publications and reports on sex education and HIV and AIDS in children.

National Spiritual Assembly of the Baha'is of the United Kingdom
Oceanair House, 6th Floor, 133–137 Whitechapel High Street, London E1
Tel. 0171 377 7539

Rape Crisis Centre
PO Box 69, London WC1X 9NJ
Tel. 0171 837 1600
Belfast: 01232 249696
Cardiff: 01222 373181
Edinburgh: 0131 556 9437
Leeds: 01132 440058
Counselling advice for women of any age who have been raped.

Relate (formerly Marriage Guidance Council)
Herbert Gray College, Little Church Street, Rugby CV21 3AP
Tel. 01788 573241
Look in the phone book for the nearest branch under Relate or marriage guidance.

Samaritans
46 Marshall Street, London W1V 1LR
Tel. 0171 734 2800
Check in the telephone directory for local branches.

Sikh Missionary Society
10 Featherstone Road, Southall, Middlesex UB2 5AA
Tel. 0181 574 1902

SPOD – The Association to Aid the Sexual and Personal Relationships of the Disabled
286 Camden Road, London N7 0BJ
Tel. 0171 607 8851

Survivors
PO Box 2470, London W2 1NW
Tel. 0171 833 3737
For male clients only who have been raped or assaulted.

Tamil Refugee Group
c/o 335 Grays Inn Road, King Cross, London W1
Tel. 0171 833 2020

Vietnamese Refugee Group
Alfreda Day Centre, Alfreda Road, Battersea, London SW11
Tel. 0171 498 9910

Visitation Committee
c/o Office of the United Synagogue, Woburn House, Upper Woburn Place, London WC1
Tel. 0171 387 4300

Women's Aid
Tel. 0272 420611 (National); 0171 251 6537 (London)
Provides support and temporary refuge for women in violent relationships – mental, physical or sexual abuse.

Women's Health
52 Featherstone Street, London EC1Y 8RT
Tel. 0171 251 6580
Can provide leaflets about women's health, disabilities and black women's health issues.

Further reading

Family planning

ALLEN, I. (1991) *Family Planning and Pregnancy Counselling Projects for Young People*. London: P.S.I. Publications.
CHRISTOPHER, E. (1987) *Sexuality and Birth Control in Community Work*. pp. 234–254. London: Tavistock.

RCN (Royal College of Nursing) (1991a) *Standards of Care in Family Planning Nursing*. Harrow: Scutari.
RCN (1991b) *Family Planning Manual for Nurses*. Harrow: Scutari.
RCN (1993) *Domiciliary Family Planning Special Needs*. London: RCN.
WHINCUP, M.H. (1982) *Legal aspects of Medical and Nursing Service*. Beckingham: Ravenswood Press.

Learning disabilities

CRAFT, A. and CRAFT, M. *Sex and the Mentally Handicapped: A Guide for Parents and Carers*. London: Routledge & Kegan Paul.
FRAZER, J. (1991) *Contraception: Birth Control, Family Planning, 'Learning to love'*. A set of simple booklets on sexuality for young people with learning difficulties who have minimal reading skills. London: Brook Advisory Service.
GUNN, M.J. (1991) *Sex and the Law: a Brief Guide for Staff Working with People with Learning Difficulties*, 3rd edn. London: Family Planning Association.
SIMS, A. and OWENS, D. (1993) *Psychiatry*, 6th edn. London: Baillière Tindall.
THOMPSON, T. and MATTHIAS, P. (1992) *Standards and Mental Handicap: Keys to Competence*. London: Baillière Tindall.

Sexual abuse

BASS, E. and DAVIS, L. (1990) *The Courage to Heal: a Guide for Women Survivors of Child Sex Abuse*. London: Mandarin.
DORKENOO, E. (1992) *Female Genital Mutilation: Proposals for Change*. London: Minority Rights Group.
FINKELHOR, D. (1984) *Child Sex Abuse*. New York: Macmillan.
LIGHTFOOT-KLEIN, H. (1991) *Prisoners of Ritual: An Odyssey into Female Genital Circumcision in Africa*. London: The Howarth Press.
LIVITNOFF, S. (1992) *The RELATE guide to Sex and Loving relationships*. London: Vermillion.
VIANO, E.C. (1992) *Intimate Violence: Interdisciplinary Perspectives*. Washington, DC: Hemisphere.

WYRE, R. and SWIFT, A. (1990) *Women, Men and Rape*. London: Hodder & Stoughton.

Cultural aspects

AHMED, L. (1992) *Women and Gender in Islam*. New Haven: Yale University Press.

HENLEY, A. (1979) *Asian Patients in Hospital and at Home*. Bath: Pitman Press.

OWEN COLE, W. (1991) *Moral Issues in Six Religions*. London: Heinemann.

RCN (Royal College of Nursing) (1994) *Female Genital Mutilation: The Unspoken Issue*. London: RCN.

THOMPSON, R. (1993) *Religion, Ethnicity and Sex Education: Exploring the Issues*. London: National Children's Bureau.

References

BENTOVIM, A. (1992) *Trauma. Organised Systems – Sexual and Physical Abuse within Families*. London: Karmac.

CARTWRIGHT, A. (1976) *How many Children?* London: Routledge & Kegan Paul.

CHRISTOPHER, E. (1980) Domiciliary family planning – a service described and assessed. *British Journal of Family Planning* 6.

COHEN, T.B., GALENSON, E., VAN LEEUWEN, K. *et al.* (1987) Sexual abuse in vulnerable and high risk children. *Child Abuse and Neglect* **11**: 461–74.

CRAFT, A. (1990) *Sex Education for Individuals with a Mental Handicap*. London: Novum.

CRAFT, A. and CRAFT, M. (1985) *Sex and the Mentally Handicapped: A Guide for Parents and Carers*. London: Routledge & Kegan Paul.

DOH (Department of Health) (1992) *The Health of the Nation*. London: HMSO.

ELLIS, D. and RYAN, J. (1987) Lawyers and Post Separation Women Abuse: The Relevance of Social Support. A report submitted to the Department of Justice: Ottawa, Canada and the Laidlaw Foundation.

ELLIS, D. and WRIGHT, L. (1987) Separation and women abuse: the impact of lawyering style. *Victimology (Ottawa)* **12**: 27–36.

HEDLEY, R. and DORKENOO, E. (1992) Child Protection and Female Genital Mutilation: advice for health, education and social work professionals. London: Forward 38 King St WC2 8JT.

HENRIQUES, L.F. (1956) *Family and Colour in Jamaica*. London: MacGibbon & Kee.

HIRO, D. (1971) *Black British, White British*. Harmondsworth: Penguin.

KALMUSS, D. and STRAUSS, M.A. (1982) Wife's marital dependency and wife abuse. *Journal of Marriage and the Family* **44**: 277–86.

KAPADIA, K.M. (1966) *Marriage and Family Life in India*. Bombay: Oxford University Press.

KOSS, M.P. (1985) The hidden rape victim: personality, attitudinal and situational characteristics. *Psychology of Women Quarterly* **9**: 193–212.

LAUNGANI, P. (1989) Asian perspectives in child abuse: a proposed paradigm shift. London: New Quest, 76.

LEATHARD, A. (1985) *District Health Authorities Family Planning Services in England and Wales*. London: FPA.

LEICESTER COUNCIL (1986) *Religious Background of Asians in Leicester*, city survey.

McGUIRE, A. and HUGHES, D. (1995) *The Economics of Family Planning Services*. London: FPA.

McLEOD, L. and CADIEUX, A. (1980) *Wife Battering in Canada: The Vicious Circle*. Ottawa.

RENVOIZE, J. (1982) *Incest: a Family Pattern*. London: Routledge & Kegan Paul.

SIMS, A. and OWENS, D. (1993) *Psychiatry*, 6th edn. London: Baillière Tindall.

THOMPSON, R. (1993) *Religion, Ethnicity and Sex Education: Exploring the Issues*. London: National Children's Bureau.

WOOLF, M. (1972) *Families Five Years On*. London: HMSO.

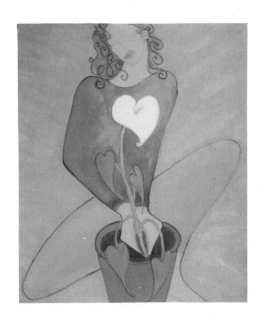

FAMILY PLANNING

6: Sexuality during and after pregnancy

Gillian Aston ◆

OBJECTIVES

After reading this chapter you will understand:

◆ how sexuality, sexual relations and sexual activity during the childbearing continuum are influenced by biological, psychological and social variables

◆ how changes in body image, especially during pregnancy, may affect sexuality

◆ that health professionals need to be aware of and address their own attitudes towards sexuality during the childbearing continuum

◆ the importance of exploring with women and their partners that there is no normal pattern of sexual behaviour during pregnancy and following childbirth

◆ that care planning should focus on the needs of the individual woman and couple.

Introduction

Childbearing is intricately bound up with a woman's sexuality and sexual health. However, the activities of sex and reproduction are surrounded by a whole series of complicated emotions and meanings. Throughout life, the way individuals respond to and feel about their sexuality changes as their lives undergo transition. The changes associated with pregnancy, childbirth and the transition to motherhood have a special significance, representing one of the most fundamental periods of change that a woman will experience. As McNeill (1994) says, 'a woman's sexual expression and sexual health is intimately linked to her self-image, her well-being, her personal circumstances and the social context in which she develops and lives'.

The relative contributions of the feelings and experiences noted above 'have not been adequately studied and thus cannot be quantified'. Nevertheless, it can be seen that central to sexual health and the childbearing continuum are individual experiences, personal histories and all the bits and pieces of our unique existences (Carter, 1979).

Biological and psychological factors influence sexuality throughout all stages of life. During pregnancy and following childbirth these factors are completely interwoven. The physical changes that occur during pregnancy and childbirth and the experiences involved while caring for a baby can, according to Alder (1994), have a considerable effect on both sexual behaviour and sexual feelings. Psychological changes in role, identity and self image also affect sexuality. These interact so that the experience of being pregnant, giving birth and breast-feeding may also depend on feelings about sexuality.

Literature for health professionals on sexuality following childbirth and during early motherhood is scarce. Fortunately more literature is available on sexuality during pregnancy but the majority, including articles from the popular media, tend to focus on and portray bleak and depressing pictures of sexual relationships. Oakley (1979) makes a similar point: 'I have tried to show the positive side, but of course it is to some extent true that the best news is bad news: happiness doesn't hit the headlines because it is boring'.

Some may feel that this chapter also perpetuates a negative image of sexuality during the childbearing continuum. However it is important for the reader to gain an understanding of the complexities involved, the need for integrated approaches as well as the need for more work on sexual health during pregnancy, labour and following childbirth.

Pregnancy: a time of transition

Pregnancy is a normal life event which involves considerable adjustment by the parents. Oakley (1979) has criticized much of the research that has focused on adjustment or 'adaptation' to pregnancy and argues that it reduces pregnancy to a symbol of conforming to cultural definitions of femininity. She suggests that it is not natural that all women should like and enjoy being mothers with all the constraints that motherhood puts on 'normal' life. Nevertheless, the transition to parenthood can be seen as a developmental crisis or a critical event in adult life (Clulow, 1982) with different degrees of stress involved. Apart from affecting the pregnant woman, the stress also affects her partner and their relationship.

A first pregnancy produces the greatest change. As Taylor (1992) pointed out, pregnancy represents the end of freedom and a dramatic change in lifestyle. It also has a dramatic effect on a couple's sense of identity, communication patterns and role behaviour. During pregnancy, concerns about finance are naturally a common problem. If the woman has been in employment she has to make decisions about whether to continue after the baby is born. There may be legitimate concern about whether the couple can afford to lose one income. Feelings of guilt can be evoked in the pregnant woman as she attempts to resolve the competing demands of career and family and listens to the conflicting advice from friends and relatives. Although a neglected area of research, evidence indicates that relationships with female friends may change during pregnancy or significantly influence the experience for the pregnant woman (Leifer, 1980).

The relationship between the pregnant woman and her partner encompasses a complex web of tangled emotions. The results of a study conducted by Taylor (1992) suggest that fears about the relationship are probably quite common experiences. Taylor reports that: 'In some cases, men feel that their relationship with their partner assumes a secondary position compared with their partner's relationship with their unborn child'.

This finding has been corroborated by other studies. Shapiro (cited in Taylor, 1992) also suggests that fear of losing this relationship plays a significant role in the tendency for some men to have an affair during their partner's late pregnancy. Feelings of rejection were cited as the main motivational factor for affairs at this stage. The ability of men to confront such fears is clearly important for both partners and for their relationship during pregnancy.

The transition and adjustments that are made during the first pregnancy are affected by the ability of both parties to come to terms with changes in their role and status. As Clulow (1982) puts it: 'the transition from wife to mother, or husband to father, is an integral part of the transition from two to three'.

Stress in pregnancy

A degree of personal stress is a common feature of most pregnancies. Anxiety, often accompanied by a revival of past conflict, depression, worries, mood lability, impaired concentration, a reawakening of early childhood relationships and experiences of mothering, as well increased dependency and altered spatial orientation have all been identified in studies of normal antenatal clinic populations (Raphael-Leff, 1991). There are a number of other factors, often unrelated to the pregnancy itself, which can affect the woman's ability to adjust and come to terms with her pregnancy. They impose added burdens and add to the stress and anxieties of pregnancy, which in turn may affect sexuality and sexual health.

Women who have to cope with moving house, changing or losing their jobs when they are expecting a baby may find it difficult to cope with the demands of pregnancy. Whilst these events would cause some anxiety and confusion in the lives of everybody, as Raphael-Leff (1991) says, 'When these life events occur alongside the emotional upheaval of pregnancy, they increase the sense of disorientation and interrupt the psychological work of pregnancy by presenting intrusive or, at times, conflicting demands for readjustment'.

Unexpected and painful distressing events can also impinge on a woman's coping ability. Bereavement in the family, eviction or dismissal as well as events associated with the pregnancy such as threatened miscarriage, negative results of a fetal diagnostic test or death of a twin *in utero*, are associated with an intrusion into the natural emotional adjustments and processes of pregnancy. Raphael-Leff (1991) suggests that these events can invoke feelings of anxiety, grief, rejection, emptiness and loss just at a time when the woman is physically and psychologically geared to receptivity, hopefulness and fulfilment. Women who find themselves alone following death, divorce, separation or abandonment by their partners are especially vulnerable. In addition to the pregnancy they are coping with an extremely distressing emotionally charged and often unforeseen life event. Women who have not chosen to become single mothers are likely to have their distress compounded by feelings of lack of control over their future destiny and dissolution of their partnership at the very time when it was about to expand into a family (Raphael-Leff, 1991).

An increasing number of women turn to complementary therapies to help them cope with stress during pregnancy and childbirth. Such therapies include massage, aromatherapy, reflexology, acupuncture, hydrotherapy and osteopathy. Counselling and advice on the many ways to reduce stress will be appreciated by both the woman and her partner and are comprehensively covered by Tiran and Mack in their book *Complementary Therapies for Pregnancy and Childbirth* (1995).

Support during pregnancy

Studies have emphasized the need for pregnant women to feel supported at home, at work and in their relationships. It has been suggested that if a woman perceives she has emotional support this then buffers the effects of life changes (Jones and Jones, 1991). Pines (1993) suggests that during pregnancy interpersonal conflicts can be exacerbated by the emotional changes that occur as a result of pregnancy. These include mood swings, introversion, extreme sensitivity and tiredness as well as changes in sexual patterns.

The father of the child is also likely to undergo emotional changes which can also affect the mother. Taylor (1992) is critical of the dearth of literature concerning men's feelings and experiences in areas related to pregnancy and states that: 'Many men are completely unprepared, both emotionally and intellectually, for the birth of their child(ren). Men have feelings and experiences in relation to issues which are often dismissed as women's matters'.

The question here then is what kind of support is he able to offer? 'The fact that a woman does have a partner, need not imply that she is supported. A husband may be present in the flesh but emotionally absent' (Raphael-Leff, 1991). Oakley (1979) demonstrated the profound emotional shock posed by the transition into first-time motherhood. The women in this study said it was good to take part in the research as they thought the process of interviewing was a socially supportive experience. Women welcomed the opportunity to talk about the things that concerned or delighted them. They also found it was a positive relief to unburden themselves of critical feelings and experiences.

It is important for health care professionals to attempt to identify women with inadequate emotional support as well as to help all pregnant women make the most of the resources available. The demands of single parenthood without adequate emotional, practical and financial support will increasingly need to be borne in mind. As Oakley (1992) points out:

> The norm that behind every pregnant woman there is a supportive husband working and ready to supply emotional companionship, domestic help and financial resources, will increasingly be a piece of cultural mythology. The old label

'marital status' is becoming a poor guide to women's living circumstances. Whether a woman is legally married or not does not inform her health care providers, either about her household arrangements, or as to the social, financial and emotional support available to her.

As we discuss later, it is also important for health care professionals not to assume that a woman is heterosexual and to expect that her main source of support during and after pregnancy will be a man. Increasing numbers of lesbian couples are choosing to become parents.

Domestic violence and pregnancy

Domestic violence has been defined as violence, physical or psychological, perpetuated by a man against a woman with whom he has or has had a sexual relationship (Bewley and Gibbs, 1994). Violence and abuse, which may be sexual, can begin within a relationship at any time. However, studies indicate that it may begin or worsen during pregnancy and that attacks on the breasts, abdomen and genitals are common during pregnancy (Bohn, 1990). On average a woman will have been attacked 35 times before she reports domestic violence and that may frequently amount to many years of torture (Byrne, 1994).

As well as the physical injuries inflicted upon women by violent men, the psychological effects of domestic violence have been shown to be profound. Anxiety, depression, shame, guilt and a low self-esteem are just some of these effects. Not surprisingly, women who are the victims of violent men 'May be quite frightened during sexual intercourse and will not be in a position to refuse unwanted activities nor will they be able to express their own needs' (Walton, 1994). Awareness of domestic violence and pregnancy has now been raised and midwives and health professionals must be alert to the problem, take heed and address the issues involved. If domestic violence is suspected then women need to be advised on the organizations and services available for practical and emotional support.

Other children

Children can bring women much happiness and joy but childrearing can also be very stressful and tiring. This can add to the complex emotional and physical adjustments a woman makes during and after pregnancy. Little or no support, shortage of money and a lack of childcare facilities to give the mother a break can result in an emotional crisis. The mother of the 1990s is more likely than her own mother to have other relatives to care for, as well as her own children. She is also much more likely to have paid employment of her own. Negotiating and resourcing childcare arrangements can be another stress and burden experienced by women during pregnancy. A mother nowadays is frequently trying to juggle the multiple roles of being a carer for elderly relatives, a loving wife or partner, a multiple orgasmic lover, a successful career woman, as well as being a devoted mother. Tiredness and looking after other children, as well as the home, may lessen sexual libido and make sexual intercourse, understandably, a low priority.

Pregnancy and sexuality

Myths and misconceptions

The relationship between sexuality and pregnancy, childbirth and the puerperium (the first six weeks after the birth) is historically replete with cultural stereotypes, false universals, myths and various 'taboos'. What is intriguing is the deep imprint these powerful and pervasive beliefs have on attitudes about sexuality during pregnancy. Kitzinger (1985) points out that pregnant women frequently fear that sexual intercourse may provoke miscarriage or premature labour or in some way damage the fetus, and as a result feel that they should abstain from sexual intercourse. She goes on to report that some men have expressed fear of breaking the 'bag of water' during sexual intercourse, whilst others believe that they could damage the baby or precipitate labour:

> It is almost as if they feel that to keep themselves under restraint will help make the pregnancy go well; as if their self control will somehow 'guard' the pregnancy. These beliefs are remarkably similar to those held in Third World societies, where taboos are enjoined on a father in order to ensure the well-being of a baby whilst it is still in the uterus.
>
> (Kitzinger, 1985)

Is pregnancy sexy? The question is an important one because within its answer lies the whole range of society's attitudes towards pregnancy, sexuality and towards women. Reamy and White (1987) stated that pregnant women are not seen as sexually attractive and societal norms stress that sexual desires, responses and activities should not occur during pregnancy. This observation is interesting as it suggests that it is not nature that makes sex and pregnancy a taboo combination, but cultural and society's attitudes towards pregnancy. Such an observation does however, need to be counterbalanced as Wallace (1989) remarks that:

> There seems to be a vast difference between what pregnant women might actually feel and what society thinks they should feel. There is an overriding ethos in our culture that pregnancy may make women feel fat, unattractive, sick, tired, fragile, neurotic or 'blooming', but the one thing that seems scarcely imaginable is that it might make us feel sexy.

Other explanations to account for the contradictory and confusing aspects of pregnancy and sexuality have been offered. Contratto (1980) argues that one of the most pervasive beliefs that still exists in Western culture, (although little information exists on who holds the belief) is that 'good mothers are generally asexual'. She suggests that many women have successfully internalized the identity of asexual motherhood. This quote from a mother of two small infants is used by Contratto to make the point: 'You're writing a paper on maternal sexuality? What in God's name is that?' Contratto proposes that many women who are pregnant or are new mothers are 'intensely uncomfortable with their own sexuality, consciously or unconsciously and as a result experience considerable psychological pain'. This could have far reaching effects on their relationships. A second explanation has been offered by Ussher (1989) to account for the confusion and contradictions regarding sexuality which women have to face when they become pregnant. She argues that it is the inevitable result of the way women are categorized:

> Individual women are inevitably positioned at either end of the dichotomy: good/bad, madonna/whore, feminine/career-orientated, and their position is often determined by their reproductive status. Thus, the woman who is pregnant or a mother cannot be a good mother and a sexual person at the same time, both madonna and whore; women's sexuality is dangerous and threatening and is therefore at odds with the stereotype of the good mother.

The preceding discussion suggests that the deep internalizing of societal attitudes and the categorization of women may affect sexuality and sexual relations during pregnancy. However, if pregnant women are not too embarrassed by cultural mores to admit it, 'their libido, sexual activity and sexual responsiveness can reach heights previously uncharted' (Black, 1994).

Sexuality issues for the pregnant woman

Pregnancy is a unique time in a woman's life. She experiences dramatic alterations in her physiology, her appearance and her body, as well as changes in her social status which all occur simultaneously. Psychic and social changes also exist for both partners in the relationship. Pregnancy can either disrupt the relationship between a couple or can deepen and strengthen it (Kitzinger, 1982). According to Kitzinger, sexual interaction is one facet of the relationship which is often affected.

Several reports describe a decrease in sexual desire, frequency and satisfaction in women during pregnancy (Bogren, 1991; Barclay et al., 1994). This decrease is usually most marked in the third trimester of pregnancy and least in the second. Masters and Johnson (1966) reported increased sexual desire and sexual satisfaction during the second trimester compared to before pregnancy. They also found that decreased desire during the first trimester was only true for women expecting their first baby.

A more recent study of pregnant women found that a large number reported a loss of libido and suggests that affection and reassurance between partners rather than physical contact is important (Jones, 1990). In this study pregnant women reported that they felt restricted because of their size and that positions for sexual activity and intercourse were limited. This observation is particularly interesting as it could indicate a lack of education from health care professionals; this problem can be overcome by discussing different positions for sex or other ways of experiencing sexual satisfaction. Researchers appear to agree that coital frequency declines during pregnancy and they link this to a woman's declining sexual interest and the discomfort caused by advancing pregnancy (Barclay, 1990). The pattern and intensity of this decline is not clear. Studies have also reported a linear decline in sexual interest and activity over successive trimesters (Alder, 1994).

Unfortunately, many studies of sexuality during pregnancy have methodological flaws. However, what is important is that there is no 'norm' of sexual behaviour, particularly with regard to pregnancy (Walton, 1994). Sexual behaviour varies between individuals. During pregnancy the desire and needs of couples for sexual intimacy and activity constantly go through a process of redefinition and change.

The physical and emotional adjustments of pregnancy can cause changes in body image, fatigue, mood swings and sexual activity. The woman's changing shape, emotional status, fetal activity, changes in breast size, pressure on the bladder and other discomforts of pregnancy result in increased physical and emotional demands. These can produce stress on the sexual relationship of the pregnant woman and her partner. As the woman's appearance and emotional status change during pregnancy, her partner may react with confusion, fear or anxiety, wondering how his relationship with her will be affected.

Being pregnant is not all sexually negative. Walton (1994) acknowledges that, freed from the fear of pregnancy, many couples find that 'it is the greatest turn-on ever. The woman feels fulfilled and magnificent and the man feels proud and protective'. A satisfying sexual relationship during pregnancy contributes to satisfaction and happiness by strengthening ties of caring, mutual respect, pleasure and intimacy.

Physiological changes

Many physiological changes occur during pregnancy. The hormones oestrogen and progesterone act together to evoke marked pelvic vasocongestion. Vaginal congestion occurs because of increased vascularity and venous stasis. The venous congestion of pregnancy can result in a heightened manifestation of all aspects of sexual intercourse. The orgasm may be heightened and the vaginal lumen become smaller, thus gripping the penis tighter (Walton, 1994). However, vasocongestion can also predispose pregnant women to discomfort during sexual intercourse. Reamy and White (1985) state that:

> The progressive deep pelvic congestion of pregnancy and its associated pressure can be aggravated by sexual intercourse; tumescence becomes increasingly exaggerated, prolonged and progressively less responsive to orgasm.

Vulval varicosities and haemorrhoids may be precipitated and aggravated by pregnancy. Labial vasocongestion and distension is also exacerbated by varicosities and by the pregnant state, making some routine activities such as walking very uncomfortable and the idea of sex seem impossible.

Body changes and body image

During pregnancy major body changes occur with startling rapidity. Such changes inevitably mean that adjustment has to be made to what constitutes a 'normal body image'. There is very little research focusing directly on women's views of their body changes or of their size during pregnancy. Nevertheless, the few studies that do exist indicate that the focus on women's physical appearance changes during pregnancy, and that they are generally viewed differently by men. For example, Price (1988) notes that there is a shift away from women being viewed as 'seducers' to being viewed as 'producers' during pregnancy. For some women body image during pregnancy is viewed in a very positive light: 'your body metamorphoses into this magnificent spectacle – loose and open and warm' (Miller, 1995).

The way a pregnant woman feels and experiences her body during pregnancy can affect her sexuality. It has been suggested that some women have very positive feelings about their bodies, whilst others are more negative, especially during the last three months of pregnancy (Raphael-Leff, 1993). Tiredness, the changes that occur in the breasts, backache, as well as frequency of micturition are just some of the physical changes that can affect sexual activity. According to Kitzinger (1985) some women have distorted views of their bodies during pregnancy: 'They feel bigger than they really are or believe that their partners must find them ugly, when in fact, men often delight in pregnant women and find their physical changes exciting and beautiful'.

However, there is evidence of considerable dissatisfaction with pregnancy due to the connotations that fatness has with being unattractive (Wiles, 1994). Such findings provide evidence of the importance of physical attractiveness in women's self-esteem. As already mentioned, women's sexual health is intimately linked to her own self-image and this needs to be acknowledged and discussed with women by midwives during pregnancy. Sexual positions to increase comfort as the pregnancy progresses as well as alternative non-coital modes of sexual expression, such as manual partner stimulation and masturbation should be explored with the pregnant woman and her partner. Women who are expecting a multiple birth may have particular concerns and anxieties about physical restrictions because of their size.

Negative feelings regarding body image during pregnancy have been identified (Jones, 1990). Yet, as Jones points out 'By paying attention to a woman's thoughts, feelings and perceptions about her body, we can help her adapt to her changing situation'.

Sexual intercourse and pregnancy

The Bible advises against it and Hippocrates maintained that it could lead to abortion (Main *et al.*, 1993). The British tradition in antenatal care in relation to intercourse in pregnancy has been one of 'avoidance' (Nicolson, 1990). Several studies have examined the relationships between sexual intercourse, uterine contractility and pre-term labour with conflicting results. Orgasm, with or without sexual intercourse, has been reported to be associated with premature rupture of membranes, especially during late pregnancy and with a slow fetal heart rate (Ekwo *et al.*, 1993). Pregnant women frequently fear that sexual intercourse may provoke miscarriage or premature labour or damage the fetus, and so feel they should abstain (Savage and Reader, 1984).

The findings of a study conducted by Mills *et al.* (1981) of the sexual activity of 10 477 women during pregnancy led them to conclude that sexual intercourse with orgasm up to term has no ill-effects on the outcome of pregnancy. Savage and Reader (1984) confirmed this, finding no significant increase of fetal distress in women who continued to be sexually active throughout pregnancy. Another finding of the study was that 27% of the women respondents noted uterine contractions following orgasm. The majority reported these as always or sometimes painful. Once painful contractions had been noted after orgasm,

women reported having sexual intercourse less frequently or ceasing altogether. The physical effects of sexual intercourse in pregnancy need to be discussed by health professionals with the woman or the couple. Any advice on sexual intercourse or abstinence during pregnancy needs to explore non-penetrative sex, sexual intercourse and orgasm. The avoidance of sexual intercourse or the avoidance of orgasm should be differentiated and explored. The warning signs indicative of abstaining from sexual intercourse and seeking professional advice also need to be discussed (Box 6.1).

Box 6.1 Indications to abstain from sexual intercourse during pregnancy (Guana-Trujillo and Higgins, 1987)

♦ Vaginal bleeding

♦ Placenta praevia

♦ Premature dilatation of the cervix

♦ Rupture of membranes

♦ History of premature delivery

♦ Multiple pregnancy

♦ Engaged fetal head.

It could be argued that more information is needed regarding the relative importance of female orgasm and sexual intercourse on uterine contractility (Main *et al.*, 1993). Nevertheless, it would seem appropriate for health professionals to suggest back massage or back rubbing as a way of attempting to relieve discomfort caused by prolonged contractions of orgasm, especially during the third trimester.

Dyspareunia in pregnancy

How frequent and problematic is dyspareunia among pregnant women? In a study conducted by Reamy and White (1985) of 52 married women throughout pregnancy, dyspareunia appears to be far from incidental and becomes increasingly prevalent as pregnancy progresses. By the third trimester of pregnancy 12% of the women were experiencing painful sexual intercourse more than half the time. Correlations were found between happiness about being pregnant, anxiety about the pregnancy or the impending delivery, and the women's perceived attractiveness to their husbands. Additionally, the authors reported that just over one-third of the women respondents reported having stopped intercourse altogether; the specific reasons for this were not identified.

Multiple physical and psychosocial factors have been identified that influence the occurrence of dyspareunia during pregnancy (Box 6.2).

Dyspareunia and avoidance of sexual intercourse demands a systematic evaluation by health care professionals. Sexual health and sexual responses are dependent upon the interaction between physiological and psychosocial systems. Reamy and White (1985) point out that pregnant women need to be given permission to feel sexual and to be sexual. They also need to know that emotional and sexual fluctuations during pregnancy are to be anticipated and are normal. Disclosure of sexual symptoms including dyspareunia, and its systematic evaluation and treatment, are important considerations during pregnancy and at any stage of a woman's life. The physical causes for the problem should not be overlooked, neither should the psychological causes be neglected.

Box 6.2 Causes of dyspareunia during pregnancy (Reamy and White, 1985)

Physical factors

◆ Pelvic vasocongestion

◆ Vaginal congestion and reduced lubrication

◆ Subluxation of the symphysis pubis and sacroiliac joints

◆ Retroverted uterus – particularly during the first weeks of pregnancy

◆ In late pregnancy weight of partner on the gravid uterus

◆ Deep engagement of the fetal head

◆ Chorioamnionitis

◆ Candidal infection

◆ Sexually transmitted *Trichomonas vaginalis*

◆ Genital herpes and genital warts.

Psychosocial factors

Intrapersonal

◆ Anxiety and fear

◆ Vaginismus

◆ General emotional state

◆ Tiredness

◆ Self-esteem

◆ Body image

◆ Sexual guilt.

Interpersonal

◆ Hurt and anger between the expectant parents

◆ Deficient communication and trust between the expectant parents.

Effects on relationships

Research into sexuality and pregnancy has predominantly focused on the female partner and ignored the male partner and the relationship. Barclay *et al.* (1994) claim that when research into sexuality ignores social context and relationships its usefulness is limited. The findings of their study of couples experiencing a first pregnancy provide an example of the effects on sexuality during the changes of pregnancy.

A substantial decline in sexual interest amongst the women, that was not matched by their male partners, was identified. This was reflected in a marked reduction in the frequency of sexual intercourse and in the range of sexual activities. Concern and guilt about the loss of sexual interest and responses to the approach of partners was expressed by some women. The need for holding, cuddling, kissing and physical affection was seen as important for a number of women. This was especially important during the later part of pregnancy. Breast tenderness, a perceived loss of physical attractiveness and their ability to maintain the interest of partners in them as women were some of the reasons articulated by the women in the study. The authors found that 76% regularly practised fellatio and cunnilingus (oral sex) and 12% of males regularly practised anal intercourse during pregnancy. Another key observation was that 28% of the men interviewed did not always achieve orgasm during sexual intercourse (Barclay *et al.*, 1994). It should be stressed to couples that the forceful blowing of air into the vagina during oral sex should be avoided particularly during pregnancy as it may cause air embolism.

These findings suggest that the mismatch of female sexual interest levels in pregnancy could present a challenge to stable partnerships (Barclay *et al.*, 1994; Taylor, 1992). During assessment and care planning maternity care professionals need to gather information about sexual activity before and during pregnancy. The comfort level around sexual activity and the interest and concerns of partners should be discussed. Guidance on the individual differences and variations in sexual response during pregnancy should be given whether asked for or not. Alder (1994) suggests that most couples will find that they have different levels of interests and patterns of sexual activity at different stages of their lives. She notes that:

> Accepting variations in sexuality would relieve the pressure to behave in what maybe perceived as the normal pattern of sexual behaviour, and allow each individual couple to find their own level of sexual activity.

By giving permission to talk about and then normalize sexual experiences, professionals can then aim to enhance the sexual experience of pregnancy and the relationship for those most intimately involved. For some women sex during pregnancy can be a more enriching and fulfilling experience: 'The necessity of finding new positions (there are plenty if you apply as much concentration as you would to finding a parking space) adds spice. And orgasms seem more intense and happen more easily' (Miller, 1995).

The findings of Barclay *et al.* (1994) highlighted that a woman's loss of self-esteem and perceptions of loss of physical attractiveness are very real to her. Black (1994) points out that:

> Knowing this, one can recommend rear-entry (a tergo) positions to the couple. As the woman's back remains slim when on view to her partners, the knee–chest position and its variants provide good support and relaxation for the pregnant body.

Research has identified that sexual functioning during pregnancy continues, albeit in varying degrees. However, it has also identified that maternity care professionals are often either inadequate in their efforts or do not provide enough information about sexual activity and sexual intercourse during pregnancy (Guana-Trujillo and Higgins, 1987; Savage and Reader, 1984). Moreover, it has been shown that women welcome information about sexual activity and sexual intercourse during pregnancy.

When planning care for pregnant women you should be able to address this need but must be aware of your own sexual feelings and attitudes towards sex during pregnancy and give accurate and informed advice. If avenues of communication are open regarding sexual intercourse and sexual activity during pregnancy, any fears and myths the pregnant woman and her partner may have can be dispelled. You can then identify areas in which more information is required and give factual, non-judgemental advice.

Assessment for care planning needs to include the biological and psychosocial variables which can affect sexuality. This includes knowledge about pregnancy and effects of pregnancy on sexuality and sexual behaviour; attitudes towards and the feelings about pregnancy; as well as attention to the concerns of the partner. Questions which could highlight some of these issues have been identified and include the following:

♦ 'What have you heard about sex during pregnancy?'

♦ 'What do you feel about sex during pregnancy?'

♦ 'How do your feelings and ideas about sex differ from your partner?'

♦ 'Most women experience changes in sexuality and their sexual relationship during pregnancy – what changes, if any, have taken place in your sexual relationship?'

Such enquiries will encourage information exchange regarding sexuality and may enable women to share their attitudes, experiences and concerns (Reamy and White, 1987).

Sexuality issues for the health professional

Pregnancy and the transition to motherhood for most heterosexual women is both the consequence of having had a sexual relationship with a man, and an enactment of ascribed gender roles. It is a manifestation of their sexuality (Nicolson, 1990). However, it is important for health care professionals to remember that not all their clients will be heterosexual. According to a study of the health care experiences of self-identified lesbians, health care professionals usually assume that their female clients are heterosexual (Robertson, 1993). Other research has indicated that this is a major hinderance in effective therapeutic communication with health care providers (Burns, 1992). In a meta-analysis of the research about lesbian health care Stevens (1993) states that: 'Lesbians believed that health care providers were generally condemnatory toward and ignorant about them . . . upon disclosure of their lesbian identity they experienced many kinds of mistreatment.'

Such findings and negative ramifications are serious issues that all health care providers must address. An increasing number of lesbian women are choosing to bear children (Kenney and Tash, 1993). There are different routes to pregnancy for lesbians but 'like any other path to parenthood, they are all emotionally intense' (Martin, 1993). Pregnancy can be a very isolating experience for lesbian women. It is often assumed that the pregnant lesbian woman is a single mother, which is a painful negation of her identity (Burns, 1992). This assumption marginalizes and negates the position of the lesbian who is supporting her partner and is going to co-parent. According to Burns (1992) 'she might well be placed in the position of the caring friend'. As with heterosexual couples, adjustment to the physical and psychological changes during pregnancy may require lesbian couples to adapt or modify their roles and relationship. Yet the lack of acknowledgement of the parental role of the non-biological parent is a poignant difference (Kenney and Tash, 1993). Maternity care professionals need to include the female partner during care provision and acknowledge the change in the life of the co-parent.

In order to provide appropriate assistance and support to lesbian childbearing couples it is important to affirm their values and relationship. It is crucial to not only learn more about their maternity and health care concerns but also to avoid acting on the assumption that all women are heterosexual. Kenney and Tash (1993) comment that:

> Lesbians would like to be understood and accepted if they reveal their identity and not feel that they might be rejected and possibly mistreated. Health care providers who adopt an open, sensitive and nonjudgemental attitude and are willing to listen to and respect lesbians as intelligent women with feelings will be sought out by this group.

The research that exists on sexuality and pregnancy and the relationship between maternity and sexuality is often confusing and contradictory. A lot of the work is anecdotal but one thing the studies all have in common is that they usually raise more questions than answers (Contratto, 1980). Many studies have documented the inadequacy of health care professionals in taking account of the sexuality of those in their care. There is also evidence of their reluctance to take an adequate sexual history (Lewis and Bor, 1994). These are important findings because childbearing is intimately bound up with a woman's sexuality and all midwives and other health care professionals must learn to address this issue if they aspire towards holistic care for their patients (Aston, 1994).

Midwives are the health professionals who are principally involved with women during the process of childbearing. Although Contratto (1980) argues that discussion of maternal sexuality makes virtually everyone anxious, Sedgwick's (1994) study of midwives challenges this view and reports that midwives felt sexual discussions with clients should be part of their normal role. The midwives also identified that it was important for them to have knowledge about the sexual aspects of the childbearing continuum. However, the majority of midwives found their training on sexual issues either inadequate or non-existent and that it had not prepared them for professional practice. Formal teaching on sexual matters to help their practice was seen as valuable by 91% of the midwives surveyed. Nevertheless, in spite of this most of the midwives did discuss sexual issues with their clients and attempted to meet the needs of women in this respect.

Sexual health problems and pregnancy

Various conditions are commonly associated with pregnancy. Although they may be perceived as 'minor ailments' they can be a source of considerable distress and adversely affect sexual health. To promote sexual health during pregnancy sensitive approaches and questioning are essential in order to minimize any embarrassment.

In this discussion the more common conditions affecting pregnant women are included. The issues surrounding HIV infection in relation to pregnancy are manifold and are not explored in this discussion (for more information see Shepherd, 1994).

Physiological vaginal discharge

Physiological vaginal discharge is the result of secretions from Bartholin's and Skene's glands and from the endocervix. Epithelium shed from the vagina and lactobacilli, the latter maintaining an acidic vaginal environment to protect against infection, are also present. The vaginal micro-environment changes with age, mostly in response to alterations in oestrogen and progesterone. An increase in vaginal secretions has been reported in pregnancy and is known as leucorrhoea. The normal leucorrhoea of pregnancy is whitish to clear in colour and should not cause soreness, irritation or an offensive odour (Walton, 1994). During pregnancy, any woman with a discharge different from leucorrhoea needs to be referred to a doctor. In pregnancy the vaginal pH is 3.8–4.4. Symptoms relating to candidiasis (thrush) occur more frequently in pregnancy due to increased vaginal glucose and glycogen and also due to the changing hormonal balance.

Candidiasis (thrush)

Candida albicans is the usual cause of 'thrush'. It is the most common fungal species found in the vagina, where it often exists commensally. Candidiasis most frequently presents as a thick, white, curd-like discharge or sometimes as a watery vaginal discharge associated with vulval irritation and vaginal soreness. Hormonal influences appear to have an important role in its occurrence and pregnant women have been reported as having a higher incidence of asymptomatic colonization and symptomatic candidiasis (Woolley, 1994). Other predisposing factors have been identified and include diabetes, broad-spectrum antibiotic therapy which can reduce commensal bacteria, especially lactobacilli, and immunosuppressive therapy (Woolley, 1994; Uthayakumar *et al.*, 1994). Women complaining of recurrent vulvovaginal candidiasis should have a thorough examination and be investigated for glucose intolerance and anaemia. Individuals with chronic mucotaneous candidiasis have been shown to have abnormal iron metabolism and low iron stores (Woolley,

1994). The woman's sexual partner should also be investigated as some men can get balanitis (Uthayakumar *et al.*, 1994).

Candida infection is characterized by severe vulval itching, which is often worse during the night. The infection can make a woman lose sleep and become exhausted and run down. On examination, the vulva and vagina appear inflamed. Although 'thrush' can be diagnosed on the basis of history alone, provided that the woman has a single stable partner, diagnosis is made on microscopy of wet preparations or Gram-staining of vaginal secretions (Uthayakumar *et al.*, 1994; Woolley, 1994). Treatment and self-help measures that the woman can use are discussed in Chapter 12 (page 295).

The urinary system

In pregnancy there are changes in the physiological and functional anatomy of the urinary system. Pelvic organs are displaced and the relationship between the bladder and the uterus and vagina are subtly altered. The changes are caused by hormonal and endocrine factors, compression of the ureters by the gravid uterus and fetus, as well as circulatory changes. These changes can predispose pregnant women to urinary tract infections (Silverton, 1993). As a result it is also common for pregnant women to have symptoms of urinary frequency and stress incontinence. Frequent nocturia can disrupt sleep patterns and affect fatigue levels and sense of well-being. Genuine stress incontinence is associated with pregnancy. The symptoms of this distressing condition may develop during the antenatal period in about 50% of women expecting their first babies and the majority of women in their subsequent pregnancies (Wallace, 1993). Pelvic floor exercises have been shown to be effective if commenced within the third trimester of pregnancy and continued after childbirth. Ideally pelvic floor exercises should continue throughout life (see also page 374).

Urinary incontinence has significant social and psychological consequences and can have a profound effect on sexuality and sexual health (see Chapter 15). Genuine stress incontinence is associated with the leaking of urine during sexual intercourse, commonly on penetration (Kelleher *et al.*, 1993). During care planning and assessment, you will need to ask your client if she leaks urine during sexual intercourse so that you can offer support and interventions, such as pelvic floor exercises. Other important factors associated with urinary incontinence and sexual health are the reaction of the pregnant women and her partner, the embarrassment, and the effect on her libido and self-esteem. Dyspareunia secondary to urine dermatitis can also add to the distress of women suffering with urinary incontinence (Kelleher *et al.*, 1993).

Haemorrhoids

Haemorrhoids are varicose veins of the anal region and are particularly common during pregnancy. They are often a joke subject to those who do not suffer from them and are not usually talked about in 'polite' company. Women with haemorrhoids may suffer in painful and embarrassed silence (Thompson, 1994) before seeking medical help. Haemorrhoids can develop during pregnancy because of venous dilatation and reduced peripheral resistance due to the hormonal influence of progesterone. Previous haemorrhoids, constipation and the woman's weight may also be contributory factors. Haemorrhoids can worsen during the second stage of labour and can also be troublesome during the puerperium.

Rectal bleeding, itching and soreness around the anus, discomfort during defecation and a mucous discharge are signs and symptoms associated with haemorrhoids. Any woman with rectal bleeding should be referred to the doctor as it may be due to other conditions. During pregnancy, women need to be advised to take appropriate action to avoid constipation (Silverton, 1993). A high-fibre diet and plenty of fluids is the best preventative action. Iron pills could be a cause of constipation. Relief may be obtained from ice cubes or ice packs or from special creams available over the counter. The discomfort and irritation of haemorrhoids may be eased by wearing loose, cotton underwear or applying a pad soaked in witch hazel.

Sexuality and pregnancy loss

Infertility

Infertility and infertility investigations can affect a sexual relationship. The need to take basal temperatures, time intercourse for the fertile period and undergo post-coital tests can be particularly disruptive (see Chapter 8). Levels of happiness and satisfaction within a sexual relationship may also vary during the various stages of infertility investigations. It has been suggested that couples with 'normal' sexual functioning prior to a diagnosis of subfertility may develop decreased coital frequency, orgasmic dysfunction or mid-cycle male impotence (Pepperell and McBain, 1985). However, there is also evidence that marital and sexual difficulties in couples undergoing infertility investigations may be relatively uncommon (Edelmann and Connolly, 1994). This finding needs to be interpreted with caution as it may be due to an element of self-selection among the client group. It may be that only couples with stable relationships get as far as seeking medical help in their efforts to conceive, and that those whose relationships are not so secure do not go so far as to seek infertility advice. Infertility may serve to improve a marital and sexual relationship by bringing a couple closer together, providing the problem is acknowledged by both partners as one that they share and which should be faced together (Edelmann and Connolly, 1994).

Miscarriage

Miscarriage is the commonest complication of pregnancy and affects 25% of all women who conceive a pregnancy. Recurrent miscarriage, defined as three or more consecutive losses of pregnancy, affects approximately 1% of all women (Clifford and Regan, 1994). The risk of a further miscarriage has been shown to increase after each successive pregnancy loss. This distressing problem can have a marked effect on sexual feelings and sexual relations. Barclay *et al.* (1994) identified that a previous miscarriage or episodes of bleeding intensified the fear of miscarriage during pregnancy. As a result, frequency of sexual intercourse and the variety of sexual activities that couples found acceptable was markedly reduced.

Fear of miscarriage can result in the pregnant woman perceiving sex as a direct threat to the baby. The partner may also feel that he poses a threat to the pregnancy. Kitzinger (1985) points out that: 'any couple who feel like this interact negatively each triggering off further anxiety in the other'. However, there is little evidence to suggest that sexual intercourse and miscarriage are related in the absence of other problems (Kitzinger, 1985). Kitzinger states that 'no studies have been done to show whether not having sexual intercourse in early pregnancy helps to avoid miscarriage, though many people think this must be so'. Pregnant women are often advised by doctors to abstain from sexual intercourse if they have previously miscarried or threaten to do so in their current pregnancy. Bleeding in pregnancy is alarming and women therefore feel safer avoiding sexual intercourse (Savage and Reader, 1984). It is important to inform pregnant women when the suspected risk period is over, so that sexual intercourse can resume. Lack of communication of this fact can result in the woman feeling guilty if she does have sexual intercourse without 'medical permission'.

Fear of miscarriage may result in the couple abstaining from sexual activity throughout pregnancy, 'assuming that a ban on intercourse means a ban on all sexual activity' (Kitzinger, 1985). Again, it will be helpful to advise women of other ways of enjoying sex without having penetrative sex.

It is important for health care professionals to be acutely sensitive to the feelings evoked by miscarriage in a subsequent pregnancy. Barclay *et al.* (1994) highlighted the deep-rooted fear that couples felt in the context of their sexual relationship. In an editorial comment on the study Black (1994) makes the point:

> Despite having assured some couples that sexual activity would be all right in this pregnancy, no amount of convincing may alter the contrary opinion of either or both partners, where there has been a previous pregnancy loss or episode of bleeding. One can only reassure such couples that if they experienced a genuinely satisfying sexual relationship beforehand, that it will return once this baby arrives safely.

Bereavement

Research on sexuality and sexual intercourse following perinatal death has largely been neglected. The difficulties of re-establishing a loving, sexual relationship following the death of a baby comes mainly from primary sources, namely mothers' personal anecdotes and experiences (Mander, 1994). Mander draws attention to the fact that enjoyment of human contact, even that quite independent of lovemaking, may be too much to ask of a grieving patient. There is evidence to suggest that following the death of a baby, sexual intercourse may not be resumed until the couple are planning another pregnancy. Mander (1994) suggests that: 'Differing patterns and rates of grieving may compound this difficulty because one partner is unable to respond to the other's tentative advances.'

Other factors also have a bearing on sexual intercourse during the process of grieving. Sexual intercourse may seem as a reminder of the birth and also of the death. Borg and Lasker (1982) suggested that the pleasure of making love may be regarded as inappropriate. This may be due to 'previous memories of lovemaking which began their baby's brief existence being a carefree and joyful time' (Mander, 1994). Couples may regret their inability to give each other intimate and loving support at this difficult time. However, the removal of anxieties about performance and conception may be a relief for some couples (Borg and Lasker, 1982).

Childbirth and sexuality

Women approach labour and childbirth with a mixture of emotions ranging from happiness and excitement about their new baby to apprehension and fear. These anxieties can cover many aspects of childbirth.

♦ Will I be alright in hospital amongst strangers?

♦ Will I be able to cope with the pain?

♦ Will I be able to remain within my birth plan?

♦ Will my new baby be normal?

♦ How will my other children left at home cope?

If there is a positive outcome to all these anxieties then a woman will often feel the whole experience of childbirth has been an enriching fulfilment of her hopes. Her relationship with her partner will be enhanced and this can facilitate attachment to her new baby.

Although labour and birth are often associated with pain and anxiety, the experiences and feelings evoked are also closely linked to sexuality and sexual health. Kitzinger (1985) described the experience of birth for some women as:

the most intensely sexual feeling a woman ever experiences, as strong as orgasm, even more compelling than orgasm. Some women find it disturbing because it is sexual and they feel out of control as the energy floods through them and they can do nothing to prevent it.

Drawing on her personal experiences, Southern (1994) also addresses the links between the process of childbearing and sexuality:

> Even if labour does not directly evoke sexual feeling in the woman, the process of childbearing must surely indirectly evoke sex. How are babies conceived? And how are they born? The reproductive organs are sexual organs and I do not believe that women can expose themselves and open up to give birth without making this connection.

Given that childbirth and sexuality are related, as well as the many personal experiences and dimensions encompassed under the term sexual health, this discussion will only focus on just some of the issues associated with women and sexual health during labour and childbirth.

Childbirth following sexual abuse

Sexual abuse is covered more fully in Chapter 5 but issues that are relevant to childbirth are discussed in this section.

One of the most consistent findings to emerge from recent work has been clear evidence of the significance of childbirth in evoking personal sexual experiences. As Southern (1994) points out: 'Some women's experiences of sex will have been invasive and traumatic as a result of rape, incest or some other sexual abuse'. In assessing this important and often neglected area of women's lives, Kitzinger's (1992) study of 39 women survivors of childhood sexual abuse draws attention to the kinds of feelings and vulnerability stirred up during childbirth. Kitzinger reported that over half of the respondents were reminded of their experiences of sexual assault by internal examinations, cervical smears, dental examinations, but of particular significance was the process of childbirth. Women explained that they had felt 'lack of control over their own bodies', 'helpless in the hands of another person', 'depersonalized' and other similar feelings during childbirth. Such feelings had reminded them of the feelings and indignities associated with

the abuse all over again. Kitzinger's analysis also acknowledged that childbirth may be a significant experience because of extra-medical factors:

> Pregnancy and giving birth involve feelings about one's body – how it looks and feels and whether it is 'good' enough. Women often feel that their body has been deformed or ruined by abuse, or that it betrayed them by attracting the abuser or sexually responding to his touch. Childbirth may either confirm or challenge these perceptions.

It is not only women who have been sexually abused who may find childbirth experiences traumatic and distressing. Other such women are those who have previously undergone invasive obstetric or gynaecological procedures (Clement, 1994). Vaginal examinations have also been identified as difficult for women with a history of miscarriages, terminations and stillbirths.

So it is important that midwives and other health professionals create an environment during pregnancy and labour that facilitates optimal conditions and the potential for a more satisfying experience for all women (Southern, 1994). Care givers will often not know of a previous experience of sexual abuse, and without individualized care and continuity of carer 'women are unlikely to disclose experiences of abuse. Even in optimal conditions, some women will choose not to share this information' (Clement, 1994).

A common thread that runs through the literature is that midwives, doctors and health professionals should ensure that the care they offer 'counteracts rather than reenacts the violation of women's bodies' (Kitzinger, 1992):

> Childbirth can be an opportunity for women to relate to their bodies in new ways, to experience them as powerful, competent and creative. Some women whom I interviewed spoke positively of the care with which midwives, doctors, and nurses responded to their needs. A gentle examination, a listening ear, and a respectful approach can all help women to overcome alienation from their bodies. Sensitivity on the part of the staff who understood and validated their distress, provided information, and offered practical support was vital in helping women through such experiences.

Female genital mutilation

Female genital mutilation damages the health of women and because it interferes with their sexuality it is a sexual health issue (see also page 105). During labour and childbirth great sensitivity as well as cultural awareness is important, in order to give appropriate care and psychological support for women who have undergone any form of female genital mutilation, especially infibulation. Omer-Hashi (1994) suggests that all infibulated women should be expected to have fears about labour and birth complications. Specialist antenatal clinic services have found that assessment prior to labour of whether problems are likely to occur during childbirth have made a significant contribution to the health and emotional well-being of women during labour and delivery. The provision of information and counselling on de-infibulation for women and their partners during pregnancy has been a crucial part of this maternity care provision (Eaton, 1993).

There is a dearth of research literature available on the sexual and psychological effects of severe forms of genital mutilation when compared to studies and case reports on the physical complications during childbirth. A syndrome of chronic anxiety and depression 'arising from worry over the state of their genitals' and other sexual health issues has been observed in many infibulated women (Toubia, 1994). When performing an examination during labour on any woman who has been mutilated, it is important that health care professionals 'should control their facial expression and shock at her distorted genitalia so as not to hurt her self esteem' (Omer-Hashi, 1994).

Vaginal examinations and other interventional procedures (such as applying fetal scalp electrodes, performing fetal blood sampling) can be difficult, painful or impossible in some cases. A normal birth may also not be possible. However, there is evidence to suggest that 'where physicians are not trained to deal with infibulated women unnecessary caesarean section which can be avoided with a simple deinfibulation performed with the woman under a local anaesthesia' is causing increasing concern (Toubia, 1994).

It is important that midwives and other health professionals are knowledgeable and comfortable about female genital mutilation, its variations and potential complications. During labour and childbirth may not be the optimal time to establish whether or not a woman has been infibulated. It is recommended that this is done:

> as soon as possible during the course of normal physical examinations. This is an ideal opportunity to provide information and non-directional counselling for the woman, together with her partner, if she has one, about the appropriate treatment at and after the birth.
>
> (RCN, 1994)

Although deinfibulation can be performed during pregnancy or labour, early deinfibulation is associated with decreased pain during labour and a shorter period of postpartum recovery (Omer-Hashi, 1994).

Men and birth

The effects of the presence of men during childbirth and the implications for sexual relationships in the short and long term is a contentious issue. Odent (1992) proposes that the father's presence at the birth has long-term implications for sexual attraction 'which needs mystery'. Shannon (1993) argues that although 90% of births are now attended by fathers 'in the midst of all the superlatives, some local difficulties are beginning to emerge'. These include pressure, guilt, trauma, fears and 'damage to the relationship between the mother and father'. Although a recent survey of 441 men who were present at birth identified that women were the biggest influence on the decision to be present during childbirth (86%), the majority (93%) of men said they wanted to be there. The experience was described as 'wonderful' by 64%; 29% described feelings of being 'scared', whilst only 9% admitted to being 'upset' by events that occurred in the delivery room (Royal College of Midwives, 1994).

There is little documented information and research in professional literature about the short- and long-term effects for both partners and their sexual relationship after a shared birth experience. However, O'Driscoll (1994) draws attention to psychosexual problems that could be traced back to men witnessing birth. Hall (1993) also points out that:

> No one should deny that childbirth is painful, and to watch someone you love in excruciating pain and be unable to do anything about it may have a devastating effect on a man. If the birth becomes complicated, as with forceps delivery, men have been known to become totally switched off sexually and need counselling for many months through fear of putting his partner (and himself) through the experience again.

The issues are complex and there are no clear answers. Yet the implications and significance for sexual relationships and sexual health must be taken into account by midwives and health professionals. Individual couples should be encouraged to discuss their fears and feelings about what is right for them as individuals, as well as what is right for them as a couple and their relationship, during labour and childbirth. O'Driscoll (1994) suggests that as: 'being present at the birth may cause long-lasting harm to the relationship men should not be coerced into staying'. She also highlights the importance of the recognition of the needs of individual men and women. She suggests that 'sexual matters with both partners should be discussed openly at preparation classes and during postnatal care' with both partners. About this last point O'Driscoll comments that: 'midwives should educate both partners about the anatomy of the vagina and its marvellous ability to stretch and return to normal size'.

In a positive vein, there is evidence to suggest that the father's presence during delivery can be beneficial and that his presence adds to the enjoyment of birth for both parents, as well as strengthening the relationship between them (Clulow, 1982). Labour and childbirth are events of pivotal significance for both partners and their psychosexual life and should be openly discussed.

Postnatal sexuality

Studies of the sexual behaviour and sexual health of women after childbirth have indicated that they are influenced by profound psychological, interpersonal, social and biological variables (Corkhill, 1996, Demyttenaere *et al.* 1995). Some of these will be raised in this discussion. Once again there is evidence that midwives and other health professionals often fail to adequately address sexuality and sexual relations following childbirth. Recent studies have shown that only 25% of men received information about resuming sexual relations following childbirth (Royal College of Midwives, 1994). Whilst another study found that although most women had been given advice about contraception after the birth (75%) only a few (24%) had the opportunity to talk about sex after childbirth during the pregnancy. Women also reported that following childbirth they had been left to deal with changes and potential problems in their sexual relations on their own without support (National Childbirth Trust, 1994).

Studies of when women resume sexual intercourse following childbirth show that this varies a great deal (Alder, 1994). The study by Robson *et al.* (1981) found that about a third had resumed intercourse by six weeks after delivery and nearly all had done so by 12 weeks after delivery. However, many women were having intercourse less frequently at 12 weeks (77%) and one year after delivery (57%) compared to before they became pregnant. This study concludes that overall, childbearing diminishes sexual activity and enjoyment for at least a year after delivery. However, positive aspects of sexual activity after childbirth have been reported as many women have described feeling that whatever time they chose to resume sex was the right time for them. Whilst others have reported improvement in their sex lives and relationships following delivery: 'My sexuality has blossomed with motherhood, my erotic responses have been enhanced not damaged' (Miller, 1995). Some of the reasons that have been offered are:

♦ Feeling less inhibited

♦ Being more relaxed

♦ Having a better body image.

In addition, women have also commented that sex may be less frequent but of better quality. This was summed up by one respondent as 'Quantity down – Quality up' (National Childbirth Trust, 1994).

Several authors have reported that women are anxious about their bodies in the early weeks and months following childbirth. This is often attributed by respondents to perineal pain, soreness, as well as a decreased sense of attractiveness (Reamy and White, 1987). The physical demands made by a new baby and the stress of new parental roles, responsibilities and fatigue place particular demands on the emotional reserves of women (Tobert, 1990) creating anxiety and frustration in a couple. Nicolson (1990) in her study of the experiences of women in the transition to motherhood reported that a reduction in intimacy and quality of adult couple relationships was exacerbated by men's perceived secondary role in childcare and their lack of understanding of their partner's daily routine combined with her increased investment in the mothering role. Tiredness can compromise the coping ability of a new mother and affect her libido. Loss of libido following childbirth is common.

For our purposes, this is important because the birth of a baby may herald a time of discord, relationship problems and sexual dissatisfaction (Reamy and White, 1987). Moreover, it has been found that sexual and marital therapists often report that their clients say that their sexual problems first became apparent at the time of the birth of their first child (Alder, 1994). It could be argued that if there was greater understanding and more realistic expectations of the demands and what is involved in becoming a parent, some of these problems could be avoided. Although Alder (1994) states that:

> When there is important change in role and accompanying physical demands it is not surprising that there may be communication problems. If the male partner feels unable to express his feelings about the baby and partners changing role and the woman is too tired and anxious about the baby to give him attention, there is ample opportunity for failure of communication.

Whilst these factors may have some relation to and impact on sexual health and the relationship between the woman and her partner following childbirth, they are not the whole story. There is also a gender issue and Van Wert (1991) reminds us that all too often the way the 'problem' of changed sexual relations after childbirth between partners is constructed, is that it is the woman's 'problem and fault':

> To hear couples tell the tale, the halt in sexual relations is usually the woman's fault. Men say they are ready, they have always been ready, but the women have changed, feel too tired or ugly, won't tolerate the barest of touches, or reject them outright. Women blame themselves as well, having succumbed to culturally instilled guilt for failing to fit the role models shown in books, movies and mass advertising.

It is clear that social and contextual factors influence the dynamics of interpersonal relationships and the sex life of a woman after having a baby (Walton, 1994). However, there are also physical causes which may affect libido and sexual health following childbirth.

Following childbirth the couple need to be advised that they may resume intercourse as soon as they feel it is appropriate. It is important to determine what knowledge and concerns the woman and her partner have about their sexual relationship. Evans (1992) suggests that:

> By establishing what knowledge the couple already have the midwife will then be able to use this as a basis for further education, to prepare parents for the physical and emotional reactions they may encounter when resuming sexual intercourse and to enable them to respond appropriately to problems.

However, midwives and other health professionals need to initiate the giving of such information as women may be reluctant to ask. Robson *et al.* (1981) found that many women did not mention sexual difficulties to their general practitioners or obstetricians during pregnancy and at three months after delivery 30% of the women respondents said that they would have liked sexual counselling and would have found it beneficial.

A discussion of the normality of fluctuations of sexual interest and enjoyment following childbirth is a crucial part of professional care planning.

> Alternative coital positions and non coital options for the intimate expression of affection and mutual pleasure can do much to enrich the quality of the pregnancy, the birth experience, and the marital and family bond.
>
> (Reamy and White, 1987)

Several factors contribute to sexual health following childbirth. McConville (1994) argues that following childbirth: 'Women are certainly under pressure to get back to "normal" (i.e. "sexual") as soon as possible after birth'. However, sexual relations and sexual activity after childbirth cannot be isolated from the psychological and sociological adjustments that are required by the woman and her partner. The effect of fatigue, as a result of coping with the demands of a new baby, on libido and sexual activity should not be underestimated. Riley (1989) reports that reduced sexual desire, resulting in lowered frequency of sexual intercourse is not uncommon following childbirth. This can result in disharmony in the relationship, which may further inhibit the resumption of satisfactory and mutually satisfying sexual activity. The common causes of concern that have been reported over the resumption of sexual intercourse include the risk of damage to a healing episiotomy scar, damage to internal organs and the abdominal wound following caesarean section, as well as the risk of infection. Riley (1989) suggests that: 'Perhaps some of the sexual and emotional problems encountered in the postnatal women can be prevented by adequate preparation'.

Postnatal women and their partners need to know what to expect when resuming sexual intercourse and how any discomfort can be prevented. They also need advice on contraception during the puerperium and safer sex. Health professionals also need to inform women and their partners what *not* to expect, for example excessive pain, persistent lack of desire, so that they will know what is abnormal and when to seek help.

Postnatal dyspareunia

Health professionals need to ask women about painful intercourse as it appears that postnatal superficial dyspareunia is not uncommon. Postnatal superficial dyspareunia has been defined as painful sexual intercourse following childbirth, excluding those women who have experienced persistent dyspareunia in their nulliparous state and/or have dyspareunia of a known psychosexual origin (Lee, 1994). The common causes are listed in Box 6.3.

Box 6.3 Common causes of postnatal dyspareunia (Lee, 1994)

◆ Decreased vaginal lubrication which may be associated with breastfeeding or with decreased sexual arousal

◆ Inflammation and infection, e.g. granuloma, Bartholin's abscess

◆ Sensitive hymenal tags/skin tags following malalignment of perineal repair

◆ Contracture/scarring of the perineum

◆ Vaginismus due to expectation of pain with intercourse.

Potential sources of discomfort should be identified, for example, an episiotomy incision or caesarean section wound. Advice on coital positions such as side-to-side and female superior positions which minimize episiotomy soreness may be helpful. Gentle insertion of a clean finger into the vagina and massage may help promote relaxation as well as enable women to check the healing process and any residual soreness. Gels for vaginal lubrication, especially for women who are breastfeeding, may be helpful, if there is vaginal dryness. Information regarding pelvic floor exercises may be beneficial, as such exercises increase cognitive awareness of vaginal sensation and tension, promote healing, strengthen the muscles and improve vaginal tone (Reamy and White, 1987). Increasing age and parity are associated with progressive denervation of the pelvic floor muscle and consequently stress incontinence and prolapse. To some degree 80% of mothers are affected and one study showed that perineal squeeze pressure had not returned to normal at eight weeks post-delivery (Smith cited in Lee, 1994). A need for the correct teaching and subsequent review of pelvic floor exercises has been identified (Lee, 1994).

Although this distressing condition progressively resolves for most women, a significant group are left with a persistent problem. Health professionals need to include the topic in parenthood and health education programmes. Myths surrounding birth may need to be dispelled to make accurate information available. It is important to listen, advise and support women and to know when to refer them for further counselling or advice.

Postnatal depression

Psychiatrists argue that postnatal depression is affected by environmental and social factors, but endocrinologists postulate that ovarian hormones may be responsible for the occurrence of depressive illness in women at times of profound hormonal change, e.g. after pregnancy, premenstrually and during the climacteric. Studd (1992) suggests that these three depressive disorders constitute a triad of oestrogen-responsive psychiatric pathology.

Postnatal depression affects one in ten women in the first year following childbirth. The condition usually begins in the first few weeks following delivery and can last for weeks, months or for more than a year (Kumar, 1994). Postnatal depression is often a silent and hidden disorder and the condition is frequently overlooked by health professionals. According to Pitt (1991) the symptoms include: 'anxiety, irritability, fatigue, and a demoralising sense of failure to cope with consequent feelings of guilt and reduced confidence and self esteem'.

Another key feature of postnatal depression is

loss of libido which may put further strain on a relationship. Pitt (1991) states that: 'There is usually little interest in sex which may further strain a marriage already overcast by the new mother's troubled preoccupation and apparent lack of responsiveness'.

A recent study has reported that fathers are more likely to have postnatal depression at both six weeks and six months postpartum if their partners also suffer from postnatal depression (Ballard *et al.*, 1994). Recent studies have shown a link between the maternity 'blues' and postnatal depression. The blues have been described as transient episodes of low mood which typically occur around the 4th or 5th day after childbirth. They occur in at least 50% of mothers and normally lift within one or two days. The blues, however, can be severe and may merge into postnatal depression (Kumar, 1994).

In order to support the woman and her partner health professionals must recognize and be able to deal with postnatal depression. This is an important part of our role as the onset of postnatal depression can be insidious and many women are not aware of what is wrong with them. It may be difficult for women to admit how miserable they are feeling due to embarrassment or feelings of guilt. Jebali (1993) suggests that: 'Guilt is very common among new mothers and is usually internalised; the woman may eventually convince herself that she is a bad mother and therefore a bad person'. According to Jebali, it is also not culturally acceptable to admit to feeling unhappy as a new mother.

As a health professional you need to ask women how they really feel, and also ask them whether they have felt depressed during the first few weeks following childbirth. The Edinburgh Postnatal Depression Scale has been found to be a valuable screening test. Treatment with antidepressants may be helpful, but more important is ensuring that the woman has sustained regular support and counselling. Pitt (1991) asserts that: 'The most important step in the provision of support is ensuring involvement of the husband, family, and if the patient agrees, friends'.

Women with severe postnatal depression have been helped with high-dose oestrogen replacement therapy and it has been shown that such therapy significantly reduces depression scores and accelerates recovery (Henderson *et al.*, 1991).

Midwives, health visitors and general practitioners as well as other health professionals are ideally placed to recognize the onset of depression in new mothers. They are also in the unique position to initiate whatever help, support, and therapy is considered appropriate.

Breastfeeding and sexuality

It has been suggested that in 'contrast to the close association between "breasts and sex", "breastfeeding and sex" are not supposed to go together . . . they are cultural chalk and cheese' (McConville, 1994). Breastfeeding women and their sexual partners may lose the desire for sex whilst others may find that breastfeeding has the effect of enhancing sex. Breastfeeding women may feel particularly fatigued and exhausted, 'which is never good for sex' (McConville, 1994). McConville comments that this can be distressing, usually for the male partner, and engender resentment, especially if the couple have had no prior warning that this may occur. Alder (1994) states that:

> Some sexual partners may find breastfeeding by their partners arousing, others will be indifferent, and a few will find it offensive. Most women enjoy the pleasurable sensation of a baby suckling but some women may feel guilty. Their partners may resent it, either because they regard the women's breasts as their property, or because breastfeeding is an activity which they cannot share.

The physiological mechanisms and the psychological experiences associated with breastfeeding can reduce sexual interest and arousal. Breast tenderness and fear of milk leakage is associated with sexual inhibitions in lactating women and may reduce sexual desire in their partners (Hames cited in Alder, 1994). Painful intercourse, which may be related to low oestrogen levels, is more common in women who exclusively breastfeed when compared to women who bottle feed their babies (Alder, 1994). Sexual arousal which can accompany breastfeeding may engender feelings of guilt and anxiety in the woman. McConville (1994) argues that 'a deep and meaningful silence about the sensual or sexual pleasure which can accompany breastfeeding' pervades.

Explanations about factors that may influence sexuality and breastfeeding need to be offered.

Sexual activity and sexual intercourse may be a low priority during breastfeeding. However, for some couples breastfeeding is 'a time to enjoy breasts and a woman's sexuality in a deeper way than ever before' (McConville, 1994).

Conclusion

Sexuality and sexual health during pregnancy, childbirth and the postnatal period is affected by many different variables and contexts. Health professionals must take into account when planning care the needs and personal experiences of the individual woman and her partner. Alder (1994) has argued that there is a wide variation of sexual behaviour and that couples should be aware that there is no normal pattern, as frequency, quality and satisfaction vary throughout the lifespan. Any notion that 'normal' sexual activity requires penetrative sex should be dispelled and alternatives ranging from kissing and cuddling to oral sex and masturbation can be discussed.

In this chapter there is a clear demonstration of the need for health professionals to address their own attitudes, knowledge and skills about and towards sexuality and the childbearing continuum, in order to provide holistic care (Curtis and Dunn, 1996). The relationship between women's sexual health and body image, especially during pregnancy is an important aspect of assessment and care planning. Health care professionals should explore the normality of the fluctuations of sexual interest and enjoyment with women during pregnancy and following childbirth. It is possible to build up a gloomy picture of sexuality in relation to the childbearing continuum, however, for many women childbirth enhances and intensifies their sexual pleasure. Health care professionals are in the unique position to care for the sexual health of women during pregnancy, childbirth and family beginnings, which should be a positive experience for all those most intimately involved.

Resources

Association for Post-Natal Illness (APNI)
25 Jerdan Place, London SW6 1BE
Tel. 0171 386 0868

Association of Breastfeeding Mothers
26 Holmshaw Close, London SE26 4TH
Tel. 0181 778 4769

La Leche League of Great Britain
BM 3424, London WC1N 3XX
Tel. 0171 242 1278

National Childbirth Trust
Alexandra House, Oldham Terrace, Acton, London W3 6NH
Tel. 0181 992 8637

Further reading

LEROY, M. (1994) *Pleasure: The Truth About Female Sexuality*. London: Harper Collins.
LITVINOFF, S. (1992) *The Relate Guide To Sex In Loving Relationships*. London: Vermillion.
MILLER, J. (1983) *Happy As A Dead Cat* London: Women's Press.
NICOLSON, P. and USSHER, J. (eds) (1992) *The Psychology of Women's Health and Health Care*. London: Macmillan.

References

ALDER, B. (1994) Postnatal sexuality. In Choi, P.Y.L. and Nicolson, P. (eds) *Female Sexuality, Psychology, Biology and Social Context*. Hemel Hempstead: Harvester Wheatsheaf.
ASTON, G. (1994) The construction of pregnant women and HIV. Paper presented at *AIDS' Impact*, 2nd International Conference on Biopsychosocial Aspects of HIV Infection, Brighton.
BALLARD, C.G., DAVIS, R., CULLEN, P.C., MOHAN, R.N. and DEAN, C. (1994) Prevalence of postnatal psychiatric morbidity in mothers and fathers. *British Journal of Psychiatry* **164**(6): 782.
BARCLAY, L. (1990) Sexuality and pregnancy. Paper presented at the International Confederation of Midwives 22nd International Congress, Kobe, Japan.
BARCLAY, L., McDONALD, P. and O'LOUGHLIN, J.A. (1994) Sexuality and pregnancy: an interview study. *The Australian and New Zealand Journal of Obstetrics and Gynaecology* **34**(1): 2.
BEWLEY, C. and GIBBS, A. (1994) Coping with domestic violence in pregnancy. *Nursing Standard* **8**(50): 25.
BLACK, J.S. (1994) Sexuality and pregnancy: an interview study. Editorial comment. *The Australian and New Zealand Journal of Obstetrics and Gynaecology* **34**(1): 1.
BOGREN, L.Y. (1991) Changes in sexuality in women and men during pregnancy. *Archives of Sexual Behaviour* **20**(1): 35.
BOHN, D.K. (1990) Domestic violence in pregnancy: implications for practice. *Journal of Nurse Midwifery* **35**(2): 86.

BORG, S. and LASKER, J. (1982) *When Pregnancy Fails.* London: Routledge and Kegan Paul.

BURNS, J. (1992) The psychology of lesbian health care. In Nicolson, P. and Ussher, J. (eds) *The Psychology of Women's Health and Health Care.* London: Macmillan.

BYRNE, J. (1994) *When Home is Where the Hurt Is.* London: BBC Radio Two Social Action Team and the Women's Aid Federations.

CARTER, A. (1979) *The Sadeian Woman – An Exercise In Cultural History.* London: Virago.

CLEMENT, S. (1994) Unwanted vaginal examinations. *British Journal of Midwifery* **2**(8): 368.

CLIFFORD, K.A. and REGAN, L. (1994) Recurrent pregnancy loss. In Studd, J. (ed.) *Progress in Obstetrics and Gynaecology,* vol. 11. Edinburgh: Churchill Livingstone.

CLULOW, C.F. (1982) *To Have and To Hold Marriage, The First Baby and Preparing Couples for Parenthood.* Aberdeen: Aberdeen University Press.

CONTRATTO, S.W. (1980) Maternal sexuality and asexual motherhood. *Signs: Journal of Women in Culture and Society* **5**(4): 766.

CORKHILL, A. (1996) Effects of the birth of a first baby on a couple's sexual relationship. *British Journal of Midwifery,* **4**(2), 70.

CURTIS, P. and DUNN, K. (1996) Sex and Sexuality. *Modern Midwife,* **6**(5), 26.

DEMYTTENAERE, K., GHELDOF, M. and VAN ASSCHE, F.A. (1995) Sexuality in the postpartum period: a review. *Current Obstetrics and Gynaecology* **5**(2), 81.

EATON, L. (1993) Going forward. *Nursing Times* **89**(46): 14.

EDELMANN, R.J. and CONNOLLY, K.J. (1994) Reproductive failure and the reproductive technologies: a psychological perspective. In Penny, G.N., Bennett, P. and Herbert, M. (eds) *Health Psychology A Lifespan Perspective.* Chur, Switzerland: Harwood Academic.

EKWO, E.E., GOSSELINK, C.A., WOOLSON, R., MOAWAD, A. and LONG, C.R. (1995) Coitus late in pregnancy: risk of preterm rupture of amniotic sac membranes. *American Journal of Obstetrics and Gynecology* **1**(1): 22.

EVANS, K. (1992) Getting back to nature. *Modern Midwife* **2**(1): 14.

GUANA-TRUJILLO, B. and HIGGINS, P. (1987) Sexual intercourse and pregnancy. *Health Care for Woman International* **8**(5): 339.

HALL, J. (1993) Attendance not compulsory. *Nursing Times* **89**(46): 69.

HENDERSON, A.F., GREGOIRE, A.J.P., KUMAR, R. and STUDD, J.W.W. (1991) The treatment of severe postnatal depression with oestradiol skin patches. *Lancet* **2**: 816.

JEBALI, C.A. (1993) A feminist perspective on postnatal depression *Health Visitor* **66**(2): 59.

JONES, A. and JONES, K. (1991) Accepting motherhood. *Nursing Times* **87**(20): 58.

JONES, K. (1990) Expectant fears. *Nursing Times* **86**(15): 36.

KELLEHER, C.J., CARDOZO, L.D., KHULLAR, V., WISE, B. and CUTNER, A. (1993) The impact of urinary incontinence on sexual function. *The Journal of Sexual Health* **3**(7): 186.

KENNEY, J.W. and TASH, D.T. (1993) Lesbians childbearing couples' dilemmas and decisions. In Stern Noera-

ger, P. (ed.) *Lesbian Health: What Are The Issues?* London: Taylor & Francis.

KITZINGER, J.V. (1992) Counteracting, not reenacting, the violation of women's bodies: the challenge for perinatal caregivers. *Birth* **19**(4): 219.

KITZINGER, S. (1982) Sexuality in pregnancy. *British Journal of Sexual Medicine* **9**: 44.

KITZINGER, S. (1985) *Woman's Experience of Sex.* London: Penguin Books.

KUMAR, R.C. (1994) Postnatal depression. *Maternal and Child Health* **19**(11): 354.

LEE, B. (1994) It all started after I had my baby. *Journal of the Royal Society of Medicine* **87**(10): 639.

LEIFER, M. (1980) Pregnancy. *Signs: Journal of Women in Culture and Society* **5**(4): 754.

LEWIS, H.S. and BOR, R. (1994) Nurses' knowledge of and attitudes towards sexuality and the relationship of these with nursing practice. *Journal of Advanced Nursing* **20**(2): 251.

MAIN, D.M., GRISSO, J.A., SNYDER, E.S., CHIU, G.Y. and HOLMES, J.H. (1993) The effects of sexual activity on uterine contractions in pregnancy. *Journal of Women's Health* **2**(2): 141.

MANDER, R. (1994). *Loss and Bereavement in Childbearing.* Oxford: Blackwell Scientific.

MARTIN, A. (1993) *The Guide to Lesbian and Gay Parenting.* London: Pandora.

MASTERS, W.H. and JOHNSON, V.E. (1966) *Human Sexual Response.* Boston: Little, Brown.

McCONVILLE, B. (1994) *Mixed Messages Our Breasts in Our Lives.* Harmondsworth: Penguin Books.

McNEILL, E. (1994) Blood, sex and hormones: A theoretical review of women's sexuality over the menstrual cycle. In Choi, P.Y.L. and Nicholson, P. (eds) *Female Sexuality Psychology, Biology and Social Context.* Hemel Hempstead: Harvester Wheatsheaf.

MILLER, L. (1995) We did it. And it was good. *The Guardian* 7 March.

MILLS, J.L., HARLAP, S. and HARLEY, E.E. (1981) Should coitus late in pregnancy be discouraged? *The Lancet* **11** (8238): 136.

NATIONAL CHILDBIRTH TRUST. VICTOR, C. and BARRETT, G. (1994) Is there sex after childbirth? *New Generation* **13**(2): 24.

NICOLSON, P. (1990) Sexuality and the transition to motherhood: an impossible dilemma? Paper presented at the 10th Annual Merseyside Conference on Clinical Psychology, Chester College.

OAKLEY, A. (1979) *Becoming a Mother.* Oxford: Martin Robertson.

OAKLEY, A. (1992) The changing social context of pregnancy care. In Chamberlain, G. and Zander, L. (eds) *Pregnancy Care in The 1990s.* Carnforth: Parthenon Publishing.

ODENT, M. (1992) It's time to let men stay away from childbirth. *London Evening Standard* 10 September.

O'DRISCOLL, M. (1994) Midwives, childbirth and sexuality 2: men and sex *British Journal of Midwifery* **2**(2): 74.

OMER-HASHI, K.H. (1994) Commentary – female genital mutilation: perspectives from a Somalian midwife. *Birth* **21**(4): 224.

PEPPERELL, R.J. and McBAIN, J.C. (1985) Unexplained infertility: a review. *British Journal of Obstetrics and Gynaecology* **92**(6): 569.

PINES, D. (1993) *A Woman's Unconscious Use of Her Body. A Psychoanalytical Perspective*. London: Virago.

PITT, B. (1991) Depression following childbirth. *Hospital Update* 17(2): 133.

PRICE, J. (1988) *Motherhood: What It Does To Your Mind*. London: Pandora.

RAPHAEL-LEFF, J. (1991) *Psychological Processes of Childbearing*. London: Chapman and Hall.

RAPHAEL-LEFF, J. (1993) *Pregnancy: The Inside Story*. London: Sheldon Press.

RCN (Royal College of Nursing) (1994) *Female Genital Mutilation. The Unspoken Issue*. London: RCN.

REAMY, K.J. and WHITE, S.E. (1985) Dyspareunia in pregnancy. *Journal of Psychosomatic Obstetrics and Gynaecology* 4(4): 263.

REAMY, K.J. and WHITE, S.E. (1987) Sexuality in the puerperium: a review. *Archives of Sexual Behaviour* 16(2): 165.

RILEY, A.J. (1989) Sex after childbirth. *British Journal of Sexual Medicine* 16(5): 185.

ROBERTSON, M.M. (1993) Lesbians as an invisible minority in the health services arena. In Stern Noerager P. (ed.) *Lesbian Health: What Are The Issues?* London: Taylor & Francis.

ROBSON, K.M., BRANT, H.A. and KUMAR, R. (1981) Maternal sexuality during first pregnancy and after childbirth. *British Journal of Obstetrics and Gynaecology* 88(9): 882.

ROYAL COLLEGE OF MIDWIVES (1994) Men at birth. News Release NR279/11/94. London: Royal College of Midwives.

SAVAGE, W. and READER, F. (1984) Sexual activity during pregnancy. *Midwife Health Visitor and Community Nurse* 20(11): 398.

SEDGWICK, L.R. (1994) Midwives' view on discussing sexual issues with clients. Unpublished BSc(Hons) midwifery dissertation. King's College University of London.

SHANNON, D. (1993) Fathers in hard labour. *Independent on Sunday* 24 October.

SHEPHERD, C.M. (1994) *HIV Infection in Pregnancy*. Hale: Books for Midwives Press.

SILVERTON, L. (1993) *The Art and Science of Midwifery*. Hemel Hempstead: Prentice Hall International.

SOUTHERN, M. (1994) Labour and sexuality. *Midwifery Matters* 61: 5.

STEVENS, P.E. (1993) Lesbian health care research: a review of the literature from 1970 to 1990. In Stern Noerager, P. (ed.) *Lesbian Health: What Are The Issues?* London: Taylor & Francis.

STUDD, J.W.W. (1992) Oestrogens and depression in women. *British Journal of Hospital Medicine* 48: 211–13.

TAYLOR, V.J. (1992) Pregnancy: a shared experience? Men's experiences and feelings about their partner's pregnancy *Journal of Advances in Health and Nursing Care* 2(2): 59.

THOMPSON, J. (1994) *Haemorrhoids The Facts*. Brentford: SmithKline Beecham, Consumer Healthcare.

TIRAN, D. and MACK, S. (eds) (1995) *Complementary Therapies for Pregnancy and Childbirth*. London: Baillière Tindall.

TOBERT, A. (1990) Sexual problems in pregnancy and the postnatal period. *Midwife Health Visitor and Community Nurse* 26(5): 177.

TOUBIA, N. (1994) Female circumcision as a public health issue. *New England Journal of Medicine* 331(11): 712.

USSHER, J.M. (1989) *The Psychology of the Female Body*. London: Routledge.

UTHAYAKUMAR, S., SHAH, P.N. and SMITH, J.R. (1994) Vaginal discharge. *Update* 49(3): 155.

VAN WERT, W.F. (1991) Sex after childbirth. *Mothering* 60 (Summer): 115.

WALLACE, R. (1989) A pregnant pause. *The Guardian* 5 December.

WALLACE, T. (1993) Management of the bladder in childbearing. *Modern Midwife* 3(1): 17.

WALTON, I. (1994) *Sexuality and Motherhood*. Hale: Books for Midwives Press.

WILES, R. (1994) 'I'm not fat, I'm pregnant': the impact of pregnancy on fat women's body image. In Wilkinson, S. and Kitzinger, C. (eds) *Women and Health Feminist Perspectives*. London: Taylor & Francis.

WOOLLEY, P. (1994) Diagnosis and management of vaginal infections. part 2. *British Journal of Sexual Medicine* 21(3): 16.

7: Unplanned pregnancy
Kati Gray

OBJECTIVES

After reading this chapter you will have considered:

♦ the practical and emotional aspects of pregnancy

♦ what is meant by an 'unplanned pregnancy'

♦ the difficulties surrounding decision-making

♦ the legal and moral considerations surrounding abortion

♦ professional dilemmas

♦ the role of the health professional.

Introduction

When a woman has an unplanned pregnancy it can be a shocking and deeply disturbing experience. An unplanned pregnancy is not a single entity in itself, but is usually preceded and followed by many incidents (of greater or lesser complexity) which together form the whole experience. This multiplicity of events, and the process of addressing and understanding them, are what will be discussed in this chapter.

Practical issues, such as giving the results of a pregnancy test, the law relating to abortion and abortion procedures, will be considered along with more emotional concerns. What an unplanned pregnancy means, how to make a decision about it and what the impact of that decision will have upon a woman's life, are not questions to which there are practical or general answers. Every woman's experience of pregnancy is a personal one. For whilst many women have unplanned pregnancies, the circumstances each of them faces, what pregnancy means to her, and what she decides to do about it, involve emotions and experiences that belong uniquely to her. Many women go through this experience in confusion and isolation, feeling desperately in need of help but not knowing where to go. The aim of this chapter is to enable you, as a health professional, to think about the practical and emotional aspects of unplanned pregnancy. Reflecting upon some of the issues discussed may facilitate and support you in your work with a woman who has, or had in the past, an unplanned pregnancy. The care of a woman in this situation can be greatly enhanced by your skilled nursing intervention, and using your skills in this area of women's health care can be a richly rewarding (albeit challenging) experience for you, too.

Defining unplanned pregnancy

When a woman has an unplanned pregnancy it is important to be clear about what this means for her as an individual. Health care workers may assume that the woman has been foolish, unlucky or careless; that her pregnancy is unwanted or that she secretly desired to be pregnant; that she ought/ought not to continue the pregnancy because of her personal circumstances; and that a decision about the pregnancy must be made quickly. On the other hand, the pregnant woman may experience a mixture of emotions such as shock, despair, anger, excitement and relief simultaneously, and consequently any hope of making a decision based on her own needs and desires may seem slim indeed.

In the midst of the potential ambivalence and confusion surrounding unplanned pregnancy it is important that you recognize that some unplanned pregnancies may have occurred 'accidentally on purpose', and that many are most definitely not unwanted. The meaning of unplanned pregnancy can only be revealed and understood in relation to an individual pregnant woman. For whilst women with unplanned pregnancies share a common reality, their experiences of that reality and their thoughts and feelings in relation to it are always deeply personal. There is no 'right' way to feel about an unplanned pregnancy. What is important is that any woman in this situation is able to discover what her feelings are.

Confirming pregnancy

A woman may suspect, feel, hope or fear pregnancy before she comes to the clinic or surgery. Often she will have used a home pregnancy testing kit, or paid a chemist to do a test for her. Therefore, when she first comes to the clinic it is helpful to establish whether a test has been done previously, and what the result was.

Obtaining this information gives the woman the opportunity to begin speaking about her reactions to being pregnant, and offers you an initial insight into her emotional response to her possible pregnancy.

In some clinics it is the policy to carry out a pregnancy test for every woman, regardless of the result of any previous test. If this is the case, it is important to explain this to her (along with the possibility of a false positive or false negative result) so that she understands the reason for the procedure. When such explanations are not given, a woman may feel that she is being disbelieved or mistrusted, or that her physical experience of pregnancy is being dismissed.

Whether a previous test has been done or not, it is necessary to inform the woman of the arrangements regarding testing (and the policy relating to giving test results) at the particular clinic she is attending. For example, whilst many clinics now offer a 'walk-in' pregnancy testing service with results available in minutes, at others it may take several days before the results can be given as the tests are sent outside the clinic to be processed.

Some clinics require the woman to make an appointment with a medical practitioner in order to be given results, whilst at others it is the nurse who fulfils this role.

Explaining the process at the outset not only avoids misunderstanding and confusion, but allows the woman to consider whether what is available at the clinic meets her individual needs.

For a number of reasons a woman may not want the result of her pregnancy test at the time she submits it. She may have come to the clinic alone but want her partner, friend or a relative to be with her when she is given the result. Or she may be on her way to work, place of study or another appointment, and not feel it is appropriate to know the result at that particular time. She may have a baby or young child in her immediate care and therefore not feel able to deal with the impact of having her pregnancy confirmed.

Alternatively, she may feel that she needs to know whether or not she is pregnant immediately and is not prepared to wait several days before the result is available.

Once the service offered at the particular clinic she is attending has been explained, the woman is in a position to choose how she wishes to proceed. You can then discuss with her the appropriate course of action. The clinic's service may be what the woman expects and wants, but if not then alternatives need to be discussed and found. Testing at another clinic, where results are available more quickly, or another appointment when her partner or friend can be present, or when she feels it would be a more appropriate time to know the result, are all possibilities that you could consider.

Unplanned pregnancy can result in a woman feeling powerless and out of control. Enabling her to exercise choice about how and when she has her pregnancy confirmed can be the first stage in the process of her regaining a sense of control within this situation, and also in her life.

Giving a pregnancy test result

When required to tell a woman what the result of her pregnancy test is, you should first give some thought to the setting. Whether a 'walk-in' service or one where she is returning for the result, the woman should be offered a quiet private space in which to sit with you. It is a courtesy to have a box of tissues available within her reach and a bin in which she can easily deposit any used tissues. If she does begin to cry tissues should not be pushed towards her as she may take it as a signal to stop crying and 'pull herself together'.

If you know in advance that the woman is coming for a pregnancy test result, extra time should be allowed. This way neither the woman nor you will be under pressure to 'get on with it' or hurry the interaction. Asking her what she thinks the result is or what she wants it to be is preferable to saying 'It's positive', 'I'm sorry to tell you . . .', 'I'm afraid that . . .', 'You're going to be a mum'. The difficulty with such statements is that they do not take account of the woman's feelings and reveal a lot about your own. For the pregnant woman, the agenda and tone of the interaction will have been set for her, rather than by her.

Alternatively, if you have already ascertained the woman's feelings about a result this will then allow her to set the agenda. She may say 'I'm terrified that . . .', 'I just know that . . .', 'I just don't know . . .', 'If I am, I'll . . .' – any of which may give you an indication of how best to continue.

The value of this approach is that you are *responding* to the thoughts and feelings of the woman rather than *leading* the interaction between you.

Once the pregnancy has been confirmed the woman should be allowed time to reflect upon this result. If she is distressed and crying she should be allowed to cry; if stunned into silence, the silence should be respected; if shouting about the unfairness or awfulness of it all, she must be allowed to express these feelings. Even for a woman who has long suspected that she is pregnant, having the pregnancy confirmed can be a shocking and extremely distressing experience. Whilst for the woman who had no idea that she was pregnant, being told that she is may make no sense to her at all. Women in this situation can need several hours or days before they are able to respond and react in any way.

Having an unplanned pregnancy confirmed means that a decision about the pregnancy has to be made. However, unless the woman is especially clear in her thoughts or has already made her decision it is always appropriate to offer her another appointment. Not only does this provide invaluable time for her to consider and reflect upon her feelings but it also provides an opportunity for her to discuss her pregnancy with her partner, family or friends. It is also a way for you to enable the woman to create space and time in which to think.

Women with unplanned pregnancies often feel very alone and that they should have already made a decision. By offering another appointment you are conveying two very important messages. First, that there is time for the woman to think about her pregnancy and to discuss her thoughts and feelings with others if she wishes. Secondly, that there is someone in a professional capacity willing to help her and therefore she does not have to manage alone.

Whilst it is often the case that a woman does not feel she wants or needs a second appointment, this in no way detracts from the value of the message conveyed when the offer is made. Moreover, given the degree of shock, disbelief and despair that the woman may experience when her pregnancy is confirmed, it is unrealistic to expect a considered decision at this stage.

The meaning of unplanned pregnancy

Before a decision can be made about her pregnancy, the woman needs to understand what becoming pregnant at this stage of her life means for her. Pregnancy may mean that contraception has failed; that a woman is fertile despite previously being told otherwise; that she had sexual intercourse when she was not expecting to and therefore was not using contraception; that she wanted to know whether she could conceive and was 'testing' her fertility; that she wants a baby; that life is chaotic and difficult and preventing pregnancy the least of her concerns.

The possible meanings of pregnancy are numerous but are always unique for the individual pregnant woman. Understanding what pregnancy means for her involves the woman being able to explore her thoughts and feelings about it, as well as the circumstances in which she became pregnant. This can be a difficult process, not least because the woman may have feelings she considers to be contradictory or mutually exclusive. It is only by acknowledging or addressing these feelings that the meaning of this specific pregnancy for this particular woman can be revealed.

The difficulty for you can be in acknowledging and tolerating the confusion and distress of the woman, whilst avoiding telling her what her pregnancy means and what she should do about it. This can be particularly difficult when the woman asks such questions as 'What do you think I should do?' or 'What's going to be best for me, please tell me?' or 'I can't decide – what would you do in my position?'

In situations such as these it is vital to remind yourself that your role is not to tell her what to do. It is to enable her to understand what her pregnancy means and then to make her own decision about it. While you can help her to explore the meaning of her pregnancy, you cannot tell her this meaning and you should not tell her what to do about it. Clearly, some women with an unplanned pregnancy will find this process much more difficult than others. Furthermore, individual life situations vary and some are far more complex than others.

A woman for whom contraception has failed within a stable, supportive relationship may feel clear about making a decision to continue her pregnancy or to have an abortion. Even so she may value the opportunity to discuss the meaning of her pregnancy, and her feelings about it, with you. She may also need practical information about antenatal care or abortion. It is important for both of you that she has, and continues to receive, the help and support she needs and is comfortable with whatever decision she has made.

Another woman may be pregnant as a result of not using contraception. This could mean that her pregnancy is the result of rape or coercive intercourse, or that she refuses or does not feel able to take control of her own fertility. She may not have any stable or supportive relationships in her life and may feel completely unable to understand or make a decision about her pregnancy.

Abortion is an issue that most people have an opinion about, but in fact nobody can be certain about their own reaction until they themselves are pregnant, and have to make a decision about whether to continue the pregnancy. Thus, a woman who has always supported a woman's right to choose an abortion and who has used contraception believing that should it fail she would choose to have an abortion, finds she cannot make that decision for herself. Similarly, a woman who has always been fiercely opposed to abortion and said that it would never be a choice she would make, can have an unplanned pregnancy and realize that abortion is the only suitable option. Another woman may say she is having an abortion because it is what her partner/mother/family or medical practitioner thinks is right for her, whilst another may simply say 'I have no choice, I have to do it'.

In these, and numerous other similar situations, it is of paramount importance that a woman recognizes she always has a choice, and that she makes that choice herself, based on her own needs and desires. For some women this is an extraordinarily difficult task and you may both recognize that the complexities involved need to be addressed before any decision about her pregnancy can be made.

If you feel it is appropriate and possible for you to address these issues with her, then it may be feasible to offer a series of appointments to explore her feelings. However, your work environment (clinic lay-out, lack of private rooms, heavy caseload, ten-minute appointments, etc.), your expertise being in other areas (e.g. practice nursing, family planning, women's health, rather than in-depth psychological and emotional counselling) and your own personal feelings may make such extended work impossible. Should this be the case, the woman should be told that although you recognize her need to discuss and try to resolve some of the complex issues, you are unable to do this with her. (This should be said using words that you feel comfortable with and are natural for you.) You can then offer to refer her to someone who has the necessary training, experience and time to do this work with her. It is helpful to have a regularly updated list of counsellors and support agencies that you can give her if, after discussion with you, a referral seems appropriate. Any cost and restrictions of the service should also be discussed prior to referral.

Referring on can be a vital aspect of the woman's care and can relieve you of a potential burden that would be impossible to cope with in your current professional role and practice.

Personal needs – professional responsibility

Unplanned pregnancy and abortion are not just professional clinical issues but also involve personal private feelings. For both male and female health care workers pregnancy, childbirth, subfertility, miscarriage, parenthood or the decision to be childless are personal issues as well as professional ones. Therefore it is of paramount importance that when working with women or couples with unplanned pregnancies you are clear about your own feelings and attitudes.

Working professionally does not mean that you are not entitled to your own views and feelings. However, it does mean that you have a responsibility to reflect upon them, and to ensure that your personal feelings neither influence nor inhibit the treatment of patients.

Clearly there are times when it may be impossible to work with women contemplating abortion. For example, if you have just had a baby, an abortion or a miscarriage; are recently bereaved; or if you are trying to conceive or are having fertility treatment, any of the above life events is likely to mean that you are very involved in your own emotional responses and possible confusion. To expect to deal with the emotions of a woman with an unwanted pregnancy who is considering an abortion is at best unrealistic, and at worst harmful for you and your patient.

The interests of the patient and yourself will best be served by referring her to someone else who is not emotionally vulnerable in the way you are at present. Not only does this ensure that the patient gets the care she needs (from someone who is able to focus on her emotional state whilst temporarily putting their own emotions to one side) but it relieves you of a potentially painful and distressing burden. When we are emotionally distraught, the emotions of others are much more difficult to tolerate and it may be impossible not to become critical and judgemental in our work.

Referring on in situations such as those mentioned above ensures you are acting professionally in the interests of the patient and also in the interest of your own well-being – which is of no less importance. It is, of course, equally important to refer on when for religious, ethical or moral reasons you choose not to become involved in the treatment of a woman seeking an abortion.

Decision-making

Counselling is an important part of the decision-making process for a woman with an unplanned pregnancy. Whilst counselling is not about giving advice, or telling the woman what to do, it does provide a space for her to explore her thoughts and feelings about her pregnancy (no matter how confused or conflicting they may seem). Thus counselling facilitates an understanding of the meaning of pregnancy for each individual woman and can provide the emotional support necessary for her to be able to make a decision.

Counselling should be offered with someone who has appropriate training and experience and who has no emotional investment in the woman's decision. Therefore, family, friends, GP, the medical practitioner agreeing to perform an abortion, reproductive health or practice nurse that the woman may know well, or any other individual with whom she has similar contact, cannot adequately fulfil the counselling role. Family and friends are likely to be emotionally involved themselves; GPs and other medical practitioners may have conflicting interests. The counsellor should be someone the woman does not know personally and to whom she feels able to speak freely, honestly and confidentially without being concerned about needing to apologize, to protect or to convince them. The skill of the counsellor lies in being able to deal with the confusion and distress of the pregnant woman, to hear the ambiguities and covert desires in what she says, and to be able to keep her or his own feelings and opinions out of the interaction between them.

The degree of distress and confusion felt by women with unplanned pregnancies varies greatly but there are few who do not welcome the opportunity of discussing their pregnancy and their feelings about it. Being someone whom the woman does not know and who will have no involvement with either her continuing pregnancy or abortion enables the counsellor to fulfil an important role that other health care professionals cannot reasonably be expected to. Counselling is offered by all the major charitable agencies and clinics (see Resources, page 149) by an increasing number of NHS services, and also by some reproductive health clinics and GP practices. It is essential that women know these services are available and that they have clear information about how to access them. A woman should be able to request, and receive, counselling as soon as she feels she needs to, and for some women several counselling sessions will be necessary before they feel able to make a decision.

No woman should proceed with an abortion unless she feels able to acknowledge that this is the choice *she*, personally, has made and feels comfortable with her decision. Once she has had an abortion she cannot alter that decision and decide to continue her pregnancy. Therefore, if there is any doubt about whether an abortion is what she wants, or feels she must choose, a woman should be offered further counselling and more time to think about her choices.

In working with women with unplanned pregnancies you may feel under great pressure to encourage or facilitate them in making a decision about whether or not to have an abortion which is an option only up to a certain stage of pregnancy for most women (see below). However, it is important to remember that a woman who ultimately cannot decide to have an abortion is making a decision to continue her pregnancy – albeit vicariously. In short, there is no necessity for a woman to be pushed or rushed into deciding to have an abortion, as her *not* making that decision could be the most important decision of all.

Abortion and the law

On 27 October 1967, royal assent was given to the Abortion Act and it became law on 27 April 1968. This act of Parliament made abortion legal only under certain circumstances (Box 7.1).

The Abortion Act of 1967 did not incorporate a time limit within which legal abortion must be carried out, but the Infant Life Preservation Act of 1929 states that it is a criminal offence to terminate a viable pregnancy. Viability was taken to be from the 28th week of pregnancy, and therefore to comply with the terms of the 1967 Act, an abortion had to be carried out before the 28th week of pregnancy.

Before an abortion could take place, the Act stated that two medical practitioners were to be in agreement that the pregnant woman's request for abortion met with one, or more, of the criteria listed in Box 7.1.

On 1 April 1991 the Human Fertilisation and

> **Box 7.1** Circumstances under which abortion is allowed under the Abortion Act 1967
> 1 The continuance of the pregnancy would involve risk to the life of the pregnant woman greater than if the pregnancy were terminated.
> 2 The continuance of the pregnancy would involve risk of injury to the physical or mental health of the pregnant woman greater than if the pregnancy were terminated.
> 3 The continuance of the pregnancy would involve risk of injury to the physical or mental health of the existing child(ren) of the family of the pregnant woman greater than if the pregnancy were terminated.
> 4 There is substantial risk that if the child were born it would suffer from such physical or mental abnormalities as to be seriously handicapped.

Embryology Act (1990) amended the 1967 Abortion Act in the following two ways:

◆ A time limit for abortion was incorporated in the Act and this was set at 24 weeks of pregnancy.

◆ The time limit stated in the Infant Life Preservation Act (which previously applied in all circumstances) was removed where there was considered to be risk to the life of the pregnant woman; risk of permanent damage to the mental or physical health of the pregnant woman; or risk that the child would be seriously handicapped.

Opponents of the legalization of abortion believe it is ethically or morally wrong, and that legalizing abortion leads to women aborting pregnancies they would otherwise carry to term. However, these beliefs are not borne out by research. Whilst the question of whether or not abortion is morally acceptable can only properly be decided by the pregnant woman; making abortion illegal does not prevent women having abortions. A report published in 1947 estimated that there were 100 000 illegal abortions annually in England and Wales (Chance *et al.*, 1947), and other researchers have drawn similar conclusions (Francome, 1977). Moreover, enquiries into maternal deaths revealed that mortality in England and Wales due to illegal abortion fell from 77 during 1961–63 to one in 1979–81, and to zero since 1981 (DOH, 1994).

It is evident that whilst making abortion legal does not interfere in any way with a woman's right to choose to continue her pregnancy, the criminalization of abortion does little to prevent a woman who does not wish to be pregnant from having an abortion, even though exercising this choice may cost her her life.

The fact that abortion in the UK has been legal for nearly 30 years does not mean that all women have equal access to NHS abortion services. The interpretation of the clauses of the Act is liberal by some medical practitioners and extremely strict by others. District Medical Officers are under no obligation to provide abortion services and this means that while in some areas women requesting abortions are seen and treated swiftly within their local NHS service, for others NHS services are at best restricted and at worst non-existent. For these women there is little choice but to consult one of the charitable or private agencies. This is not only costly in financial terms (the lowest current fee for early abortion being £300) but often involves the women travelling many miles to the nearest charitable or private clinic.

In spite of the often expressed contrary view, there is no such thing as 'abortion on demand' in the UK. To have a legal abortion means the criteria of the Abortion Act have to be fulfilled and that two medical practitioners have to consent to a woman's request for an abortion. For women in areas where there is no NHS provision of abortion services, it also requires a considerable financial outlay and a great deal of determination to find the appropriate agencies.

Abortion procedures

When a woman has had her pregnancy confirmed, received counselling, had medical consultations and had time to consider the choices available to her, she may decide to abort her pregnancy. Where NHS services are available, this can be done at a local hospital. Where there is not adequate NHS provision or when a woman has the financial resources to allow her to choose where to be treated, she may be seen by one of the charitable or private clinics. Whether in the NHS or private sector, the method by which the abortion is carried out is usually defined by the gestation of her pregnancy (Box 7.2).

> **Box 7.2** Methods of abortion
>
> *Early abortion*
> ♦ Suction termination of pregnancy (STOP)
> ♦ Medical termination of pregnancy (MTOP).
>
> *Mid-trimester and late abortion*
> ♦ Dilatation and evacuation (D and E)
> ♦ Prostaglandin abortion.

Suction termination of pregnancy (STOP)

This procedure is similar to a dilatation and curettage (D and C) (see Chapter 17). A STOP can be carried out under local or general anaesthesia and is usually a day-case procedure up to around 12 weeks of pregnancy.

The woman is admitted to the hospital or clinic having had nothing to eat or drink for at least six hours. She is taken to the operating theatre where either local anaesthesia is administered to the cervix (this is not usually offered after nine weeks of pregnancy) or she has a general anaesthetic. The surgeon then dilates the cervical canal sufficiently to allow insertion of an aspiration cannula into the womb. Vacuum aspiration is then used to remove the pregnancy, but it is not necessary to perform a D and C at this stage of pregnancy. The procedure takes approximately ten minutes and is followed by a four-hour recovery period prior to being discharged. There is rarely any necessity for the woman to remain at the hospital or clinic overnight, but she will be advised to rest for 24–48 hours afterwards.

There should be no major pain or discomfort following the procedure, but mild analgesia is usually prescribed for uterine cramp or pain, should it occur. On the day of the operation, or the following day, 95% of women will bleed, but this should not be heavier or last longer than a normal menstrual period. If the bleeding becomes heavy or prolonged, the vaginal discharge begins to smell offensive, there is a sudden rise in body temperature or the symptoms of pregnancy persist, the woman should consult a medical practitioner at the hospital or clinic where the abortion took place, or at her GP practice, or local casualty department. Routine medical follow-up after the procedure is advisable to establish that a successful recovery has been made and to give the woman the opportunity to ask any questions that are important for her, now that the physical process is complete.

Most women feel physically able to resume their usual daily activities 48 hours after the operation. However, emotional recovery can take longer and some individuals might need more time before resuming work, study, childcare etc.

Medical termination of pregnancy (MTOP)

Since 1991 it has been possible for women in the UK to have medical abortions. Although at present this option is not widely available in the NHS, it is offered by the majority of charitable agencies and private clinics. Medical abortion is commonly known as taking 'the abortion pill' or RU 486.

For MTOP to be an option a woman must be:

♦ under 35 years old;

♦ a non-smoker, generally fit and healthy; and

♦ her last menstrual period must be less than 63 days prior to treatment.

Having had counselling and medical consultations the woman is given three tablets of mifepristone 200 mg (Mifegyne) to take whilst at the hospital or clinic. She is then able to go home. Two days later she returns to the hospital or clinic and is given a single vaginal pessary containing prostaglandin. Mifepristone acts by blocking the effects of progesterone (a hormone necessary for the continuation of pregnancy) and the prostaglandin pessary causes the cervix to soften and dilate, the uterus to contract and the pregnancy to be expelled.

Having taken the three original mifepristone tablets, the woman can spend that day and the following one in her usual way – working in or outside the home, or studying. When she returns to the hospital or clinic 48 hours later for the pessary insertion, she will have to remain there until the medical abortion is complete. It will usually take 4–6 hours before vaginal bleeding starts and the process is complete. She is then able to go home.

For many women, being able to continue their usual daily activities having taken the tablets, and the process being complete without the need for anaesthesia or surgical intervention, makes MTOP particularly acceptable. It is a relief for them not to have to wait for, and then undergo, a minor operation and they usually feel much more in control of what is happening during the abortion than women who have a surgical termination.

Although it seems unlikely to become the treatment of choice for the majority of women seeking abortions, MTOP is a valuable addition to the options available to women with unwanted pregnancies. As with any treatment option, women need to be informed, not only about the potential advantages, but also of the potential problems with MTOP (Box 7.3).

Box 7.3 Potential problems with MTOP

♦ There is a 5% chance that the procedure will be unsuccessful and therefore that a surgical abortion will be necessary.

♦ A third of women experience extreme discomfort, having had the vaginal pessary and may require strong analgesia.

♦ Sometimes women find seeing the expelled contents of the womb distressing.

However, once she has been told about these factors, and possible outcomes, a woman is then free to make an informed choice about whether this particular method of abortion is acceptable to and appropriate for her.

MTOP enables a woman to obtain an abortion in the very early stages of pregnancy and is ideal for a woman who is clear about not wanting to continue her pregnancy. This factor can greatly reduce both the impact of an unwanted pregnancy on day-to-day living and the emotional burden of unwanted pregnancy. It is regarded as a valuable development in women's health care by both the providers and the users of abortion services.

Mid-trimester and late abortion

Mid-trimester abortions are those carried out between 13 and 18 weeks and late abortions are those which take place from 19 weeks onwards. Although they account for less than 13% of all abortions performed in England and Wales, approximately 20 000 women each year have a mid-trimester or late abortion (Figure 7.1).

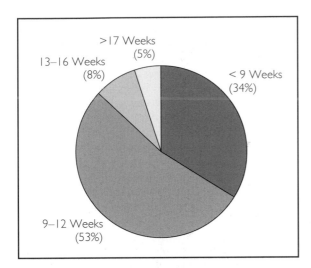

Figure 7.1 *Percentage of abortions by gestation weeks, residents of England and Wales. 1985–1991. (Data taken from OPCS, 1994).*

For most of these women, for some reason there has been a delay in recognizing their pregnancy (Box 7.4).

Box 7.4 Reasons for delay in recognizing or acknowledging pregnancy

♦ Young women may be unaware of where to go for help when they first realize they are pregnant, or else may be too frightened or embarrassed to seek help.

♦ Older women can assume that missed periods mean the beginning of the menopause rather than the beginning of pregnancy.

♦ Sometimes women fail to acknowledge pregnancy because of their precarious or unstable life situations.

♦ Women may bleed slightly during early pregnancy and wrongly assume that this is a normal period and not realize they are pregnant.

However, there are other factors that can contribute to women seeking abortions after 12 weeks of pregnancy:

♦ Lack of access to reproductive health services

♦ Poor access to general health care services

♦ Unsympathetic GPs (who may refuse to refer a woman for an abortion)

♦ Poor local resources for addressing the needs of a woman with an unplanned pregnancy

♦ Insufficient information about services and options available

♦ Where ante-natal screening has detected a fetal abnormality

♦ Where the woman has recently been given medical information about her own health, e.g. positive HIV result or cancer.

A study published by the Royal College of Obstetricians and Gynaecologists in 1984 revealed that 21% of women having NHS abortions after 20 weeks of pregnancy, and 39% of those having an abortion between 15 and 16 weeks, had been referred before they were 13 weeks pregnant (Alberman and Dennis, 1984). Women awaiting results of tests for major fetal abnormality also present for mid-trimester, rather than early, abortions and may require considerable skilled counselling both before and after an abortion.

The decision to end a pregnancy is one that few women reach easily. Whilst early abortion can be difficult to decide upon and come to terms with, the more advanced a woman's pregnancy, the greater the potential difficulties she is likely to experience – both emotional and physical.

A woman having an abortion because of fetal abnormality is likely to have planned her pregnancy and wanted the baby. The knowledge of a fetal abnormality means that she is faced with difficult and painful decisions: to continue her pregnancy, knowing her baby will be severely mentally and/or physically handicapped and may even die shortly after birth, or to abort this planned and wanted pregnancy and with it all the desires, plans and love that she has attached to it. Whether there is fetal abnormality or not, a woman having a mid-trimester or late abortion has been pregnant for several months and may even have felt the fetus moving inside her uterus. These factors add to the emotional difficulty of deciding to have an abortion as she may feel by this stage she is aborting a baby and not just a pregnancy.

Physical complications arising from abortion increase after 15 weeks of pregnancy (Clayton *et al.*, 1986) and it is not usually possible for the abortion to be done as a day-case procedure, so a longer stay is required in the hospital or clinic.

Having had counselling and medical consultations and decided that she wishes to proceed with an abortion, the woman will be admitted to the hospital or clinic. All of the standard pre-operative tests will have been carried out prior to admission, together with a pelvic ultrasound scan to establish the precise gestation of her pregnancy. There are two procedures for performing mid-trimester and late abortions: dilatation and evacuation (D and E) and prostaglandin abortion.

Dilatation and evacuation (D and E)

Prior to going to the operating theatre the woman is given a prostaglandin pessary to soften her cervix, thereby making dilation easier. Once she has been given a general anaesthetic the surgeon gently dilates the cervix and then the contents of the womb are evacuated. When this procedure is carried out, the surgeon is careful to ensure that all fetal and placental material is removed, as retained products can cause haemorrhage and infection. This procedure is usually followed by an overnight recovery period at the hospital or clinic. As long as post-operative complications do not develop, follow-up can be with the woman's GP or local reproductive health clinic.

Complications can occur at the time of surgery from perforation of the uterus or tearing of the cervix during the procedure, and post-operatively due to retained products of conception, or infection. In the longer term, damage to the cervix during the operation can lead to cervical incompetence during future pregnancies, thus increasing the risk of miscarriage.

Prostaglandin abortion

Prostaglandin abortion may be performed on a young woman in the second trimester of pregnancy (whose cervix is soft and therefore more susceptible to tearing and damage), or an older woman whose pregnancy is advanced by more than 18 weeks. This is administered in the form of vaginal pessaries or via an intravenous infusion.

A woman undergoing a prostaglandin abortion will usually be admitted to the hospital or clinic mid- to late morning. After the usual admission procedures have been carried out the gynaecologist will begin the administration of the prostaglandin.

If she is having prostaglandin pessaries, these are given four-hourly for a maximum of five doses. If an intravenous infusion is used prostaglandin is given via this route.

During these procedures the woman is cared for by skilled nursing staff. Observations of pulse, blood pressure, uterine contractions and cervical dilation are maintained. Analgesia is offered if the woman finds the process painful or too uncomfortable, and she will usually be offered fluids orally.

It is not possible to predict for an individual woman how long it will take before the prostaglandin causes uterine contractions strong enough to expel the pregnancy. However, most women are expected to abort within 12–20 hours and, once the pregnancy has been expelled, she will be taken to the operating theatre for a dilatation and curettage under general anaesthesia. This ensures that there are no retained products of conception.

The reason for beginning the prostaglandin treatment during the afternoon or early evening is so that the process hopefully will be completed during the night or early hours of the morning, allowing the woman to have her D and C during the morning theatre list. Following this she will have a recovery period at the hospital or clinic before being discharged. As with surgical abortion, routine follow-up can be with her GP or reproductive health clinic.

The procedure for mid-trimester and late abortion varies from district to district and hospital to hospital. There are some gynaecologists who are willing (and, more importantly, skilled enough) to perform mid-trimester and late abortions vaginally, whilst the woman is under general anaesthesia. For the majority of women this is understandably the treatment of choice. However, this procedure requires considerable skill on the part of the surgeon and particular dedication on the part of all staff working in the operating theatre. Whilst it may make the process easier for the pregnant woman, these late surgical abortions can undoubtedly be far more demanding and distressing for health care staff to witness.

Post-abortion follow-up

Many women choose follow-up care with their GP practice or reproductive health clinic rather than returning to the hospital or clinic where they had their abortion. This may be because a woman prefers to be seen by someone she knows in familiar surroundings. Alternatively there may be reasons for her not wanting to return to the place where her abortion was carried out:

♦ If she felt she was treated unsympathetically or disrespectfully it is unlikely she would wish to return.

♦ If the process was painful, complicated or distressing she may be reluctant to seek further care from that source.

♦ If the hospital or clinic was a great distance or difficult to reach from her home it may be impractical for her to return.

Conversely, a woman who has had a positive experience with staff and an uncomplicated treatment from a local service may also be unwilling to return for follow-up care. She may find it just too painful to return to the building where her abortion was performed and she may fear either the memories it could evoke, or being overwhelmed by sadness or grief. She may also dread a re-emergence of the physical symptoms of pregnancy, or even a more or less temporary desire to still be pregnant; whilst for a woman for whom the decision to have an abortion was particularly difficult, going back to the hospital or clinic could be like 'returning to the scene of the crime'.

So for all these reasons, and more, you may find yourself in your clinical setting being responsible for the follow-up care of a woman who has recently had an abortion. Of course her physical recovery or lack of it is a medical matter, but by asking about her health, whether the post-abortion bleeding has stopped, and if the symptoms of pregnancy have abated, you could help to establish whether or not further medical intervention is necessary. If it seems clear that her pregnancy has ended and that there are no physical complications following the abortion, you could then ask the woman how she is feeling generally. For some women, this invitation to speak about how they are feeling is a vital aspect of follow-up care. It may also be the first time anyone has asked her how she is feeling.

A woman who has post-operative complications may feel physically unwell, confused and angry. She may not understand what is happening and could believe that her physical complications are due to something she has done, or failed to do.

The opportunity to talk about her feelings and to have the necessary explanations about the problems she is experiencing, and their treatment, is extremely valuable.

No matter how clear a woman feels about her decision to have an abortion, post-operative complications often give rise to feelings of guilt and self-doubt. 'Did I do the right thing?' 'Is this my punishment for having an abortion?' 'Am I still pregnant?' are all questions that a woman may repeatedly ask herself, and ask you. They are not questions you should attempt to answer (except perhaps the one about remaining pregnant) but you should allow the woman the opportunity to talk about her own responses to her questions. For example, how does she judge whether or not she did the right thing, and what does that judgement mean for her? Or, if she does feel she is being punished for having an abortion, why does she think she should be punished, and by whom? It is through exploring the meaning of her questions with her (as opposed to giving your own answers to them) that the woman will be able to find an emotional context in which to place her experience of abortion.

Whether she has complications or not, a woman may find it extremely helpful to discuss her feelings after having an abortion (even though she may not request, or require, formal post-abortion counselling). An appointment for a post-abortion medical check, for contraceptive supplies or a cervical smear can all provide an opportunity for you to discuss with her whatever feelings about her abortion she may have.

In the days immediately afterwards many women feel extremely sad and tearful and often talk about feelings of emptiness, or of feeling nothing. In talking with these women, you may discover that in their own individual ways they are engaged in the process of mourning. Freud in 1915 wrote that when we suffer a loss we mourn, and mourning involves feelings of loss, grief and sadness, losing interest in the world around us, being preoccupied with whatever (or whoever) is lost and constantly seeking its (or their) return. The statement that 'Those who mourn may mimic madness to the observer's eye', aptly expresses not only the feelings of the woman who is mourning, but also those of people who come into contact with her at this time. Yet this is no madness. The fact that abortion is a loss which the woman has chosen in no way mitigates her feelings of loss and sadness. The emotional well-being of each one of us is dependent upon being able to mourn during times of loss (see also page 61). It is a slow, painful process, but for most it reaches an end, and the woman is able to resume day-to-day living, having ceased to mourn.

Sadly, for some grief does go wrong, and mourning can become depression. If a woman is still struggling with feelings of loss and grief many weeks or even months after her abortion, she should be offered referral to a formal counselling service. This will give her the opportunity to discuss her feelings with someone who is trained for this work, and able to offer the time and support she requires.

Of course, it may not always be immediately obvious that a woman is having emotional difficulties following an abortion, but these difficulties may be expressed in other ways. For example, a woman may be reluctant to have a pelvic examination or a cervical smear taken. She may not come for, or may cease requesting, contraceptive supplies, and she may become overanxious about vaginal infections or pelvic pain and discomfort. Sensitive questioning may reveal that she is having problems maintaining a sexual relationship (or has even stopped any kind of sexual activity altogether) since her abortion. At the time of requesting an abortion, or immediately afterwards, it is very common for a woman to say she does not want contraceptive supplies because she does not ever intend having sexual intercourse again. Happily, for most women this is not an intention that endures! For those who have not felt able to resume sexual relationships, referral to a counselling service may be the most appropriate and helpful form of treatment.

In the longer term, unresolved grief and sadness about an abortion may re-emerge during a later pregnancy; at the time of her first child's birth; pre- or post-hysterectomy; during the menopause and following a daughter's pregnancy, abortion or first child being born. A woman receiving treatment for gynaecological cancer may have her recovery impeded by unresolved feelings about a previous abortion or abortions. She might have subconscious thoughts that she is being punished, or that she was damaged in some way by the abortion procedure. Such thoughts can be deeply troubling to her, especially if she has not had children at the time of her diagnosis and treatment. The anniversary of her abortion, or the expected birthday of her potential baby, are dates a woman may remember many years later and, in some cases, for the rest of her life.

This may mean that a woman attending a reproductive health clinic, an antenatal clinic, a well-woman clinic or GP surgery may need the issue of past abortion to be addressed, regardless of how long ago it was, and of her age and her current reason for attending the clinic. The fact that unresolved grief does not go away (thus a woman may continue to suffer many years later) means that the grief is accessible, can be worked with and the woman helped. Your awareness of this, together with sensitive picking up on clues about sexual difficulties, depression, etc. can be the first step toward a woman being able to overcome her difficulties following an abortion – no matter how long after this may be.

Professional dilemmas

If for personal, religious or ethical reasons you feel unable to actively participate in the care of a woman undergoing an abortion you still have a professional responsibility to ensure that the woman receives the nursing care and help she requires. Abortion is always a regrettable and sober matter, for pregnant women and health care professionals alike. It is undertaken for reasons which are considered and deeply personal for the woman concerned, and believed to be serious and proper by those providing abortion services. However, there are some circumstances where you may feel the understandable dilemmas about abortion to be greater than usual (Box 7.5).

> **Box 7.5** Some situations in which professional dilemmas may arise
>
> ♦ Repeat abortions
> ♦ Abortions for young women under 16
> ♦ HIV positive women and abortion
> ♦ Abortion following subfertility treatment
> ♦ Abortion for fetal abnormality.

Repeat abortions

Women who have repeated abortions present perhaps the greatest challenge of all. You may feel angry at what you believe to be their irresponsibility, frustrated because they fail to use adequate contraception and distressed because there appears to be little that you (or anyone else) can do to help them avoid unwanted pregnancy.

One unwanted pregnancy may be considered a mistake, two seen as unfortunate but, after that, compassion and empathy often begin to run out. It is even believed that women who have several abortions are simply using abortion as a form of contraception. Sadly for the minority of women (and in the UK they are a minority) who present for repeat abortions, little in their lives tends to be simple.

Some women have repeat abortions because they have repeated failures with contraception. The pill does not suit them, the IUD caused pelvic problems, they conceived whilst using the diaphragm, their partner is allergic to rubber, etc. As we approach the end of the twentieth century it is a regrettable fact that we still do not have safe, reliable contraception for every woman who wants it.

Other women have repeat abortions because each time they become pregnant their relationship founders and they do not feel able to continue a pregnancy unsupported. Some women conceive as a result of forced intercourse within an abusive relationship. They did not want or plan to have sexual intercourse and therefore were not using (or were prevented from using) contraception. There are also women who repeatedly become pregnant because they never use contraception, and who then go on to have abortions because they have no wish to have a baby or to be a mother. The desire to be pregnant (whether conscious or unconscious) is not necessarily the same as the desire to have a baby and to be a mother. Whilst acknowledging and understanding this difference is a complex and difficult process, it is worth while remembering that for some women this difference does exist.

Another reason why some women repeatedly become pregnant whilst not using contraception is that for them life is a chaotic and constant struggle. Taking control in any area of their lives may feel impossible and that often includes control of their fertility. There is no single reason why women are willing to risk pregnancy but have no wish to have a baby, or why chaos and struggle are the ruling forces of women's lives. What individuals in these situations need is skilled help to enable them to begin to understand what their repeat pregnancies

and abortions may mean. Through understanding what is being expressed by her actions, a woman will hopefully be enabled to discover that she can make other choices, including the choice to control her fertility or to allow herself to become a mother.

Whilst it may not be possible for you to address these complex issues, an awareness of them (together with an effort to see the woman you are working with as an individual whose personal and unique life experiences have brought her into your care) may enhance your capacity to engage professionally with a woman requesting repeat abortions.

Under-16s

When a young woman who is not yet 16 becomes pregnant there are legal considerations as well as medical ones that have to be taken into account. Legally, a young woman under 16 cannot become pregnant. In reality, for some sexual activity begins long before they are 16 and, unfortunately, this may result in an unplanned pregnancy. Before any decisions are made about her pregnancy a young woman should be offered counselling with a trained counsellor. The paradox of a 'child' making a decision about an 'adult' predicament has to be accepted by the counsellor, and the wishes of the young woman must be seen as paramount. It may take several counselling sessions before the fear, confusion and distress felt by the young woman can be worked through. At all times her right to confidentiality must be respected and she should be assured that contact will not be made with parents/guardian, GP or anyone else, without her consent.

The circumstances in which she became pregnant, whether she has a regular partner and what support (if any) she currently has, must all be addressed, together with what it is she wants to do now that she is pregnant. Every pregnant woman has the right to choose whether to continue her pregnancy or to have an abortion, and this right applies equally to those under 16. If the wishes of her parents/guardian conflict with her own, then the counselling process must address this. If she does not want her parents/guardian to know about her pregnancy and decides to have an abortion, this can be legally carried out as long as the medical practitioner is satisfied that she/he has done all that is possible to encourage parental involvement, and that the young woman is mature enough to understand the consequences of her choice and the abortion procedure.

Young women often present later in pregnancy (see page 141) and therefore clear information about what abortion entails and what to expect afterwards is an important aspect of care. This may be part of the role you are called upon to fulfil. Therefore ensure you have all the necessary information to hand when seeing her. Ask if there are any questions she wishes to ask and do not be afraid to check whether she feels she has had enough time to discuss things with a counsellor, doctor or anyone else involved in her care. It may be worth while suggesting that she asks a parent/guardian, partner or friend to go with her to the hospital or clinic, and encourage them to ask questions on her behalf, if necessary.

The experience of pregnancy and abortion may leave a young woman feeling different to and separate from her peer group and thus unable to utilize her usual support network. Therefore, a follow-up appointment is an important opportunity for her to be able to discuss her feelings. If you are offering the follow-up care, be aware that young women do not mourn or grieve any less than older women, and that because they have returned to school or college after an abortion it does not mean that life is 'back to normal'.

A young woman may feel she has to protect her family, friends and others from her grief, or else she may feel so guilty and embarrassed herself that she does not want others to see her emotions. A follow-up appointment allows you to establish whether she is physically and emotionally well after her abortion, as well as to address the important issue of future contraception. If you do not feel that the service in which you work is able to meet the needs of a young woman pre- and post-abortion, she can always be referred to a dedicated young person's reproductive health service (see Resources, page 150).

Finally, it can be very difficult to work with a pregnant under-16 year old, particularly if you have teenage children yourself. Parental emotions may take over and you find yourself asking 'What would I do in this situation?' or feeling that 'I'd want to know', 'I'd want to help'. However, it is not as a parent that this young woman is seeking your help but as a professional upon whose skills

and objectivity she is depending. If you find the conflict between your experience as a parent and your professional role too great, you should not attempt to work with this young woman. Referring her to someone else at the initial stages will be the best thing for both of you.

Women who are HIV positive

It is not within the scope of this chapter to address all the health issues relating to a woman being HIV positive, however a brief consideration of some issues concerning pregnancy is appropriate.

When a woman who is HIV positive has an unplanned pregnancy, she faces all the dilemmas that any other woman in this situation may experience, but in addition, her pregnancy raises issues concerning her own health and the health of her baby (if she decides to continue her pregnancy).

Every woman who has an unplanned pregnancy has a right to receive the help and support relevant to her, to enable her to make a decision about her pregnancy. A woman who is HIV positive may assume (and may find that others assume) that she has to have an abortion, and therefore that there is no decision-making process to be gone through. This assumption is not justified on medical grounds, and it is likely to inhibit the pregnant woman's exploration of her thoughts and feelings about her pregnancy. A woman who is HIV positive may need your time and support, in the same way any other woman with an unplanned pregnancy does. However if she has specific concerns about the effects of pregnancy upon herself, and her potential baby, she should be referred to specialist services.

Someone who is HIV positive may already be in contact with health professionals, and may wish to seek information and support from them, as part of the decision-making process in relation to pregnancy. In addition there are self-help groups and organizations that she could contact.

Whilst an important factor in the decision-making process, a positive HIV status should not be seen by you as *the* issue in your work with this woman. Like any other woman with an unplanned pregnancy, she may be shocked, distressed, need time to think and need to speak with a partner, family or friends (as well as needing sound impartial medical information) before a decision can be made. Moreover, like every other pregnant woman, the decision whether (or not) to continue the pregnancy must be hers.

Abortion following subfertility treatment

Occasionally, a woman who has been receiving treatment for subfertility problems will become pregnant, only to request an abortion. Whatever her personal reasons for this request, it is clearly an indication that something, somewhere is wrong.

It may be that in the months or years since treatment began her desire in relation to having a baby has lessened or ceased. The idea of pregnancy and motherhood may have been attractive but the reality much less so. A woman may become pregnant with someone other than her regular partner and, in spite of her desire for a child, feel unable to continue this particular pregnancy. The pregnancy may have occurred at a time when she was relinquishing all hope of pregnancy or when she (or her partner) were about to change jobs, home, country of residence, or face some similar major life-upheaval.

Whatever the reason for her abortion request the woman must also reassess her desire for future pregnancy. If the probability of future conception is low, is abortion the right thing for her? Once the forthcoming life-events have taken place, is not being pregnant going to be what she wants? Do she and her partner need to reassess their desire for a child? Should she continue with fertility treatment? Addressing these issues while she is still pregnant will enable the woman to make a clear informed choice about this particular pregnancy and about future treatment and conception.

Liaison with the hospital or clinic that she attends for fertility treatment may be valuable for her, as could joint appointments for her and her partner. It may take more than one appointment before she (or they) can begin to think clearly about her current situation and the implications of her request for an abortion. Do not hesitate, therefore, to offer more than one appointment with you or, if you feel her particular situation requires more formal help, to suggest referral for counselling.

Fertility treatment is about becoming pregnant; abortion is about ceasing to be pregnant. For a woman who is in receipt of the former to be requesting the latter, indicates that somewhere

between the two, things have become very confused. Your willingness to recognize this and the offer of time for discussion could enable a woman to begin to address, and perhaps resolve, some of that confusion.

Abortion for fetal abnormality

A woman who has decided to have an abortion because of fetal abnormality is likely to be in the second or third trimester of her pregnancy. She is also probably choosing to abort a pregnancy that was planned and a baby that was wanted. This can only add to the difficulties and distress involved in reaching the decision to have an abortion.

Where there is a known risk of abnormality or hereditary life-threatening disease a woman and her partner may have received genetic counselling. However, this does not mean that the emotional aspects of abortion will have been addressed. Knowing the risks involved and the chances of carrying a healthy pregnancy to term does not make the choices a woman faces any easier, or mean that an abortion has been prepared for. You should be aware that this may not be the first time this woman has become pregnant, only to be told that her pregnancy is not healthy and thus decided to have an abortion.

In addition to the guilt she may feel for wanting to 'keep on trying' to have a healthy baby, a woman also has to deal with the loss of her unhealthy ones. This loss is not only physical but is also a loss of her hopes, her plans and of her 'family' – that she may in fact never have. For all women pregnancy is a symbolic as well as a physical and emotional experience. The symbolism of a deformed, disabled or diseased baby is extremely powerful and distressing and, for a woman who may never be able to have the healthy baby or family she desires, it may feel symbolic of a whole aspect of her life, and of herself.

The fact that a woman at risk of having a pregnancy with a fetal abnormality may be seen in designated ante-natal clinics or diagnostic units, does not mean that she is any less in need of your skilled help than other women before or after an abortion. Indeed, she may greatly value the opportunity to speak with someone whom she may see as being less focused on the process of testing and diagnosis, and therefore more able to discuss feelings, rather than facts, about her pregnancy.

Fostering and adoption

An unplanned pregnancy may be unwanted but unwanted pregnancy does not always result in abortion. For many reasons a woman may not wish, or feel able to, care for a baby but she may also know that abortion is not an option for her. Continuing pregnancy to term and giving up the baby for fostering or adoption is a choice few women make since the Abortion Act became law. It does, however, remain an option that is open to women with an unplanned pregnancy and for some it is the choice they make.

A woman considering continuing her pregnancy and then having her baby fostered or adopted needs to ask questions and to know facts. Therefore, it is vital that she discusses these options with social workers, childcare and legal professionals. She needs to know what the process involves, what her rights are throughout (and afterwards, in relation to her child), and how to halt the process once it has begun, should she choose to.

Having an infant fostered or adopted is a serious step to take. A woman may not realize that she is ultimately relinquishing all her rights in relation to her child and she needs time to consider the impact of this choice upon her own life, as well as her child's.

In your work with women with unplanned pregnancy, fostering and adoption are options that you should bear in mind and may perhaps choose to raise with some women. Any woman who then wishes to give serious consideration to these choices should be referred to the appropriate agencies and charities in the first instance (in order that she gets adequate accurate information), and then to the appropriate professionals.

When working with older women across the spectrum of women's health care, it is important to remember that any one of them who had an unplanned pregnancy before the 1967 Abortion Act may have given up a child for adoption, not out of choice but rather because there was no other option available at that time. For these women grief about their lost – usually first – child is often compounded by the awfulness of not knowing anything about their son or daughter – where they are or who they have become. A woman who has had this experience may be in no less need of help than a woman who has had an abortion.

Contraception

Any woman requesting an abortion does so because she feels unwilling or unable to continue her pregnancy and/or care for a baby. With the possible exception of women who have been raped and those for whom fetal abnormality was detected, this usually means that the woman neither wishes to be pregnant at the present time, nor in the near future. In order that she receives complete care at this time the issue of contraception must be addressed.

At what stage this issue is raised, and by whom, is a moot point, and it would be inappropriate to lay down hard and fast rules, as clearly contraception is not just a practical matter. The circumstances in which a woman became pregnant, how she feels about her decision for an abortion and the existence (or not) of a current sexual relationship, will all affect her thoughts and feelings about contraception. It would be negligent in the extreme for contraception not to be discussed at some point during the process of confirming an unplanned pregnancy and having an abortion. However, for the individual woman the appropriate time for this discussion varies greatly.

Before the decision about her pregnancy has been made; when she is emotionally distraught; or immediately before or after the abortion procedure are times when a discussion about contraception is wholly inappropriate. At any other stage of the process the issue may be raised, and not infrequently it is the woman herself who raises it. Deciding on a method of contraception means that clear information must be available, together with specialist help and advice (see Chapter 9). If it is a professional who raises the issue, this should always be at a time appropriate to the individual woman and in the form of an offer of help (as opposed to a requirement of the referral to the hospital or clinic, or the abortion being carried out). For whilst it is an essential aspect of her care at this time, it is one which needs to be approached with sensitivity and great skill.

Conclusion

An unplanned pregnancy can cause confusion and despair in pregnant women and health care professionals alike. Pregnant women may despair of ever getting the support and care that they need; the professionals may feel confused by their emotional response to this situation, and wonder what help they can usefully give. Yet, a willingness by you, the professional, to honestly reflect upon your own feelings whilst allowing those of the pregnant woman to be central, can enable this confusion and despair to be transformed. Using your skills to facilitate the woman's thinking and speaking about the dilemma she is currently facing, and ensuring that she has all the factual information she wants, can bring relief and promote well-being where previously there seemed to be only pain and anguish.

An awareness of the practical issues, together with a determination to avoid assumptions, decision-making on the woman's behalf and judgements about her and her situation, can facilitate a potentially disastrous life-experience becoming one that is negotiated without long-term suffering. It can be a demanding area of work, and you should refer on without hesitation if the impact upon you feels too great, or the situation too complex. Yet it is also a field where your skills are invaluable, and using them can be a rewarding and fulfilling experience for you; whilst for your patient, the efforts made on her behalf bring benefits both profound and enduring.

Resources

Charitable abortion services

London

British Pregnancy Advisory Service
7 Belgrave Road, London SW1V 1QB
Tel. 0171 828 2484 (Central London); 0171 602 3804 (West London); 0181 809 6600 (North London)

Marie Stopes
108 Whitfield Street, London W1P 6BE
Tel. 0171 388 2585

Pregnancy Advisory Service
11–13 Charlotte Street, London W1P 1HD
Tel. 0171 637 8962/0500 400973

Nationwide

British Pregnancy Advisory Service
(Head Office, Solihull, West Midlands Tel. 01564 793225 for full details of branches throughout the country)
Birmingham Tel. 0121 643 1461
Glasgow Tel. 0141 204 1832
Liverpool Tel. 0151 709 1588

Marie Stopes
Leeds Tel. 01132 440685
Manchester Tel. 0161 832 4260

Counselling and advisory services

A = Advice
C = Counselling

Abortion Anonymous (C)
Tel. 0171 350 2229
Free telephone counselling service

Asian Family Counselling Service (C)
Equity Chambers, 40 Piccadilly, Bradford BD1 3NN
Tel. 01274 720486

British Association for Counselling (C)
1 Regent Place, Rugby, Warwickshire CV21 2PJ
Tel. 01788 578328 (information); 01788 550899 (office)
Can provide details of counsellors nationwide

Citizens Advice Bureaux (A)
(Details of local services are in telephone directories, Yellow Pages etc)

Dublin Well Woman Centre (A & C)
35 Lower Liffey Street, Dublin 1
Tel. 0103531 728051/728095

Family Institute Barnados (C)
Ben Kennedy, 105 Cathedral Road, Cardiff CF1 9PH
Tel. 01222 226532

Healthrights (A)
157 Waterloo Road, London SE1 8XS
Tel. 0171 633 9377

Irish Family Planning Association (C)
5–7 Cathal Brugah Street, Dublin 1
Tel. 0103531 727363

Ulster Pregnancy Advisory Service (A)
719A Listown Road, Belfast BT9 7GU
Tel. 01232 381345 (A & C)

United Kingdom Council for Psychotherapy (C)
Regent's College, Inner Circle, Regent's Park, London NW1 4NS
Tel. 0171 487 7554
Can provide details of registered counsellors and psychotherapists throughout the UK

Women's Counselling & Resource Centre (A & C)
1st Floor McIver House, Cadogan Street, Glasgow G2
Tel. 0141 227 6006/6020

Women's Health (A)
52–54 Featherstone Street, London EC1Y 8RT
Tel. 0171 251 6580

Contraception services

For further details see resource list of Chapter 9 (p. 216)

Young people's services

Brook Advisory Centres
National Office: 0171 713 9000 will provide details of local clinics nationwide providing contraception, abortion advice, pregnancy testing, counselling and health information

Brook Advisory Helpline
Tel. 0171 617 8000 (24 hour nationwide information and advice helpline)

National Association of Young People's Counselling and Advisory Services
Magazine Business Centre, 11 Newmarket, Leicester LE1 5SS
Tel. 01162 558763
Referral can be made to a service for young people in areas throughout the UK

Rape crisis centres

Rape Crisis Centre
PO Box 69, London WC1X 9NJ
Tel. 0171 837 1600

24 hour crisis line for women and girls who have been raped. Also have details of Rape Crisis Centres throughout the UK

Rape and Sexual Abuse Support Centre
PO Box 908, London SE25 5EL
Tel. 0181 688 0322 (Helpline)

Fetal abnormality

Support around Termination for Abnormality
73–75 Charlotte Street, London W1P 1LB
Tel. 0171 631 0280/0285
Pre and post abortion advice and support

Adoption and fostering

British Agencies for Adoption and Fostering
11 Southwark Street, London SE1 1RQ
Tel. 0171 407 8800
Information about adoption and fostering and details of agencies nationwide

Post Adoption Centre
8 Torriano Mews, Torriano Avenue, London NW5
Tel. 0171 284 0555

Support for continuing pregnancy

Department of Social Security
Tel. 0800 666555 – Freephone
Confidential information and advice about welfare benefits

Gingerbread
16 Clerkenwell Close, London EC1R 0RA
Tel. 0171 336 8183/8184
Self help groups for one-parent families plus information about groups nationwide

Life
83 Margaret Street, London W1N 7HB
Tel. 0171 637 1529
This is an anti-abortion agency but they offer free counselling and advice to women who are willing to continue their pregnancy. Have centres nationwide

Lifeline
1st Floor, Ruskin Building, 191 Corporation Street, Birmingham B4 6RP
Tel. 0121 233 1641

National Childbirth Trust
Alexandra House, Oldham Terrace, London W3 6NH
Tel. 0181 992 8637
Antenatal classes, postnatal support groups, information, advice and counselling. Nationwide groups.

National Council for One Parent Families
255 Kentish Town Road, London NW5 2LX
Tel. 0171 267 1361
Information and advice on housing, welfare benefits and all other aspects of single parenthood

Scottish Council for Single Parents
13 Gayfield Square, Edinburgh EH1 3NX
Tel. 0131 556 3899
Advice and information

References

ALBERMAN, A. and DENNIS, K. (eds) (1984) *Late Abortions in England & Wales: Report of a Confidential Study*. London: Royal College of Obstetricians and Gynaecologists.

CHANCE, J. *et al.* (1947) *Backstreet Abortion?* London: Abortion Law Reform Association.

CLAYTON, S.G., LEWIS, T.L.T. and PINKER, G.D. (eds) (1986) *Gynaecology by Ten Teachers*. London: Edward Arnold.

DOH (Department of Health) (1994) *Report on Confidential Enquiries into Maternal Deaths in the United Kingdom*. London: HMSO.

FRANCOME, C. (1977) Estimating the number of illegal abortions. *Journal of Biosocial Science* **9**(4): 467–79.

FREUD, S. (1915) *Mourning and Melancholia* Standard edition Vol XIV, London: Hogarth Press.

OPCS (Office of Population, Censuses and Surveys) (1994) *Abortion Statistics, Series AB, 1985–1991*. London: HMSO.

8: Fertility problems
Mary Power ◆

OBJECTIVES

After reading this chapter you will understand:

◆ the many causes of subfertility

◆ the investigations required to establish a cause

◆ the many complex assisted reproduction techniques that are available

◆ how the stress of subfertility can affect a relationship.

Introduction

Couples are classified as subfertile if pregnancy has not occurred after one year of regular, unprotected intercourse. About one in six couples seek specialist help because of difficulty in conceiving, although this figure includes some trying for a second pregnancy (Hull *et al.*, 1985; Randall and Templeton, 1991).

As women become older their fertility decreases, and as they are born with their eggs already *in situ* in their ovaries, a woman of 40 years is therefore releasing eggs which are also 40 years old. These eggs may be of poor quality, with reduced capacity for fertilization and implantation. Sperm, on the other hand, are being produced all of the time from puberty and generally take about three months to mature, thus men tend to remain fertile until a much later age.

In general, human fertility is relatively inefficient, largely being a matter of chance. Like trying to throw a six with a dice, you may be lucky first time but there is no guarantee that you will succeed, even after many attempts. Therefore, many couples who have been trying to conceive for only a year or two actually have normal fertility and will eventually conceive without help. It is important to understand that 80–90% of fertile couples will have achieved a pregnancy after 12 months, and 95% will have done so within two years (Cooke *et al.*, 1981; Vessey *et al.*, 1986). Others will have a real cause for their subfertility, however, and therefore all deserve to be investigated. It is thought that one-third of subfertility problems are attributed to the female, one-third to the male and one-third to both of them.

Subfertile couples are under tremendous pressure and are by nature secretive, considering their problems to be very personal. This is exacerbated by the fact that some of them suffer from unexplained subfertility, which probably constitutes between 20 and 25% of all cases of subfertility. This lack of explanation can become a nightmare for both the couple and their clinician. Thus the couple, desperate for a baby, are often beset by feelings of inadequacy and guilt and many are subjected to pressures from both family and friends. They frequently have to endure comments from relatives and colleagues such as, 'So, when are you going to start a family?' and are often unsupported in coping with the emotional trauma and upset of such remarks. As their problem becomes more long-standing they may begin to blame one another, with consequent marital disharmony. Subfertility, therefore, is not only a physical disease but also a social one, affecting both individuals and society in general.

Normal physiology

Semen needs to be ejaculated close to the cervix. Sperm penetrate the cervical mucus, leaving the seminal fluid behind in the vagina. The sperm are stored in the mucus in the cervical canal for a day or two, and released in a steady stream to swim towards the Fallopian tube to meet the egg. When the egg follicle in the ovary is fully grown it ruptures to release the egg, which had previously been loosely attached to cells lining the follicle. The egg is picked up by the finger-like fimbria of the tube and is guided along the tube between the folds of its lining, which has microscopic cilia which beat towards the uterus.

Fertilization of egg and sperm occurs within the tube and the newly fertilized egg, now called an embryo, begins to divide and subdivide into 2, 4, 8 cells, etc. It remains in the tube for several days before reaching the uterus and, once there, it begins to implant itself in the endometrium, approximately seven days after ovulation. Following implantation, the embryo is then able to grow in size.

Soon after implantation, the hormone HCG (human chorionic gonadotrophin) from the embryo can enter the woman's bloodstream and so stimulates the ovarian follicle (now called a corpus luteum) to continue functioning and producing the hormone progesterone. This in turn continues to support the endometrium and prevents menstruation occurring, at which time a pregnancy test can detect the presence of HCG.

Causes of subfertility (Figure 8.1)

Female problems

Female problems may be due to failure to produce eggs, or irregular release of eggs from the ovary. Abnormal or blocked Fallopian tubes, endometriosis or hostile cervical mucus are other frequent causes of subfertility.

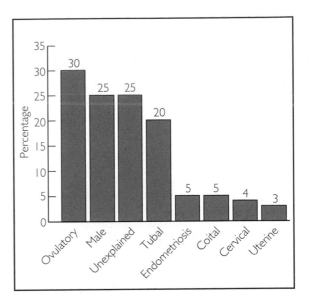

Figure 8.1 *Causes of subfertility. Note that the numbers do not add up to 100% because some couples will have more than one cause. Source: Lister Hospital.*

Ovulation

Overall, ovulatory problems are the commonest cause of subfertility. These usually arise as a result of hormonal imbalance either within the hypothalamus, the pituitary gland or in the ovaries. Common causes of this include stress, excessive exercise, weight loss, excessive prolactin production and polycystic ovarian disease.

Follicular development in the ovary is dependent upon the pituitary gland secreting the hormone FSH (follicle-stimulating hormone). If the pituitary gland is failing, for whatever reason, then follicular development will cease. This could be due to pituitary tumours or, very rarely, to pituitary infarction following post-partum haemorrhage.

Polycystic ovarian disease is a common condition in which there are a number of small cysts on the surface of the ovary, and also a hormonal imbalance. It is associated with absent or irregular periods, but may also occur in women with a normal menstrual cycle. It has been estimated that approximately 22% of all women with regular menstrual cycles have polycystic ovaries and, in fact, about 85% of women with irregular periods will have polycystic ovaries, and 93% of those with hirsutism as well as irregular periods will suffer from polycystic ovarian disease.

The major problem with polycystic ovaries is that instead of one dominant follicle developing, multiple small follicles try to develop but none of them reach maturity. This is associated with an increased level of the hormone LH (luteinizing hormone). There could also be an elevation in the level of male hormones. This condition is associated with infrequent ovulation, poor quality oocytes and a higher miscarriage rate.

Ovarian failure affects 1% of the female population under the age of 40 years. This condition could be primary ovarian failure, as in Turner's syndrome or ovarian dysgenesis, in which a woman is born without any ovarian function. These women are normally diagnosed early in life as there will be no secondary sexual development. Secondary ovarian failure may be due to a premature menopause or may occur following surgery (bilateral oophorectomy), chemotherapy or radiotherapy.

Women with anovulatory subfertility may present with amenorrhoea (primary or secondary), anovulatory menses (oligomenorrhoea or irregular cycles) or luteal insufficiency, with regular menstrual cycles but low or undetectable serum progesterone in the luteal phase. The causes of ovulatory failure are summarized in Box 8.1.

Box 8.1 Causes of ovulatory failure

Primary ovarian failure

♦ Genetic, e.g. Turner's syndrome

♦ Premature menopause.

Secondary ovarian failure

♦ Diseases of gonadotrophin regulation
  - hyperprolactinaemia
  - weight loss
  - exercise

♦ Gonadotrophin deficiency
  - pituitary tumour
  - pituitary infarction

♦ Polycystic ovarian syndrome

♦ Bilateral oophorectomy

♦ Chemotherapy

♦ Radiotherapy.

Tubal blockage

Tubal blockage can occur as a result of any infection which ascends into the Fallopian tubes, or which descends to the tubes from other sites in the peritoneal cavity, such as the appendix. It may also arise as a result of sterilization procedures or from other previous abdominal surgery.

The Fallopian tubes have a delicate internal structure which, if damaged, may impede the transport of the egg, thus preventing fertilization. If the fimbrial end of the tube is affected, the pick-up of the egg may be impaired. More extensive damage to the tube may result in complete blockage.

Salpingitis may occur following sexually transmitted diseases such as chlamydial infection or gonorrhoea and can also follow puerperal sepsis (a common cause in the Third World). Tuberculosis may lead to shortened malfunctioning Fallopian tubes. Severe endometriosis is also associated with tubal damage and impairment.

Hostile cervical mucus

Only at the time of ovulation will the cervical mucus allow the free passage of sperm. At all other times, this passage is obstructed by hormonally induced changes in the mucus. Some women have antibodies against sperm within their mucus and in these women, even at times of ovulation, sperm are often unable to pass through the cervical canal. The most common cause of poor cervical mucus is, in fact, infrequent ovulation.

Uterine conditions

There are several uterine factors which can interfere with sperm transport and the secure implantation of the fertilized egg. These include fibroids, polyps or an abnormally shaped uterus. The uterus may be bicornuate or it may contain a septum, and all of these may inhibit implantation or cause a high rate of miscarriage. Tuberculosis and other chronic infections may affect the endometrium and thus prevent implantation.

Endometriosis

Endometriosis arises when tissue which normally lines the uterus (endometrium) is found in other sites in the pelvis (see also page 415). At the time of menstruation, bleeding occurs from this tissue and can give rise to pain and dyspareunia. The presence of spots of endometriosis in the peritoneal cavity does not in itself constitute a cause for subfertility. With moderate and severe endometriosis, however, there does seem to be a connection and these cases are linked with a disruption of the anatomy of the Fallopian tubes and ovaries, due to the presence of scar tissue. Endometriosis is also associated with cysts on the ovaries, and these may prevent ovulation from occurring.

Male problems

Abnormalities in the semen are primarily due to a defect in sperm production by the testicles. The cause is usually unknown, but occasionally may be associated with previous infections, excessive drinking or smoking, or simply to stress. The presence of a varicocoele, a condition in which there is an increase in the blood flow around the testicles due to dilated veins, may lead to a rise in the temperature around the testicles, affecting sperm production and motility. Failure to produce sperm is occasionally hormonal and this is normally associated with the absence of secondary sexual characteristics and impotence.

Certain drugs and the administration of radiotherapy may also have a detrimental effect on the production of sperm, as can severe viral infection such as mumps.

Obstruction or absence of the vas deferens is an important cause of male subfertility. In this situation, sperm and semen production are normal but there will be no sperm in the ejaculate. Obstruction of the vas may follow infection such as tuberculosis, and may also follow trauma to the testicle. There is also an association between congenital absence of the vas and cystic fibrosis.

Antisperm antibodies may be present in the semen, and these attack the sperm and inhibit their motility. This condition commonly occurs following reversal of a vasectomy, but may also be related to previous infections or injury.

Sexual problems

The couple may not be making love very frequently due to pressure of work, stress or other factors. Vaginismus or even non-consummation of the relationship may be causes, or there may even be serious psychological factors involved which need

to be identified and treated with as much understanding and sensitivity as the physical problems that are more generally found.

Basic investigations

A couple who are concerned should be seen and counselled, regardless of the duration of their subfertility. Very often, couples who present at an early stage have particular concerns or they themselves perceive they have a problem which is worth discussing. Seeking help is often a very difficult step for them, and it may take a lot of courage to discuss something about which they feel deeply embarrassed or upset. Patients are all different in their needs, some merely require reassurance that they are doing everything correctly, whereas some want active treatment. If the woman is over 37 years, however, it is advisable to refer them to a specialist centre sooner rather than later, as time may be at a premium.

General indications for referral to a specialist clinic are listed in Box 8.2.

Box 8.2 Indications for referral to specialist clinic

♦ Women over 35 years with 6–12 months' subfertility

♦ Women with a one year history of subfertility

♦ Elevated FSH ovarian failure

♦ Failure to respond to clomiphene

♦ Possibility of tubal or pelvic disease

♦ Abnormal semen analysis

♦ Negative post-coital test.

History and examination

A full medical history should be taken from both partners, and this should include any previous history of pregnancy or miscarriage. Previous methods of contraception will also need to be recorded. The menstrual history is of great importance and the length of time between each menstrual period should be noted, as should the frequency of intercourse. Even questions as basic as, 'Are you making love?', 'How often?' and 'Do you know when your fertile period is?' should always be asked and can help give a better overall view of the problem.

A general examination of the woman should include weight, height, blood pressure and abdominal examination. A cervical smear and *Chlamydia* titres should be performed where appropriate, along with a pelvic examination. HIV testing for couples undergoing infertility investigations is left to the discretion of the individual unit. A couple where one or both partners are HIV positive may find it difficult to find a unit to treat them due to the moral, ethical and legal implications.

Lesbian women who are wishing to become pregnant face additional problems as infertility treatment for them is controversial and not necessarily every unit will consider their needs a priority. However, in units that do treat lesbian women with donor sperm (either from a known or an anonymous donor) counselling is mandatory as in any other situation where donors are used to provide either eggs or sperm.

Hormonal profile

Preliminary investigations should be organized for the woman, the most important being to confirm ovulation by taking blood in the mid-luteal phase of her cycle for assay of progesterone. If the cycle is irregular, varying from 28 to 50 days, then weekly plasma progesterone estimations should be carried out starting on day 21. However, it should be emphasized that these results can only be interpreted in relation to the timing of the next menstrual cycle (see also page 393).

Temperature charts are of limited use, and couples should be discouraged from completing them. They may or may not provide evidence of ovulation, but many couples experience unnecessary anxiety and worry because their temperature charts do not follow the textbook pattern, despite the fact that there is a normal menstrual cycle and proven ovulation.

Another method of detecting ovulation which has gained popularity recently, is the use of commercially available LH urine testing kits. These are simple to use home kits similar to pregnancy test kits, and testing is normally performed around the time of expected ovulation in order to detect the early signs of mid-cycle LH rise.

In women with amenorrhoea, the important investigations are measurement of serum FSH, prolactin levels and an oestrogen assay. The main purpose of a serum FSH measurement is to exclude primary ovarian failure, in which FSH concentrations are invariably elevated.

A common cause of secondary amenorrhoea is hyperprolactinaemia, therefore a serum prolactin is also vital. Stress may result in transient and, in some cases persistent hyperprolactinaemia, therefore further measurements should be undertaken. If hyperprolactinaemia is confirmed, underlying causes including primary hypothyroidism should be excluded, therefore the TSH (thyroid-stimulating hormone) should be evaluated. Finally, it may be necessary to perform a CT scan to eliminate a pituitary tumour.

Where the woman is complaining of irregular cycles it is necessary to carry out an LH assay, which is characteristically high in women suffering from polycystic ovarian disease.

Ultrasound scan

A pelvic ultrasound scan is now a mandatory investigation in the treatment of subfertility. It allows for accurate assessment of the size and shape of the uterus and ovaries, and polycystic ovaries are mainly diagnosed using this procedure. Other ovarian cysts can also be demonstrated, e.g. chocolate cysts, which are associated with endometriosis. A scan can also detect the presence of uterine fibroids, polyps and other uterine abnormalities.

Semen assessment

Semen analysis forms a fundamental part of the assessment of the subfertile couple. As male subfertility constitutes at least a third of all causes of subfertility, this simple test should be performed at the very beginning of subfertility investigations, although there is still uncertainty about the minimum values associated with fertility or with the ability to fertilize human oocytes. The World Health Organization's standards for 'normal' semen samples, and the minimum parameters which should be reported are listed in Box 8.3.

> **Box 8.3** WHO criteria for minimal normal semen parameters
> ♦ Volume 2–5 ml
> ♦ Concentration greater than 20 million/ml
> ♦ Motility greater than 40% motile
> ♦ Morphology greater than 40% normal forms
> ♦ White blood cells less than 1 million/ml.

Volume

Seminal fluid makes up the vast proportion of the ejaculate and is composed of secretions mainly from the prostate gland and the seminal vesicle. If the volume is exceedingly low (< 0.5 ml) part of the ejaculate may be entering the bladder (retrograde ejaculation). In this case, a post-ejaculatory urine sample should be obtained, centrifuged and examined for the presence of spermatozoa.

Concentration

The number of sperm present is a good indication of spermatogenesis. Concentrations below 10 million are associated with marked impaired fertility.

Motility

Recently ejaculated spermatozoa are actively motile and able to swim with a forward progressive motion. However, motility decreases with time after ejaculation, therefore the time at which the sample is produced is relevant to the assessment. If all of the sperm are immotile, the use of lubricants for producing the sample or exposure to excessively high temperatures, should be excluded. Agglutination or clumping of the spermatozoa may be due to the presence of antisperm antibodies.

Morphology

Samples of semen with large numbers of poorly structured spermatozoa have reduced fertilizing capacity, and are associated with subfertility.

White blood cells

Samples with an increased white cell count should be screened for infection.

Sperm mucus interaction

Sperm mucus interaction can be tested by performing a PCT (post-coital test), and this is a valuable screening test for sperm function and mucus receptivity. The PCT is technically simple to perform, but timing and experience are needed for it to be reliable and therefore it should be performed in a specialist fertility unit. The mucus must be obtained in the pre-ovulatory phase if the test is to give valid information.

The couple are asked to come to the clinic, having had intercourse 6–8 hours earlier. A sample of mucus is removed from the cervical canal and placed on to a glass slide. Whilst this is being done, the stretchability of the mucus is noted, as is the amount of sperm present. A completely normal post-coital test will show very flowing, 'stretchable' mucus containing a significant number of moving sperm.

The most common cause for a poor post-coital test is inaccurate timing in the cycle, and the diagnosis of a poor or negative test should only be made after serial investigations in at least two consecutive cycles. Only in the presence of good mucus production and normal semen analysis can poor sperm penetration be diagnosed.

Hysterosalpingogram

The patency of the Fallopian tubes can easily be checked by performing an HSG (hysterosalpingogram), which is carried out on an outpatient basis. An HSG is an X-ray during which a dye is passed through the cervix, uterus and Fallopian tubes. If the dye is seen to pass easily into the abdominal cavity, then the tubes are said to be clear. It has the advantage of outlining the uterine cavity, allowing for the diagnosis of intrauterine fibroids and adhesions. The test does not, however, provide any information about the relationship between the tubes and ovaries. Nor does it identify the presence or absence of pelvic adhesions.

Laparoscopy

Once the couple have been referred to a specialist fertility centre, any remaining investigations not already performed can be arranged. When no abnormality has been detected on the initial investigations of either partner, a diagnostic laparoscopy is often carried out. This is an important part of a thorough investigation, and should not be delayed but should be regarded as a primary investigation, where indicated. The great advantage of a laparoscopy is that it allows the surgeon to obtain a direct view of the pelvic organs, thereby permitting a much more accurate assessment of their condition. The patency and integrity of both Fallopian tubes is determined under direct vision and a dye test performed (see page 428). The presence of adhesions around the tubes and ovaries can be easily detected, and their significance assessed. Other problems such as endometriosis and fibroids will also be revealed, and definitive therapeutic procedures can be performed under direct vision using the laparoscope. Such procedures include the removal of adhesions, ablation of endometriotic spots and drilling of the ovarian capsule in patients who suffer from polycystic ovarian disease.

Hysteroscopy

Examination of the uterine cavity with a hysteroscope is a valuable investigation where there is a history of repeated miscarriage or where the HSG suggests that the shape of the cavity is irregular. During this procedure, a good view of the uterine cavity is obtained. Both tubal openings are seen, and any intrauterine abnormalities can be diagnosed. In some cases minor surgical procedures can also be performed under direct vision, such as the removal of intrauterine polyps or the resection of intrauterine fibroids. Intrauterine adhesions can also be removed.

Unexplained subfertility

When investigations have been completed and no satisfactory explanation for a couple's subfertility has been found, the couple is said to be suffering from unexplained subfertility. A high standard of investigation is required, and the diagnosis should only be suggested when all standard investigations have been completed.

The other aspect of unexplained subfertility is that there are factors which affect the subfertile couple which are either still unknown to medicine or are untestable using all conventional methods for investigating fertility. Although there may be evidence of ovulation occurring, such as an elevated serum progesterone or a rise in basal body temperature, the egg may still be retained within the corpus luteum. In this condition, all signs of ovulation will be positive yet the oocyte will not reach the site of fertilization and as yet, it is not easy to detect this condition.

The testing of tubal patency by HSG or even laparoscopy only informs us that the woman has patent tubes, but it does not confirm that the oocyte pick-up mechanism of the Fallopian tubes is intact. Knowledge of this pick-up mechanism is very limited, and there is no suitable way yet to test for it.

Treatment

If the primary investigations are normal, couples should be encouraged by an explanation of the normal chances of conception, and they should be given advice on the correct timing of intercourse and how to detect pre-ovulatory cervical mucus. At the time of ovulation, due to increasing oestrogen levels, the mucus is a very profuse, clear, watery secretion and many women are aware of these changes. If the woman is unable to detect mid-cycle cervical mucus, ovulation may be predicted with the help of a urinary LH kit.

Apart from the problem of ovarian failure virtually all ovulation disorders are treatable with drug therapy, the most commonly used being clomiphene. Treatment starts within the first five days of the period, and continues for five days. Ovulation will usually occur 5–13 days after the last tablet of clomiphene has been taken.

If a pregnancy does not occur following 3–6 months of clomiphene therapy or where the level of oestrogen is low, the treatment of choice is HMG (human menopausal gonadotrophin), for example, Pergonal (Serono, UK). This is administered by intramuscular injection, and careful assessment of the ovarian response to therapy must be made in specialist centres. The objective of this form of treatment is the production of one or two mature follicles. In patients treated with HMG, careful monitoring by means of ultrasound scan is important to detect hyperstimulation and, therefore, prevent multiple pregnancies.

Patients with tubal blockage may be advised to

have tubal microsurgery, or else be referred directly for *in vitro* fertilization.

Endometriosis can be treated either surgically through the laparoscope, or by using medication. The objective of drug treatment in endometriosis is to induce a period of amenorrhoea, which will hopefully give the condition time to heal. The most commonly used drugs presently are LHRH analogues i.e. Zoladex (Zeneca, UK).

Couples whose infertility is caused by a male factor may be referred to an andrologist to further investigate causes of semen abnormality. In some cases, minor surgical procedures or drug treatment may help to improve semen quality. Assisted conception in the form of intrauterine insemination (IUI), *in vitro* fertilization (IVF), gamete intra-fallopian transfer (GIFT) or micromanipulation remains the only treatment available for the majority of patients with male factor subfertility.

Human Fertilisation and Embryology Authority (HFEA)

People who are considering infertility treatment are often faced with a difficult decision about which treatment centre to go to. The HFEA provides a valuable source of information for prospective patients, as well as patients already undergoing treatment. The HFEA was set up in August 1990 as a result of the Human Fertilisation and Embryology (HFE) Act 1990 in order to monitor the treatment and research carried out in centres performing IVF. It does this by means of a licensing system, and each unit is inspected annually to ensure that the service provided adheres to a Code of Practice set out by the HFEA itself.

The Authority publishes a range of information leaflets on: *Egg Donation*, *Sperm and Egg Donors and the Law*, *In vitro Fertilisation*, and *Treatment Clinic: Questions to Ask*, and has recently published a *Patient Guide to In-Vitro Fertilization and Donor Insemination*. It has published results for individual centres, and these results were adjusted for common factors which might affect the outcome of treatment, such as age and parity. There was a wide variation in the results between different centres, but the overall take-home baby rate was 14.1%. The guide also contains advice to prospective couples about the questions they should ask and the information that should be made available to

them, to enable them to decide on which clinic to choose for their treatment. It is emphasized that pregnancy and take-home baby rates alone do not constitute a successful and popular clinic – friendly, compassionate and professional staff providing an excellent overall standard of care, can make a huge difference to the patients who enter into this field of medicine.

NHS or private treatment

There are many excellent NHS clinics offering infertility investigations and treatment but unfortunately many of these clinics have long waiting lists and do not necessarily offer the full range of treatment options. Fertility treatment is not perceived as needing extra government funding and this situation is unlikely to change in the foreseeable future. There are far more private clinics offering advanced infertility management than there are NHS programmes. Increasingly many NHS units are now offering some forms of treatment privately as well as within the public sector. Any profits made are ploughed back into the public sector which can then be used for the benefit of all the patients.

A number of women, particularly the older woman for whom time is at a premium, may be tempted into the private sector where they can be seen without a long wait for a first appointment and without lengthy delays for subsequent appointments.

Private treatment can be very expensive and is rarely covered by private health insurance and, of course, there is no guarantee that the outcome will be successful. When choosing a clinic, women should check on success rates that a clinic has with achieving a pregnancy, although all results must be looked at with caution as they might compare different age groups of women.

Assisted reproduction techniques

The advent of assisted conception techniques has dramatically changed the treatment of prolonged subfertility. Since the birth of the world's first baby following *in vitro* fertilization and embryo transfer in 1978, IVF has been improved and simplified.

Other forms of assisted conception such as intrauterine insemination (IUI), gamete intra-fallopian transfer (GIFT) and zygote intra-fallopian transfer (ZIFT) have also been developed. The general principles involved in all these techniques are as shown in Box 8.4.

Box 8.4 General principles of assisted conception techniques

♦ Induction of multiple follicular development

♦ Preparation of a sperm sample of reasonable count and mobility

♦ Bringing the gametes together in order to enhance the chance of fertilization.

The factors responsible for increased success in the course of the last decade are better ovulation induction regimens, improved ultrasound-guided oocyte recovery, optimal embryo culture conditions and finally, the facilities of cryopreservation. Although a success rate very close to that of natural conception can be achieved, there still remains a higher risk of spontaneous abortion in pregnancies achieved by these means. Even so, assisted conception has brought new hope to childless couples who have no natural prospects of achieving a pregnancy, and for whom all other measures have failed.

There is an increased demand for assisted conception. The factors contributing to this are:

♦ a trend towards childbearing at a later age, which increases the span of years of exposure to toxins or infections, as well as an age-related reduction in fertility;

♦ a greater public awareness of the availability and scope of such services; and

♦ the availability of new technology and drugs for the treatment of previously hopeless cases of subfertility.

Pre-treatment assessment

Adequate time for consultation of both partners is important to decide upon the best available options and to assess the most suitable treatment for the individual couple. It is important that they fully understand not only their chances of success, but also the possibility of unsatisfactory response to medication and, therefore, cancellation of the cycle. They must also appreciate that there is a possibility that the eggs may fail to fertilize, that the embryos may fail to implant and that even if a pregnancy does result, this may sadly end in miscarriage.

Intrauterine insemination (IUI)

Intrauterine insemination (IUI) involves the injection of washed sperm into the uterine cavity via the cervix, using a fine plastic catheter. It is a painless procedure which takes only a few minutes, and is performed on an outpatient basis.

Currently, there is a renewed interest in IUI in many cases of subfertility. This is due to improved methods of sperm preparation in assisted conception units, and better ovarian cycle monitoring facilities.

IUI is useful when:

♦ the female partner has a cervical mucus problem – the mucus may be scanty or hostile to the sperm and with IUI the sperm will bypass the cervix and enter the uterine cavity directly;

♦ the male partner suffers from retrograde ejaculation, in which the semen travels backwards into the bladder instead of through the penis – with IUI, a sample of urine is collected and the sperm removed and prepared for insemination;

♦ the male partner suffers from impotence or anatomical abnormalities of the penis such as an uncorrected hypospadias, or if the man is paraplegic;

♦ there is unexplained subfertility, since the technique of IUI increases the chances of the eggs and sperm meeting – this is also an inexpensive alternative to GIFT, especially for younger couples, and is a reasonable first choice of treatment; or

♦ the couple is using donor sperm.

The insemination cycle

Insemination may be carried out in a natural menstrual cycle, but by combining it with ovarian stimulation it is often possible to achieve a higher pregnancy rate per cycle. This involves taking fertility drugs to stimulate the ovaries to produce more than one egg. The growth of the egg follicle is monitored by ultrasound and when it has reached the appropriate size, ovulation is triggered by administering HCG (Profasi, Seroni, UK 10 000 units or Pregnyl, Organon 10 000 units). The intrauterine insemination is then performed some 36–40 hours following administration of the HCG.

The insemination procedure

It is necessary to prepare sperm prior to IUI, as 'neat' untreated semen contains prostaglandins which can be highly irritant to the uterus and can cause a 'shock-like' reaction, resulting in severe abdominal pain and collapse.

Sperm for IUI is prepared by either simple washing or by using a sperm separation technique to isolate the motile fraction. The final preparation is drawn into a sterile catheter and introduced into the uterus via the cervical os.

Success rates with IUI

Generally, the chance of conceiving in one treatment cycle is approximately 10–15%, and the cumulative conception rate is approximately 40% over five or six treatment cycles. The success rate depends upon several factors. First, the cause of the subfertility problem is important; for example, men with a normal sperm count who are unable to have intercourse have a much higher chance of success than couples who are undergoing IUI with poorer sperm counts. If the woman is 35 years of age or more, the chance of a successful pregnancy is significantly reduced. If IUI is going to prove successful, it usually does so within six treatment cycles. If a pregnancy has not resulted in this time, the chance of IUI working is remote, and the couple should be encouraged to explore other possibilities. IUI is a relatively simple and inexpensive form of treatment, and is often attempted before moving on to more expensive and invasive options. Repeated cycles of insemination without success can prove extremely stressful to couples, however, and close support for them is essential.

Donor sperm

The use of donor sperm is an option which should be offered when the semen characteristics of a male presenting with subfertility are such that it is unlikely a pregnancy will be achieved.

It is used to treat couples in which the male partner has either no sperm, or a very low sperm count. It is also recommended in cases where the male partner is known to be a carrier of a hereditary disease. Couples in which the male partner has a low sperm count are currently being offered micromanipulation as a primary course of treatment with increasingly successful outcomes. Some couples, however, opt to use donor insemination for either financial or ethical reasons.

The couple may be acutely distressed by the knowledge of abnormal semen results, thus it is most important that counselling is made available.

Counselling

It is most important that the medical, legal and emotional implications of donor insemination are fully understood by the couple undergoing the treatment. Counselling gives the couple an opportunity to explore their feelings in relation to the male partner's subfertility, and its implication on their relationship. The couple will also need to consider telling the child of its origins, at what age this might be done and how it might be best presented. It is important to ascertain if they have already confided in friends or relatives about their condition, and what their plans might be to discuss it in the future with others. It is entirely up to the parents to tell the child the circumstances of its birth, however, there is always the burden of secrecy which the parents have to bear for the rest of their lives. The current trend is to encourage openness, as secrets are difficult to keep and it can also be argued that it is the child's right to know of its origins, but still many parents choose secrecy. Patient support groups can be useful to couples in this situation, as they can share experiences and develop an understanding of each other's problems.

A group called DI Network (see Resources, page 172) has been formed to help couples undergoing donor insemination treatment and has produced a book entitled *My Story* in order to help parents tell their children of their origins.

Laws governing donor sperm

This treatment is governed by the HFEA, which requires that all sperm donors and couples receiving donor sperm, are registered with the Authority.

The sperm donor has no parental rights or legal obligations towards any children resulting from treatment using his sperm. Couples undergoing donor insemination are required to sign a consent form prior to treatment, in which the male partner acknowledges that he is the legal father of any child born as a result of donor insemination.

Recruitment, selection and screening of donors

Most sperm donors are recruited from medical schools, local colleges and businesses, and, according to the Human Fertilisation and Embryology Act must be aged between 18 and 55 years. All potential donors are required to complete a questionnaire giving details about their physical characteristics as well as data about their medical and family history. Subject to the information acquired, a semen sample will then be required for analysis and if this specimen reaches the required standard, it will be cryopreserved – all semen used for donor insemination is quarantined for a minimum of 180 days prior to use.

Urethral cultures are performed for gonorrhoea and *Chlamydia*, and serological tests are carried out for HIV-1, HIV-2, hepatitis B surface antigen, hepatitis C, syphilis and cytomegalovirus. Live births from any one donor are restricted to ten under HFEA regulations, in an effort to reduce the risk of consanguinity.

A recent survey (Golombok and Cook, 1994) revealed that only 25% of all men wishing to become sperm donors are accepted, and that the most common reason for rejection is suboptimal semen analyses. A payment of up to £15.00 per donation as well as reasonable expenses is currently allowed under HFEA guidelines, and it is interesting to note that Golombok and Cook report a widespread feeling amongst fertility centres that should these payments cease, approximately 80% of sperm donors would be lost.

Method of treatment

The method of treatment with donor sperm depends on the cause of subfertility. If there is no evidence of a fertility problem with the woman, then IUI may be a suitable form of treatment. However, there may also be indications for GIFT or IVF.

Psychological effects

Couples undergoing donor insemination often have psychological reactions which can be difficult to cope with. The sense of isolation is even more than with other forms of subfertility, since many couples do not tell anyone they are undergoing donor insemination. The male partner may feel inferior, insecure and jealous, and even wonder whether he will be able to 'father another man's child'. The female partner may in turn be resentful about having to undergo treatment for a problem which is medically not her own.

The involvement of a completely unknown third party in the form of the donor sperm can make coping with the pregnancy especially difficult. Fantasies may occur about the unknown donor, and anxieties may arise as to whether the child will be normal and what it will look like. It is therefore important that the couple do not rush into treatment with donor sperm, but also explore the alternative options.

In vitro fertilization (IVF)

In vitro is the Latin term for 'in glass', which quite literally describes the technique of IVF: fertilization performed outside the body in a Petrie dish. It first reached public awareness in 1978 with the birth of the first so-called 'test tube baby', Louise Brown. It is a process in which the woman's eggs are collected from her ovaries, fertilized in the laboratory with her partner's sperm and, when normal embryo development has occurred, replaced in her uterus.

In early days, the indications for IVF treatment were absent, blocked or irreparably damaged Fallopian tubes. Subsequent developments led to IVF also being used to help couples with other problems such as male subfertility, endometriosis, unexplained subfertility and cervical factors. Essentially, IVF may be an option for any subfertile couple in whom less aggressive forms of subfertility therapy have been unsuccessful.

Finally, IVF may also be employed as a means of obtaining diagnostic information in severe forms of male subfertility as well as idiopathic subfertility, as it is the ultimate test to assess a couple's potential to achieve fertilization. No other test is currently available to determine this potential.

When IVF was first used successfully, a single egg was obtained during a natural menstrual cycle, without the use of drugs to stimulate follicular development. It was later found that the pregnancy rate was higher when several, rather than just one embryo was transferred. Since then, it has become standard practice in most IVF centres to give the patients medication to stimulate the ovaries, in order to allow the development of more than one follicle.

The basic steps in the performance of IVF are ovarian stimulation, egg collection and embryo transfer.

Ovarian stimulation

Medication starts early in the cycle to enhance the growth and development of the ovarian follicles which have been naturally selected for that cycle. The medication is administered over a period of 10–12 days, and the ovaries are scanned at regular intervals during this time to ensure that they are responding to the medication. Hormone assays for oestradiol may also be performed to indicate oocyte maturation. When specific criteria have been met, HCG 10 000 units is given to encourage final egg maturation and induce ovulation. Egg retrieval is performed 36–40 hours later.

Ovarian stimulation is initiated with a variety of different medication protocols. Those commonly used are human menopausal gonadotrophins (Pergonal, Serono; Humegon) and follicle- stimulating hormone (Metrodin, Serono) as well as LHRH (luteinizing hormone-releasing hormone) analogues (Suprefact, Suprecur). The function of the LHRH analogue is to take complete control of the woman's ovarian function, by preventing her from producing FSH and LH naturally. It also prevents a pre-ovulatory LH surge from occurring, and therefore avoids spontaneous ovulation.

There are two protocols for the administration of the LHRH analogue. In the 'long' protocol, the analogue is given for approximately 10 days to desensitize the pituitary gland. Once this has occurred, daily injections of HMG are commenced to stimulate the ovaries. Both the LHRH analogue and the HMG are continued until the eggs are mature enough for egg collection to be undertaken. In the 'short' protocol, both the analogue and the HMG are started together at the beginning of the menstrual cycle. This protocol is suitable for patients who have a previous history of poor response to the medication. The analogues are available either as a nasal spray or a subcutaneous injection.

HMG and FSH are available only in the form of intramuscular or subcutaneous injections. It may in some cases be appropriate to teach the woman herself how to administer the injection, and some partners may be willing to participate. Couples who do their own injections tend to find the whole procedure less stressful, as this avoids the inconvenience of their visiting the clinic or attending their GP surgery on a daily basis, therefore diminishing the intrusion of the treatment in their normal daily lives.

Unfortunately, not all patients respond ideally to a given medication protocol. If the ultrasound and hormone monitoring reveal a suboptimal response in terms of follicular development, the cycle may be cancelled as the chances of pregnancy will be reduced. The medication protocol may be adjusted, and a new cycle can be attempted at a later date. If the couple feel very strongly about proceeding even when it is likely that only one or two eggs will be collected, however, they will be allowed their right to go ahead with the treatment.

Possible side-effects of the drugs. Whilst taking the drugs, some women experience mild unpleasant symptoms, but these are normally short-lived and are no cause for concern. They can include hot flushes, headaches, irritability and feelings of depression.

Despite careful monitoring, a small percentage of women may develop a mild or severe form of overstimulation to the drugs, where too many follicles may develop. The ovaries will be enlarged and symptoms such as nausea, vomiting, abdominal pain and swelling may occur. Under these circumstances the cycle should be abandoned, and the woman should be carefully monitored by a fertility specialist.

Very rarely, in about 1% of cases, a more serious form of hyperstimulation may occur, where the woman notices a reduction in urine output and shortness of breath along with the previously mentioned symptoms. These complications require hospital admission to restore fluid balance and to monitor progress.

Egg collection

Egg collection may be performed through a laparoscope or vaginally using ultrasound guidance, which is now the most favoured technique. This may be performed whilst the patient is under a general anaesthetic, or it may be carried out with the patient only mildly sedated.

In ultrasound-guided procedures, an ultrasound probe is inserted into the vagina in order to visualize the ovaries, and a fine hollow needle is then guided directly into the ovaries and the eggs are aspirated.

A laparoscopic egg collection may be required in certain cases where it is difficult to access the ovaries from the vaginal route.

Egg identification and insemination. As the follicles are aspirated, the follicular fluid obtained is immediately taken to the laboratory where it is examined, and the eggs identified. Once evaluated for the level of maturity, the eggs are transferred to a special culture medium in preparation for insemination. In the meantime, a sample of the partner's sperm is prepared by a washing technique to remove the seminal plasma and separate out the healthy sperm.

About 100 000 motile sperm are added to each egg approximately 4–6 hours following egg collection, to allow fertilization to take place. The exact length of time the eggs are incubated before the sperm are added depends upon the maturity of the eggs. Generally, 80% of mature eggs will be fertilized in the absence of a male problem. Fertilization should occur within 18–24 hours of insemination.

Once fertilization has occurred two pronuclei can be identified; however, the embryos are allowed to continued developing to a two-cell or four-cell stage before transfer back into the uterus (Figures 8.2 and 8.3).

Embryo transfer (ET)

Embryos are transferred though the cervix into the uterus using a fine plastic catheter 48 to 72 hours after egg collection. This is a painless procedure, and no anaesthetic is required. Usually, two or three embryos are transferred in order to increase the chances of pregnancy but under HFEA guidelines, clinics are not allowed to transfer more than three embryos – this is to reduce the risk of multiple pregnancy.

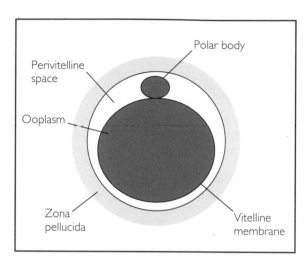

Figure 8.2 *Diagram of an oocyte (egg).*

Following embryo transfer the woman is allowed to carry on with her normal routine, as there is no evidence to suggest that resting increases the chances of becoming pregnant. Embryo transfer is often regarded as the culmination of many weeks of treatment, and the emotional significance of it to the couple should not be ignored.

Embryo freezing

In many cases, more than three embryos are collected and fertilized. Those embryos not transferred may be cryopreserved and stored for future treatment should the first attempt be unsuccessful, or indeed to try to achieve a second pregnancy. These embryos may be transferred at the appropriate time in a natural cycle, without the need for

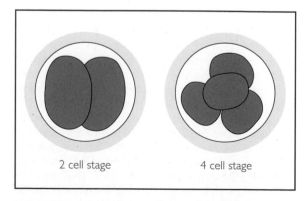

Figure 8.3 *Embryos two days after egg collection.*

drugs and surgery, and are replaced 2–3 days following natural ovulation.

The chance of success using frozen embryos is less than when using fresh, as some or all of the embryos may not survive the freezing/thawing process. It is therefore important that the couple are carefully counselled on the chances of conception and the costs involved. They are also required to sign a consent form giving the clinic permission to freeze their embryos and also to determine the fate of these, should anything happen to either or both partners.

Embryos can legally be kept in storage for only five years, except in exceptional circumstances.

Gamete intra-fallopian transfer (GIFT)

GIFT offers an alternative treatment to IVF for women who have patent Fallopian tubes. The first stages of the treatment are similar to those for IVF, namely ovarian stimulation with hormone treatment, monitoring of follicular growth and administration of HCG to induce final maturation of the eggs. It is from here on that the GIFT procedure differs from IVF.

The eggs are collected laparoscopically. They are examined for maturity, and the three most mature eggs are mixed with the prepared sperm and drawn separately into a fine catheter, then immediately transferred into the fimbriated end of the Fallopian tube. Fertilization therefore occurs in the Fallopian tubes as with normal conception, rather than in the laboratory. The fertilized egg then travels through the tube to the uterus for implantation, as in normal reproduction. Gametes will be transferred only if the Fallopian tubes appear healthy and if they are not, IVF will be attempted instead of GIFT.

This procedure is primarily used for patients who suffer from unexplained subfertility and cervical hostility. Many centres claim a higher success rate using this method of treatment.

Although GIFT has the advantages of fertilization and early embryo development occurring in the normal environment, in the absence of a successful outcome, the fertilizing capacity of gametes remains unknown. To overcome this deficiency, the surplus oocytes may be fertilized *in vitro* and then cryopreserved. This 'back-up' IVF has a diagnostic value of confirming fertilization, and also has a therapeutic role which allows transfer of cryopreserved embryos at a later date.

Zygote intra-Fallopian transfer (ZIFT)

Following egg collection and successful fertilization, embryos may be transferred into the Fallopian tubes through the laparoscope. The concept of tubal transfer arises from higher success with GIFT than IVF/ET, implying that the tubal environment is preferable for gametes and embryos. This treatment combines the best features of both IVF and GIFT, in that fertilization is known to have occurred and the embryos have the opportunity of entering the uterine cavity naturally.

Micromanipulation

Until recently, the treatment for couples with severe male factor problems was extremely limited; therefore most couples in this situation were forced to consider either the use of donor sperm or else the prospect of remaining childless. Micromanipulation is a relatively new technique which allows the embryologist to perform very precise surgical procedures upon eggs and embryos with the use of a micromanipulator. This is a very high-powered microscope with robotic arms, which enables the operator to perform extremely delicate manoeuvres using eggs and sperm which are normally not even visible to the naked eye. This facility is also capable of allowing the embryologist to withdraw as little as one cell from an embryo for research purposes and to look for the presence of genetic diseases such as cystic fibrosis – such research is not widely available at the present time, but it must be regarded as the way forward holding, as it does, vast scope for knowledge within the field of genetic engineering.

Several micromanipulation techniques have been devised to help the sperm pass through the zona pellucida – the tough outer coating of the egg, which is thought to be the main barrier to the penetration of sperm. In cases of male factor subfertility, the ability of sperm to penetrate the zona may be reduced. At present, these methods are being tried in cases of severe male subfertility and when conventional IVF has failed.

Two main groups of patients suitable for

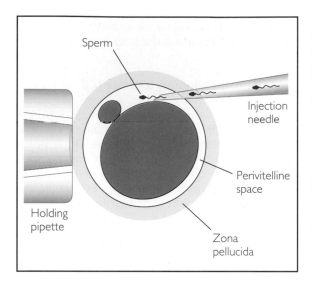

Figure 8.4 *Subzonal insemination (SUZI). The holding pipette keeps the egg in place. The injection needle is loaded with a number of sperm which are injected into the perivitelline space between the zona and the vitelline membrane.*

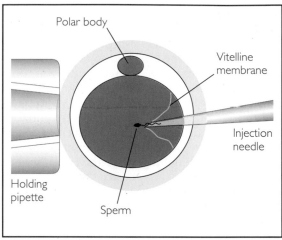

Figure 8.5 *Intracytoplasmic sperm injection. The holding pipette keeps the egg in place. The injection needle is loaded with one sperm which is injected directly into the centre of the egg. The needle is then withdrawn, leaving the sperm behind.*

micromanipulation are those couples who have either very poor or no fertilization with a good number of eggs (i.e. four or more), or those couples whose semen contains very low numbers of sperm.

These procedures can also be used to help men who have obstruction of the vas (the tube which connects the testicle to the base of the penis). Sperm can be surgically removed from the epididymis (the area on top of the testes in which sperm are maturing) or directly from the testicle itself.

Subzonal insemination (SUZI)

This method involves the direct insertion of between three and ten sperm under the outer layer (zona pellucida) of an egg (Figure 8.4). The egg is cleared of surrounding cells, and placed into a solution which causes it to temporarily shrink away from the zona pellucida, thus enlarging the space between the zona and the egg itself, and making it easier for the embryologist to carefully pass a needle through the zona without directly touching the egg. A hollow needle is used to select the previously prepared sperm, and this is then passed through the outer barriers. The sperm are gently deposited into the enlarged space and then left to penetrate the egg's membrane by natural

means. From 12 to 18 hours following the initial insemination, the eggs are checked for fertilization and any resulting embryos are then transferred into the uterus as in a standard IVF procedure.

One of the difficulties with SUZI is that the number of sperm needed to fertilize a particular patient's eggs is unknown. This can result in too few sperm being injected with no consequent fertilization, or too many sperm being injected with fertilization of each egg with more than one sperm. This makes the outcome of SUZI difficult to predict.

Intracytoplasmic sperm injection (ICSI)

In this method, a single sperm is injected into the centre of an egg (Figure 8.5). The sperm which is selected for injection is ideally one of normal shape, morphology and motility, and it is immobilized by having its tail touched with the microneedle before being picked up. The egg is held in place whilst the needle is passed through its outer layer, and the needle is then brought into contact with the egg's membrane. The membrane is carefully penetrated and the centre of the egg reached, then the sperm is injected and the needle is gently withdrawn, care being taken to leave the sperm within the egg.

The advantages and disadvantages of ICSI are outlined in Box 8.5.

Box 8.5 Advantages and disadvantages of ICSI

Advantages of ICSI over SUZI
1 ICSI can be performed on patients who have almost no sperm in their semen.
2 ICSI can be performed on patients whose sperm have no activity (often in these cases, only one sperm in a few hundred thousand may be moving).
3 ICSI has a higher fertilization rate than SUZI, therefore couples have a resultant higher number of embryos to transfer.
4 ICSI has a higher pregnancy rate than SUZI.
5 ICSI reduces the chances of overfertilization.

Disadvantages
The technique may damage the eggs in one of the following ways:
1 The piercing of the egg's membrane may lead to damage, and this will be evident either during or after the procedure. These damaged eggs will not be used in treatment, and approximately 15% of the eggs will be lost in this way.
2 It is possible that a small amount of material from inside the eggs could be drawn into the injection needle, and therefore be removed from the egg. It is theoretically possible that this could cause a loss of, or damage to, genetic material of the egg and lead to the development of an abnormal embryo. Such damage will not be obvious. Nevertheless, there are no data to suggest that children born from this technique have a higher abnormality rate than those conceived naturally.

The risk of fetal abnormality

The ICSI and SUZI methods of assisted fertilization must be considered to be novel procedures which carry an unknown risk of abnormality. At this point in time, the risk of having an abnormal child using the above techniques is uncertain. The number of children born as a result of ICSI is very small and as yet, the worldwide survey of such children has not been completed, but of the children born from such a procedure the incidence of major abnormality is only 2.4%, compared to a 2% rate of abnormalities found in children born from natural conception. Couples contemplating such techniques are advised to undergo pre-natal diagnostic procedures to detect the chances of fetal abnormalities.

All centres performing micromanipulative procedures have a responsibility to their patients and to the medical profession as a whole, to record the progress and ultimate development of all children resulting from this treatment.

Chances of success with assisted reproductive techniques

Whilst IVF has enabled many couples to have children, the treatment is more likely to be unsuccessful than successful in any individual cycle. Perhaps the best measures of success in IVF are therefore the cumulative conception and the cumulative live birth rates – these describe the likelihood of a woman becoming pregnant or having a live birth after a specific number of cycles of treatment.

There are many factors which affect the pregnancy rates, the most important being the age of the woman, the subfertility cause and the quality of the semen. For example, a 30-year-old woman whose only indication for subfertility is a tubal factor, will have a higher probability of achieving a pregnancy than a 40-year-old woman who has

Table 8.1 *Pregnancy and delivery rates in women under the age of 38 years old, Lister Hospital, 1988–95*

	CYCLES	PREGNANT	DELIVERED
IVF	2085	679 (33%)	465 (22%)
GIFT	1378	467 (34%)	314 (23%)
ICSI[a]	715	227 (32%)	185 (26%)

[a] Cases between October 1993 and December 1995.

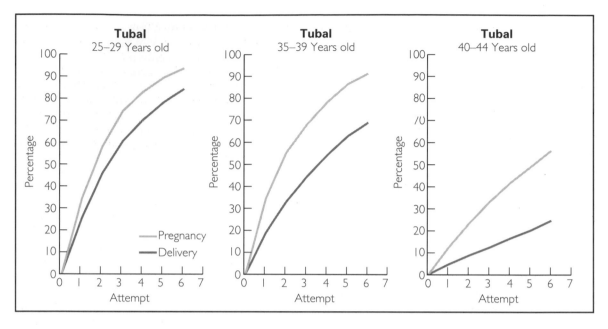

Figure 8.6 *Cumulative pregnancy and delivery rates for IVF. Source: Lister Hospital.*

extensive endometriosis and whose husband has a male factor. It is therefore important for couples to understand the meaning of reported statistics, and to know how these apply to their individual circumstances. Generally speaking, although the chances of success per cycle are only approximately 30%, repeated attempts at treatment are likely to result in a pregnancy.

Table 8.1 shows a general overview of the IVF/GIFT/ICSI pregnancy rates for the IVF Unit at Lister Hospital, and Figure 8.6 shows the cumulative pregnancy and delivery rates for IVF.

Ovum donation

Sperm donations for infertile couples have been practised for over 100 years. The use of donor eggs is a natural extension of the IVF process, and recent advances have opened up hope for women who are either unable to produce eggs or fail to achieve a pregnancy using their own eggs. It is now an established part of assisted conception, used primarily for women who have suffered premature ovarian failure (Box 8.6).

Couples undergoing treatment with egg donation require extensive counselling prior to commencing treatment, particularly in cases where

the donor is known to the recipients. Close attention must be paid to the long-term attitude towards the child, as well as the proposed definition

---

Box 8.6 Conditions treated by ovum donation

Women with ovarian function
Women for whom ovum donation may be suitable include those:

♦ carrying an inheritable genetic disorder such as haemophilia,

♦ who repeatedly fail to respond to ovarian stimulation in IVF programmes,

♦ whose apparently normal eggs repeatedly fail to fertilize in IVF programmes,

♦ who may be carriers of disorders such as Tay–Sachs disease, Huntingdon's disease, cystic fibrosis, thalassaemia or sickle-cell disease, or

♦ who have a history of recurrent miscarriage.

Women without ovarian function
These include women:

♦ suffering from Turner's syndrome,

♦ suffering from premature menopause, and

♦ with ovarian damage following surgery, radiation or oophorectomy.

of future interaction and their relationship with the child.

Source of egg donors

Egg donors were originally recruited from women receiving assisted conception treatment, who wished to donate extra eggs for altruistic reasons (Trounson *et al.*, 1983). This source of donors has decreased since the introduction of embryo freezing, as most couples opt to store their embryos for a future attempt at treatment. By far the most successful method of recruiting egg donors is to encourage all recipients joining an ovum donation programme to help in recruiting their own donor. These donors may either be known to the recipient, or they may remain anonymous.

There is a tremendous demand for egg donation treatment and most centres have a waiting list, as it is not easy to maintain a large pool of egg donors. Also, with the present state of technology, because eggs cannot be easily cryopreserved, 'egg banks' do not exist in the same way as 'sperm banks'. It is important to note that all donors are registered with the HFEA Central Registry, which takes great care to protect their anonymity and retain confidentiality. The recruitment of egg donors raises many ethical, moral and emotional issues; however, the increasing demand for oocytes requires that this controversial issue be discussed and possible solutions be found (Burton *et al.*, 1990).

A survey of donors was performed in 1990 (Power *et al.*, 1990), to try to ascertain exactly why these women donate, and it was found that over 90% of them made the donations simply because they felt the need to help other women.

Donor criteria

The potential donor must be under the age of 36 and have preferably completed her family, although this is not essential. She will be carefully screened for HIV, hepatitis and venereal disease, and a full medical and family history will be recorded to ensure that there are no known genetically inheritable diseases or defects present.

Physical characteristics are recorded such as nationality, skin, hair and eye colour, height and build, to ensure that every care can be taken to find the most suitable donor for each recipient. Recipients of donor eggs frequently enquire about the donor's interests, pastimes, religion and educational qualifications, the answers obtained helping to alleviate their curiosities and fantasies about the potential child. As much information as possible should be made available to them. Frequent questions asked are: 'Is the donor an animal lover?' 'Is she artistic or sporty?' 'Is she intelligent?' 'Does the donor have children and are they healthy?'

All of this information is hand-written by the donor herself, at which time she has an opportunity to write a personal message to the child which may evolve as a result of her donation. When any resulting child reaches the age of 18 years, it is then legally able to acquire this paperwork and read for itself the message left for it by its genetic mother so many years before.

Donors are counselled to ensure that they understand all of the implications and issues involved with egg donation. The donor relinquishes all rights to the egg, and has no responsibility towards any resulting children. The Human Fertilisation and Embryology Act states that the mother of a child is the woman who actually gives birth to it (HFEA, 1990).

The difficulty and challenge of egg donation revolves around matching the ovulatory cycle of the donor with the appropriate endometrial maturation of the recipient, as a fresh embryo replacement with donor/recipient synchronization is the ideal situation for achieving a pregnancy. The recipient is commenced on hormone replacement therapy in order to synchronize her cycle with that of her donor, as well as for optimal endometrial development. In women with normal ovarian function, the LHRH analogue can be used to suppress the natural cycle. If cycles cannot be synchronized, the eggs can be fertilized and frozen for use in a future cycle.

The donor undergoes a similar stimulation protocol to that described in an IVF cycle, with egg recovery usually being performed vaginally. Following fertilization of the donor eggs, the embryos are transferred to the uterus or the Fallopian tubes.

Egg donation can be an extremely successful method of treating infertility, with a mean pregnancy rate of 27% (as in IVF, the success rate depends upon the cause of subfertility). Patients with primary ovarian failure tend to have a better outcome than those with secondary ovarian failure, and the pregnancy rate in patients with Turner's syndrome is almost 50% (Abdalla *et al.*, 1990).

Surrogacy

Surrogate parenthood is a highly controversial and emotive issue, and very few fertility centres in the United Kingdom currently provide this facility.

Surrogacy involves a fertile woman having a baby, whom she consents to hand over to an infertile couple at birth, and this requires one of two procedures to be performed. In the first, the surrogate mother is artificially inseminated with the sperm of the husband of the infertile woman. In the second, the infertile woman undergoes an IVF procedure whereby an egg is removed from her ovary, fertilized with her husband's sperm and the resulting embryo is then placed in the uterus of the surrogate mother, who carries the baby throughout pregnancy, gives birth and then hands the baby over to the commissioning couple, i.e. a husband and wife who have arranged for a surrogate mother to carry a child for them using their eggs and/or sperm. This latter procedure is called 'host surrogacy'.

Surrogacy is fraught with all kinds of problems, and commercial surrogacy is illegal in most countries. The difficulties include those of a legal nature, such as who determines the pregnancy outcome if fetal abnormalities are detected early on, who bears the responsibility of caring for the surrogate mother and her family if she has medical problems as a result of the pregnancy, who looks after the child if it is born with a defect, and what happens if the surrogate mother forms a strong bond with the baby and refuses to hand it over to the infertile couple.

Until recently, the commissioning couple were required to go through an adoption procedure to ensure the legality of the child, but in December 1994 the HFEA introduced new regulations which make it much easier to transfer legal parenthood to the commissioning couple. These parents will therefore no longer need to go through the full adoption procedure.

Adoption

Adoption means to become the legal parents of a child whose biological parents have decided to give up all legal rights over that child.

As a result of improved family planning methods and the availability of abortion, the numbers of children available for adoption are considerably fewer than the number of prospective parents. Therefore realistically, only a small number of couples are successful in adopting a child and it often means they have to accept an older child rather than a baby.

The child-free option

One of the most common fears that women express when considering a child-free life is that they may regret this decision when they are older, and that they may end up lonely and frustrated. However, there is a difference between choosing to remain child-free and having childlessness forced upon you.

After many years of fertility investigations and treatment, it is very difficult to accept childlessness and focus upon the positive aspects of life without children and some couples might need the help and support of a counsellor to enable them to 'let go' of their quest for a baby and accept their infertility. Initially they may be overwhelmed with feelings of bereavement (as in the death of a relative) which are not visible to others around them, and consequently they do not receive the support and empathy they require.

Couples who perhaps initially postponed trying to conceive or who felt ambivalent about becoming parents often find that once they have taken the decision to cease treatment, it is possible to pick up their lives again, and may well be able to rediscover the values which once took priority over having children. There are real advantages in leading a life without children – more personal freedom and more time and energy to invest in one another and in shared interests. Acceptance of subfertility should therefore mark the beginning of a new lifestyle, with new goals and ambitions to strive towards.

Subfertility and sexuality

Subfertility brings about many changes in a couple's relationship. It may bond them closer together in a mutual show of support and understanding for one another, but it may on the other hand bring out feelings of guilt, resentment and despair. Couples must expose the most intimate aspect of their lives – their sexual relationship – in their desire to have children.

In many cases, failure to conceive destroys self-esteem and self-worth. Sex often becomes a chore with a single-minded purpose, and it loses its association with fun and pleasure. It may be useful to seek counselling at this stage to help the couple to separate sex from reproduction.

It is also not uncommon, when faced with the diagnosis of subfertility, for a woman to feel 'less of a woman' and that she has failed to fulfil her role as a woman. These feelings of inadequacy are enhanced during the investigation and diagnosis of her condition.

Procedures such as the post-coital test, although painless, intrude greatly on a couple's intimate relationship. They are required to 'perform' at a specific time, arrive at the clinic at the appointed time and face fear of failure if they do not 'pass the test'.

Men, too, feel that their masculinity is on the line when asked to produce a semen sample, and it is not uncommon for a man to become impotent for a short period whilst undergoing investigation. It is important for all health professionals concerned in the couple's treatment to be aware of and to identify the emotional problems which their condition may well create, and offer as much support, sensitivity and understanding as possible.

Support groups

A support group provides a safe, comfortable environment in which couples can share their experiences with people who truly understand them – nobody understands subfertility as clearly as those who have been affected by it. Meeting and talking to other couples in a similar situation is a good way of breaking down the barriers of isolation which often accompany this problem, and can help couples to realize that they are not alone in their dilemma. It is also a useful forum in which to exchange ideas and obtain information.

Many couples are reluctant to join such groups as they fear that such gatherings may encourage them to dwell even more on their fertility but in reality, subfertility can affect every aspect of their lives, and trying to shut out painful feelings will only make them worse. In many cases, frank discussion with non-medical people is often a tonic in itself, a place in which fear, pain and distress can be released, experiences both happy and sad can be shared, and where empathy and support will always be forthcoming.

Most fertility units will have their own support group but in the absence of this, they will certainly have details of appropriate bodies. A national support network exists for this exact purpose and is called ISSUE, providing practical information, care and support for subfertile couples (see Resources, page 172).

The future

Assisted conception techniques have opened up an exciting new world for both patients and medical practitioners. Research is mainly focusing on the field of pre-implantation diagnosis at present. Increasing numbers of inheritable disorders may well be identified in the embryos before their transfer back to the uterus, with the obvious aim of reducing the incidence of fetal abnormality, as well as the incidence of miscarriage. This same technique could also be used for sex determination, with a view to preventing the inheritance of sex-linked disorders.

Another new and exciting facet of this research is maturation of oocytes *in vitro*. In this situation, a woman's ovaries may be removed and the immature oocytes frozen, to be matured *in vitro* at a later stage. This technique would be of major benefit to women suffering from leukaemia who need to undergo total body irradiation prior to bone marrow transplant.

In a similar vein, women undergoing elective surgery to remove their ovaries may eventually have the option of donating these, and oocytes removed from them could be used to treat other women with subfertility problems. As with all new developments in the field of assisted conception, these remarkable possibilities stimulate wide-ranging discussion of the ethical and social implications of these new techniques.

Conclusion

In summary, the incredible advances in the treatment of subfertility over the last few years have dramatically altered the lives of many couples who had hitherto been regarded as having untreatable problems, and have opened the doors of medicine to a world full of recently unimagined possibilities. No facet of this area of medicine will be left unexplored, and the limits of what we can achieve are unbounded. Those couples who have lived with subfertility and its associated pain applaud the advent of these treatments and the medical staff who work so hard to improve them. Those staff who work within fertility units and watch the progress of medical science at close range are privileged and honoured to be able to witness its advances, and humbly bring its many benefits to those who need them.

Resources

British Agencies for Adoption & Fostering (BAAF)
Sky-Line House, 200 Union Street, London SE1 0LX
Tel. 0171 593 2000

British Infertility Counselling Association
10 Alwyne Place, London
Tel. 0171 354 3930

CHILD
Charter House, 43 St Leonards Road, Bexhill on Sea, East Sussex, TN40 1JA
Tel. 01424 732361
Support for those with infertility problems.

COTS (Childlessness Overcome Through Surrogacy)
Loandhu Cottage, Gruids Lairg, Sutherland, Scotland IV27 4EF
Tel. & Fax. 01549 402401

DI Network
PO Box 265, Sheffield S3 7YX

Human Fertilisation & Embryology Authority
Paxton House, 30 Artillery Lane, London E1 7LS
Tel. 0171 377 5077

ISSUE (The National Fertility Association) Ltd
509 Aldridge Road, Great Barr, Birmingham B44 8NA
Tel. 0121 344 4414; Fax 0121 344 4336

Multiple Births Foundation
Institute of Obstetrics & Gynaecology, Queen Charlotte's & Chelsea Hospital, Goldhawk Road, London W6 0XG
Tel. 0181 740 3519

Further reading

READ, J. (1995) *Counselling for Fertility Problems*. Sage Publications.
SNOWDEN, R. and E. (1993) *The Gift of a Child – A Guide to Donor Insemination*, 2nd edn. Exeter: University of Exeter Press.
TAN, S.L. and JACOBS, H.S. (1991) *Infertility – Your Questions Answered*. New York: McGraw-Hill.
WINSTON, R. (1993) *Getting Pregnant*, Revised edn. London: Pan.

References

ABDALLA, H., BABER, R., KIRKLAND, A., LEONARD, T., POWER, M. and STUDD, J. (1990) A report on 100 cycles of oocyte donation: factors affecting the outcome. *Human Reproduction* **5:** 1018.
BURTON, G., ABDALLA, H. and STUDD, J. (1990) Ethical problems of recruiting oocyte donors. Editorial. *British Journal of Hospital Medicine* **44:** 239.
COOKE, I.D., SULAIMAN, R.A., LENTON, E.A. and PARSONS, R.J. (1981) Fertility and infertility statistics: their importance and application. In Hull, M.G.R. (ed.) *Clinics and Obstetrics and Gynaecology*. London: W.B. Saunders, pp. 531–48.
GOLOMBOK, S. and COOK, R. (1994) A survey of semen donation: Phase I – The view of UK licensed centres. *Human Reproduction* **9:** 882–88.
HFEA (1990) *Human Fertilisation and Embryology Authority Code of Practice*. London: Human Fertilisation and Embryology Authority.
HULL, M.G.R., GLAZENER, C.M.A., KELLY, N.J. *et al.* (1985) Population study of causes, treatment and outcome of infertility. *British Medical Journal* **291:** 1693–97.
POWER, M., BABER, R., KIRKLAND, A., LEONARD, T. and STUDD, J.W. (1990) A comparison of the attitudes of volunteer donors and infertile patient donors on an ovum donation programme. *Human Reproduction* **5:** 352–55.
RANDALL, J.M. and TEMPLETON, A. (1991) Infertility: the experience of a tertiary referral centre. *Health Bulletin (Edinburgh)* **49:** 48–53.
TROUNSON, A. and MOHR, L. (1983) Human pregnancy following cryopreservation, thawing and transfer of an 8 cell embryo. *Nature* **305:** 707–709.
TROUNSON, A., LEETON, J., BESANKO, M., WOOD, C. and CONTI, A. Pregnancy established in an infertile patient after transfer of a donated embryo fertilised in vitro. *British Medical Journal* **286:** 835–38.
VESSEY, M.P., SMITH, M.A. and YEATES, D. (1986) Return of fertility after stopping oral contraceptives: influence of age and parity. *British Journal of Family Planning* **11:** 120–24.

9: Contraception

Suzanne Everett

OBJECTIVES

After reading this chapter you will understand:

♦ the different types of contraception and how they work

♦ the problems encountered by clients in trying to choose a method of contraception and the possible solutions

♦ the sexual anxieties encountered with clients

♦ how to identify and correct the misconceptions often held by clients.

Introduction

For thousands of years women and men have attempted to control their fertility using a variety of methods. Few people realize that the name of the condom originated from the Earl of Condom, personal physician to King Charles II, who tried to protect the king from syphilis in the seventeenth century. In the past, women have used oiled rags and halved lemons as diaphragms and men have used condoms made of linen, silk and animal gut. A famous exponent of the condom was Casanova who called it his 'English riding coat' (Durex, 1993). Other methods for preventing pregnancy have been the consumption of mercury by Chinese women and the use of elephant faeces as a vaginal pessary by Arab women.

In the twentieth century we have developed these ideas into more consumer-friendly methods, but there are still many traditional homeopathic remedies in use. For example, women in Sri Lanka eat green papayas to prevent pregnancy, as they contain an enzyme which disables progestogen. Perhaps information such as this will help us with the development of new contraceptive methods for the future.

In the UK, contraception is easily and widely available. Barrier methods can be bought at many retail outlets including chemists, supermarkets, petrol stations and public toilets, or are provided free of charge at family planning clinics, youth advisory services, genito-urinary medicine clinics and some GP surgeries. Other methods of contraception are available from the latter sources and there are no prescription charges for contraception in the UK. A woman is entitled to obtain contraception from any GP who is on the contraceptive list; this GP does not need to be the GP with whom she is registered.

In this chapter we discuss all the methods available in detail and outline their advantages and disadvantages.

Safer sex

When discussing the issues of safer sex with clients, it is important to distinguish between 'safe sex' – i.e. sexual activities that carry minimal or no risk of acquiring or spreading HIV – and 'safer sex' – i.e. sexual activities that reduce the risk of transmitting HIV but are not completely safe.

Any sexual activity that includes penetrative sex carries the risk of acquiring or spreading HIV. '*Safe sex*' involves activities other than penetrative sex to provide satisfaction and enjoyment, and can include kissing, massaging, masturbation, using sex toys and watching or reading erotic material.

If there is penetrative sex, whether oral, vaginal or anal, then clients should be encouraged to practise '*safer sex*', by using condoms to protect themselves from HIV and other sexually transmitted diseases. A wide variety of types of condom are easily available and genito-urinary medicine clinics can provide a wider selection for certain uses, including dental dams for protection during oral vaginal intercourse. Extra strong condoms are the only type suitable for anal intercourse.

It is recommended, and is becoming increasingly common, to use the 'double Dutch' method, i.e. a condom for protection against HIV and sexually transmitted diseases and an additional method such as the Pill or an IUD to provide contraception. Nevertheless, comments such as 'it will never happen to me' or 'I can trust him' are not uncommon and in these situations it can be difficult for you to persuade your client that there is a risk in her sexual behaviour. Women should be encouraged for their personal protection to:

♦ be determined to resist the desire to have penetrative intercourse and to practise safe sex instead;

♦ inform a new partner as early as possible in the relationship that intercourse will not be allowed without a condom; and

♦ be prepared and always carry condoms.

Avoiding the issues of safer sex can be dangerous and it is important that you raise the subject with your clients, as they are frequently unable to voice their anxieties with you for fear of being labelled either sexually deviant or at risk of already having a sexually transmitted disease.

Barrier methods of contraception

Barrier methods of contraception used to be thought of as 'old fashioned' but due to the advent of HIV and AIDS and with substantial government funding to promote their importance they are now being used more extensively.

Barrier methods include the male condom, the female condom, the diaphragm and cervical caps. They are called barrier methods because they not only provide a physical barrier, preventing the sperm from meeting the ovum, but they also give protection (particularly the condom) from sexually transmitted diseases. All users of barrier methods of contraception should be given information about emergency contraception in case of failure in use.

Condoms

Often referred to as 'johnnies', 'rubbers', 'French letters', sheaths, condoms. Condoms are a barrier form of contraception. They prevent pregnancy by stopping the sperm from being released into the vagina, and thus prevent fertilization. Condoms are 85–98% effective in stopping pregnancy and they are also effective in protecting against sexually transmitted diseases and HIV (Box 9.1).

Types of condoms

There is a large and bewildering choice of condoms available. They may have different textures (ribbed) to heighten sensitivity, and different colours ranging from gold, black, coral, red, blue to luminous. Unlubricated flavoured condoms are available for oral intercourse, and hypo-allergenic condoms for those with allergies. There is a wide range of strengths, the thicker condoms will decrease sensitivity and help the man maintain his erection longer, and also give greater safety against breaking. Extra strong condoms are the only condoms suitable for anal intercourse. Clients can choose lubricated or unlubricated condoms, the lubricated condoms can contain either a non-spermicidal lubricant or a spermicide and this will be advertised on the packet. Occasionally men or women are allergic to spermicides; in this case a non-spermicidal lubricant should be used. Condoms containing the spermicide Nonoxynol 9 may help to protect against sexually transmitted disease and HIV. You should recommend that your clients use condoms that have the British standards kitemark or the European CE marking which means that they have been tested and fulfil certain regulations.

Teaching clients how to use condoms

Many female clients need and appreciate specific factual advice about how to use condoms so that they can teach their partner and integrate condom use effectively into sex. When discussing the wide variety of condoms available you should also explain about expiry dates, BSI kitemarks, and storage at normal room temperature should also be mentioned. Women and men may feel embarrassed and inhibited when purchasing condoms so may be very grateful for advice you can give them.

If a model is available for teaching the application of condoms then this will aid learning, otherwise fingers can be used as a replacement. The client should be shown how to open a condom packet (using an actual packet) by teaching them to push the condom inside the packet away from the end that will be opened to avoid tearing the condom. The condom should be squeezed out of the packet, taking care not to tear it with long finger nails or rings.

The condom should be unrolled over the demonstration model or your fingers holding the teat with the other hand. Any air should be squeezed out, and the condom should look smooth. Your client may now have gained enough confidence to try applying the condom herself on to the model. A condom should be applied to an erect penis, but it is important that the penis does not come into contact with the vagina before the condom is applied, as semen containing small amounts of sperm is present before ejaculation occurs. Once the man has ejaculated he should hold on to the end of the condom when withdrawing. Clients should only use condoms for one episode of sexual intercourse and should dispose of them carefully after use.

Common problems

♦ *'It came off'* Condoms usually only fall off when the man loses his erection and withdraws without holding on to the condom, leaving the condom in the vagina. The man should be advised to hold on to the condom when he withdraws.

♦ *'It burst'* Condoms burst if they are put on incorrectly, for example if there is an air bubble in the teat or if they have been put on inside out. They also burst if oil-based lubricants are used: baby oil, Vaseline, body oil, massage oil, ice cream, butter and margarine, etc. (Durex, 1988).

Certain vaginal and rectal preparations also cause condoms to burst: e.g. Nystan cream®, Orthodienoestrol®, Premarin®, Nizoral®, Gyno-daktarin®, Gyno-pevaryl®, Cyclogest®, etc. You should always advise your clients about products which cause condoms to break.

♦ *'He says he can't feel anything'* Clients who complain of loss of sensitivity can try ribbed or thinner makes of condoms. 'Gel-charging' –

using a non oil-based lubricant inside the condom – can heighten sensitivity for the man.

♦ '*The condoms are too small for him*' '*He's too big*' Condoms can accommodate any penis size and different varieties may be more comfortable, e.g. flared or contoured.

Condoms and sexuality

Clients use condoms for a variety of reasons; they can be used for a 'one night stand' and in long-term relationships. Many couples have used nothing else for years, and use the application of the condom as part of foreplay with either partner applying it. Increasingly more clients are using the 'double Dutch' method, using one form of contraception, such as the combined pill, to give contraception and using a condom for protection against sexually transmitted diseases and HIV.

The condom is one of the few forms of contraception which gives the man an active part in preventing pregnancy. It also gives both men and women the opportunity to discuss their relationship and contraception. Couples often progress on to other methods after initially starting with the condom. Condoms can be seen as giving a woman permission to touch her partner's genital area, and the idea of helping to apply the condom may feel a 'safer' form of foreplay at first.

Myths and the media

With the advent of AIDS and HIV, condoms have had considerable coverage in the mass media. 'Safer sex' is promoted and condom use is an integral part of this message. Condoms are easily available, and they have been successfully marketed at both men and women. The design of discreet packaging aimed at women has enabled many women to feel comfortable about purchasing and carrying condoms.

The media has created a new image for the condom which shows the condom user to be a sensible and caring individual. This has also advanced the variety of choice available, from flavoured condoms to blue condoms, and all in easy reach of the buyer!

The diaphragm

Women can be influenced tremendously by the nurse who is teaching her about the diaphragm. All your personal feelings can be conveyed at the initial consultation and if these are helpful and positive they will certainly influence her decision. Conversely if you convey negative messages then your client picks these up and her commitment to the method may be less than ideal.

The first consultation can be very time consuming, but it can help to educate women not only about this form of contraception but also about their bodies. Many women do not realize where their cervix is, and find that the fitting of a diaphragm can help to give them permission to understand and examine their bodies.

The diaphragm (Figure 9.1) is a barrier method that many women find simple and easy to use. Often referred to as 'the cap' or the 'Dutch cap', it offers effective contraception without any hormonal effects. It works by acting as a barrier to the cervix, stopping the sperm and ovum from meeting and therefore preventing fertilization. Box 9.2 summarizes the advantages, disadvantages and contraindications of using the diaphragm.

When used with a spermicide, the diaphragm is between 82% and 90% safe or effective in preventing pregnancy this figure increases to between 92% and 96% safe with careful and consistent use (Bounds, 1994). It is thought that the lower safety rate may be due to the lack of experience of the woman in the first year. As women under the age of 25 years are more fertile they should be advised of their increased risk of pregnancy if they require this method and of the need for careful use. However for the conscientious woman it can be a very safe and effective form of contraception without any hormonal effects.

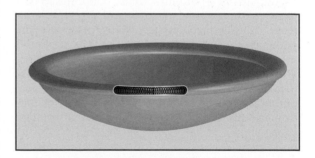

Figure 9.1 *Diaphragm.*

Box 9.2 The diaphragm: advantages, disadvantages and contraindications

Advantages

♦ Under the control of the woman

♦ Has no systemic or unwanted side-effects on the body

♦ May help to protect the cervix against sexually transmitted diseases and cancer by acting as a barrier, and the spermicides may help by killing bacteria

♦ Can be inserted in advance of sexual intercourse

♦ Can be used when a woman is menstruating

♦ When used correctly, an effective method of contraception.

Disadvantages

♦ Needs to be inserted prior to sexual intercourse and requires forethought

♦ Sometimes can cause increased cystitis and urinary tract infections, as it may irritate the bladder and urethra through pressure

♦ Needs to be used with a spermicide to be fully effective and this can be perceived as messy

♦ May cause vaginal irritation.

Contraindications

♦ Congenital abnormalities, e.g. septal wall defects (where a woman has an extra vaginal wall separating the vagina into two), two cervices

♦ Poor muscle tone

♦ Allergy to rubber

♦ Inability to touch the genital area through personal choice or religious reason

♦ An already present infection (either vaginal, cervical, or pelvic should be treated first)

♦ Undiagnosed genital tract bleeding should be investigated prior to diaphragm fitting

♦ Past history of toxic shock syndrome. This is rare but has been noted in women who left their diaphragms in for longer than 30 hours

♦ Lack of personal hygiene

♦ Vaginal prolapse

♦ Virgo intacta. This is a term used for a woman who has not had sexual intercourse and has an intact hymen. A diaphragm may be fitted after intercourse has taken place.

Types of diaphragm

A diaphragm should be fitted by a family planning trained nurse or doctor and it can take up to 30 minutes to instruct a woman how to insert and use one. The session should be held in a warm, private room, free from interruptions where the woman will feel comfortable. The diaphragm is made of latex rubber and there are three types:

♦ coil spring;

♦ flat spring; and

♦ arcing spring.

The flat spring and coil spring diaphragms are made in sizes 55–95 mm (rising by 5 mm each size). The arcing spring diaphragm is made in sizes 60–95 mm (rising in 5 mm sizes). The coil spring diaphragm may be suitable for women with a shallow symphysis pubis, while the flat spring diaphragm is ideal for women with an anterior or mid-plane positioned cervix. The arcing spring diaphragm is ideal for women whose cervix is in a posterior position and who find it difficult to feel their cervix and therefore check that it is covered by the diaphragm.

Fitting the diaphragm

When a woman has chosen to use a diaphragm, a vaginal examination needs to be performed to check the position of the cervix. It may be anterior and near the bladder and easy to feel, or posterior near the rectum, or between the two in a mid-plane position. From this examination it is also possible to check vaginal muscle tone to exclude vaginal wall prolapse and note the retro pubic ridge.

This examination is important for assessing the size of diaphragm required and which type of diaphragm is most suitable. You should measure from the posterior fornix (the area immediately behind the cervix) to the symphysis pubis (the bone in front of the bladder) using your index and middle fingers (Figures 9.2 and 9.3). It can be helpful to measure your fingers so you know approximately what size of diaphragm may be needed, but with practice this is easily learnt. Once the correct size is fitted the client should be unable to feel the diaphragm *in situ*. If she bears down and you can feel the diaphragm protruding forwards into the introitus, then the diaphragm is too big.

Teaching a client how to fit a diaphragm

In an ideal clinical situation, two sessions should be allowed to fit a diaphragm and to teach the

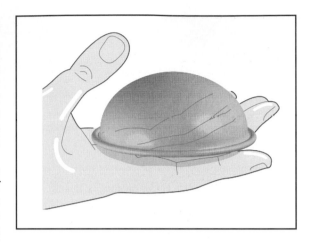

Figure 9.3 *Size of diaphragm on hand.*

woman how to use it and care for it. In practice, however, you may be able to merge these two visits into one.

First clinic visit

Sometimes it is helpful to show a woman a pelvic model or draw a diagram, so that she can understand exactly what you are trying to teach her. In practice many women find it difficult to insert their diaphragm correctly at the initial consultation.

With the diaphragm in place, first ask your client to feel inside her vagina to check the position of the diaphragm and feel her cervix. She can do this either by putting one foot on a chair or by squatting down. Women who use tampons may find it easier to assume the position used for inserting these. It is important for a client to be able to feel her cervix, so that she is able to check her diaphragm is fitted correctly. The cervix is frequently described as a fleshy lump feeling a bit like the end of a nose, and a woman often needs some time to get used to feeling inside her body in what can be an embarrassing and awkward situation. An empathetic nurse should create an atmosphere that feels comfortable and 'safe' as this may be the first time the client has felt inside her vagina and her success will depend on you and your attitude. This is often the longest part of the consultation. Once the client is able to feel her cervix, ask her to remove the diaphragm by slipping her finger over the anterior rim of the diaphragm and pulling downwards. If a client has difficulty doing this, ask her to bear downwards, which often makes it easier.

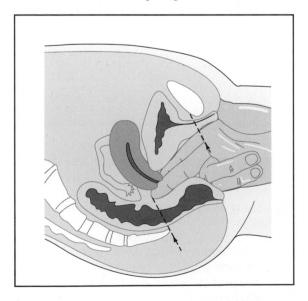

Figure 9.2 *Assessing the size of diaphragm required.*

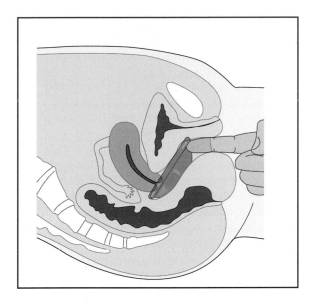

Figure 9.4 *Diaphragm fitted correctly.*

Next get the client to insert the diaphragm herself. She should hold it firmly (she may need to use two hands at first), squeezing the two sides together, and insert it into the vagina as far as it will go. Then she pushes the anterior part of the diaphragm up behind the supra pubic ridge. Once she feels she has positioned the diaphragm correctly, the client should check to feel that the cervix is covered. The diaphragm should be checked by you to see that it is fitted correctly, while the client is in the supine position (Figure 9.4).

When the client can fit and remove the diaphragm correctly, give her a diaphragm to practise with over the next week. This practice should include insertion and removal, as well as use during sexual intercourse, sleeping, passing urine and having her bowels open, so that if she has any problems these can be discussed at the next visit. It is important that the client uses another form of contraception until then. A little spermicide on the rim of the diaphragm helps insertion at this stage, but the full use of spermicide is best left until the diaphragm can be handled with dexterity.

Second clinic visit

After a week of practising with the diaphragm, whilst using another form of contraception, the woman returns with her diaphragm *in situ* to be checked. At this visit she should be given the opportunity to discuss any problems she has encountered.

Check that the diaphragm has been fitted correctly and that the cervix is covered. Occasionally the woman will be more relaxed on a subsequent visit and may require a larger diaphragm to be fitted. Revision of the care and use of the diaphragm and spermicides should be given. The client should be weighed and the importance of this discussed. If a woman's weight goes up or down by 3 kg she may need a larger or smaller diaphragm.

There is a great deal of information that you need to give your client about the use of the diaphragm and it is vital that you back up this information with leaflets.

Using spermicides

There is little research on the effectiveness of diaphragms used without spermicides, so you should advise your clients always to use a spermicide. Two 2-cm strips of a spermicidal cream or gel should be squeezed on to each side of the diaphragm before it is inserted. This will give protection for up to three hours. If sexual intercourse takes place after three hours, a spermicidal pessary should be inserted 5–10 minutes beforehand.

How long to leave the diaphragm in

The diaphragm should be left in for a minimum of six hours after sexual intercourse but no longer than 24 hours. If sexual intercourse occurs again before six hours have elapsed, a spermicidal pessary should be inserted to provide additional spermicidal cover.

Care of the diaphragm

The diaphragm should be washed after use with warm water and mild soap, dried carefully with a soft towel and bent back into shape. This is also a good time to check it for holes. Diaphragms should be stored in their cases in a cool, dry place. They should not be stored on radiators or sunny window sills as they can perish in such conditions. Disinfectants, detergents and talcum powder should not be used on diaphragms.

Follow-up visits

Diaphragms should be checked every six months, or annually in those women who are long-term users. Additional checks are advisable in the following circumstances:

♦ If the woman's weight alters by 3 kg

♦ Following any pregnancy

♦ If the woman contracts a vaginal infection (This is necessary to prevent re-infection once the infection has been treated.)

♦ If the diaphragm shows signs of deterioration or has a hole in it.

Common problems

♦ *'I can't find my cervix'* If your client cannot feel her cervix, suggest that she bears down, which pushes the cervix downwards. If this does not help, try fitting her with an arcing spring diaphragm, which will automatically cover the cervix if inserted correctly. Alternatively, teach the woman's partner to check that her cervix is covered.

♦ *'It doesn't cover my cervix'* This may mean that the diaphragm is too small or that the cervix is in a very posterior position and that an arcing spring diaphragm might be more suitable.

♦ *'It's too messy'* There may be many reasons for this complaint and changing the spermicide used may help. Some women find cream spermicides easier to use than a clear gel, which tends to be more runny. You could recommend she uses gel or cream spermicide on the side which will be next to her cervix and the use of a foam which comes in an aerosol container with an applicator and is applied once the diaphragm is in place. Bear in mind that a complaint about messiness may indicate underlying feelings about sexual intercourse being messy and dirty. It is important to deal with the problem with understanding and to come up with some

solutions. Ask your client how she and her partner feel about using the diaphragm and whether she is having any problems with sexual intercourse in general. Given time, she may be able to express some of her anxieties. The women may well feel more comfortable complaining about her diaphragm than looking at more personal problems.

♦ *'My partner can feel the diaphragm'* This may indicate that the diaphragm is too big or that it has been incorrectly fitted. If the problem remains after changing the size, it may be worth trying a different type of cap.

♦ *'I find it difficult to remove'* Remind your client that the diaphragm cannot get lost and that it is important to try not to panic. If she feels upset, she should leave it in and wait until she feels relaxed. Sometimes it helps to take it out in the bath or she could ask her partner to remove it.

♦ *'I keep getting cystitis'* Recurrent cystitis indicates that a different type of cap should be fitted that is less likely to press on the bladder and urethra. Encourage your client to empty her bladder completely prior to sexual intercourse.

Disabled clients

If a disabled woman finds difficulty in fitting her diaphragm, you may like to suggest that her partner should be taught how to insert it.

Diaphragms and sexuality

The diaphragm can give women permission to touch and explore their bodies. Women have often used other methods of contraception before, and will choose the diaphragm because they feel it is free from side-effects and remains under their own control.

A barrier for many women in choosing and using the diaphragm is ignorance of their body and their fear of expressing this. In a clinical setting it is important for you to allow time for these feelings to be expressed and it may also allow any sexual problems to be discussed and any sexual barriers to be dismantled. Comments from clients such as 'does it get lost?' and on seeing their new diaphragm 'am I that big?' are frequently heard.

Choosing the diaphragm as a method of contraception can signify a woman's ease with her own body and with her sexuality.

The cap

Although this type of cap has been used for decades it is often referred to as 'the new cap'. The cap is smaller than the diaphragm and only covers the cervix itself, being held there by suction. It is made of rubber and works in the same way as the diaphragm in that it stops the sperm from meeting the ova and thus prevents fertilization. It is vital that the client is able to locate her cervix if she is to be able to use a cap.

In order to optimize its effectiveness, the cap should be used in conjunction with a spermicide. This should fill one-third of the cap but should not be used on the rim as this would affect the suction. The same care and precautions apply to the cap as the diaphragm, and its advantages and disadvantages are listed in Box 9.3.

There are three types of cap in common use today. These are the cervical cap (prentif cavity rim), the vault cap (Dumas cap) and the vimule cap (Figure 9.5).

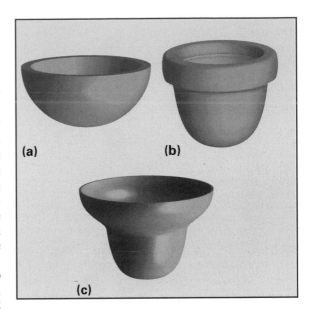

Figure 9.5 *(a) Vault cap; (b) cervical cap; (c) vimule cap.*

Cervical cap

The cervical cap is thimble-shaped with a wide rim. It comes in sizes from 22 to 31 mm in 3-mm steps. The size to use is determined by measuring the base of the cervix. This type of cap is best for women with a long, parallel-sided cervix as it fits snugly around the base of the cervix (Figure 9.6). It is not suitable for a flat or short cervix.

Dumas cap

The Dumas or vault cap is shaped like an upsidedown bowl and comes in sizes from 50 to 75 mm in 5-mm steps. It is suitable for women with healthy, short cervices which allow the rim of the cap to adhere to the vaginal wall (Figure 9.7).

Vimule

The vimule is somewhere between the Dumas and the cervical cap in shape and comes in sizes 45, 48 and 51 mm. It clings by suction to the vaginal wall and is suitable for women who have problems using other types of cap or diaphragm because of poor vaginal muscle tone.

Box 9.3 The cap: advantages and disadvantages

Advantages

♦ All the advantages listed for the diaphragm in Box 9.2

♦ Suitable for women with poor pelvic muscle control

♦ Less pressure on the urethra and so less tendency to cause cystitis

♦ Less spermicide used so perceived as 'less messy'.

Disadvantages

♦ All the disadvantages listed for the diaphragm in Box 9.2

♦ More difficult to fit and remove

♦ Not suitable for women unable to locate their cervix.

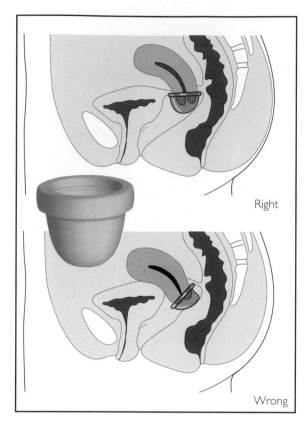

Figure 9.6 *The cervical cap in position.*

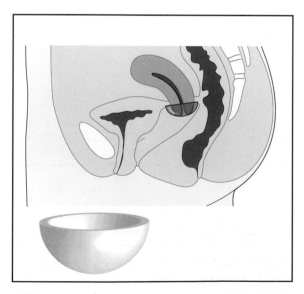

Figure 9.7 *The Dumas (or vault) cap in position.*

Teaching a client how to fit a cap

A woman should be taught how to insert and remove a cervical cap as she would a diaphragm. It is important that she feels confident at locating her cervix so that her cap can be inserted correctly. Many women who use the cap have previously used a diaphragm and are familiar with their own anatomy.

The sponge

The sponge, often referred to as the 'Today sponge' and available over the counter, is no longer being manufactured because of a change in production requirements.

The polyurethane sponge, impregnated with a spermicide, was a useful additional choice for women wishing to use a barrier method of contraception. It was easily obtained, simple to fit and could be used for more than one episode of sexual intercourse. However the efficacy of the sponge was only between 83% and 89% (Trussel *et al.*, 1993).

Femidom

The Femidom is a polyurethane condom with a non-spermicidal lubricant and is the only female condom available in the UK. It has two small rings, one which aids insertion into the vagina like a tampon, and the second to keep it in place on the outside of the genital area (Figure 9.8).

The Femidom acts as a barrier preventing sperm from fertilizing the ovum and is as effective as the male condom, which is between 85 and 98% effective in preventing pregnancy. Its advantages and disadvantages are summarized in Box 9.4. It has recently (Trussel *et al.*, 1994) been found that the use of the Femidom appears to have the potential to reduce the risk of a woman acquiring HIV.

Problems with Femidom

It is possible for the man to insert his penis between the vaginal wall and the Femidom, so you should

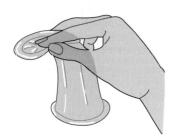

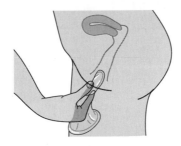

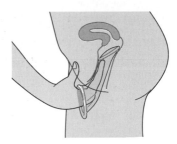

1. The small ring which lies within the closed end of the condom helps to insert Femidom much like a tampon and holds the the condom in place in the vagina. To insert, firmly hold the small ring between the thumb and middle finger.

2. Find a comfortable position; either lying down, sitting with the knees apart, or standing with one foot up on a chair. Insert the squeezed ring into the vagina pushing it inside as far as possible.

3. Put a finger inside the condom and push the small ring inside as far as it can go, like a tampon. Most women do not feel the inner ring once Femidom is inserted. Some may find that insertion is fully completed by the penis when it enters the vagina. There is no need for Femidom to be fitted over the cervix.

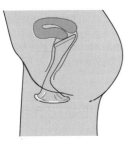

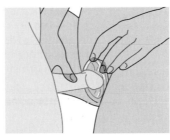

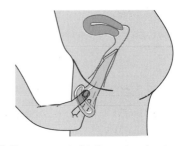

4. It is normal for part of the condom to hang outside the body. The outer ring helps keep the condom in place and will lie flat against the body when the penis is inside the condom. Most couples do not feel the outer ring during use.

5. The penis should be guided inside the condom. As long as the penis remains inside the sheath and the outer ring remains outside the body, then Femidom is working.

6. To remove, twist the outer ring to contain the semen and gently pull Femidom out. Femidom must be removed before risk of spilling any ejaculate, immediately after loss of erection.

Like male condoms, Femidom can only be used once, and must not be flushed down the toilet.

Figure 9.8 *Guide to inserting female condom – Femidom. (Reproduced with permission of Chartex International plc.)*

advise your clients to be aware of this possibility and help their partner with insertion.

Femidoms are made of polyurethane, which is stronger than condoms and can make a 'rustling sound'. You can advise women that using extra lubrication eases this problem.

Spermicides

Spermicides prevent pregnancy by killing sperm and by changing the pH in the vagina so that the environment is unfavourable for sperm. It is difficult to assess how effective spermicides, if used on

---

Box 9.4 Femidom: advantages and disadvantages

Advantages

♦ Easily obtained and used

♦ Not damaged by oil-based lubricants

♦ Protects against most sexually transmitted diseases and HIV

♦ Possible protection against cervical neoplasia

♦ Use can be alternated with male condom, thereby enabling both partners to take responsibility for contraception.

Disadvantages

♦ May be perceived as disrupting sexual intercourse

♦ Needs to be inserted prior to sexual intercourse

♦ Can only be used once

♦ Expensive

♦ 'Hangs down' outside the vagina.

---

their own, are in preventing pregnancy as research is limited. Usually spermicides are used in conjunction with another method like the diaphragm or condom. Some advantages and disadvantages are listed in Box 9.5.

Spermicides are available in a variety of forms: pessaries, gels, creams and foams. Creams are thicker and white in colour, whereas gels are clear

---

Box 9.5 Spermicides: advantages and disadvantages

Advantages

♦ Increase efficacy of other methods

♦ No systemic effects

♦ Easy to obtain and use

♦ Provide lubrication

♦ May give some protection against sexually transmitted diseases and HIV.

Disadvantages

♦ Low efficacy rate

♦ Local allergic reaction

♦ May be perceived as messy.

---

and slightly runnier and personal choice will determine the type used. Pessaries take ten minutes to dissolve; creams, foams and gels can be inserted into the vagina using an applicator similar to a tampon applicator. Most spermicides contain Nonoxynol 9 which has shown to be active against HIV *in vitro* (Bird, 1991). Hypoallergenic spermicides are available for people who find they are allergic to other spermicides. Complaints of 'messiness' can be combated by changing to creams or foam instead of gels.

The combined oral contraceptive pill

Often referred to by women as 'the Pill', the combined oral contraceptive pill (COC) contains the two hormones: oestrogen and progestogen. It works in three ways by: (1) stopping ovulation; (2) thickening cervical mucus to stop sperm from entering the uterus; and (3) helping to prevent implantation by alteration of the endometrium. It is between 97% and 99% effective in preventing pregnancy, although the failure rate can be higher with poor compliance. The advantages and disadvantages of using the Pill are listed in Box 9.6.

Absolute contraindications

See Box 9.6.

Relative contraindications

With certain women extra care needs to be given when prescribing the combined oral contraceptive pill. Women with any of the conditions listed below may be prescribed the combined pill, but will require further counselling and increased supervision.

♦ Diabetes mellitus with no complications

♦ Long-term immobilization

♦ Severe depression

♦ Using enzyme-inducing drugs to treat epilepsy and tuberculosis. These can reduce the safety of the combined pill. Another form of contraception may need to be considered or they can use a higher dose of combined pill

♦ Sickle cell anaemia

♦ Chronic renal disease

♦ Crohn's disease

Box 9.6 The Pill: advantages, disadvantages and contraindications

Advantages

♦ High efficacy

♦ Easy to take, convenient, and easily reversed

♦ Reduces dysmenorrhoea and menorrhagia

♦ Less risk of anaemia because of lighter periods

♦ Pelvic inflammatory disease reduced

♦ Protection against osteoporosis

♦ Less benign breast disease

♦ Reduces pain from endometriosis

♦ Fewer ovarian cysts

♦ Protects against cancer of the ovary and endometrium

♦ ? Reduced risk of underactive and overactive thyroid disease.

Disadvantages

♦ Needs to be taken regularly.

♦ Does not protect against sexually transmitted diseases and HIV

♦ Increased risk of circulatory problems, including migraines, hypertension, deep vein thrombosis, pulmonary embolism and myocardial infarction

♦ Increased risk of liver disorders, such as cholestatic jaundice, gallstones and liver adenoma.

Absolute contraindications

♦ Pregnancy

♦ Breastfeeding – the combined pill will inhibit milk production

♦ Undiagnosed genital tract bleeding

♦ Focal or crescendo migraines

♦ Blood lipid disorder with family history of parent with heart disease below 45 years of age

♦ Hypertension

♦ Previous or present circulatory problems (particularly deep vein thrombosis, pulmonary emboli, transient ischaemic attacks)

♦ Liver disorders or impaired liver function tests (the combined pill may be started three months after liver function tests have returned to normal), including gallstones and porphyrias.

♦ Aged 35 or over and a smoker

♦ 50% above ideal weight for height

♦ Diabetes mellitus with severe complications, e.g. renal impairment

♦ Oestrogen-dependent cancers, e.g. breast cancer

♦ Previous serious illness when taking the combined pill, including: hypertension, otosclerosis, pemphigoid gestationis and trophoblastic disease.

♦ Treatment for cervical intraepithelial neoplasia (CIN)

♦ Young first-degree relative with breast cancer.

Types of combined oral contraceptives

These days, most women take a monophasic pill which contains the same pill dose for 21 days. The monophasic pill is less complicated to take, particularly if she forgets a pill or wishes to delay a withdrawal bleed.

There are biphasic pills which include two types of pill with different doses of oestrogen and progesterone, and triphasic pills which include three types of pills with different dosages – it is important to take these pills in the correct order. These pills were introduced in an effort to mimic the varying hormone levels in the normal menstrual cycle. Every day (ED) combined pills are rarely used in Britain but are used widely in Europe and Australia. An ED packet contains 28 pills and includes 7 inactive pills. ED pills are useful for those women who find it difficult to remember to restart their pill after the 7-day break.

What type of 'pill'?

There are many different types of combined pill available (see Table 9.1). It is good practice to start a client on a low-dose pill when they are first given this method of contraception; 30 µg or less of oestrogen is considered low dose.

The oestrogen in combined pills is ethinyloestradiol and they contain different types of progestogen (see Table 9.1). It can be seen that there are several different groups of the combined pill. If a woman is started on a low-dose combined pill and this does not suit her, then she can be changed to another low-dose pill from another group or she can be prescribed a slightly higher dose pill.

New research has shown that for women taking combined pills containing levonorgestrel or norethisterone (see Table 9.1) the excess risk of a venous thromboembolism is 1 per 10 000 per year, but for women taking pills containing the progestogens gestodene and desogestrel the excess risk doubles to 2 per 10 000 per year. For women taking combined pills containing the progestogen norgestimate there is insufficient information as to whether there is also an increased risk of venous

thromboembolism (Committee on Safety of Medicines, 1995).

Women who have the following risk factors for a venous thromboembolism should be given a low dose combined pill containing either levonorgestrel or norethisterone types.

Risk factors for venous thromboembolism include:

♦ family history of venous thromboembolism

♦ varicose veins

♦ obesity – this is considered if the body mass index (BMI) is over 30 kg/m^2

♦ NB. A previous history of venous thromboembolism is an absolute contraindication to any combined pill.

Women who take gestodene or desogestrel containing pills and are intolerant to other combined pills because they have previously experienced side effects on them, may continue if they are prepared to accept the slightly increased risk of venous thromboembolism. Her informed choice should be documented.

Gestodene, desogestrel and norgestimate containing pills have been shown to have a 'slightly more beneficial effect on lipid metabolism' (Robinson, 1994) compared to other combined pills. The clinical significance of this is uncertain, but this is likely to be an area for future research.

Women are often unaware that pregnancy has a higher incidence of venous thromboembolism, 6 per 10 000 per year in full term pregnancy (Department of Health, 1995), and this information can help to balance the risks of the combined pill. When counselling women it is important that you discuss current research so that they are able to make an informed choice, and give updated literature.

A first visit

Often women will have decided that they want to start taking the combined pill before coming to see you. It is useful to find out how much they already know and you can then build upon this information.

Topics to be covered on a first visit include:

♦ Past and present medical history to discover any absolute or relative contraindications.

♦ Any current medication that may interfere with the effectiveness of the combined pill.

Table 9.1 *Combined oral contraceptives available in the UK*

PILL TYPE	PREPARATION	MANUFACTURER	OESTROGEN (mcg)	PROGESTOGEN (mg)	
Combined					
Ethinyloestradiol/	Loestrin 20	Parke-Davis	20	1	norethisterone acetate
norethisterone type	Loestrin 30	Parke-Davis	30	1.5	norethisterone acetate
	Conova 30	Searle	30	2	ethynodiol diacetate[a]
	Brevinor	Roche	35	0.5	norethisterone
	Ovysmen	Janssen-Cilag	35	0.5	norethisterone
	Neocon 1/35	Janssen-Cilag	35	1	norethisterone
	Norimin	Roche	35	1	norethisterone
Ethinyloestradiol/	Microgynon 30	Schering HC	30	0.15	
levonorgestrel	Ovranette	Wyeth	30	0.15	
	Eugynon 30	Schering HC	30	0.25	
	Ovran 30	Wyeth	30	0.25	
	Ovran	Wyeth	50	0.25	
Ethinyloestradiol/	Mercilon	Organon	20	0.15	
desogestrel	Marvelon	Organon	30	0.15	
Ethinyloestradiol/	Femodene (also ED)	Schering HC	30	0.075	
gestodene	Minulet	Wyeth	30	0.075	
Ethinyloestradiol/	Cilest	Janssen-Cilag	35	0.25	
norgestimate					
Mestranol/	Norinyl-1	Roche	50	1	
norethisterone	Ortho-Novin 1/50	Janssen-Cilag	50	1	
Biphasic & Triphasic					
Ethinyloestradiol/	BiNovum	Janssen-Cilag	35	0.5	(7 tabs)
norethisterone			35	1	(14 tabs)
	Synphase	Roche	35	0.5	(7 tabs)
			35	1	(9 tabs)
			35	0.5	(5 tabs)
	TriNovum	Janssen-Cilag	35	0.5	(7 tabs)
			35	0.75	(7 tabs)
			35	1	(7 tabs)
Ethinyloestradiol/	Logynon (also ED)	Schering HC	30	0.05	(6 tabs)
levonorgestrel			40	0.075	(5 tabs)
			30	0.125	(10 tabs)
	Trinordiol	Wyeth	30	0.05	(6 tabs)
			40	0.075	(5 tabs)
			30	0.125	(10 tabs)
Ethinyloestradiol/	Tri-Minulet	Wyeth	30	0.05	(6 tabs)
gestodene			40	0.07	(5 tabs)
			30	0.1	(10 tabs)
	Triadene	Schering HC	30	0.05	(6 tabs)
			40	0.07	(5 tabs)
			30	0.1	(10 tabs)

[a] Converted (>90%) to norethisterone as the active metabolite
Source: Reproduced with permission from *MIMS. Monthly Index of Medical Specialities.* London: Haymarket Publishing Services, July 1996. Updated monthly.

♦ Blood pressure, weight and height.

♦ Smoking history: what, how many and for how long?

♦ Previous contraceptive history: what methods previously used and problems encountered? This could indicate a relative contraindication, and may help in deciding which combined pill to prescribe.

♦ Methods of contraception used recently. Does she need emergency contraception?

♦ Date of last menstrual period. Was it a normal period? This will eliminate pregnancy.

♦ Date of last cervical smear, if she has had one. What was the result? Have previous smear results been normal? If the client does not know or has had a previous abnormal smear (and there is no smear result available), or it is now three years since the last smear then a smear will need to be performed at a convenient date.

♦ Any bleeding after sexual intercourse – known

as post-coital bleeding (PCB). If there is, a cervical smear will need to be performed with bimanual examination. PCB has a number of causes including cervical ectopy, polyps, infection and malignancy.

♦ Any change in normal vaginal discharge. Does it smell? What does it look like? If there are any doubts it is worth screening for infection.

♦ Breast awareness. Does she check her breasts regularly for lumps or changes?

♦ Sexual anxieties and problems. Towards the end of the consultation the client is hopefully feeling more relaxed and able to share any anxieties or problems. Is intercourse painful? If it is can she tell you more about the pain?

Having found out about your client's medical history and discussed any problems, you should go on to give clear information about the advantages and disadvantages of the combined pill and about how to take the Pill, when to start, and when to use extra precautions, for example after forgetting a pill, after diarrhoea and vomiting or whilst taking other drugs.

Minor problems a woman may encounter when

Box 9.7 Minor problems encountered when starting the Pill

♦ *Nausea* This normally settles after three packets. It can be avoided by taking the pills with food or after a meal.

♦ *Forgetting to take the pills* Many women find it difficult to remember to take their pills before they get into a regular routine. Helpful tips include:

  – Take the pill on waking or going to bed
  – Take the pill when cleaning teeth
  – Keep the packet in your handbag or by your alarm clock
  – Set your digital watch as a reminder
  – Keep the packet in your coffee jar or tea caddy.

♦ *Breakthrough bleeding* This may occur in the first couple of months. If the pills have been taken correctly, your client's contraception will remain effective.

♦ *Breast tenderness or bloatedness* Normally these symptoms disappear after three packets.

Box 9.8 Reasons for changing the combined pill

♦ *Continuing breakthrough bleeding* First check the client is taking her pills correctly and has had no diarrhoea, vomiting or drugs that may interfere with the pill. If it is a new problem then get the client to keep a diary and review the bleeding in a couple of months. Check that a recent smear and vaginal examination have been performed to exclude infection and disease. If necessary, change to a higher dose pill or try a different progestogen.

♦ *Breast tenderness* Examine breasts. The client may find that taking evening primrose oil or vitamin B6 one week before the symptoms helpful. If necessary, change pill to a lower dose of oestrogen or a different progestogen.

♦ *Vaginal dryness* Is there an underlying sexual anxiety or problem. Try changing pill.

♦ *Nausea* Advise your client to avoid taking the pill on an empty stomach. Change pill.

♦ *Spots and acne* Try changing pill to a different progestogen.

♦ *Weight gain* A small weight gain may be noticed initially. If weight gain continues and a woman's diet is healthy, try changing pill.

---

starting the pill are outlined in Box 9.7. You should discuss these thoroughly so that she is prepared for them and to prevent unnecessary worry. It is not advisable to change to a different pill within the first three months as a response to any of these minor symptoms. Changing pills may perpetuate the symptoms, and the initial problems normally settle on their own after the first three packets. If, after the first three months, problems persist, it will be worth considering a change to a different pill (Box 9.8).

It is important to point out to your client that problems sometimes occur for which she should seek medical attention. These include:

♦ Pain or swelling in the calf

♦ Chest pain

♦ Shortness of breath

♦ Increasing headaches

♦ Episodes of loss or disturbance of vision

♦ Pain, tingling or weakness of an arm

♦ Jaundice

♦ Prolonged bleeding or post-coital bleeding.

You should also advise her to return to you if, despite taking the pills correctly, she does not have a withdrawal bleed. It is unlikely that she is pregnant but this should be excluded.

Always discuss how the risks of the Pill (e.g. cardiovascular disease) are increased by smoking. If a smoker gives up, these will reduce to the same as those for a non-smoker.

Remind your client that the Pill does not protect against HIV or other sexually transmitted diseases. To reduce the risk of contracting these, her partner will need to use a condom.

Leaflets containing all this information should be given to back-up your discussion. You should also hand out the telephone numbers of your clinic and emergency advice centres in case she needs further information, and where and when to obtain emergency contraception information.

Follow-up and subsequent visits

It is important to find out how your client has got on with the combined pill and if she has experienced any problems including increased headaches or migraines. It is a good idea to start by asking an open ended question such as 'how have you got on?' and encourage her to talk about anxieties she may have.

Always check blood pressure and weight at each visit to make sure these are within normal limits. If a client smokes it is good practice to check this is not increasing and encourage cessation.

Check that a cervical smear has been performed and is up to date, and that the client knows when this needs to be repeated. This is also a good time to check when the client's last menstrual period was, and whether she has any bleeding at any other time. Does she have any problems with her periods?

The first follow-up visit is an important time to check that your patient is taking the pill correctly and knows what to do if she forgets a pill. Information should be given about emergency contraception.

If there are no problems your client will be given a prescription for six months' supply of the combined pill, encouraged to use condoms if necessary, and given another appointment. It is a good idea to encourage women to return before they run out of supplies, and if possible to keep a spare packet of pills for emergencies.

A woman who is happy with the combined pill and has no complications or contraindications can continue using this method until she reaches the perimenopause.

How to take the combined pill

These instructions are the same for all combined 21-day pills (whether they are monophasics, biphasics, or triphasic pills). When starting for the first time, if the Pill is started on the first day of the period, no additional contraception is required. If started at any other time in the cycle then additional contraception should be used for 7 days. Take the pill every day at roughly the same time for 21 days following the arrows on the packets. This 21 days of pill taking is followed by a 7-day break during which a period or withdrawal bleed will be experienced. The next packet of pills after the 7-day break should be started on day 8. Some women get confused trying to remember when to start a new packet. It is always helpful to remind them that all new packets should be started on the same day of the week as when they first started the pill.

When the combined pill is not effective

The Pill has reduced effectiveness when:

♦ A client has forgotten to take a pill and is more than 12 hours late

♦ Vomiting occurs within three hours of taking the pill

♦ Severe diarrhoea occurs

♦ Certain drugs are taken (Table 9.2).

Instructions for a missed pill (see Figure 9.9)

If a forgotten pill is remembered within 12 hours of when the woman normally takes the pill, then she should take the pill and no other extra precautions are necessary.

Table 9.2 *Drugs that affect the efficacy of the combined pill*

GROUP	DRUG
Anticonvulsants[a]	Phenytoin
	Primidone
	Carbamazepine
	Barbiturates
Antitubercle[a]	Rifampicin
Diuretics[a]	Spironolactone
Hypnotics[a]	Dichloralphenazone
Tranquillizers[a]	Meprobamate
Antifungal treatments[a]	Griseofulvin
Broad-spectrum antibiotics[b]	Ampicillin
	Tetracycline
	Cephalosporins

[a]These are all liver enzyme-inducing drugs which increase the metabolism of the combined pill and, as a result, decrease the contraceptive effectiveness.
[b]These affect the bowel flora and consequently the absorption of the combined pill.

If, however, it is more than 12 hours from when the pill is normally taken, then the pill should be taken and another contraceptive method used (e.g. condoms) for the next seven days. Meanwhile the woman should continue taking her pills and once she has taken seven consecutive days then the pill will be effective. If there are not enough pills in the packet and the client is taking a monophasic pill then she will need to continue on to another packet without a break and avoid having a withdrawal bleed. If the client is taking biphasic or triphasic pills and does not have seven days' worth of pills left in the packet then she will need to take enough pills from the end of another packet to make seven days, but they must be of the same colour and same dose.

Women are safe to have sexual intercourse in the seven-day break as long as they do not lengthen this gap any longer than seven days. If a client forgets the last pill of the packet and then continues to have a seven-day break then she is at risk of ovulating and becoming pregnant. So if a client forgets the last pill of the packet she should be advised to then only have a further six-day break of the pill so that in total the client only has a seven-day gap.

If she forgets the first pill of a new packet then she will have had a total of eight days break from the pill. She should be advised to take seven days

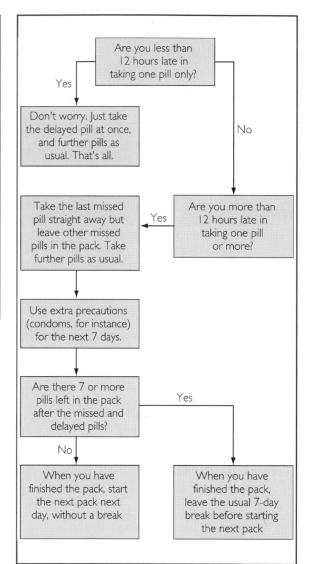

Figure 9.9 *Instruction for missed pills (21-day packaging).*

of consecutive pills before considering her contraception safe. In the meantime she should be advised to use a condom.

Diarrhoea and vomiting

When a client has severe diarrhoea and or vomiting then her contraception will not be effective. In this situation the client needs to use another form of contraception (e.g. condoms) until the diarrhoea has finished, meanwhile she should continue taking her pills. Once the diarrhoea or vomiting has finished then she should be advised to continue using condoms until she has taken a further seven days of consecutive pills after which she will be safe to use the combined pill on its own.

Drugs

The drugs that affect the efficiency of the combined pill are summarized in Table 9.2. Some of these, such as spironolactone (a potassium-sparing diuretic), dichloralphenazone (used for insomnia) and meprobamate (an anti-anxiety drug), should be avoided altogether with combined oral contraceptive use. Others, such as long-term antibiotics, should be used in conjunction with extra precautions for the first two weeks to avoid conception.

If anticonvulsants or liver enzyme inducers are being taken, a woman will need to be given a pill with an increased level of oestrogen of 50 μg and/or to be instructed to tricycle her pill.

Long-term use of anticonvulsants or liver enzyme inducers will mean that the client should be encouraged to consider another form of contraception, such as an IUD or Depo-Provera at a shortened 8-week interval. When enzyme inducers are discussed with the woman, she should be advised that it can take many weeks for liver metabolism to return to normal, and she must wait at least 4–8 weeks before returning to a standard low-dose COC.

Tricycling

In tricycling, three or four packets of monophasic pills are taken without a gap and the woman has her pill-free week at the end of the three months instead of monthly. Tricycling may be recommended for problems which occur in the pill-free week; by reducing the number of pill-free weeks in a year the amount of suffering is reduced. It is important to check that the problem only occurs in the pill-free week. This can be done by asking the client to keep a diary of her symptoms and when they occur.

The main reasons for tricycling are as follows:

♦ Headaches during the pill-free week sometimes occur due to a decrease in hormone level. So long as these headaches do not cause focal disturbances – an absolute contraindication to the combined pill – then tricycling will reduce the number of headaches.

♦ Premenstrual symptoms may occur during the pill-free week and tricycling can be effective.

♦ Recurring vaginal thrush often happens when a period is due and the vaginal pH balance is changed. Tricycling pills may reduce the episodes of thrush.

♦ Enzyme-inducing drugs (e.g. anticonvulsants, antifungal, antitubercle) will reduce the efficacy of the combined pill. Tricycling is used to increase safety and the pill-free week is reduced to 4 or 5 days.

♦ At the woman's choice to avoid bleeding.

The combined pill and sexuality

The combined pill is one of the safest, most reliable and easily reversible forms of contraception. It has given women over the years the power to choose when they get pregnant. For some women this control has become difficult to handle, the pill is in some ways too effective and the decision to come off the pill and start a family can seem very calculated. All this has led to many women postponing pregnancy and starting families later. Women sometimes feel confused and ask for your advice as they feel guilty about avoiding pregnancy but enjoy their freedom. They may also be anxious about whether their fertility is in jeopardy for taking the pill for many years.

Conversely, women who have been on the pill for a number of years and then discontinue in order to become pregnant become very anxious if this does not happen immediately, and tend to blame the pill for their failure to conceive.

Alternatively there are some women who frequently forget their pill or continually find new problems with the pill and as a result have tried most brands. These women are not only unhappy with their pill but may also be trying to tell you there is something wrong with their lives, perhaps really wanting to get pregnant but unable to admit it to herself or her partner. The client who constantly finds problems with her pills may have other underlying problems not directly related to contraception but having an effect on her sexuality which you may be able to uncover with sympathetic questioning.

Myths and the media

There are many myths surrounding the combined pill. It is often felt that it is not natural to suppress ovulation, yet it is forgotten that in many countries women spend most of their fertile years suppressing ovulation through pregnancy and breastfeeding. It could be argued that it is not natural to ovulate every month.

Another myth is that the pill causes breast cancer which is regularly reinforced by the media and new 'scare' stories. The incidence of breast cancer is high and inevitably will develop in women whether or not they take the COC. However, results from the UK National Case Control Study Group (UKNCCS, 1989) found that the slight increase in breast cancer with the combined pill was duration dependent particularly in young women. Today's modern low-dose COCs seem to have a lower risk of breast cancer. What the media do not mention is how much the pill protects women from getting cancer of the endometrium and ovaries.

That the pill is dangerous is a misconception held by many people. In fact it is a very safe form of contraception that is highly acceptable to large numbers of women. Perhaps it should be put another way that smoking can be dangerous, but if you smoke and take the combined pill it is the smoking and not the pill that is dangerous. Smoking is considered a risk to your health because of the damage it causes to your circulatory system. If you do not smoke and there are no other contra-indications then there is no reason why you cannot take the combined pill indefinitely.

Progestogen-only pill

The progestogen-only pill, commonly known as the 'mini pill', is not to be confused with the low-dose combined pills. Often abbreviated to the POP, the progestogen-only pill prevents pregnancy in four ways, by (1) making the cervical mucus impenetrable to sperm, (2) making the endometrium less favourable for implantation, (3) occasionally suppressing ovulation in some women, and (4) reducing Fallopian tube function. The progestogen-only pill is 96–99% effective in preventing pregnancy. Its advantages, disadvantages, absolute and relative contra-indications are outlined in Box 9.9.

Types of progestogen-only pill

There are six progestogen-only pills on the market (Table 9.3). It is now believed that if you weigh more than 70 kg the progestogen-only pill may be less effective, so it is recommended that such a woman takes two pills a day.

What reduces the effectiveness of the progestogen pill?

The effectiveness of the progestogen-only pill will be reduced if:

Table 9.3 *Progestogen-only pills available in the UK*

PILL TYPE	PREPARATION	MANUFACTURER	OESTROGEN (mcg)	PROGESTOGEN (mg)	
Norethisterone type	Micronor	Janssen-Cilag	–	0.35	*norethisterone*
	Noriday	Roche	–	0.35	*norethisterone*
	Femulen	Searle	–	0.5	*ethynodiol diacetate*[a]
Levonorgestrel	Microval	Wyeth	–	0.03	
	Norgeston	Schering HC	–	0.03	
	Neogest	Schering HC	–	0.075	*norgestrel*

[a] Converted (>90%) to norethisterone as the active metabolite
Source: Reproduced with permission from *MIMS. Monthly Index of Medical Specialities*. London: Haymarket Publishing Services, July 1996. Updated monthly.

Box 9.9 The progestogen-only pill: advantages, disadvantages and contraindications

Advantages

♦ Does not inhibit lactation, therefore suitable for breastfeeding women

♦ No evidence of increased circulatory disease or malignancy

♦ Can be given to women who have side-effects with the combined pill, e.g. headaches, weight gain, reduced libido

♦ Can be given to women over 35 who smoke

♦ Can be given to hypertensive women.

Disadvantages

♦ Needs to be taken reliably and regularly

♦ Not as effective as the combined pill

♦ Irregular bleeding pattern

♦ Small number of women may develop symptomatic functional ovarian cysts

♦ Slight increase in ectopic pregnancy if the pill fails to be effective.

Absolute contraindications

♦ Past or present severe arterial disease

♦ Liver adenoma, cholestatic jaundice, or present liver disease

♦ Pregnancy

♦ Undiagnosed genital tract bleeding

♦ Serious side-effects with the combined pill, not linked to oestrogen

♦ Trophoblastic disease

♦ Past history of an ectopic pregnancy in a nulliparous woman.

Relative contraindications

The progestogen pill may be given to women with relative contraindications but will need extra monitoring

♦ Functional ovarian cysts

♦ Sex steroid cancers

♦ Focal migraines, hypertension, lipid abnormalities

♦ Relevant interacting drugs and severe malabsorption.

♦ A woman has severe diarrhoea

♦ Vomiting occurs within three hours of taking the pill and the woman fails to retake it

♦ A woman takes drugs which are enzyme inducers, like rifampicin, griseofulvin or anticonvulsants. In this situation an injectable form of contraception is preferable. If this is unsuitable she may need to increase the dose of progestogen she takes to 3–4 pills a day. The efficacy of this regime is unknown

♦ Weight is above 70 kg, in which case two pills a day may need to be taken.

Teaching a client how to take the POP

The client should start the progestogen-only pill on the first day of her period, and will need no extra precautions. She should take it every day at around the same time. If the client takes her pill more than three hours late then the pill's effectiveness will be reduced and she will need to use another form of contraception for seven days. In the meantime she should continue taking her pills and once she has taken seven consecutive days, then the pill will be effective again.

The progestogen-only pill is taken continuously; there is no gap between packets. Periods will usually be similar to her previous cycle, but occasionally they can be irregular with spotting and sometimes stop altogether.

As the progestogen-only pill mainly stops pregnancy through thickening cervical mucus its effectiveness will be greatest a few hours after ingesting the pill, and lowest when a new pill is due to be taken. You should advise your clients to take the progestogen-only pill a few hours before the time when regular sexual intercourse takes place, so that the effect on cervical mucus is at its optimum, e.g. early evening on the assumption that most couples have intercourse late evening.

When should the POP be started after pregnancy?

If a woman is not breastfeeding she may start the progestogen-only pill on day 21 after birth; no extra precautions are needed. If a woman is breastfeeding she can start the progestogen-only pill four weeks after delivery with no extra precautions. The POP does not affect lactation nor does it affect the baby.

Problems encountered

No menstrual bleed

Irregular bleeding is common with the POP, but some women find that their menses cease altogether. As long as pregnancy has been excluded, then she can be reassured that in fact the POP is working even more effectively and stopping ovulation as well as thickening cervical mucus.

Breakthrough bleeding

If a woman complains of breakthrough bleeding with the POP it is important to check that she is taking her pills correctly and not taking pills late, thereby causing reduced effectiveness. If this is not

the problem it may be a good idea to change her to a different progestogen pill (Table 9.3), and ask her to keep a diary of the bleeding and review in three months.

Care of a client taking the progestogen pill

Initial visit

◆ Explain how to take the POP, its advantages and disadvantages.

◆ Check the client is not taking any drugs that will reduce the effectiveness of the POP.

◆ Take a full case history so that any contraindications can be ascertained.

◆ Check blood pressure and weight.

◆ Discuss smoking cessation if she smokes – although smoking is not contraindicated in the POP at any age.

◆ Check that a recent cervical smear has been performed.

◆ Discuss safer sex.

◆ Discuss emergency contraception.

◆ Back-up verbal information with leaflets and relevant telephone numbers.

◆ Give the client three packets of pills and arrange a review before the end of the third packet.

Follow-up visits

These sessions are to ascertain whether a client has any problems with the POP. It is important to find out if she is having a regular bleeding pattern, with no breakthrough bleeding or amenorrhoea, and investigate accordingly. Blood pressure and weight should be checked, and cervical smears should be performed as required. If a client has no problems she can be prescribed further supplies of the progestogen-only pill and reviewed at six-monthly intervals.

Myths and the media

The media always seems to focus its interest towards the combined pill, and as a result the POP is largely a forgotten method of contraception. Many women still refer to the POP as the 'mini pill', resulting in the belief that it is not very safe. In fact, if taken correctly it is a very effective form of contraception. Nowadays the newer combined pills are referred to as lower dose pills, resulting in even more confusion as women will come in asking for the 'new mini pill'.

POP and sexuality

Women may be prescribed the POP because they have contraindications to the combined pill. This may mean that the POP is not their first choice of contraception, and they may be more easily dissatisfied with it. As the POP is not as effective as the combined pill there can be anxiety over unwanted pregnancies. It is important to discuss the reduced effectiveness of the POP and women may choose to use spermicides or condoms as well as the POP to increase effectiveness.

Women who frequently say 'I can't remember to take my pill' may subconsciously be hoping to become pregnant, but not ready yet to admit this to themselves. If given time they may be able to discuss what makes it difficult for them to remember to take it, and how they feel about becoming pregnant. The acceptability of the POP depends very largely on your attitude and the confidence with which you talk to your clients about the method.

Injectables

Depo-Provera is the most widely used injectable contraceptive in the UK. It is often shortened by clients to 'Depo'. Injectables prevent pregnancy primarily by stopping ovulation. As with other hormonal methods they thicken cervical mucus preventing sperm penetration, and cause the endometrium to become less favourable to implantation.

Depo-Provera and Noristerat are 99–100% effective at preventing pregnancy and are the most effective reversible methods of contraception. Their advantages, disadvantages and contraindications are listed in Box 9.10.

Box 9.10 Injectables: advantages, disadvantages and contraindications

Advantages

♦ Effective, does not require the client to remember to take daily pills, so has a very low user failure rate

♦ Less pre-menstrual tension in some women

♦ Reduced dysmenorrhoea and menorrhagia

♦ Suitable for breastfeeding women

♦ Free of oestrogen-related side-effects

♦ Beneficial in endometriosis

♦ Method of choice in sickle cell disease.

Disadvantages

♦ Delay in return of fertility for up to a year

♦ Irregular bleeding and spotting

♦ Amenorrhoea

♦ Increase in weight due to increased appetite

♦ Galactorrhoea

♦ Depression and loss of libido have been reported but it is difficult to know whether they are due to the injection or other circumstances

♦ ? Possible increased risk of osteoporosis.

Absolute contraindications

♦ Present or past severe arterial disease, or high blood lipid levels

♦ Pregnancy

♦ Undiagnosed genital tract bleeding

♦ Trophoblastic disease

♦ Serious side-effects with the combined pill which are not oestrogen related.

Relative contraindications

Injectables may be given to women who have the following problems, but only under specialist supervision and close observation.

♦ Liver disease

♦ Sex steroid-dependent cancers

♦ Past history of severe depression

♦ Obesity.

Types available

Depo-Provera

This is a 150 mg injection of depot med-roxyprogesterone acetate, which is given every 12 weeks by deep intramuscular injection into the buttock. The ampoule should be shaken thoroughly before use. The injection site should not be massaged afterwards as this shortens its duration of effectiveness.

Noristerat

This is a 200 mg injection containing norethist-erone oenanthate, which is given every eight weeks by deep intramuscular injection into the buttock. The ampoule should be warmed to body temperature before administration as the solution is thick and oily, and the injection site should not be massaged afterwards.

Care of a woman having injectables

Initial visit

It is important that the woman is aware of the advantages and disadvantages of injectables. Once the injection has been given it cannot be removed, so the client should be especially aware of possible menstrual irregularity, amenorrhoea, and delay in return of fertility.

Routine blood pressure and weight should be recorded. Weight measurement is important and can be useful at a later date when clients may feel they have increased in weight and tend to blame the injection.

A full past and present medical history should be taken to exclude any contraindications. A cervical smear test should be performed if necessary. Smoking cessation and breast awareness should be discussed where applicable. Leaflets backing up verbal information and emergency telephone numbers should be given.

The first injection should be given within the first five days of the menstrual cycle. If given on the first day no extra contraception is required but if given between days 2 and 5 extra contraception for seven days should be used.

Women who wish to have the injection follow-ing birth should wait 5–6 weeks after delivery, to reduce the risk of menorrhagia.

Subsequent injections and visits

Noristerat should be given every eight weeks, and the client should be warned of the importance of not delaying her injection.

Depo-Provera should be given every 12 weeks and again it is important to stress the necessity of not being late with repeat injections. These injections can be given earlier if necessary if holidays etc. are planned to coincide with appointment dates. At each visit blood pressure and weight measurements should be taken. Time should be given to the client so that any anxieties or problems, e.g. about irregular bleeding, may be discussed. Clients should be aware when future injections are due.

If a woman wishes to become pregnant she should be advised that it may take up to a year from the last injection to conceive.

Drugs which reduce the effectiveness of the injectable

Enzyme-inducing drugs may reduce the effectiveness of the injectable so the frequency should be increased. Depo-Provera should be given every ten weeks or earlier at eight weeks if rifampicin is prescribed. Noristerat should be given at six-week intervals.

Some common problems

Irregular bleeding

The injections can cause irregular bleeding, although any undiagnosed genital tract bleeding should be investigated before starting injections. If there is excessive bleeding injections can be given earlier, but not less than four weeks from the last injection. Oestrogen may be prescribed to treat bleeding if not contraindicated.

Myths and the media

Many women are concerned about the effect the injections have on their menses. 'What happens to the blood?' 'Doesn't it all build up?' and 'Isn't it harmful not to have a period?' are questions that are frequently asked. At the moment the long-term implications of amenorrhoea are not fully understood, and research into the possible risk of osteoporosis is being undertaken.

Sexuality and injectables

For many women the injectable is the answer to a prayer. They may be unable to take the combined pill because of contraindications, be anxious about the reduced effectiveness of the progesterone-only pill, and be unhappy with other methods. The injectable is very effective, and if a woman is not planning to become pregnant in the near future, and is happy with the possibility of irregular bleeding this may be an anxiety-free method that is exactly what she needs and wants.

Many women, once established on the injection, are very reluctant to change their method as they are happy with amenorrhoea and the increased freedom that they feel this method gives them.

Other women may choose the injectable so that they do not have to think about contraception. It is easy, quick and only has to be given every 8–12 weeks and is almost 100% effective. It may help postpone or avoid the decision of permanent contraception like sterilization. 'I can never decide whether I want to be sterilized or not, because then I have to decide if I definitely don't want more children'. So by continuing with the injection the decision can be delayed, sometimes indefinitely!

Implants

Norplant is the first implant used in the UK. It consists of six capsules made of a rubber called elastomer containing the progestogen hormone levonorgestrel. These capsules are inserted into the inner aspect of the upper arm in a fan-shaped pattern under local anaesthetic and the contraceptive effect lasts for five years (Figure 9.10).

Norplant stops pregnancy by: (1) preventing ovulation in 50% of women (Population Council, 1990); (2) thickening cervical mucus and making it impenetrable to sperm; and (3) making the endometrium unfavourable to implantation.

Norplant is nearly 100% effective at preventing pregnancy in the first year and 98% effective over the remaining four years. The advantages,

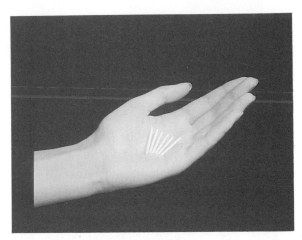

Figure 9.10 *Norplant capsules.*

disadvantages and contraindications are outlined in Box 9.11.

What you need to tell your client

Your client must use contraception up to the time of fitting to exclude pregnancy. If possible she should have her Norplant inserted on the first day of her menstrual period, as it is effective immediately and no extra precautions will be required. Otherwise Norplant should be inserted during the first five days of a period. If Norplant is inserted at any other time in her cycle pregnancy must first be excluded and she will need to use an additional contraceptive method for seven days. The Norplant can remain *in situ* for five years.

It is important that your client is fully aware of the disadvantages of the implant, such as irregular bleeding, and is prepared to accept this. This menstrual irregularity is similar to that of the progestogen-only pill, i.e. irregular periods, spotting or amenorrhoea, but this should settle after the first year. Recent research has found that women who receive implant counselling are more likely to continue with this form of contraception despite menstrual irregularities (Mascarenhas, 1994).

The implant is inserted under local anaesthetic in the inner aspect of the upper arm using a sterile technique. A small incision is made where the capsules are inserted (Figure 9.11). Steri-strips are applied to the incision and may be removed after three days. A compression bandage is applied over the incision which can be removed after 24 hours.

Once the capsules have been inserted they are

Box 9.11 Implants: advantages, disadvantages and contraindications

Advantages

♦ Very effective and lasts five years

♦ Once removed fertility returns to normal within hours

♦ Free from oestrogen-related side-effects

♦ Once in place, nothing to remember.

Disadvantages

♦ Has to be inserted under local anaesthetic by trained professional

♦ Irregular bleeding particularly during the first year

♦ Slightly increased risk of ectopic pregnancy

♦ Slightly increased risk of asymptomatic functional ovarian cysts

♦ Occasional problems with headaches, acne, weight gain, hirsutism, nausea and mastalgia.

Absolute contraindications

♦ Pregnancy

♦ Allergy to levonorgestrel

♦ Present liver disease or neoplasm

♦ Undiagnosed genital tract bleeding

♦ Sex hormone-related neoplasia

♦ Past or present history of cardiovascular/thromboembolic disease

♦ Present or past history of severe arterial disease or raised lipid profile

♦ Trophoblastic disease.

Relative contraindications
These clients require closer observation.

♦ Hypertension

♦ Epilepsy

♦ Migraines

♦ Diabetes

♦ Benign breast disease

♦ Depression

♦ Severe anaemia.

not visible unless the woman is very thin, but she will be able to feel them to reassure herself. The insertion procedure usually takes 10–15 minutes in experienced hands.

Unlike the oral contraceptive pill there is no reduced effectiveness of Norplant with severe diarrhoea, as it is absorbed directly into the bloodstream. Antibiotics, with the exception of rifampicin and griseofulvin, do not reduce the effectiveness of Norplant.

Drugs which reduce the effectiveness of Norplant

The effectiveness of Norplant is reduced by certain anticonvulsants (phenytoin, primidone, carbamazepine, barbiturates), and also by the antibiotics rifampicin and griseofulvin, and the anti-inflammatory drug phenylbutazone.

Follow-up of a client with an implant

As with any hormonal method of contraception, clients should be seen three months after insertion for routine blood pressure and weight check. If there are no problems they should be seen at six-monthly intervals to check any bleeding irregularities and for blood pressure and weight measurements. Obviously, you should encourage a client to seek further advice if she has a problem in between clinic visits.

Removal procedure

The removal of the capsules takes slightly longer than the insertion. It is also carried out under local anaesthetic, and an incision is made at the previous insertion site for removal. New capsules can be inserted after removal through the same incision but pointing in a different direction (downwards).

Myths and the media

It was originally felt that this method of contraception would be suitable for older women who had completed their families. However, from current usage in the UK and experience from abroad

Figure 9.11 *Norplant insertion procedure. (Reproduced with permission of Roussel.)*

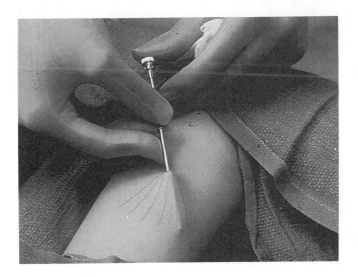

it seems that younger women are choosing this method if they definitely want to postpone a pregnancy, because of its convenience, effectiveness and its easy reversibility.

Implants and sexuality

This method gives women freedom from taking pills, using condoms, etc. yet is very effective and easily reversible. 'What's the catch?' clients ask, as for many this appears to be an ideal method of contraception and is just what they have been waiting for. It helps give women who are unable to take the combined pill another choice, and also gives women time to decide on a more permanent form of contraception.

Emergency contraception

Emergency contraception, or post-coital contraception, is often referred to as the 'morning after pill', which is an unfortunate misnomer as it can be taken up to 72 hours after unprotected intercourse.

It is unclear precisely how emergency contraception works but it is thought to prevent implantation of the ovum (which occurs five days after ovulation if fertilization has occurred). Implantation is prevented by making the endometrium unsuitable to support a developing blastocyst. If emergency contraception is given prior to ovulation it may postpone or prevent ovulation. If it is given after ovulation it may prevent pregnancy by blocking progesterone and oestrogen receptors, and interfere with the ovum transport mechanism.

The hormonal method of emergency contraception is about 95% effective with mid-cycle exposure and around 99% effective at other times, whilst the intrauterine device is almost 100% effective at preventing pregnancy.

The advantages, disadvantages and contraindications of emergency contraception are outlined in Box 9.12.

Emergency contraception is available from:

♦ Any GP who provides contraceptive services

♦ Any family planning clinic

♦ A young persons' clinic or Brook Advisory Centre

♦ Some hospital accident and emergency departments

♦ Some genito-urinary medicine (GUM) clinics.

Types of emergency contraception

The two main types of emergency contraception are: (1) the insertion of an intrauterine device, and (2) the hormonal Yuzpe method. If there are

Box 9.12 Emergency contraception: advantages, disadvantages and contraindications

Advantages of the IUD and Yuzpe method

♦ Effective in preventing pregnancy

♦ IUD may be kept *in situ* and provide continuing contraception

♦ Extended time span (up to 5 days) allows women the opportunity to obtain emergency contraception, e.g. weekends

♦ Unrelated to partner.

Disadvantages

The IUD:

♦ Increased risk of pelvic infection

♦ Minor 'surgical' procedure

♦ Complications related to IUD insertion, e.g. pain, expulsion, perforation and infection.

The Yuzpe method:

♦ Does not provide future contraception

♦ Nausea and sometimes vomiting

♦ Next menstrual period may be delayed

♦ Failure rate approximately 1–5%.

Absolute contraindications

The IUD:

♦ Pregnancy

♦ Active pelvic or sexually transmitted infection

♦ Undiagnosed genital tract bleeding

♦ Past history of an ectopic pregnancy, although an IUD may be inserted but removed following the next menstrual period.

The Yuzpe method:

♦ Pregnancy

♦ More than 72 hours has elapsed since unprotected sexual intercourse

♦ Absolute contraindications to oestrogen-related contraception, e.g. past history of thromboembolism

♦ Current focal migraine

absolute contraindications to these two methods then other hormonal methods may be used.

Intrauterine device

A copper-bearing IUD is fitted up to five days after the calculated date of ovulation. Almost 100% effective in preventing pregnancy even in cases of multiple exposure, the IUD works primarily by blocking implantation.

Yuzpe method

Four tablets containing a high oestrogen dose (50 µg) and progesterone are given in batches of two pills, 12 hours apart, within 72 hours of unprotected sexual intercourse. This is available as Ovran or the specially formulated package Schering PC4. It prevents pregnancy by delaying or preventing ovulation if given prior to this, or by blocking implantation if given after ovulation.

Other methods

Other methods are suitable for women who have absolute contraindications to the insertion of an IUD or the Yuzpe method, but their disadvantages are that they involve high doses of hormones with more complicated regimes and are currently unlicensed for emergency contraceptions.

1 Levonorgestrel 0.6 mg (e.g. 20 Microval tablets) given within 12 hours of unprotected sexual intercourse. 97% effective in preventing pregnancy.

2 Levonorgestrel 0.75 mg for two doses 12 hours apart has been shown to be at least as effective as the Yuzpe regime (Ho and Kwan, 1993) although the time limits (48 hours instead of 72 hours) from unprotected sexual intercourse to first dosage is more restrictive. Further studies progress.

3 Mifepristone. Two initial studies (Webb *et al.*, 1992 and Glasier *et al.*, 1992) using 600 mg as a once-only dose within 72 hours of unprotected sexual intercourse showed no ongoing pregnancies and greatly reduced side-effects, but there were problems with altered bleeding patterns. Further studies continue.

4 Conjugated equine oestrogens (e.g. Premarin) given at high doses three times a day for five days.

History taking

It is important when clients attend for emergency contraception that you are able to put them at their ease, as information about their sexual activity is very personal and the situation can feel threatening and embarrassing. Clients will often remember and talk about the most recent act of sexual intercourse, but may forget about unprotected sexual intercourse earlier in the month, thinking they would have been 'safe' then. Earlier unprotected sexual intercourse beyond 72 hours will contraindicate the Yuzpe method, but it may be possible for the woman to have an IUD inserted within five days of the calculated date of ovulation, thereby preventing pregnancy from previous exposures. It is helpful to chart the first day of the last menstrual period and episodes of unprotected sexual intercourse on a menstrual calendar, as this will make it easier to calculate when ovulation may occur. A full medical history should be taken to eliminate any contraindications and weight and blood pressure measured.

Often women will tell you they either did not use contraception or that there was an accident with the method they used. Common statements about the condom are: 'It came off!', 'It burst!', and about the oral contraceptive 'I ran out of pills', 'I forgot to take them' or about the diaphragm 'I forgot to put it in', 'I found it had a hole when I took it out afterwards' etc. If the client does not volunteer whether she used contraception or not, it is important to ask as this is an ideal time to discuss and advise on future contraception. In a recent survey (Durex, 1994), 43% of adults having unprotected sexual intercourse were aged between 18 and 24 years of age. Anyone (male or female) who has unprotected sex puts themselves at risk of a sexually transmitted infection, including HIV, and should be advised about their local genitourinary medicine (GUM) clinic.

Information the client needs to know about the Yuzpe method

The client should take two tablets of the prescribed pills with a further two tablets 12 hours later. The first two can be taken in the evening before going to bed as long as this is still within 72 hours of unprotected sexual intercourse. The tablets may cause nausea so you should advise your client to avoid taking them on an empty stomach, and either take them with or after food or else with a medication which prevents travel sickness. If she vomits within three hours of taking the first dose she should take the second dose immediately and return for more pills. If she vomits within three hours of taking the second dose she will need to return for further pills. The Yuzpe method will not protect the client from becoming pregnant for the rest of the month so she will need to abstain from sexual intercourse or use a condom. If a client wishes to start the combined oral contraceptive pill she could be given a packet to commence on the third day of her next menstrual period, but would need to use further contraceptive cover for the first seven days of pills.

The advantages and disadvantages should be discussed and this information should be backed up with suitable leaflets.

Information the client needs to know about the IUD

The IUD will give the woman contraception for rest of the month. If she wishes, the IUD can be left *in situ* after her next period or she may wish to have it removed at that time.

You should show your client how to check her IUD threads, and warn her that she may get period-like pains after it is fitted. If she experiences persistent pain she should seek medical attention to exclude an ectopic pregnancy.

The advantages, disadvantages and insertion procedure should be discussed and relevant leaflets given.

IUD insertion

Prior to fitting an IUD *Chlamydia* screening should be performed. These results will not be back before fitting the IUD in cases of post-coital contraception and some doctors will prescribe prophylactic antibiotics. Analgesia (e.g. mefenamic acid) may be given prior to fitting the IUD if the client prefers. Follow-up is essential.

Follow-up visit

Your client should return 3–4 weeks later with details of her first period after having emergency contraception. If she has not had a period a pregnancy test can be performed. The first period after emergency contraception may be earlier or slightly later and should seem like a normal period to the woman. If the period seems shorter or lighter than normal a pregnancy test should be performed. It is important to find out whether the client had any problems with her emergency contraception, e.g. vomiting, abdominal pain etc., to exclude any reduced effectiveness. You should also check at this visit if she is happy with her chosen method of contraception, and if she has decided to take hormonal contraception (COC or POP) that this is being taken correctly.

Myths and the media

Originally emergency hormonal contraception was advertised as the 'morning after pill'. This gave the impression that it could only be taken the morning following unprotected sexual intercourse and prevented many women from seeking advice and help. As a result of this, the name was changed to emergency contraception but many women are still unaware of the two main types of emergency contraception or the length of time available.

Many women are unsure where to obtain emergency contraception, and are unaware of how it works and wrongly believe that it is inducing an abortion. The effectiveness and availability of post-coital contraception should be more widely advertised. Debate continues over whether it may be possible for women to buy the Yuzpe method over the counter at chemists without a prescription.

Emergency contraception and sexuality

The request for emergency contraception may be the first time a woman consults you for contraceptive advice, so the impression you give can encourage or discourage their attendance in the future. Often women attend expecting to be chastized for their failure to use contraception correctly and will relax visibly in the chair when they realize someone is going to help and support them. After all we are all human! Clients who frequently attend for emergency contraception may need time to discuss problems they have with their chosen method of contraception. If they choose to use no contracep-

tion but attend for emergency contraception only, this may illustrate poor self-esteem and their feelings of powerlessness over their lives.

The intrauterine device

The intrauterine device (IUD) or intrauterine contraceptive device (IUCD) is often referred to as 'the loop' or 'the coil'. It is a device which is inserted into the uterus through the cervical canal. It may have copper wrapped around the body (Figure 9.12) or it may contain the hormone levonorgestrel. Roughly the size of a 50p piece, the IUD has threads which hang down into the vagina, so that women are able to reassure themselves and check it is still *in situ*.

The IUD prevents pregnancy by: (1) preventing implantation – this is the main mode of action; (2)

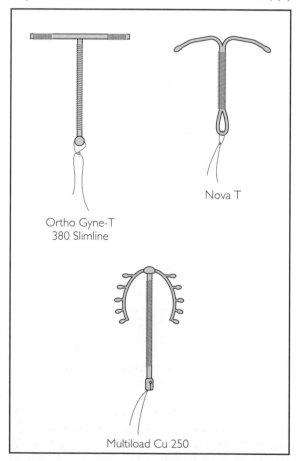

Ortho Gyne-T
380 Slimline

Nova T

Multiload Cu 250

Figure 9.12 *Three different intrauterine devices.*

Box 9.13 The IUD: advantages, disadvantages and contraindications

Advantages

♦ Safe and immediately effective, no extra contraception required

♦ No drug interactions

♦ Long lasting

♦ Once inserted the woman does not have to remember to do anything else

♦ Not related to sexual intercourse.

Disadvantages

♦ Menorrhagia and dysmenorrhoea

♦ Slight increased risk of ectopic pregnancy

♦ Increased risk of pelvic infection

♦ Expulsion of the IUD

♦ Perforation of the uterus, bowel and bladder

♦ Malposition of the IUD

♦ Pregnancy caused by expulsion, perforation or malposition of the IUD.

Absolute contraindications

♦ Previous ectopic pregnancy in a nulliparous woman

♦ Abnormalities of the uterus, e.g. bicornuate uterus

♦ Pelvic or vaginal infection: once treated an IUD may be fitted

♦ Pregnancy

♦ Undiagnosed genital tract bleeding; once the cause has been diagnosed and treated an IUD may be inserted

♦ Allergy to components of IUD, e.g. copper

♦ Wilson's disease

♦ Heart valve replacement because of the increased risk of infection

♦ HIV and AIDS because of the reduced immune system and increased risk of infection from the IUD.

Relative contraindications

♦ History of pelvic infection

♦ Fibroids, endometriosis

♦ Nulliparity

♦ Diabetes

♦ Dysmenorrhoea and or menorrhagia

♦ Penicillamine treatment may reduce the effectiveness of copper.

altering uterine and Fallopian tube fluids, thereby impeding the meeting between sperm and ovum and preventing fertilization; and (3) causing a foreign body reaction, with increased leucocytes and phagocytosis.

The IUD is between 98 and 100% effective in preventing pregnancy; after the first year of use it is almost 100% effective. The advantages, disadvantages and contraindications are listed in Box 9.13.

When should an IUD be inserted?

The IUD is usually inserted at the end of a menstrual period as the cervix is fractionally more dilated then therefore making insertion easier. But an IUD can be inserted any time up to day 19 of a 28-day cycle, which is particularly useful for post-coital insertion.

Before insertion of IUD

Prior to insertion of an IUD a full explanation of the advantages and disadvantages should be discussed, with a leaflet backing up the verbal information. The insertion procedure should be explained.

Analgesia, e.g. mefenamic acid may be prescribed and given 20–30 minutes before insertion to help reduce pain from period-like cramps. It is a good idea to encourage clients to eat something an hour or so before insertion, as it has been found that clients who miss meals are more likely to faint. Immediately prior to IUD insertion the woman should be encouraged to empty her bladder, as a full bladder can prevent the uterus being felt abdominally and makes the procedure more uncomfortable.

All women should be screened for *Chlamydia* prior to IUD insertion. This should be performed preferably one week before insertion, so that treatment may be given. If this is not possible then *Chlamydia* screening may be performed at insertion with treatment given as a prophylaxis. A review (Farley *et al.*, 1992) of the incidence of pelvic inflammatory disease and IUDs showed that it was strongly related to the insertion process and sexually transmitted disease history. It showed that the risk of pelvic infection was six times higher during the first 20 days – indicating how important it is to screen for infection prior to insertion. Because of the increased risk of pelvic infection at insertion it is important that IUDs are left *in situ* for their recommended time rather than changed at the whim of the client.

Care of client and insertion procedure

During insertion of an IUD the client will need support; she may want someone to hold her hand or want someone to talk to her and tell her what is happening. This can be by far the most important part of an IUD insertion; it can make the procedure easier for the client by reducing anxiety and as a result pain, and also can be supportive to the person inserting the IUD.

The skill and expertise of the inserter will help to reduce insertion problems and side-effects. If a client has had problems with IUD insertions in the past or feels she would like stronger analgesia, then local anaesthetic may be used to reduce pain. This can be with lignocaine cream or a paracervical lignocaine block and referral may be necessary to a hospital clinic which specializes in difficult insertions and removals.

Prior to insertion a bimanual examination is carried out to ascertain the size, position and direction of the uterus and that there is no tenderness.

Insertion is by a 'no-touch' technique, so a clean (not sterile) pair of gloves are needed after the bimanual examination. A sterile speculum is inserted into the vagina and the cervix located. The cervix is cleaned with antiseptic solution and cottonwool balls, a uterine sound is inserted through the cervical canal into the uterus to ascertain the patency of the cervical canal and the length and direction of the uterus. The cervix may be stabilized with Allis forceps or a tenaculum so that the IUD can be inserted more easily, although these can cause some discomfort as the cervix can be very sensitive. The IUD is inserted and IUD threads shortened so that they can be tucked up behind the cervix. If there are any problems with insertion of an IUD then the client should be referred to a gynaecologist.

Once the IUD is inserted the client should lie down and rest for a few minutes; analgesia may be given for period-like cramps. If a client gets up too quickly she may feel faint. A sanitary pad may be required as she may bleed slightly. This is a good time to remind her of any initial problems she may have with period pains and bleeding. If a client has persistent pain or change in her normal vaginal discharge she should be advised to telephone for advice and return for an examination. The woman should be shown what the threads feel like by showing her those that have been trimmed earlier and should be encouraged to feel her IUD threads at the top of the vagina once a month after a period in case the device has been expelled during heavy menstruation. No extra contraception is required as the IUD is effective immediately. The actual IUD insertion procedure takes about ten minutes.

Vasovagal attacks and anaphylaxis

Although vasovagal attacks and anaphylaxis following IUD insertion are rare, equipment should be readily available for an emergency and should include clear guidelines on how to manage such a crisis. The woman may become pale, sweaty and complain of feeling faint or sick and have a slow pulse. If not completed, the insertion procedure should be stopped and the client laid in the supine position, the head lowered and the feet raised. If bradycardia persists then slow intravenous atropine 0.3–0.6 mg may be required. If she has difficulty breathing and there is loss of consciousness and absence of a carotid pulse, her airway should be maintained with a Brook airway or Laerdal pocket mask, and emergency help sought. The client should be laid in the left lateral position; if there is no central pulse then 1/1000 of adrenaline 0.5–1.0 ml may be given by deep intramuscular injection. If there is no improvement, this may be repeated at ten-minutes intervals to the maximum of three doses. If required, cardiopulmonary resuscitation should be commenced.

Follow-up

A follow-up visit should take place 4–6 weeks after insertion so that the IUD can be checked and any problems discussed. At this session you should check that the woman is happy with her method of contraception, her bleeding pattern has been satisfactory, she can feel the threads and they do not cause any problems to her partner. The woman should be examined using a speculum so that the IUD threads can be observed, any signs of infection can be assessed, and a cervical smear can be taken if required. Following a speculum examination a bimanual examination should be performed. Occasionally the tip of the IUD can be felt at the cervical os which might not have been seen on speculum examination. If the tip is felt then the IUD is too low in the uterine cavity and should be removed and a new IUD inserted. This is also a good opportunity to check for any cervical excitation, by moving the cervix

gently from side to side. If any pain or discomfort is felt then the woman may have an infection or an ectopic pregnancy.

If there are no problems then the IUD should be checked every six months.

Lifespan of an IUD

The officially approved lifespan of an IUD varies from 3 to 8 years. Any device inserted after the age of 40 years may be left in place until the menopause but should be removed one year post-menopause (Szarewski and Guillebaud, 1991).

Removal of the IUD

The IUD can be removed at any time but if a client does not wish to become pregnant then another form of contraception should be provided first. This may mean starting an oral contraceptive pill or learning how to use a diaphragm before removal. The IUD is removed by inserting a speculum into the vagina. Spencer Wells forceps are applied to the IUD threads and gentle traction is applied. The IUD should slowly begin to descend into the vagina. If the IUD does not descend then it may have become embedded inside the uterus and the woman may need referral to a doctor who is skilled in difficult removal procedures. Sometimes the IUD removed is an old device, which has long since ceased manufacture and has not been in use for many years in the UK. If the IUD has been inserted abroad it can be very interesting to compare the different shapes, sizes and materials used!

Problems with IUDs

Lost threads

If you or your client are unable to locate the IUD threads then you should advise that she uses an alternative form of contraception as she is at risk of becoming pregnant. Lost threads can indicate that the IUD has been expelled or that the IUD has moved within the uterus or perforated the uterus, taking the threads with it. She may already be pregnant so it is important to exclude this possibility. Details of last menstrual period and symptoms of pregnancy should be obtained, and a bimanual examination and pregnancy test performed. If a client is pregnant and wishes to continue, the IUD may be left *in situ*, as it would be difficult to remove with absent threads, but she should be advised of the increased rate of spontaneous abortion, antepartum haemorrhage, premature labour and stillbirth, and the IUD should be located after the birth if there are no complications.

If the client is not pregnant, the threads may be retrieved with Spencer Wells forceps or thread retrievers by an experienced nurse or doctor. If this is unsuccessful then the woman should have an ultrasound performed to locate the exact position of the IUD. If this shows the IUD to be correctly positioned in the uterus then no other further action will be necessary. If, however, no IUD is seen in the uterus then a straight abdominal X-ray will need to be performed to exclude perforation.

Perforation

This usually occurs at insertion or shortly afterwards and is extremely rare. It most commonly happens when an IUD is inserted post-partum in a lactating woman. For this reason a client should always be advised to return if she is suffering from persistent abdominal pain. The IUD can perforate the bowel or the bladder and will need to be located by ultrasound and X-ray and removed by laparoscopy.

Infection

A client should return to see you if she has increased vaginal discharge, which may be of a different colour or odour, or cause itching and pain. If full screening for *Chlamydia* and other sexually transmitted diseases is unavailable then she should be referred to her local genito-urinary medicine clinic.

To reduce the risk of infection and increase the efficacy of the IUD, particularly mid-cycle, a client may wish to use spermicides. The spermicides will act as a germicide, killing bacteria.

Ectopic pregnancy

If a client complains of persistent localized abdominal pain then an ectopic pregnancy may be the cause. A pregnancy test and bimanual examination will be performed to confirm diagnosis. If the client has a positive pregnancy test and pain she should be referred to her local hospital for prompt emergency treatment. If the pregnancy test is negative then an ultrasound may be performed to further exclude any likelihood of an ectopic pregnancy.

Pain or bleeding

If a woman complains of continuing pain or bleeding then she should be examined to exclude infection, perforation and an ectopic pregnancy. A full history of the pain and pattern of bleeding needs to be taken and the relevant tests performed such as ultrasound, infection screening, pregnancy test, bimanual examination and cervical smear test. If the pain continues and there is no evidence of infection, perforation and ectopic pregnancy then appropriate analgesia should be given. Sometimes removal of the existing IUD and then refitting with another type of IUD after a few weeks is an appropriate solution.

Actinomyces

Actinomyces is a bacteria found occasionally in women with IUDs *in situ*, and is usually diagnosed by cytologists when a cervical smear test is performed. If a client is not complaining of any pelvic pain, dyspareunia, or increase in vaginal discharge then the IUD may be removed and sent for culture minus the threads and a new IUD inserted. If the culture returns negative to *Actinomyces* then a follow-up smear should be performed. In asymptomatic women this standard replacement with subsequent cytology is very reassuring. However, if the culture is positive to *Actinomyces* then the client will need antibiotic therapy – the microbiology department will advise on which antibiotic to use and the duration of treatment.

Levonorgestrel intrauterine system (IUS)

The levonorgestrel IUS is a T-shaped IUD containing the progestogen levonorgestrel in a sleeve around its stem (Figure 9.13). It is inserted and removed by the same method as other IUDs, and is marketed in the UK under the name 'Mirena'.

This type of IUD prevents pregnancy in the

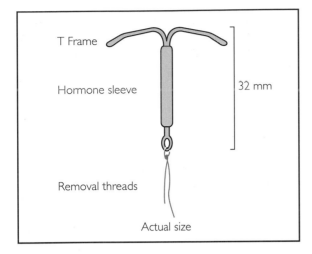

Figure 9.13 *Levonorgestrel IUS.*

same way as a standard IUD but has the added benefit of the levonorgestrel, which is released at 20 µg a day. This helps to make the cervical mucus impenetrable to sperm, the endometrium less favourable for implantation, and causes a reduction in Fallopian tube function. In some women it may also prevent ovulation.

The levonorgestrel IUS is 99.5% effective in protecting against pregnancy. It provides most of the benefits of both hormonal and intrauterine contraception without any of the disadvantages of either and is becoming a popular form of contraception. It is currently licensed for three years although this may well be extended to five years.

Box 9.14 Levonorgestrel IUS: advantages and disadvantages

Advantages

♦ High safety rate

♦ Reduced risk of infection

♦ Reduced dysmenorrhoea

♦ Oligomenorrhoea and amenorrhoea.

Disadvantages

♦ Intermenstrual bleeding

♦ Amenorrhoea

♦ Expensive

♦ Body of IUS is wider than other IUDs, therefore the cervix may need some dilatation.

The advantages and disadvantages are listed in Box 9.14.

The levonorgestrel IUS is currently licensed only for contraceptive use in the UK but research in Scandinavia shows there are other gynaecological and non-contraceptive benefits that make it a particularly interesting system. It is ideal for the older perimenopausal woman who wants to start hormone replacement therapy (HRT) but still requires contraception. In the future, if research in the UK proves satisfactory, then women who are already established on HRT may find this method of administering progestogen more convenient than having to take regular systemic progestogen to protect the endometrium from hyperplasia. The levonorgestrel IUS would also be particularly suitable for women with menorrhagia and may reduce iron deficiency anaemia and the need for a hysterectomy.

Sexuality and IUDs

Many women chose the IUD because 'once in, it can be forgotten!'. Although an IUD may cause some problems many women see these as minor relative to the convenience of the IUD. Once an IUD is inserted no additional contraception is required, and in effect it can be forgotten, it cannot be felt *in situ*, and there is nothing to remember prior to intercourse which would interrupt spontaneity.

A large majority of women who choose this type of contraception are in stable relationships, have completed their families and perhaps this is why they see the risks of the IUD as relative.

Myths and the media

The IUD is frequently portrayed as an abortifacient by the media, nursing and medical professions. This mistaken and ignorant view unfortunately prevents many women from choosing this method. Women are often given the impression that the IUD is 'bad news' with a painful insertion, painful heavy periods, and a high risk of infection. Unfortunately women have only heard bad news about an IUD from one source and may need reminding of the many thousands of women who are delighted with this method of contraception. However with the development of new improved IUDs, and the opportunity of pre-insertion analgesia and local anaesthetic, a painful insertion and menorrhagia are less likely to occur.

Fertility awareness

Common names

Fertility awareness is also known as natural family planning, the 'rhythm method' or 'the safe period'. There are four main methods that a woman should be taught so that she can more accurately calculate when to avoid intercourse. These are (1) the calendar method, (2) the temperature method, (3) the cervical mucus method or Billings method, and (4) the sympto-thermal method or double check method.

Fertility awareness is a way of predicting ovulation and the information can be used by the client as way of either *preventing* or *achieving* pregnancy. Ovulation usually takes place 14 days before the first day of the next menstrual period and not 14 days after the last menstrual period as many women think. So, for example, a woman with a regular 28-day cycle would be likely to ovulate around day 14 and a woman with a regular 30-day cycle would ovulate on day 16. An ovum can live for up to 24 hours, whereas sperm can live in the female body for up to 7 days. It is this estimation of ovulation and sperm survival time which indicates the fertile time (Figure 9.14).

The efficacy of fertility awareness varies from 80 to 98%. The sympto-thermal method is considered the safest of the four methods. The advantages and disadvantages are summarized in Box 9.15.

The calendar method

A woman is taught to calculate when she ovulates by looking retrospectively at at least six menstrual cycles, and calculating ovulation as 14 days before the first day of when her next menstrual period is due. As stress and illness can cause cycle irregularity this is considered the least safe of the methods, but is useful to teach clients when they are fertile if they are trying to become pregnant.

The temperature method

A woman can calculate her day of ovulation by taking her temperature daily either vaginally or

---

> **Box 9.15** Fertility awareness: advantages and disadvantages
>
> *Advantages*
> ♦ No side-effects
> ♦ Under the control of the couple
> ♦ Acceptable to certain religious beliefs, for example Roman Catholics
> ♦ Once taught no further expense or follow-up required
> ♦ Can help couples plan a pregnancy.
>
> *Disadvantages*
> ♦ Requires motivation
> ♦ Requires commitment
> ♦ Requires daily observation and record keeping.

---

orally, but it must be the same route each day. Her temperature is taken for a minimum of three minutes on waking and should be done before getting out of bed and before having a drink or cigarette as this will affect the accuracy of the result. After she ovulates her basal body temperature (BBT) will go down slightly and then rise by 0.2°C and stay up until the next period. A special thermometer needs to be used for this measurement, and the results are plotted on a chart. Basal body temperature can increase with infections, making it harder to estimate ovulation.

Cervical mucus method

A woman is taught to observe her cervical mucus by looking at the texture, colour and amount. Prior to ovulation, under the influence of oestrogen, cervical mucus looks like raw egg white and is stretchy, transparent and glossy – this is called spinnbarkeit mucus. After ovulation, cervical mucus becomes thick and dry under the influence of progesterone. This method of looking at cervical mucus is affected by vaginal infections, arousal and sexual intercourse. The increase of vaginal mucus that occurs at arousal can look similar to ovulatory mucus.

Sympto-thermal method

This is a combination of the above methods and is considered the safest. A woman may use some or

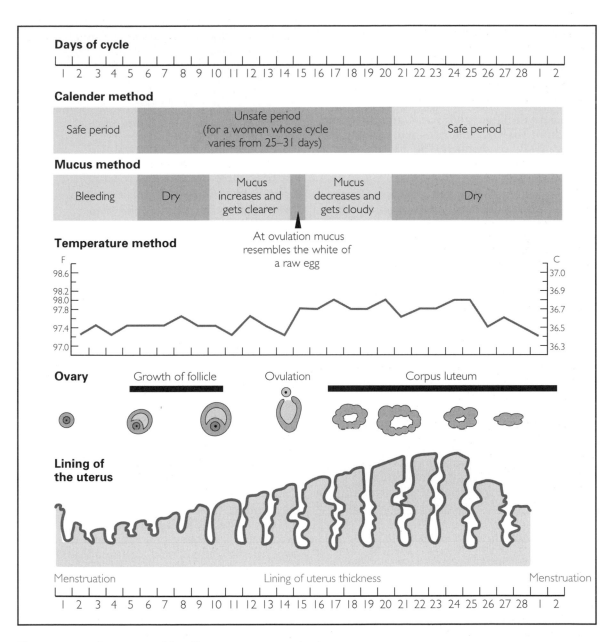

Figure 9.14 *Summary of fertility awareness methods.*

all of the above methods to estimate her fertile period, plus the measurement and consistency of the cervix, the observation of mittelschmerz (ovulation pain) and cyclic changes such as breast tenderness, etc. A woman is taught how to locate her cervix and measure its position every day, and to assess the softness and opening of the cervical os. When a client is about to ovulate the cervix rises in the vagina and is almost out of reach of her finger, becoming soft with the cervical os opening slightly.

Teaching fertility awareness

A woman will need careful explanation of how these methods can be used, with the aid of diagrams and appropriate leaflets. Learning how to use and interpret this method takes place over a period of time under supervision, where women record details of their cycle, vaginal mucus, cervical position and temperature. The Natural Family Planning Service of the Catholic Marriage Advisory Council will teach Catholic and non-Catholic women throughout the UK, and personal teaching may also be arranged through The Natural Family Planning Centre (see Resources, page 216).

Fertility awareness and sexuality

Women who use fertility awareness as a way of preventing or achieving pregnancy find their increased knowledge encourages them to listen to their bodies and interpret its signals. Women are often unaware of how much their cervical mucus changes in their cycle, mistaking any changes for infections. Fertility awareness can help to inform them and alleviate anxiety.

Fertility awareness will become more sophisticated when the 'Personal Contraceptive System' is launched onto the market. Such a system will reliably identify the fertile phase in a woman's menstrual cycle. This is achieved by a small hand-held electronic monitor which interprets assay test sticks which are briefly held in a stream of early morning urine and signals changes in estrone-3-glucuronamide (E3G) and luteinizing hormone (LH) levels. The personal monitor indicates a woman's fertile status by a red or green light and adapts to each individual woman by referring to the last six months of her stored data.

Coitus interruptus

Coitus interruptus, or withdrawal, where a man controls his ejaculation during sexual intercourse and ejaculates outside the vagina, is often referred to by clients as 'being careful' and some women may say that their partners 'look after things'. Many euphemisms are used, such as 'getting off a stop too early'. Coitus interruptus is about 90% effective at preventing pregnancy. Failure of this method tends to arise as small amounts of semen are leaked before ejaculation takes place. The advantages and disadvantages are listed in Box 9.16.

Box 9.16 Coitus interruptus: advantages and disadvantages

Advantages

♦ Free of charge

♦ Empowering the couple to choose either full intercourse or coitus interruptus.

Disadvantages

♦ Important to have a good control of ejaculation, therefore will be unsuitable for men with premature ejaculation.

♦ Maybe dissatisfying for the couple

♦ Increased anxiety for the man to withdraw before ejaculating and for the woman that he withdraws 'in time'.

♦ Under the control of the man.

Myths and the media

Coitus interruptus is more widely used than is generally thought and is the oldest form of contraception. It is referred to in the Bible, and is used widely throughout the world by different cultures.

Female sterilization

Female sterilization involves the blocking or excision of the Fallopian tubes, thereby preventing the ovum from meeting the sperm and fertilization taking place. Women often refer to being sterilized by saying 'I've had my tubes tied'. It is 99.4–99.8% effective in preventing pregnancy and the advantages, disadvantages and contraindications are listed in Box 9.17.

Procedure

Female sterilization can either be performed under local or general anaesthetic and it can be performed abdominally by laparoscopy or laparotomy or through the vagina by culdoscopy. The Fallopian tubes can be excised or blocked by: (1) applying a Hulka or Filshie clip which flattens and occludes the Fallopian tube; (2) drawing up and applying a Falope ring to a section of the Fallopian tube; (3) cauterization and diathermy; (4) excising and ligating the Fallopian tube (Figure 9.15).

Box 9.17 Female sterilization: advantages, disadvantages and contraindications

Advantages

♦ High efficacy

♦ Permanent

♦ Effective immediately.

Disadvantages

♦ Not easily reversed

♦ Involves anaesthetic and surgical procedure.

Contraindications

♦ Indecision over operation by either partner

♦ Relationship problems

♦ Ill-health or disability which may increase risk of operation

♦ Psychiatric illness.

Post-operative care and advice is similar to laparoscopic procedures mentioned in Chapter 17.

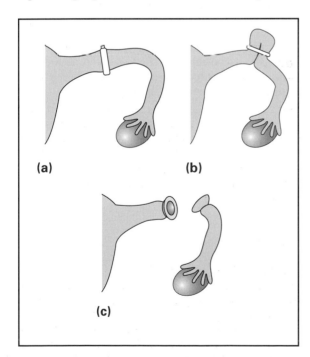

(a)   (b)

(c)

Figure 9.15 *Female sterilization techniques. (a) Filshie clip; (b) Falope ring; (c) tying the ends after the tubes have been cut.*

Counselling a client

As this procedure is permanent and has to be considered irreversible, it can take women some time to decide whether or not to proceed. They also need time to discuss sterilization with their partner. It is important that they think about how they would feel if they lost their present partner, and met someone new – would they like to have children with a new partner or would they feel too old? Many women are certain that they would not want more children, but how would they feel if they lost a child? If a woman has not had children is she sure that she might not change her mind in the future? These are occasionally difficult areas to discuss and there are no set answers for all the questions, but it is important that the client and her partner think through the issues involved. It is easy to influence clients with your own views about these situations, but it is important that women and their partners are given unbiased counselling, as sterilization should be looked upon as irreversible.

It is useful to discuss with the client whether she suffers from menorrhagia or dysmenorrhoea as these will continue following sterilization, and a hysterectomy may be a more appropriate option. In the past many women complained that being sterilized increased menorrhagia and dysmenorrhoea, but it is more likely this was due to the fact they had used a method of contraception like the COC which caused light and pain-free periods and they reverted to their true cycle following sterilization. The woman should be advised to continue to use her method of contraception until after the procedure, so that she is not pregnant that cycle. If a woman has an IUD then she should also use condoms for the menstrual cycle prior to surgery to ensure that no sperm are in the Fallopian tubes which could fertilize an ovum that is released shortly after surgery thereby causing an ectopic pregnancy.

Side-effects

Female sterilization is relatively free of side-effects. Pregnancy is very rare but if it does occur there is a higher risk of an ectopic pregnancy. Occasionally women regret their decision and loss of fertility, although counselling prior to the operation should reduce this. Women should be offered post-operative counselling if they are encountering problems. Sterilization should not be performed at a termination of pregnancy or following childbirth as the failure rate is higher due to increased vascularity of the tissues involved.

Reversal of female sterilization

Although female sterilization should be considered irreversible, it can occasionally be successfully reversed. Two factors are important at determining the success of the reversal. First, the type of surgical procedure originally used and secondly, the skill of the individual surgeon at delicate reversal techniques. The most easily reversible methods are the Hulka and Filshie clips as these flatten the Fallopian tube which can then be reinflated. Cautery and diathermy are used less often these days as it is easy to damage other organs and they are hardest to reverse. The Falope ring can cause a section of the Fallopian tube to necrose. There is an increased risk of an ectopic pregnancy following a sterilization reversal. The success of the operation in achieving a pregnancy can be between 50 and 90%, depending on the original method used.

Sexuality and female sterilization

Many women feel liberated once they have been sterilized. They no longer have anxieties about having to rely on a method of contraception that they may not have been particularly happy with, and concerns about pregnancy diminish to become a remote possibility. This new found freedom from anxiety enables many women to explore their own sexuality and enjoy sex in a way they have not previously been able to.

Male sterilization

Male sterilization, or vasectomy, is often referred to as 'having the chop' or 'having the snip'. It involves the excision or removal of part of the vas deferens which is the tube which transports sperm from the testes to the penis (Figure 9.16).

Male sterilization is 99.9% effective in preventing pregnancy. Its advantages, disadvantages and contraindications are listed in Box 9.18.

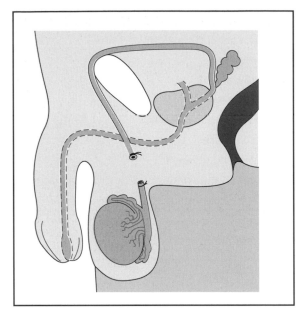

Figure 9.16 *Male sterilization.*

Procedure

A vasectomy can be performed under local or general anaesthetic. An incision is made on either side of the scrotum and the vas deferens located, excised and ligated. Men should wear a scrotal support and be encouraged to take things gently

---

Box 9.18 Male sterilization: advantages, disadvantages and contraindications

Advantages

♦ Permanent

♦ Highly effective.

Disadvantages

♦ Not effective immediately – can take up to three months

♦ Not easily reversed

♦ Minor surgical procedure.

Contraindications

♦ Indecision about operation by either partner

♦ Relationship problems

♦ Psychiatric illness

♦ Present urological problems.

for the first week following a vasectomy by avoiding strenuous exercise, heavy lifting and sexual intercourse.

It takes about three months for a man's ejaculate to be clear of sperm, and he cannot consider it safe to have sexual intercourse without contraception until he has had two consecutive clear sperm counts.

Counselling a client

When counselling men who are considering a vasectomy, it is important that they are given unbiased advice and information. Men should be encouraged to consider how they would feel if their present relationship ended and they found a new partner, or if one of their children died – would they want more children? Men are often anxious about vasectomy and keen to know if they will notice any change in their libido, or whether they will still be able to ejaculate properly. You should advise them that everything will remain the same, the ejaculate will look the same but will not contain sperm but this is not detectable to the human eye.

While discussing a vasectomy many men will ask about the risk of testicular and prostate cancer and whether there is any increase in incidence. It may be that men who have had vasectomies are more aware of their testicles and seek advice more quickly if they find a problem. At the moment there is no definite proof of a link between prostate cancer and vasectomies, and if there is it is very small. It is not known what the cause of prostate cancer is, but clients should be advised that smoking increases all forms of cancer.

Side-effects

A vasectomy is a very safe form of contraception with relatively few side-effects: infection, haematoma and sperm granuloma. Infection should be treated with antibiotics, and a haematoma with analgesia and support. Haematoma usually occur if the client has not given himself time to rest and recuperate. A sperm granuloma occurs when sperm leaks into the surrounding tissue from where the vas deferens has been incised. This can be asymptomatic but can also cause pain and localized swelling and may need excision.

A small number of vasectomies fail, even after negative sperm counts. This is thought to be due to re-canalization of the vas deferens and all men should be warned about the small failure rate.

Reversal of a vasectomy

Reversal of a vasectomy is easier than reversal of a female sterilization, but may be only 50% successful in achieving a pregnancy. The main problem in reversing a vasectomy is due to the development of anti-sperm antibodies in some men. Re-anastomosis of the vas may be successful but antibody production may mean that the sperm count is very low and a pregnancy difficult to achieve.

Sexuality and male sterilization

For many clients this decision has taken a great deal of time and thought. It may cause arguments between a couple – 'I feel it's his turn to do something' – and sex can be used as a weapon to emotionally influence the decision – 'we're not doing anything until he does something'. There can be an element of self-sacrifice and martyrdom about the decision which may continue to cause conflict in the future.

Many couples may postpone the final decision of sterilization, but a pregnancy 'scare' will suddenly make both partners seek a more permanent method of contraception.

Many men feel only too happy to have a vasectomy – 'It's my chance to do something' – especially if their partner has had a difficult time with finding a satisfactory method of contraception. Some men, however, feel that a vasectomy will affect their ability to function as a man and see it as tantamount to castration.

After a vasectomy, a man may subconsciously suffer from grief – of loss of fertility, of opportunity and of sexuality. On the other hand sterilization can also help cement the relationship if it is a shared decision, and can give the couple freedom to enjoy sexual intercourse without the anxiety of pregnancy.

Myths and the media

Sterilization has become a more popular choice of contraception in recent years. More men are choosing to have a vasectomy; not only has it become fashionable but it coincides with the 'new sharing/caring male image' created by the media. However misconceptions still exist and it is still commonly believed that male sterilization causes impotence and sexual dysfunction.

Contraceptive problems

The younger client

By the time many young women consult you requesting the combined oral contraceptive pill, they will usually have started having sexual intercourse and hopefully will have used a condom. Their first visit to discuss contraception will often coincide with a condom failure or having had unprotected sexual intercourse and requesting emergency contraception. The young woman often expects to be reprimanded for her mistake, and may come to the consultation 'quaking in her shoes'. If given time and non-judgemental counselling, it is likely that she will continue to consult in the future. Many young women feel that the confidentiality they are entitled to will be betrayed, but this should be respected unless the health, safety or welfare of someone other than the woman is at serious risk (BMA, GMSC, HEA, BAC, FPA and RCGP, 1993).

Occasionally young clients are being physically abused, although this may not come out on an initial consultation. If a rapport is allowed to develop and the young woman trusts you she will return and may begin to confide in you. You will then have to decide what to do with this information you have been trusted with and refer on for further counselling or advise the child protection agencies if necessary.

However young the woman is, it is surely preferable that she has an effective method of contraception rather than an unplanned pregnancy. It is also important to discuss the issues surrounding HIV and safer sex, and two methods of contraception may be required: one to help prevent pregnancy, like the COC, and a second method to protect against HIV, like condoms. Such a method is known as the 'double Dutch method' as it is widely practised in the Netherlands. It is important to give young women highly effective contraception if they do not wish to become pregnant as they are very fertile in this age group. The combined pill may be the method of choice and they should be commenced on a low-dose pill. Many young women are anxious that their parents remain unaware of the fact that they are sexually active. The pill in such cases may be difficult for them to keep secret in case the packet is noticed. In such cases an injectable method may be chosen. For further information see Chapter 4.

Contraception following pregnancy

Women who have had a baby are often anxious to avoid becoming pregnant again too soon. They may remember the delivery vividly and be unwilling to repeat such an event – this is frequently the time when clients say 'never again'.

Breastfeeding alone does not give complete protection against pregnancy although many new mothers mistakenly believe this to be the case and do not use a form of contraception whilst lactating. They assume their amenorrhoea is due to breastfeeding and are unaware that it might be due to another pregnancy. Such women who have had unprotected intercourse need careful questioning about other symptoms of pregnancy and a pregnancy test performed if necessary. Ovulation may occur by about day 28 after delivery so early contraception is vital for the postnatal woman who does not want to become pregnant.

If the woman is breastfeeding, the COC should not be used as it inhibits lactation and enters the milk in small quantities. The progestogen-only pill, however, is perfectly safe in breastfeeding women as it does not affect the supply of breast milk and only an insignificant amount enters the milk. If the POP is used it should be started four weeks after delivery in breastfeeding women. In women who are not breastfeeding, the COC or POP should be started three weeks after delivery. If the woman wishes to use an injectable form of contraception this should be given six weeks following delivery to reduce the risk of irregular bleeding, whether she is breastfeeding or not.

An IUD may be inserted at six weeks postpartum and extra care is needed to avoid perforation as the uterus is still soft following delivery – particularly so in a woman who is breastfeeding. Caps and diaphragms need refitting 5–6 weeks following delivery (even after a Caesarean section) as a different size may be required. Fertility aware-ness methods are difficult at this time due to the fluctuating hormone levels and lack of a regular cycle. Condoms should be used until other meth-ods are established.

Ovulation may occur as early as ten days fol-lowing an abortion. Hormonal methods of contra-ception can be commenced on the same day as the abortion or an IUD may be inserted at the end of the surgical procedure. Sterilization is not usually recommended to be performed at the same time as an abortion due to the extra operative risks and the emotional trauma that may be involved.

The older woman

In the past, sexuality was a subject often avoided, but with wider media coverage men and women now expect to be having and enjoying sexual relationships regardless of their age. This is often a time when women have a 'stronger sense of themselves', their children are growing up and they now have greater freedom to do what they want.

Women are sometimes unaware that contra-ception is still required in their forties and fifties. It is recommended that contraception is continued for two years after her last menstrual period if this occurs when a woman is under 50 years old, and for one year after her last menstrual period if this occurs when she is over 50 years old.

When discussing contraception with the older woman it is important that you assess her individ-ual needs and health. If she is over 35 years old and smokes then the combined oral contraceptive pill will be contraindicated. Many women who are non-smokers will want to continue with the COC, particularly if they have been happy with this method in the past. The combined pill of choice is a 20 µg pill, and it is possible for a woman with no contraindications to stay on this until the meno-pause providing she is regularly and carefully mon-itored. Longer lasting methods like injectables, IUDs, implants, may be preferred by clients as they take away the anxiety of pregnancy, and may give greater freedom. Those peri-menopausal women who have already started HRT must be advised on the continuing need for contraception. They should not use a hormonal method but should continue with barrier methods or an IUD (see Chapter 14).

Disabled clients

It is important that each client is treated as an individual, as an absolute contraindication to a method of contraception may become a relative contraindication if pregnancy is considered detri-mental to the woman's health. If a client wishes to use a diaphragm or a cervical cap but is unable to fit it herself then her partner can be taught this simple procedure. Involvement of the partner can not only increase the choices available to your client, but may also give you the opportunity to counsel the couple about any problems they may be experiencing in their sexual relationship. They may well appreciate advice you can give them about different sexual positions and that sex need not be penetrative for both of them to gain plea-sure. Partners of clients who have become disabled through illness, e.g. myocardial infarction, pros-tate problems, etc., may feel angry, guilty and even suffer grief. They may find it difficult to discuss their emotional and sexual needs with their part-ner, and as a result may be unaware of what is possible sexually, and how they can initiate it. Sensitive counselling by you will enable them to explore these other possibilities.

Clients who have mental disabilities may have had little opportunity in the past to discuss sexual intercourse and contraception, and may require more frequent consultations with you, particularly if their memory is poor. Always try and involve the partner if there is one.

If a woman is wheelchair-bound then COC is not suitable due to increased risk of deep vein thrombosis etc. However the injectable method may be very suitable as this will produce amenor-rhoea and may be very acceptable to the woman.

For further information, see Chapter 5.

The future

What does the future hold for the professional working in the contraceptive field? Two major changes which will hopefully occur in the near future will be nurse supplying or prescribing contraception and the opportunity for women to purchase emergency hormonal contraception over the counter at chemists. For clients this will widen the choice of people to consult and will reduce waiting times at clinics as hopefully more nurse-led clinics will result. By allowing women the opportunity to purchase emergency hormonal contraception it is felt that the incidence of unwanted pregnancies will be reduced, although buying over the counter will reduce the opportunity for counselling about safe sex and alternative methods of contraception etc.

What does the future hold for developments in contraception? Research is being carried out into biodegradable implants and also smaller single rod implants containing different progestogens. New formulations of oral contraceptive pills are unlikely but the hormonal IUD may be developed to contain different hormones. Trials are still taking place on a vaginal ring which will release progesterone, and with the advent of HIV it is likely that improvements in male and female condoms will be made. Perhaps in the future we will see flavoured spermicides and disposable diaphragms impregnated with spermicide. We may start taking our hormonal contraception via a patch or nasal spray or perhaps the combined oral contraceptive will become available in the form of an injectable. One thing is for certain: women are choosing to have children later in life and are having smaller families, therefore the need for new research into highly effective methods of contraception is increasing.

Resources

Brook Advisory Centres
165 Grays Inn Road, London WC1X 8UD
Tel. 0171 713 9000

Family Planning Association
2–12 Pentonville Road, London N1 9FP
Tel. 0171 837 5432 switchboard
0171 837 4044 general helpline

Family Planning Association in Northern Ireland
113 University Street, Belfast BT7 1HP
Tel. 01232 325488

Family Planning Association in Scotland
2 Claremont Terrace, Glasgow G3 7XR
Tel. 0141 211 8156

Family Planning Association in Wales
4 Museum Place, Cardiff CF1 3BG
Tel. 01222 342766

Margaret Pyke Centre
73–75 Charlotte Street, London W1T 1LB
Tel. 0171 530 3600
Advice sister available 9 am–4 pm on weekdays.
Tel. 0171 530 3636

Marie Stopes
153–157 Whitfield Street, London W1P 5PG
Tel. 0171 574 7400

National Association of Nurses for Contraception and Sexual Health (formerly NAFPN)
19 Whitacre Road, Knowle, Solihull, West Midlands B93 9HW
Tel. 01564 770032

National Association of Natural Family Planning Teachers (NANFPT)
Natural Family Planning Centre, Birmingham Maternity Hospital, Queen Elizabeth Medical Centre, Edgbaston, Birmingham B15 2TG
Tel. 0121 627 2698

Natural Family Planning Service of the Catholic Marriage Advisory Council
Clitherow House, 1 Blythe Mews, Blythe Road, London W14 0NW
Tel. 0171 371 1341

Further reading

BELFIELD, T. (1993) *FPA Contraceptive Handbook. The Essential Reference Guide for Family Planning and other Health Professionals.* London: FPA.

CHALKER, R. (1987) *The Complete Cervical Cap Guide.* New York: Harper & Row.

CURTIS, H., HOOLAGHAN, T. and JEWITT, C. (1995) *Sexual Health Promotion in General Practice.* Oxford and New York: Radcliffe Medical Press.

FLYNN, A. and BROOKS, M. (1988) *Natural Family Planning.* London: Unwin Hyman.

GUILLEBAUD, J. (1993) *Contraception: Your Questions Answered*, 2nd edn. Edinburgh: Churchill Livingstone.

KLEINMAN, R. (ed.) (1988) *Family Planning Handbook for Doctors*, 6th edn. London: IPPF Medical Publications.

KLEINMAN, R. (ed.) (1991) *Intrauterine Contraception*, 5th edn. London: IPPF Medical Publications.

LOUDON, N. (ed.) (1991) *Handbook of Family Planning*, 2nd edn. Edinburgh: Churchill Livingstone.

MONTFORD, H. and SKRINE, R. (eds) (1993) *Contraceptive Care: Meeting Individual Needs*. London: Chapman and Hall.

SZAREWSKI, A. and GUILLEBAUD, J. (1994) *Contraception: a User's Handbook*. Oxford: Oxford University Press.

WHITEHEAD, M. and GODFREE, V. (1992) *Your Questions Answered: Hormone Replacement Therapy*. Edinburgh: Churchill Livingstone.

References

BIRD, K.D. (1991) The use of spermicides containing nonoxynol 9 in the prevention of HIV infection. *AIDS* **5:** 791–96.

BMA, GMSC, HEA, BAC, FPA and RCGP (British Medical Association, General Medical Science Committee, Health Education Authority, Brook Advisory Centres, Family Planning Association and Royal College of General Practitioners) (1993) Joint guidance note. *Confidentiality and People under 16.*

BOUNDS, W. (1994) Contraceptive efficacy of the diaphragm and cervical caps used in conjunction with a spermicide – a fresh look at the evidence. *The British Journal of Family Planning* **20:** 84–87.

COMMITTEE ON SAFETY OF MEDICINES (1995) Combined oral contraceptives and thromboembolism, letter. London: CSM.

DEPARTMENT OF HEALTH (1995) The response for doctors to the committee on safety of medicines, letter. FPA and Faculty of Family Planning and Reproductive Health Care of the Royal College of Obstetricians and Gynaecologists: London: HMSO.

DUREX (1988) *Oil-based Lubricants and Ointments can Damage Condoms and Diaphragms*. London: Durex Information Service for Sexual Health.

DUREX (1993) *History of the Condom*. London: Durex Information Service For Sexual Health.

DUREX (1994) *The Durex Report. A Summary of Consumer Research into Contraception*. London: The London Rubber Co.

FARLEY, T., ROSENBERG, M., ROWE, P., CHEN, J-H. and MEIRIK, O. (1992) Intrauterine devices and pelvic inflammatory disease: an international perspective. *Lancet* **39:** 785–88.

GLASIER, A., THONG, K.J., DEWAR, M., MACKIE, M. and BAIRD, D.T. (1992) Mifepristone (RU486) compared with high-dose oestrogen progestogen for emergency post coital contraception. *New England Journal of Medicine* **327**(15): 1041–44.

HO, P.C. and KWAN, M.S.W. (1993) A prospective randomised comparison of levonorgestrel with Yuzpe regimen in post coital contraception. *Human Reproduction* **8**(3): 389–92.

LLEWELLYN SMITH, J. (1994) New lessons from old wives. *The Times* 28 July.

MASCARENHAS, L., NEWTON, P. and NEWTON, J. (1994) First clinical experience with contraceptive implants in the UK. *British Journal of Family Planning* **20:** 60.

POPULATION COUNCIL (1990) *Norplant Levonorgestrel implant: a Summary of Scientific Data*. New York: The Population Council.

ROBINSON, G.E. (1994) Low dose combined oral contraceptives. *British Journal of Obstetrics and Gynaecology* **101:** 1036–41.

SZAREWSKI, A. and GUILLEBAUD, J. (1991) Regular review: contraception: current state of the art. *British Medical Journal* **302:** 1224–26.

TRUSSELL, J., STRICKLER, J. and VAUGHAN, B. (1993) Contraceptive efficacy of the diaphragm, the sponge and the cervical cap. *Family Planning Perspectives* **25**(3): 100–5, 135.

TRUSSELL, J., STURGEN, K., STRICKLER, J. and DOMINIK, R. (1994) Comparative contraceptive efficacy of the female condom and other barrier methods. *Family Planning Perspectives* **25**(2): 66–72.

UKNCCS (UK National Case-Control Study Group) (1989) Oral contraceptive use and breast cancer risk in young women. *Lancet* **i:** 973–82.

WEBB, A.M.C., RUSSEL, J. and ELSTEIN, M. (1992) Comparison of Yuzpe regimen, danazol and Mifepristone (RU486) in oral post-coital contraception. *British Medical Journal* **305:** 927–31.

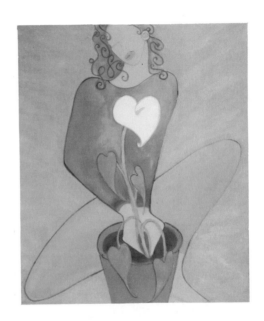

WOMEN'S HEALTH ISSUES

10: Breast screening and breast disorders

Gay Curling and Karen Tierney

OBJECTIVES

After reading this chapter you will understand:

♦ the importance of promoting breast health awareness for women

♦ the structure and function of the healthy breast

♦ the epidemiology and risk factors for breast cancer

♦ what happens in a breast screening unit, covering clinical examination, breast awareness and diagnostic investigations

♦ the role of surgery, radiotherapy and chemotherapy in the treatment of breast cancer

♦ the need for psychological and social care for the woman with breast cancer

♦ the need for symptom control in the palliation of metastatic disease.

Introduction

Breasts are an obvious indication of femininity and are seen by both men and women as symbols of womanhood, fertility and motherhood. In Western society the breast is associated with sexual attractiveness and sexual stimulation, whereas in many other cultures the breasts' purpose is purely functional and utilitarian – feeding babies.

Women tend to be very conscious of their breasts. Breast problems and anxieties account for a large number of consultations in GP surgeries, family planning and well-woman clinics. Nurses are in the 'front line' in many of these consultations and so it is important that they have up-to-date information and are aware of the psychological aspects of breast disease.

This chapter will focus on some of the problems associated with benign breast disease and breast cancer and will provide an insight into all aspects of breast care. There is so much to learn about breast screening and breast disorders that it is impossible to cover the subject in finite detail in a chapter of this nature. It is therefore suggested that the reader should refer to the further reading list and references at the end of the chapter if they need more information.

Anatomy and physiology of the breast

The breast is a glandular organ which lies over the 2nd to 6th ribs on the chest wall. During fetal development an ectodermal ridge (milk line)

extends from the axilla to the groin bilaterally; in time this disappears, leaving a pair of breasts in the position described above. During puberty, breasts increase in size, connective tissue increases, the ducts lengthen and breast lobules are formed.

The ductal system of the breast extends from the nipple to the lobule (Figure 10.1). There are approximately 15–20 ducts which open on to the nipple. From the lobule, which ends in 100 or so tiny bulbs called acini – where milk is produced – the ducts extend towards the nipple and enlarge, where they are called the lactiferous sinuses. It is these that open on to the nipple for the secretion of milk. The nipple is surrounded by the areola, which may vary in colour from pinkish to dark brown. It contains small elevations which are known as the tubercles of Montgomery, and these help to lubricate the area during breastfeeding.

Apart from lobules and ducts, the breast contains fat and blood vessels, predominantly from branches of the internal mammary artery and from branches of the lateral thoracic artery. Major lymph drainage is to the axilla and internal mammary chain. The lymph drainage system is thought to be important in relation to the spread of malignant disease. The breast tissue is held in position by Cooper's ligaments – fibrous bands which run from the fascia between the lobes to the skin and extend up towards the armpit, forming the axillary tail. Two muscles lie beneath the breast – the pectoralis major and pectoralis minor.

Breast structure varies considerably. At the time of menarche the breasts begin to grow rapidly under the influence of sex hormones. Each month, when a woman approaches menstruation, the size of the breasts may fluctuate. This is in preparation for a possible pregnancy. If a pregnancy does occur, then the breast enlarges even more and the acini multiply. By the end of pregnancy the breast is almost entirely a glandular structure.

Following pregnancy these changes subside and the breast becomes less glandular. As the woman grows older the lobules and acini begin to decrease and fatty tissue increases. This is accelerated with the menopause.

Oestrogen and progesterone produced by the ovaries influence the initial growth and subsequent development of the breast. The proliferation and development of the mammary tissue during pregnancy is stimulated by oestrogen and progesterone produced by the corpus luteum and the placenta. Other hormones believed to be involved are prolactin and the adrenal corticosteroids. It has been surmised that the high levels of sex steroids present during pregnancy inhibit the action of prolactin on breast tissue. After the separation of the placenta at delivery there is rapid fall of oestrogen and progesterone production, the inhibitory effect is lifted, and milk production is stimulated. Prolactin levels rise rapidly during breastfeeding, thus stimulating additional milk production. In the absence of breastfeeding, prolactin levels drop to a normal non-pregnant state within seven days after delivery (DiSaia, 1993).

Epidemiology and risk factors for breast cancer

Epidemiology is the study of the distribution of diseases in a population. Breast cancer is the

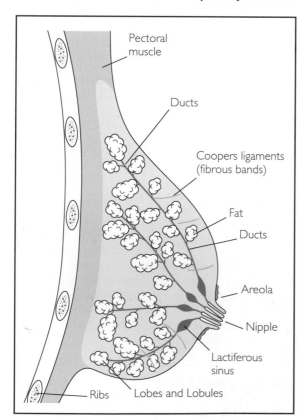

Figure 10.1 *Sagittal section of the breast.*

Pectoral muscle

Ducts

Coopers ligaments (fibrous bands)

Fat

Ducts

Areola

Nipple

Lactiferous sinus

Ribs   Lobes and Lobules

commonest malignancy in the female population worldwide (Parkin *et al.*, 1984), and is the commonest cause of death in women between the ages of 44 and 50. In the UK 1 in 12 women develop breast cancer. The incidence of breast cancer is ideally measured by population-based cancer registries which record all new diagnoses of cancer in a given population in a given time period (Chamberlain, 1993). In most countries breast cancer is increasing in frequency, the increase being most marked in previously low-incidence developing countries, and least in countries like the US which have been affluent over several decades (Kalache, 1990).

Risk factors

Family history

The most common risk factor is a history of breast cancer in a first-degree relative on the maternal side. This risk nearly doubles if the relative was pre-menopausal and almost trebles if the cancer was bilateral, or there was more than one first-degree relative who was pre-menopausal. In certain families it is clear that breast cancer is hereditary. In 40% of these families there is a mutation in a gene known as *BRCA1* located on chromosome 17 (Dixon and Sainsbury, 1993). In addition a further gene, *BRCA2*, has been isolated.

Women with a family history of breast cancer may be fortunate enough to be referred to one of the few early diagnostic or screening units in the UK. There are relatively few such units at present but hopefully more will be opening in the future.

Menstrual history

An early menarche before 12 years and a late menopause after the age of 55 years increases a woman's risk factors. Women who have had a pre-menopausal oophorectomy are at a substantially reduced risk of developing breast cancer.

Age

Age is another very important factor, with older women being at a much greater risk than younger women. The increase of risk rises steadily from the age of 40.

Reproductive history

Nulliparous women are at greater risk than those who have had children, but another important risk factor is a woman's age at her first full-term pregnancy. The risk of breast cancer in women who have their first child after the age of 30 is about twice that of women who have their first child before the age of 20. Women who have their first child after the age of 35 appear to be at even higher risk than nulliparous women (Dixon and Sainsbury, 1993).

Breastfeeding

Results of studies on lactation and breast cancer are confusing although breastfeeding appears to be protective against the development of breast cancer, particularly in young women (Chilvers *et al.*, 1993). This study also demonstrated that the risk decreases with increasing duration of breastfeeding, with breastfeeding each baby for three months or longer giving greatest protection.

Oral contraception

Numerous case-controlled studies have been done comparing use of the oral contraceptive pill in breast cancer cases and age-matched controls. It has been established that there is no association between use of oral contraception and breast cancer amongst women in their late twenties and thirties after one or more pregnancies; moreover oral contraception seem to have a protective effect against benign breast disease (Chamberlain, 1993). In other studies, in women who have used oral contraception at a young age the risk of breast cancer does increase, particularly if used continuously for several years (UK National Case-Control Study Group, 1989).

Hormone replacement therapy (HRT)

The benefits of HRT are well-known, i.e. protection against cardiovascular disease and osteoporosis as well as an increased quality of life in women suffering from menopausal symptoms. With regards to the breast cancer risk most studies have shown a slightly increased risk in long duration of use (i.e. more than 10 years). Duration of treatment is more important than dose used. However, it appears that if breast cancer is diagnosed in women who are already taking HRT then it will be picked up at an earlier stage, it tends to be of a lower grade and with a relatively good prognosis.

Exposure to radiation

Follow-up of survivors of the nuclear bombings in Japan has demonstrated an increased risk of breast cancer in those exposed. A number of other studies of women who received large doses of ionizing radiation for medical reasons have also shown an increased risk (Chamberlain, 1993).

Diet, weight and alcohol

Fat consumption has been investigated, but no definite conclusion can be drawn from available data although it has been shown that obese women are at a greater risk than slim women. Alcohol has been associated with a moderately increased risk of breast cancer, particularly in thin, pre-menopausal women (IARC, 1988).

Interestingly, cigarette smoking is *not* related to an increased risk of developing breast cancer.

Geographic variations

There is marked variation in the incidence of mortality of breast cancer between different countries

(Figure 10.2). In families migrating from Japan – a low-incidence country – to the US – a high-incidence country – studies show that second-generation women acquire the same incidence as the host country.

Clinical examination

It is very important to take a detailed history before performing a clinical examination. If any of the risk factors mentioned earlier are present then these must be taken into account. It is important, if the woman is pre-menopausal, to determine the start of her last period because this may necessitate bringing her back for a further examination at a different time in her cycle as breasts are frequently tender and lumpy premenstrually.

Obviously symptoms noted by the woman herself are important:

♦ If the patient has found a lump in her breast, has it changed in size, become larger or smaller? Is it tender?

♦ Has one breast increased or decreased in size? Most women have one breast slightly larger than the other and this sometimes becomes more obvious if the patient has put on weight. Many women, however are unaware of this

Figure 10.2
International breast cancer rates. (Reproduced from Cancer Research Campaign *Factsheet 6.3, 1991.)*

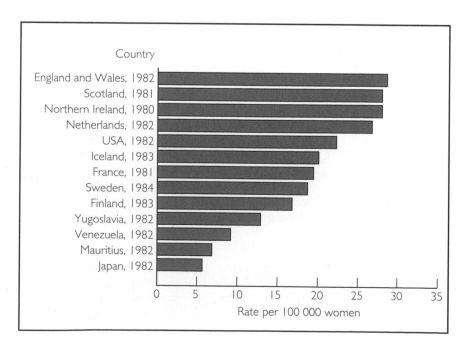

asymmetry and 'my husband has never noticed' is a frequently heard comment.

♦ Has there been any nipple discharge? This is particularly significant if it occurs spontaneously. Was the discharge blood-stained? Has there been any nipple change? Has the nipple started to retract, or does it appear to be pointing in a different direction?

♦ Is there any nodularity or thickening in one area? This can be just as important as a lump.

♦ Has the woman noticed a dimple or crease, and what position was she in when she noticed this? For instance, was she looking down on her breasts or was she looking in the mirror, and what position were her arms in at the time? If she was looking down, then the examiner should look at the breasts in the same position, i.e. from behind the patient and looking down.

♦ Any other symptoms? Many patients do not have a definite symptom but state that they have an 'increased awareness' of one breast.

Examination of the breasts should always be performed in two parts: either *looking* and then *feeling* or vice versa. If you are looking first then the patient should sit on the side of the couch, facing you and you should stand back to see if there is any difference in size or shape. As mentioned earlier, it is very common to have one breast slightly larger than the other and the woman may be unaware of this and ask if it means something is wrong. She needs to be re-assured and it must be stressed that this is a common occurrence. Asking if her bra seems to have always been slightly tighter on one side can sometimes confirm this. If not, then particular attention should be paid when examining this breast. The woman should then be asked to raise her arms above her head for you to observe any dimples or creases, then she should place her hands on her hips, push in and bring the elbows forward. At this point, it may be necessary to bend down and look at the breasts from beneath – there are not many breast sizes that you can see the lower part of the breast without bending down. The woman should then put her hands on the side of the couch keeping the arms straight and pushing down and then lean forward. Again you must bend down to observe the lower part of the breast. Women feel reassured if you always explain what you are doing and what you are looking for.

These three positions that the woman is asked to adopt – with hands raised, with hands on hips, and leaning forward – are very important when looking for a dimple or crease because they may only appear in one of the three positions. When documenting findings it is essential that if a dimple or crease has been observed, then the position the woman was in must be stated, i.e. dimple only seen with hands on hips. If an abnormality has been noted, it is sometimes helpful to mark the area so that when physically examining the patient attention can be paid to this area with regards to identifying any nodularity, thickening or lump which may be associated with the dimple or crease which has previously been observed.

Scenario

Doreen, aged 66, had been routinely screened at a diagnostic unit for many years. She had no family history of breast cancer. At one routine screening appointment, when a detailed history was taken, she reported that her left nipple was becoming more retracted than had previously been noted. There were no problems with her right breast.

Before starting a clinical examination, it was noted that Doreen had a slight crease in the inner central area of the right breast which Doreen had not noticed. On examination, an area of discrete nodularity was noted. The left breast, which Doreen was more concerned about, was normal. On sitting, the crease was again observed in the right breast. No actual clinical mass was felt.

Because of these findings Doreen was sent for a mammogram. The report stated that there was a carcinoma in the right *breast and that Doreen's left breast was normal.*

This was an impalpable cancer in a large breast – 42D – that was detected only because of the observed crease.

Whilst the woman is in the sitting position, the supraclavicular fossa can be palpated, either standing in front of the patient or from behind. The infraclavicular area can also be felt by running the hands down from the clavicle to the breast. Then the axilla should be palpated by feeling high up into the axilla with the flats of the fingers and bringing them down towards the axillary tail.

On completion of this part of the examination, the woman should then be asked to lie down. The arm should be raised above the head on the side of the breast which is to be examined first. The clinical examination should be performed with the flat of the fingers and a systematic examination should be carried out. If an abnormality is detected then the fingertips are used to determine consistency, size and mobility. The clinical examination must cover the whole breast and not forget the axillary tail and beneath the nipple. After examining both breasts individually, then the patient should be turned on her side in the oblique position, with her arm raised above her head. This positioning allows for a more thorough examination of the outer quadrant of the breast, particularly in the larger breasted patient and quite often a lump which was not felt with the patient lying on her back can be very obvious in this position.

If a suspected abnormality is found as mentioned earlier in the case of a crease, then all the characteristics must be noted and documented and the position of the abnormality accurately stated. Figure 10.3 shows the most common sites for breast cancer.

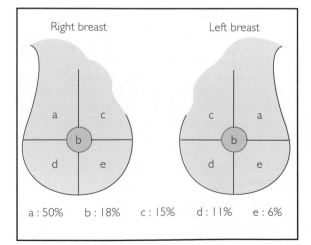

a : 50%   b : 18%   c : 15%   d : 11%   e : 6%

Figure 10.3 *Most common sites for breast cancer.*

Scenario

Annie, aged 61, had been routinely screened at a diagnostic unit for 12 years. Her maternal aunt had breast cancer.

Annie presented for a routine screening appointment. She was asymptomatic and had been taking HRT for four years. On clinical examination, she was found to have a cystic feeling nodule adjacent to the areola in the right breast. She was sent for an ultrasound which reported a highly suspicious 0.9-cm nodule in the right breast. Because of this report, she was sent for a mammogram which stated that she had no radiologically sinister features on either side.

Aspiration cytology was performed on the lump, which felt gritty to the needle. Cytology report was C4, suspicious of cancer and this was confirmed by biopsy.

Breast awareness and breast care advice

There has, and probably always will be, controversy surrounding the issue of breast self-examination. It has been stated that self-examination causes unnecessary anxiety, and that finding a cancer in the breast will not necessarily alter the course of the disease. On the other hand, it could be argued that even if it does not alter the course of the disease, perhaps the initial treatment need not be so aggressive.

Many women have made statements to the effect that it was nursing a close relative with breast cancer that made them anxious in the first place. Whatever the reasons, if a woman is going to perform self-examination then she needs some guidance about how and when to perform it. It can be helpful to explain the basic anatomy and physiology of the breasts, so that women understand why their breasts might feel lumpy premenstrually – particularly in the upper outer quadrants.

Nowadays breast self examination has been overtaken by the concept of 'breast awareness' which is what all health care professionals should be promoting in their advice to women. The difference between the two is subtle as women are still being asked to look at and feel their breasts but not in such a ritualistic way as with breast self examination. Women should be encouraged to become familiar with how their breasts normally look and feel and how this can vary at different times of the month. They are not being asked to look specifically for lumps but just to notice any *change* from their normal. Helpful guidance can include such tips as:

1 Don't feel the breasts before a period
2 Use the flat of the fingers and not the fingertips
3 Don't feel the breasts between the thumb and forefinger
4 Remember that 9 out of 10 breast lumps are *not* cancer.

There are two distinct parts to being breast aware: *looking* and *feeling*.

Looking

♦ Note any change in the shape of the breast looking down and looking in the mirror.

♦ Note any puckering or dimpling of the skin. A crease in the skin can also be important.

♦ Note any change in the nipple, i.e. if the nipple starts to go in, or points in a different direction; if the nipple becomes reddened, and perhaps moist.

Any change should be reported.

Feeling

The most important aspect of feeling is for women to get to know what is normal for them, and then to notice if there is any change from this normality. A lump in the breast should never be ignored, and any change in the way the breast normally feels should be followed up – that is why being breast aware just before a period is due is not sensible, and can give rise to unnecessary anxieties. However, women who are breast aware will appreciate that such changes are normal for them and not be alarmed at pre-menstrual lumpiness and tenderness.

The flat of the fingers should be used when checking the breasts, either in the bath/shower with a soapy hand or lying on the bed using talcum powder. Starting at the 12 o'clock position, move the fingers, pressing gently down around the outer circumference of the breast, and then in ever decreasing circles towards the nipple – making sure that

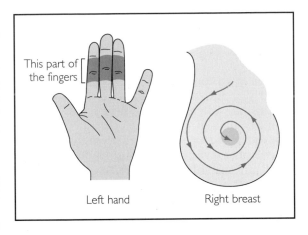

Figure 10.4 *Area of fingers to be used in breast awareness and circular method of self-examination.*

all areas of the breast have been examined. Finally gently press down on the nipple (Figure 10.4).

If a woman finds anything that is different (i.e. a lump, puckering, nipple change, etc.) or is anxious or worried about her breasts then she should be advised to see her doctor for an examination, (Box 10.1).

> **Box 10.1** Breast awareness: a summary
> Women should be aware of:
>
> ♦ Change in breast shape or size
>
> ♦ Any dimpling/puckering or creases in the skin
>
> ♦ Any lump or thickening in the breast
>
> ♦ Any alteration in the nipple, whether it starts to go in, or starts pointing in a different direction
>
> ♦ Any discharge from the nipple.

Scenario

Annette is a regular attender at a diagnostic unit. For years she has had multiple cysts and she was breast aware. She returned between appointments because she had felt a lump in the breast that felt different to her more usual cysts – this was, in fact, a carcinoma.

Breast care advice

Brassieres

Women often complain of breast discomfort, particularly premenstrually, and one of the reasons for this can often be an ill-fitting bra. Women should be advised to be correctly fitted – most large department stores have experienced staff who can measure and give advice on this. Underwired bras which are not fitting properly can often cause discomfort in the outer quadrant of the breast; if this only happens premenstrually, then wearing a bra without a wire at this time should resolve the situation. Underwired bras are unsuitable for pregnant women.

Intertrigo

A rash in the inframammary fold is common in women with large breasts and is usually due to not drying the area thoroughly after a shower/bath. Excessive perspiration can also cause a rash and advice about wearing a cotton bra can be helpful. Talcum powder should not be applied. Calamine cream or lotion can be applied, but if the area becomes inflamed then hydrocortisone cream which can be obtained from the chemist should be applied sparingly.

Hairs

Hairs may be removed from the areola with tweezers. These can be removed permanently by electrolysis but only by a trained professional. Depilation creams should not be used on the breast.

Inverted nipples

Inverted nipples are normal and are often bilateral but maybe unilateral. They should be kept clean, by gently using a cottonwool bud. Any change in nipple inversion must be reported to her GP.

Spots

Spots should not be squeezed, as this may lead to an infection.

Breast discomfort (mastalgia)

Breast discomfort can often be helped by taking vitamin B_6 50 mg with one multivitamin daily. Evening primrose oil or starflower oil (containing gamolenic acid) can also be helpful; the recommended dosage should be obtained from the packet. A stronger preparation of evening primrose oil (Efamast®) is available but only on prescription and has proved effective in helping many women with cyclical and non-cyclical mastalgia (Mansel, 1994).

Reducing or abstaining from caffeine can also be helpful, as can reducing salt intake when preparing food.

Occasionally with fluid retention a diuretic may be prescribed.

Breast pain, of any type, is a rare symptom of breast cancer, and only 7% of patients with breast cancer have mastalgia as their only symptom.

Diagnostic investigations

Mammography (breast X-ray)

Mammography is an X-ray technique used to visualize the internal structures of the breast. The National Breast Screening Programme has been phased in since 1986 by the Department of Health following the Forrest Report (DHSS, 1986) and aims to screen asymptomatic women between the ages of 50 and 64 by inviting them to attend for mammography every three years. The aim of the NHS breast screening programme is to reduce mortality from breast cancer by 25% in the population of women invited to be screened.

The recommended view chosen for mammography screening is the mediolateral oblique as this single view demonstrates the maximum amount of breast tissue. The axillary tail, pectoral muscle and inferior portion of the breast are visualized. Most abnormalities are found in the upper outer quadrant and such a mammogram clearly demonstrates this area (Yeowell, 1993). It has recently been advocated that a cranio-caudal view should also be performed on the first screening visit. This view demonstrates whether abnormalities are medial, central or lateral to the nipple. Both these mammograms are obtained by the breast being compressed between two plates whilst the exposure is made. The procedure may be uncomfortable but should not be painful. Suspicious mammograms will prompt a recall to the screening unit, causing much anxiety to the woman, but further investigations may show nothing abnormal. It is hoped that taking two mammograms as a routine will reduce the number of recall visits and minimize stress and needless worry.

The practice nurse, by being a member of the primary care team, is in an ideal setting for encouraging women in this age group to attend for screening by providing information and counselling related to all aspects of the programme. It must be stressed that women should not be made to feel guilty if they are reluctant to attend for screening. In an ideal world there should be 100% uptake but the actual uptake for screening is slightly more than 70% in most centres. A woman may not want to attend because a previous mammogram was painful or because a relative or a friend's breast cancer was detected on a screening test. There is also the common underlying fear of all women that they may have breast cancer themselves and they do not want to know about it.

There is no current evidence to support screening in women under the age of 50 years. This is due to the poorer sensitivity of X-ray in the more dense breasts of a pre-menopausal woman, and the fact that breast cancer incidence is less common in younger women. At present there is a two-centre trial being conducted in women from 40 to 47 and initial results should be available shortly. Women over the age of 65 will not be routinely screened but can be given a mammogram on request, but not more than once every three years.

Mammographic screening of asymptomatic women can pick up small impalpable tumours and microcalcification which may be the only indication of early disease such as ductal carcinoma *in situ* (DCIS). In symptomatic women it is a technique used for problem-solving, although it must be remembered that 5–10% of cancers are not detected by mammography due to the density of the cancer being less than the glandular tissue (Yeowell, 1993). This can usually be resolved by clinical examination, ultrasound and fine needle aspiration. In the case of an impalpable lesion or suspicious grouped microcalcification where surgery has been recommended then the woman will go to the X-ray department for needle localization before she goes to theatre (see page 236).

Ultrasound (sonomammography)

Breast ultrasound is now widely accepted as a valuable adjunct to mammography and is more useful in the younger woman. High-frequency sound waves are beamed through the breast using a handheld 7.5 MHz transducer. Images are built on a screen which are then frozen and a picture can be printed. The use of ultrasound in the clinical area can be very helpful for distinguishing between cystic and solid lesions. If there is any doubt with regards to the interpretation of any abnormality then the woman would be referred for detailed ultrasound in a diagnostic imaging unit.

Ultrasound can also be used for obtaining cells from an impalpable lesion by performing guided needle aspiration. The lesion is visualized on the screen and a needle is introduced into the breast. The needle is guided into the lesion by watching the screen, cells are withdrawn and sent for cytological examination. This is not a painful procedure and takes only a few minutes.

Cytological investigations (Box 10.2)

Fine needle aspiration cytology

Fine needle aspiration cytology (FNAC) has become an accepted diagnostic procedure in outpatients departments and specialist centres. The test should only be performed by professionals trained in the procedure. The advantages of the test are that it is simple, quick and relatively painless, and in a rapid diagnostic unit results are obtained whilst the woman is in the clinic, thereby making further visits to obtain results unnecessary. If a cancer diagnosis has been made then staging investigations and treatment can be discussed at that visit. If the woman is to have a mammogram then this should be undertaken before FNAC or cyst aspiration is performed as the oedema or small haematoma caused will obscure detail and give rise to a false-positive diagnosis. Ideally, mammograms should be left for two weeks after FNAC if this procedure has been performed first (Tucker, 1993).

The thought of having a needle inserted into the breast to most women is very frightening. It must be explained that it is very rarely painful and the majority of women admit afterwards that it was nothing like they thought it was going to be. Most women appreciate a hand to hold whilst the test is being performed. This may sound simplistic but

---

Box 10.2 Cytological investigations
Cytological investigations are carried out on the following:

♦ *Nipple discharge* If a discharge is elicited by gently squeezing the nipple then it should be tested to see if it is blood-stained. A slide should be gently drawn across the nipple to obtain a smear. If two slides are obtained then one is wet-fixed with cytofixative and one is air-dried. This is because of the different staining techniques used by the cytologist. The slides must be clearly marked with the woman's name, hospital number (if applicable), which breast side and whether wet-fixed or air-dried.

♦ *Cyst aspiration* The fluid obtained from the cyst is discarded, but if the aspiration is blood-stained then the contents in the syringe should be emptied into a universal container and sent for cytological examination.

♦ *Solid nodule or nodular area* Fine needle aspiration is performed to obtain cells from the appropriate site for diagnostic purposes. It is now becoming an accepted practice in younger women to leave fibroadenomas *in situ* once a diagnosis has been established.

---

put yourself in their position and maybe you will understand.

Stereotactic FNAC

This is a diagnostic technique used in the X-ray department. A needle is guided into an impalpable lesion or an area of grouped microcalcification under X-ray control and cells are obtained for cytological examination. The advantage of this test is that it avoids unnecessary biopsies. This procedure is not available in all breast cancer centres as it requires the cytopathologist to be present and to have special X-ray equipment in addition to the standard mammography machine.

Trucut biopsy

This test is performed when a histological diagnosis is required. Local anaesthetic is infiltrated into the skin and the breast where the core of tissue is to be removed. A small incision is made in the skin and a narrow-bore cutting needle which has been inserted into a mechanical biopsy gun is then inserted through the incision and guided to the area to be sampled. A core of tissue is obtained which is then fixed in formalin. The test should not be painful, but the slight noise of the needle action should be demonstrated first so that the woman is prepared. Firm pressure should be applied over the area for a few minutes afterwards to prevent bleeding, then an occlusive dressing applied.

Problems

Complications which may occur after fine needle aspiration, although fortunately fairly rare, include the following:

♦ *Haematoma or bruise* This can occur if a large vessel is punctured during aspiration and the procedure may have to be abandoned and pressure applied, or it may occur if pressure is not applied correctly after completion of aspiration. An explanation to the woman that bruising may appear which will resolve in time will relieve the anxiety if this does happen. Occasionally a mild analgesic may be appropriate.

♦ *Pneumothorax* This is a rare complication and may go undetected if the pneumothorax is small. Subtle clues such as sharp pain, coughing or a hiss of air on withdrawing the needle without evidence of air in the syringe, may occur (NHSBSP, 1993).

A woman should be advised to see her GP if she is concerned about unexpected pain, bruising or oedema after any of the above procedures.

Benign breast disorders

Cysts

Cysts are basically fluid-filled sacs which are found most commonly in the 40–60-year age group. They can vary enormously in size, depending upon the amount of fluid in the sac. On clinical examination cysts can feel soft and mobile and are often described as a lax cyst. A tense/tension cyst can feel round and hard, and can clinically resemble a carcinoma. Cysts are frequently multiple in nature, and can also be bilateral.

Symptoms of tension cysts include pain and tenderness. Cysts can also fill rapidly, which of course can be very frightening to a patient, but this is something which you should explain when discussing breast awareness with your patient.

Cysts usually subside or disappear with the menopause unless the woman is taking HRT when they may persist.

Treatment

A mammogram may be performed to rule out an incidental carcinoma. Ultrasound, if available, should be performed, although occasionally some cysts can create echoes which are produced by the turbid contents of the cyst.

Needle aspiration of a cyst should be performed if the cyst is causing pain, is very large, or if it is worrying the patient. The fluid from a cyst can vary tremendously in colour – clear, green, straw-coloured, milky, chocolate-coloured, or blood-stained. The fluid is not usually sent for cytology, unless it is evenly blood-stained.

After aspiration of the cyst the patient should be re-examined to determine whether there is any residual mass. If there is, then repeat needle aspiration should be performed and the cells sent for cytology to check for an underlying cancer.

Fibroadenomas

Fibroadenomas are the most common benign lumps in younger women and usually occur between the ages of 20 and 30 years. A fibroadenoma is a solid, fibrous nodule which is histologically composed of glandular elements and connective tissue. On clinical examination a fibroadenoma is usually well-circumscribed, firm and mobile, and is often referred to as a 'breast mouse' because of its mobility. Methods of diagnosis are clinical examination, ultrasound and fine needle aspiration cytology.

Fibroadenomas may increase in size, may stay the same, or disappear. If ultrasound is performed then a measurement can be taken, and when the patient is re-assessed at a later date the ultrasound and measurement may be performed again to see if there is any change in size. If the above tests have been performed and it has been established that the lump is indeed a fibroadenoma, then the patient can be given the option of excision or observation. If the above tests are not available, then excision is usually performed to exclude malignancy. Fibroadenomas regress with age, and a coarse nodular

calcification due to necrosis will appear on a mammogram. This is known as a degenerating fibroadenoma, and no treatment is necessary.

Giant fibroadenomas

When a fibroadenoma exceeds 5–6 cm in size it is referred to as a giant fibroadenoma. These are most commonly seen in adolescent and young Afro-Caribbean women, and the usual course of treatment is removal.

Phyllodes tumour

Phyllodes tumour is rare and used to be known as cystosarcoma phyllodes, which is a misnomer because most of these tumours are benign. However, there is a risk of malignancy and treatment is by wide local excision.

Mondor's disease

Caused by superficial thrombosis of a vein in the breast, Mondor's disease can present as a pain with a crease in the skin. Malignancy should always be excluded, but apart from this no treatment is necessary as the condition usually resolves within six months.

Tietze's syndrome

Tietze's syndrome is not common, but occurs when the costal cartilages become enlarged, painful and tender. If it is persistent then treatment with local anaesthetic and steroid injections is effective.

Gynaecomastia

Gynaecomastia is an abnormal development of male breast tissue and is therefore outside the scope of this book on women's health.

Galactocoele

A galactocoele is a cystic lesion in women which can occur during or after pregnancy or during breastfeeding. Treatment is by aspiration. This may have to be performed on several occasions in order to allow the walls of the cyst to adhere to one another, thus obliterating the space (McKinna, 1983).

Fat necrosis

Fat necrosis was originally thought to be caused by trauma. However, Haagensen (1986) described only 32% of patients who gave a history of previous trauma. Fat necrosis presents as a painless mass which is ill-defined, and can often be mistaken for a carcinoma. Diagnosis is by clinical examination, mammography and fine needle aspiration cytology. If malignancy cannot be excluded, then biopsy is indicated. Otherwise management should be by observation.

Duct papilloma

Duct papillomas are very common and may be single or multiple. They are caused by solitary papillary benign lesions growing in one of the main ducts close to the nipple. Presentation will be with nipple discharge, which may be serous or blood-stained. Occasionally a palpable mass may be felt at the areolar margin. Treatment is usually excision of the offending duct – microductectomy.

Duct ectasia

Duct ectasia is due to dilatation of major or minor ducts within the breast which leads to the retention of secretions within them. If the secretion leaks from the duct it may cause an inflammatory reaction.

Symptoms can be nipple discharge, nipple retraction and/or a palpable mass. Investigations performed are mammography, clinical examination and fine needle aspiration cytology and, if necessary, excision biopsy.

Lipoma

Lipomas, fatty growths, may be found in the breast and can be mistaken for cysts because on physical examination they are mobile and smooth. Ultrasound and FNAC will establish a diagnosis.

Intramammary lymph nodes

Occasionally intramammary lymph nodes can be felt in the outer quadrant of the breast. On clinical examination they can feel firm and mobile. Fine needle aspiration will usually establish a diagnosis.

Breast cancer

Breast cancer is a serious problem in the UK. One woman out of every 12 will develop breast cancer, and every year 26 000 women will be diagnosed with the disease. Despite the surgeons' and the oncologists' best efforts many women will die of breast cancer (CRC, 1991; McPherson *et al.*, 1994). Much can be done to help these women, particularly in the early stages of their diagnosis and treatment. As mentioned before, women 'at risk' can be identified and screened earlier than ever. For those women who have a positive diagnosis there is a bewildering range of available treatments which can cause confusion for her, her family and other health professionals with whom she may wish to discuss the issues.

It was felt appropriate to include a substantial section on the treatment of breast cancer and chemotherapy in this chapter as a significant number of women will undergo this form of treatment and will often seek physical and psychological care and advice from those not directly involved in their immediate treatment. This section is written as a guide to what is currently available so that you, as a nurse, will be able to understand the range of treatment options your patients are faced with when coping with a diagnosis of breast cancer.

Types of breast cancer

Breast cancers develop from the epithelial lining cells of the terminal duct lobular unit (see Figure 10.1). The cancer cells that remain within this structure are termed as non-invasive or *in situ*. Cancer cells that have the ability to disseminate outside the basement membrane of the ducts and lobules are described as invasive (Sainsbury *et al.*, 1994).

It is important to define the type of cancer as this will determine the future treatment for the woman. Types of breast cancer are now defined by their growth patterns and other cellular characteristics.

Ductal carcinoma in situ

Ductal carcinoma *in situ* is characterized by a proliferation of malignant epithelial cells that remain confined to the terminal duct lobular unit. Until recently, the standard treatment for ductal carcinoma *in situ* (DCIS) was the removal of the affected breast by mastectomy. Now, mastectomy is usually only considered if the disease extends over a wide area of the breast. There is currently a nationwide study which is attempting to show the best treatment for DCIS by comparing:

♦ Local surgery removing a small part of the breast containing the DCIS

♦ Local surgery followed by a course of radiotherapy

♦ Local surgery plus taking the oestrogen-blocking drug tamoxifen daily for five years

♦ All of the above, i.e. local surgery plus radiotherapy and tamoxifen.

Women who have DCIS are invited to join this randomized trial unless they have strong preference for a particular treatment. This type of breast disease is not considered a true cancer but the issues involved in choosing the treatment can involve the same anxiety. Considerable support may be needed whilst the woman is making up her mind about whether she should have her treatment randomized or not (Page *et al.* 1995; Thornton, 1993).

Infiltrating breast cancer

Infiltrating carcinoma can escape from the structures of the breast. It has also been described as ductal or lobular carcinoma. This cancer has the potential to metastasize, or spread through the body, although it does not do so in every case. Other variants of breast cancer include Paget's disease of the breast and inflammatory breast cancer. It is not within the remit of this section to discuss the rarer cancers, but more information can be obtained from the reading list at the end of the chapter.

Paget's disease

The incidence of this breast cancer is low, representing 0.5–3.2% of all breast cancers (Fowble *et al.*, 1991). It usually involves the nipple epidermis and the woman often presents to her GP with a nipple discharge, eczema-like skin changes, nipple retraction and sometimes an underlying thickening of the breast tissue. Treatment depends on what the woman will accept and the particular surgeon's choice. Either excision of the nipple and underlying tissue with post-operative radiotherapy, or a mastectomy is usual. If treated correctly the woman has a good chance of being cured of the disease, but the extent of the surgery will mean that she requires similar support to women who have the more common types of breast cancer.

Inflammatory breast cancer

About 4% of all breast cancers are diagnosed as inflammatory. The woman presents with a breast that is swollen and red, and has skin oedema with induration of the underlying breast tissue (peau d'orange). The overall survival of these patients is particularly poor. Radiotherapy and chemotherapy are the mainstays of treatment but if a woman's tumour responds particularly well then surgery may be added, to give the woman the best possible chance of local control and survival.

Clinical staging

Before the surgeon and the woman decide on the most acceptable surgical intervention for breast cancer the disease should be staged as accurately as possible. With information from cytology, mammography, ultrasound imaging and a full clinical examination the surgeon will be able to choose the best operation for the size of lump and its location in the breast. Because breast cancer has the ability to spread via the blood vessels and the lymphatic system supplying the breast, further staging investigations can be performed according to the treatment policy of the unit.

Clinical staging tests include:

♦ Blood tests (full blood count and liver function biochemistry)

♦ Bone scan

♦ Chest X-ray

♦ Liver ultrasound.

Whilst the staging investigations are taking place, the woman can be under extreme stress. It is essential that the nursing and medical staff recognize this. Support should be offered by contact with a specialist breast care nurse, giving telephone numbers of various support agencies, and by listening to the woman's hopes and fears. No assumptions should be made about how the woman is feeling at such a time. Because of initial shock she may have little opinion at all about what is happening to her, or she may have previous experience of cancer which could be positive or negative. Some breast cancers have a genetic basis and the woman may have already nursed a mother or sister through the disease. For this reason it must be emphasized that each cancer experience is different and that treatments are constantly changing for the better. Some women will wish to discuss the elements of their treatment slowly, with careful thought, before considering what comes next, while others are keen to know straight away what could be ahead of them.

Waiting for the outcome of bone scan or liver ultrasound tests can be an excruciating time for these women: 'It's the waiting for results I can't stand. I want to know what I'll be dealing with and get on with it', is a comment frequently heard from such women.

Surgery

Once all the information about the woman's breast disease has been collected, the date will be set for surgery. There is some controversy surrounding surgical options for breast cancer and there has been a considerable change of opinion over the past few years. A survey carried out in 1983 showed that mastectomy was the most commonly performed operation for breast cancer with only 18% of surgeons undertaking conservative treatment (Gazet *et al.*, 1985). By 1989 64% of surgeons were performing conservative surgery (Morris *et al.*, 1989). Work carried out in Milan between 1973 and 1980 comparing radical mastectomy for breast cancer with wide local excision of the disease plus an axillary lymph node dissection and radiotherapy showed clearly that there was no difference in survival between the two groups receiving the different treatments, thus providing solid evidence for the effectiveness of breast conserving surgery.

The surgeon will recommend the type of surgery offering the best chance of successful treatment, depending on the size and location of the lump. Mastectomy is usually required if the tumour:

♦ is more than 4 cm in size;

♦ has invaded the underlying muscle of the chest wall;

♦ is directly beneath the nipple; or

♦ is multi-focal;

♦ or if the breast is small.

However, if the tumour can be excised without major disfigurement, which principally relates to the size of the tumour relative to the breast, the surgeon should recommend wide local excision. Surgeons may feel that by offering to preserve a woman's breast they are lessening her trauma. Offering the woman choice has been shown not to reduce the psychological morbidity (Fallowfield *et al.*, 1990). In fact, when women are given the choice of surgery some do not automatically choose to retain their breast, and feel that they are better off without the affected part (Wilson *et al.*, 1998).

Assumptions about what the woman wants should not be made. She should be at the centre of the team involved in her care, and her needs taken into account at every stage of the decision-making process. For some women, however, this responsibility and choice proves too much and they ask the team to make the decision for them.

The timing of surgery during the menstrual cycle

Pre-menopausal women have circulating unopposed oestrogen (i.e. not opposed by progesterone) between days 3–12 after their last menstrual period (LMP). For the rest of the cycle these hormones are low (0–2 days) or high (13–28 days). There is a small body of evidence to suggest that unopposed oestrogen at the time of surgical intervention may encourage dissemination of micrometastases (the shedding of cancer cells). Studies are continuing in this area to refute or to confirm the findings but there is no firm conclusion as yet (Badwe, 1993).

Mastectomy

A mastectomy is the surgical removal of the breast. This can mean several different operations, ranging from those that remove the breast, chest muscles and axillary lymph nodes, to an operation that only removes the breast itself.

Mastectomy may be radical, modified radical or simple (Figure 10.5).

♦ *Radical mastectomy* This removes the breast, the pectoralis major and minor muscles, all the axillary lymph nodes, and some additional fat and skin. This procedure is also known as a Halsted mastectomy. It is an extensive operation which leaves a long scar on the chest wall and a hollow chest area. The removal of all the lymph nodes may lead to arm swelling or lymphoedema, some loss of muscle power in the arm and restricted shoulder movement. Intensive physiotherapy may be needed after surgery.

♦ *Modified radical or Patey mastectomy* This removes the breast, the axillary lymph nodes and the lining of the chest wall muscles. Sometimes the pectoralis minor muscle is removed or divided, to allow access to the axilla. Because the pectoralis major muscle is maintained, the strength of the arm is also maintained, and swelling of the arm is less likely. Breast reconstruction will be easier to achieve because more skin is left compared with a radical mastectomy.

In either of the above procedures, where the axilla is dissected to remove nodes, numbness in the inner aspect of the upper arm results from division of a nerve (the intercostobrachial) which traverses the axilla.

♦ *Simple or total mastectomy* This removes only the breast. Sometimes a few of the axillary lymph nodes are removed to give an indication of whether the cancer has spread. The advantage is that the chest muscles are not removed and arm strength is not diminished. Because most of the axillary lymph nodes remain, the risk of loco-regional recurrence is slightly higher than if the whole breast and axillary nodes are removed.

Quadrantectomy

A quadrantectomy removes the tumour plus a wedge of normal tissue surrounding it. Some axillary nodes are removed or 'sampled' to check for spread. This procedure should be followed by radiation therapy to ensure equal local control of the disease compared to mastectomy (Veronesi *et al.*, 1990). Quadrantectomy has the advantage for the woman of breast conservation. However, if the woman has medium or small-sized breasts, this procedure can noticeably change the breast shape. If radiotherapy is then given to both the breast and axilla the risk of lymphoedema is increased (Kissin *et al.*, 1986).

Wide local excision (lumpectomy)

In a lumpectomy only the breast lump is removed and usually the whole breast is irradiated. Surgeons may also remove some of the axillary nodes. The tissue removed will be examined after the surgery to ensure that all the margins around the cancer were clear of tumour. If this was not the case the woman would be strongly advised to undergo further surgery to remove the residual tumour. The breast is unlikely to be greatly altered in shape unless the lump was large and the breast

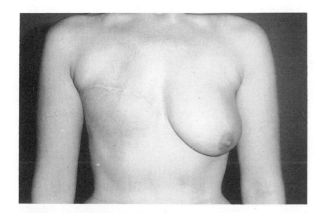

Figure 10.5 *Mastectomy scar.*

small. There would be some scar tissue from this procedure which might make it difficult to examine the breast at a later date.

Needle localization

Sometimes a breast lesion is seen on mammogram but cannot be felt by palpation. Often areas of microcalcification can be seen on the X-ray film indicating disease. This area needs to be removed for diagnostic reasons. The radiologist will be involved to locate the area for the surgeon. Using local anaesthetic, a fine guidewire is inserted into the woman's breast indicating the suspicious area. The area is also located with a mammogram. The woman is then sent to theatre with the needle in place, taped to the skin. The surgeon, using the needle and the mammograms as guidance excises the area. The removed tissue is X-rayed whilst the woman is under the anaesthetic to check that the affected area is totally removed. Further excision will be needed if any residual disease is left behind.

Reconstructive surgery

If a woman's breast has to be removed at the surgeon's recommendation or because the woman herself wishes the breast to be removed, there can be the option of breast reconstruction. This surgery is not a skill that all surgeons have, but can be explained to the woman as an option even if referral to a more specialized unit is required. Women need to be told about their treatment options as information about the disease and its subsequent treatment can give the woman more control over a frightening situation. A breast care nurse could prove invaluable as the woman's advocate, presenting her needs and expectations regarding her treatment to the doctor concerned.

There are some contraindications to reconstructive surgery:

♦ If the woman has a large invasive tumour

♦ If there are chest wall metastases

♦ If there is extensive disease involvement of other body systems (distant metastases).

When discussing reconstructive surgery it must be made clear that breast and nipple sensation will not be restored. The aim of surgery will be to retain the shape and form of the breast mound but the reconstructed breast will not be the same as the breast that has been lost.

There are several methods of reconstructing a breast. The simplest is when the surgeon working at the site of the mastectomy scar lifts muscle and fascia away from the chest wall to create a pocket for an implant. The surgeon then inserts the implant into the formed pocket and stabilizes the pocket with sutures to prevent upward or lateral movement (Solomon, 1986). The implant can be silicone, or a silicone capsule filled with silicone gel (Figure 10.6). There has been considerable controversy recently concerning silicone and its possible leakage causing auto-immune diseases and cancer. There is little evidence to support this claim but implants containing saline in a silicone envelope can be used instead of solid silicone. These implants are filled with saline injected through a device attached to the implant, the filling port. The advantage of this type of implant is that it consists largely of saline rather than possibly harmful silicone gel (see Figure 10.7). This implant can be filled over a period of time, from a few weeks to a couple of months, slowly stretching the skin which overlaps the implant. The implant can be overfilled and then deflated slightly, stretching the skin to achieve the drop or ptosis of a normal breast. Once the final shape and volume are attained, the filling port on the

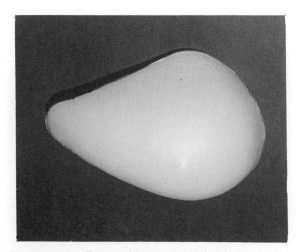

Figure 10.6 *External breast prosthesis.*

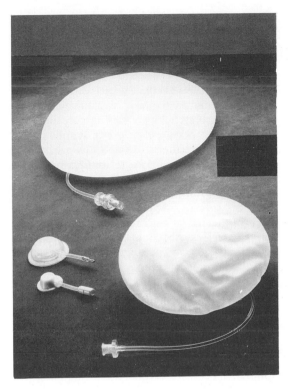

Figure 10.7 *Silcone implant with filling port.*

implant is removed as a day-case procedure under a light general anaesthetic.

For women with larger breasts, the more complex latissimus doris (LD) flap procedure can be used. The LD muscle, which runs from the broad origin on the back to insert in the upper arm, is partially dissected to fill the space of the missing pectoralis muscle. The surgeon takes a flap of skin from the back to reconstruct the new breast. The skin and muscle has an intact blood supply and is rotated from the back to the front of the chest at the incision of the mastectomy scar. The surgeon can then place an implant under the muscle, shaping the rotated flap around it.

The most complex breast reconstruction is the rectus abdominis flap. With this procedure the surgeon is able to transpose a large amount of tissue so that no implant is needed. An ellipse of skin and muscle is raised from the upper abdomen or the suprapubic region. The flap raised is the whole width of the rectus muscle; the distal end of the muscle flap is transected and the flap is rotated

up into the mastectomy defect (Ward, 1987; Watson *et al.*, 1995).

For both the LD and rectus abdominis flap repairs there are scars on the part of the body from where the flaps are raised. The woman should be counselled carefully before consenting to such an operation so she knows what is involved. Photographs of the surgeon's previous work are useful to explain the surgery, and information booklets or leaflets are helpful to reinforce what has been explained. The decision for such surgery needs considerable thought as there are drawbacks with these types of breast reconstruction. These include capsular contraction around the implant, flap necrosis and gel 'bleed'. There may be disparity between the colour of the transplanted skin and the woman's other breast, and the new breast may not have the same shape as the original breast. It is not within the context of this chapter to give further detail but more information can be found in the reading list at the end of the chapter.

Nursing care following surgery

Unless really extensive, breast surgery needs little post-operative care. Drains from the wound site are removed 24–48 hours post-surgery. Drains inserted into the axillary wound stay in for a few days or until the sero-sanguinous fluid reduces significantly. Physiotherapy can start 24 hours post-operatively and the woman will be taught a selection of exercises to improve her arm movement. Often an information booklet is provided by the hospital to encourage the woman to continue the exercises whilst at home. Additional exercises are taught according to the operation and individual requirements.

Dressings should be light and non-occlusive and replaced only if soiled. The woman's sensitivities should be taken into account when considering the type of dressing used. She may prefer that the wound is covered up securely until she is ready to look for herself.

Immediate post-operative complications may include the formation of a haematoma if there has been insufficient cautery of the smaller blood vessels at the time of surgery. The woman may have to return to the operating theatre for drainage of the haematoma and re-cautery of blood vessels.

Seroma formation is always a risk after axillary surgery. Sero-sanguinous fluid collects beneath the wound and can be aspirated with a needle and syringe as a simple outpatient procedure. These aspirations will continue until the fluid stops collecting.

The woman should be encouraged to look at her scar whilst in hospital. The first time she looks can be an extremely traumatic moment for her but the shock can be lessened with an understanding and supportive approach to her care. A nurse should be present when a woman looks at her scar for the first time and should encourage the woman to discuss what she is feeling about the way she looks. The woman may wish for her partner to be present although she may want to come to terms with the scar herself before exposing herself to another person. This 'coming to terms' with her body image can be a slow and painful process, which will be helped by continuing support from the nursing team and the woman's family and friends. This is a time when the provision of telephone support numbers, details of support groups, and contact with a specialist breast care nurse is especially important. The woman should be encouraged to ask for help from whichever agency she feels is appropriate for her needs.

If the woman has had a mastectomy she should be fitted with a soft breast form into a supportive bra or 'crop top' before she leaves the ward. This soft breast form or 'comfie' will not irritate the stitch line but will give the woman some equality of shape before she faces the outside world. An arrangement for a more permanent breast prosthesis should be made for 6–8 weeks after surgery. The restoration of the woman's external body image can be associated with her ability to cope and adjust to her diagnosis of cancer (Denton and Baum, 1983).

Lymphoedema

Lymphoedema is caused by an excessive collection of lymph in the tissues, and when it occurs can cause discomfort and pain, altered body image and a lack of mobility. There are two main categories of lymphoedema:

◆ *Primary* This is when the structure of the lym-

phatic system has not developed properly, and is a congenital problem.

◆ *Secondary* This is when the lymphatic system is damaged by surgery, radiotherapy or by disease infiltration.

The breast is particularly well-supplied with lymphatic channels which drain largely into the axillary lymph nodes. From there, lymph drains into the supraclavicular fossa and low neck.

Surgical intervention for a malignant breast lump may involve an axillary dissection. This may remove a large number of the lymph nodes, depending on the level of dissection undertaken, thereby compromising the lymphatic system. 15% of women will be at risk of developing arm swelling after this procedure has been performed, and this risk increases to 25% if the axilla is then treated with radiotherapy (Kissin *et al.*, 1986). The woman can develop lymphoedema of the arm soon after surgery but it is more likely to develop after several months. Infection or trauma of the arm can precipitate swelling.

Advice about reducing the risk of lymphoedema can start whilst the woman is still in hospital (Box 10.3).

Treatment of lymphoedema

Treatment for lymphoedema should follow the well-established guidelines of the British Lymphology Interest Group. The recommendations in-

---

Box 10.3 Advice to give on reducing the risk of lymphoedema

◆ Avoid injections on the affected arm

◆ Continue the exercises taught by the physiotherapist

◆ Use gloves when gardening to avoid cuts and abrasions and the risk of local infection

◆ Do not have blood pressure taken on the affected arm

◆ Do not lift heavy weights

◆ Keep the skin on the arm in as good condition as possible

◆ Seek medical attention promptly if the arm starts to feel tight or look swollen.

clude re-education about skin care and an explanation of why the lymph fluid is accumulating. Prompt referral to a specialist will ensure that the woman gets the right advice and education about her condition. Measurement of the limb provides a baseline for any future interventions and when compared to the measurements of the unaffected arm will give an indication of how swollen the arm has become. Exercises for the swollen limb to help mobilize lymph fluid will be taught and the fitting of an appropriate compression sleeve will further assist the drainage of fluid. Simple self-massage of the remaining lymphatic system can also be taught. Enabling the woman to take some control of her condition can help to lessen the distress from this unfortunate side-effect of breast cancer and its treatment. For a chronically swollen arm, bandaging carried out daily for a prolonged period can help to reshape the limb prior to fitting a compression sleeve. Community nurses can take over this treatment successfully.

Useful information about lymphoedema can be found by contacting the Lymphoedema Support Network or the British Lymphology Interest Group (see Resources, page 255).

Management of inoperable breast cancer

If the patient presents with a locally advanced breast cancer, surgery is not the best option and primary medical treatment must be considered. A locally advanced breast cancer is defined as having the following characteristics:

♦ Overlying, widespread oedema, and/or ulceration

♦ Chest wall fixation

♦ Skin nodules

♦ Disease-infiltrated axillary nodes

♦ An inflammatory component

♦ Supraclavicular nodal spread.

The treatment of choice depends on the menopausal status of the woman, the extent of the disease, and the woman's wishes. Treatment will normally involve radiotherapy plus hormone manipulation, with or without chemotherapy.

Nursing care of fungating breast cancer

Some women present with locally advanced disease which has ulcerated due to infiltration of the skin of the breast. Care of lesions of this sort will involve careful assessment and skilful choice of dressing.

Ulcerated lesions always grow some organisms, usually skin commensals, but sometimes pathogenic organisms can colonize the wound. Swabs should be sent for microbiological culture, and systemic or topical antibiotics given as necessary. It is usual to clean the wound with normal saline or, if it is large, it can be cleaned with a shower attachment. Useful topical applications, depending on the exact nature of the ulcer, include 'Scherisorb', 'Kaltostat' and other calcium alginate preparations, 'Metrotop', and charcoal dressings.

For wounds that smell particularly offensive, live yoghurt applied and left for 30 minutes and then washed off can be beneficial. When planning care it is important to ensure that dressings are not too bulky, that they are comfortable, and will remain in place. Every effort should also be made to preserve the woman's dignity.

Pathological staging

Clinical staging of the breast cancer takes place prior to surgery and is based on the size of the tumour, any palpable lymph nodes and any evidence of metastatic disease. A preliminary TNM (tumour node metastases) classification would have been assigned to the woman's disease. The pathological staging follows surgery and uses the histological details from the excised tissue.

Breast cancer cells are graded from I to III, where I is a well-differentiated cell which looks very similar to the tissue from which it originated, and III is undifferentiated, retaining few of the characteristics of the cell of origin. The higher the grade, the more likely the cells are to have spread through the body, either through the lymphatic system or via the bloodstream (Fowble et al., 1991). Systemic treatment will be based on the size of the tumour, the histological grade, menopausal status, age and the axillary nodal status (i.e. the number of nodes positive to cancer cells) of the patient (Richards, 1991). This adjuvant treatment must be explained and discussed carefully with the woman in order to lead her gently on to the next phase of her treatment.

The woman is likely to receive her definitive diagnosis and plans for future treatment whilst she is in hospital, or at her first follow-up visit. The wait can be a trying and nerve-wracking time both for her and also for her partner and family. The extent to which the axillary lymph nodes are invaded is a prognostic factor and the details of cell type will also show if the cancer is aggressive. The woman will have her cancer 'staged' according to the size of the breast cancer, the involvement of the axillary nodes and the presence of distant metastases.

Breast cancers are usually staged by the TNM classification as outlined in Box 10.4.

During her first follow-up clinic appointment the movement of the arm will be assessed and arm exercises reinforced. If the woman is not able to move her arm with ease then further physiotherapy should be arranged. Women often develop 'cording', thought to be where the axillary wound scarring causing tightening of the lymphatic vessels which can be felt running down the underside of the arm. The physiotherapist will concentrate on trying to break these cords with gentle exercise.

Scenario

Elizabeth, a 40-year-old, had accepted and *understood the reasons for surgery. She needed a wide local excision and follow-up radiotherapy treatment. After the surgery the histology showed a grade III, high-grade tumour, and 4 out of 20 lymph nodes were positive. Elizabeth was pre-menopausal and was advised to have adjuvant chemotherapy (in addition to the surgery). She was initially very upset by the suggestion of an additional six months of chemotherapy. She felt she had 'paid the price' of her breast cancer already and now wanted to recover physically and mentally from the surgery and radiotherapy. With careful explanation and supportive counselling Elizabeth gradually accepted the need for systemic treatment as the cancer had already demonstrated the ability to spread (metastasize). Elizabeth was*

introduced to other women who had undergone similar treatment and found their support invaluable.

Chemotherapy

Breast cancer not only has the ability to spread to the axillary nodes but also to distant sites throughout the body via the lymphatics and the bloodstream. A percentage of women who present with breast cancer will already have microscopic cancer cells in other parts of their body. If left untreated these cells would almost certainly grow into metastases despite the original breast cancer being excised. Adjuvant chemotherapy or hormone therapy will be offered to these women to prevent or delay the development of this metastatic disease. A 'meta-analysis' published in the *Lancet* looked at a large number of trials and showed that chemotherapy given to a woman with early breast cancer meant a longer (statistically significant) time to recurrence and a small but significant increase in time of survival. This overview also showed that women whose biopsied lymph nodes were negative, 30% of whom develop metastases, would also benefit from adjuvant, systemic therapy (EBCTCG, 1992). This is compelling evidence for offering some systemic treatment following surgery. A combination of chemotherapy drugs is usually given. Chemotherapy is started a few weeks after surgery and is usually given in divided doses over a six-month period. There are trials looking at peri-operative chemotherapy, i.e. chemotherapy given before and after the surgery, but this is not a usual option.

In order to understand how chemotherapy works it is necessary to understand how the cell grows and divides. The phases of cell growth are shown in Figure 10.8. They are defined as follows:

G_1 – During this phase, cells carry out their routine functions; the centrioles replicate.
S – This starts with synthesis of DNA and ends when the DNA has been replicated.
G_2 – This is a short phase during which materials needed for cell division are synthesized.
M – During this phase the cell physically divides.
Interphase – This is a resting, i.e. not dividing, phase. Also known as G_0

Box 10.4   TNM classification (UICC, 1987)

TX   Primary tumour cannot be assessed
T0   No evidence of primary tumour
Tis Carcinoma *in situ*: intraductal carcinoma, or lobular carcinoma *in situ*, or Paget's disease of the nipple with no tumour

Note: Paget's disease associated with a tumour is classified according to the size of the tumour.

T1   Tumour 2 cm or less in greatest dimension
    T1a 0.5 cm or less in greatest dimension
    T1b More than 0.5 cm but not more than 1 cm in greatest dimension
    T1c More than 1 cm but not more than 2 cm in greatest dimension
T2   Tumour more than 2 cm but not more than 5 cm in greatest dimension
T3   Tumour more than 5 cm in greatest dimension
T4   Tumour of any size with direct extension to chest wall or skin

Note: Chest wall includes ribs, intercostal muscles and serratus anterior muscle but not pectoral muscle.

    T4a Extension to chest wall
    T4b Oedema (including peau d'orange), or ulceration of the skin of the breast, or satellite skin nodules confined to the same breast
    T4c Both 4a and 4b, above
    T4d Inflammatory carcinoma

Note: Inflammatory carcinoma of the breast is characterized by diffuse, brawny induration of the skin with an erysipeloid edge, usually with no underlying palpable mass. If the skin biopsy is negative and there is no localized, measurable primary cancer, the T category is pTX when pathologically staging a clinical inflammatory carcinoma (T4d).

When classifying pT the tumour size is a measurement of the *invasive* component. If there is a large *in situ* component (e.g. 4 cm) and a small invasive component (e.g. 0.5 cm) the tumour is coded pT1a. Dimpling of the skin, nipple retraction or other skin changes, except those in T4, may occur in T1, T2 or T3 without affecting the classification.

N – Regional lymph nodes
NX   Regional lymph nodes cannot be assessed (e.g. previously removed)
N0   No regional lymph node metastasis
N1   Metastasis to movable ipsilateral axillary node(s)
N2   Metastasis to ipsilateral axillary node(s) fixed to one another or to other structures
N3   Metastasis to ipsilateral internal mammary lymph node(s)

M – Distant metastasis
MX   Presence of distant metastasis cannot be assessed
M0   No distant metastasis
M1   Distant metastasis (includes metastasis to supraclavicular lymph nodes)

The category M1 may be further specified according to the following notation:

Pulmonary	PUL	Bone marrow	MAR
Osseous	OSS	Pleura	PLE
Hepatic	HEP	Peritoneum	PER
Brain	BRA	Skin	SKI
Lymph nodes	LYM	Other	OTH

The length of the cell cycle varies with different cell types, G_1 phase being the longest and most variable phase. Most chemotherapy agents prevent the cell from dividing in some way and are grouped accordingly (Table 10.1). Adjuvant regimes given for breast cancer are usually a combination of several types of chemotherapy agents that act in different ways to effect greater cell kill. Some common regimes are shown in Table 10.2.

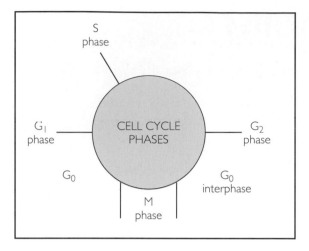

Figure 10.8 *Cell cycle phases.*

Depending on the treatment centre other regimes may include cyclophosphamide, Adriamycin or epirubicin. The optimal drug combination, treatment frequency and how long the chemotherapy should be given has not been firmly established yet. Combining several drugs is thought to lower the likelihood of drug resistance and to potentiate cell kill (Harris *et al.*, 1993; DeVita *et al.*, 1993).

Adjuvant chemotherapy is usually given as an intravenous (IV) injection in an outpatient oncology clinic. The implications of receiving chemotherapy should be carefully explained to the woman. The necessity for chemotherapy and its effect on a woman's life can cause a range of feelings. Fear and anxiety about whether the cancer has spread further than the breast are common emotions. Every woman must evaluate the known side-effects of the chemotherapy and discuss this with the medical and nursing team before making a decision about her treatment. Because research in this area is continually ongoing the woman may be asked to enter a trial which could include randomization to different treatment regimes. Again details of the trial and its consequences should be made clear to the woman before she gives consent. Several visits to the medical oncologist and input from nurse specialists may be necessary before the woman feels confident to make a decision. Information leaflets can be useful to facilitate this decision-making process and these are often available from the oncology unit. The woman's lifestyle may have to change dramatically to fit in with the administration of the treatment and its side-effects.

Primary medical therapy

Some women will present with large breast tumours which are inoperable because of the extent of disease, or because the size and location of the breast lump make a mastectomy inevitable. By giving these women chemotherapy or endo-

Table 10.1 *Groups of chemotherapy agents*

GROUP	MODE OF WORKING	EXAMPLES
Anthracyclines and antibiotics	Intercalate with DNA and prevent the DNA from untangling prior to replication	Adriamycin epirubicin, mitozantrone and bleomycin
Antifolates and antimetabolites	Prevent the constituents of DNA being synthesized	Methotrexate, 5-fluorouracil
Alkylating agents and vinca alkaloids	Prevent the cell from being replicated	Cyclophosphamide, vincristine
Antimitotic agents	Prevent the cell from physically dividing, i.e. mitosis	Vinblastine, actinomycin D
Miscellaneous	Prevent the cell from growing and dividing	Taxol

Table 10.2 *Common chemotherapy regimes for breast cancer*

DAY	DRUG	DOSE	ROUTE
CMF[a]	(28-day cycle)		
1–14	Cyclophosphamide	100 mg/m^2	Oral tablets
1 & 8	Methotrexate	40 mg/m^2	IV bolus
1 & 8	5-FU	600 mg/m^2	IV bolus
CAF	(21-day cycle)		
1	Cyclophosphamide	600 mg/m^2	IV bolus
1	Adriamycin	50 mg/m^2	IV bolus
1	5-FU	600 mg/m^2	IV bolus
MMM[b]	(6-week (42-day) cycle)		
1	Mitomycin C	7 mg/m^2	IV bolus
1 & 22	Mitozantrone	7 mg/m^2	IV bolus
1 & 22	Methotrexate	35 mg/m^2	IV bolus
ECF	(21-day cycle (of E & C))		
1	Epirubicin	40 mg/m^2	IV bolus
1	Cisplatin	60 mg/m^2	IVI + pre- and post-hydration
All of the regime	5-FU	200 mg/m^2/day	continuous IVI for 6 months

[a] There are many other versions of CMF, including cyclophosphamide given by injection every 21 days.
[b] If the patient develops mucositis during the first cycle folinic acid 15 mg × six tablets orally can be given as an antidote to the action of the methotrexate starting at 24 hours after the chemotherapy has been given. Some protocols use 8 mg/m^2 of mitozantrone and mitomycin C.

crine treatment first it may be possible to shrink the tumour to make surgical intervention less invasive, or, indeed, to prevent the need for surgery (Mansi *et al.*, 1989).

Primary medical therapy is an area of current research. Several chemotherapy regimes have been used, often using an anthracycline-based drug. Usually six cycles are given before further surgery or radiotherapy is given. If the tumour does not shrink at all in response to two cycles of treatment the women will probably be considered for surgery.

Scenario

Patricia presented with a large inoperable tumour in her right breast. She had had a mammogram *whilst she was working abroad the previous year and the result was clear, so the positive diagnosis from a biopsy performed on the lump in her right breast was a great shock.*

The medical team caring for Patricia suggested that she undergo primary medical therapy to shrink the tumour and then receive a course of radiotherapy if the tumour had regressed sufficiently. Patricia needed a lot of time with the medical and nursing teams before she felt able to accept the need for treatment. She was quite surprised that the treatment was not conventional surgery although the need for medical treatment was explained. Formalized counselling was commenced with the nurse counsellor and Patricia asked if her partner could be present at these sessions. After some considerable thought and consideration Patricia decided that she felt able to agree to the chemotherapy and felt she understood the implications of her treatment. She was introduced to another woman undergoing the same treatment and they were able to offer each other mutual support. Because the tumour shrank successfully Patricia underwent a course of radiotherapy to the breast and was commenced on the anti-hormone drug tamoxifen.

Figure 10.9 *The Hickman catheter.*

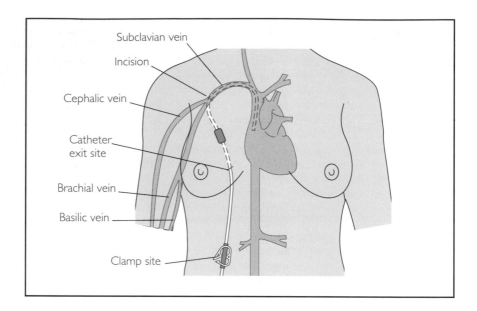

Subclavian vein

Incision

Cephalic vein

Catheter exit site

Brachial vein

Basilic vein

Clamp site

Administration of chemotherapy

There is a basic principal when administering chemotherapy that the more chemotherapy that is administered over time the more cells are likely to be killed (DeVita *et al.*, 1993). For this reason some primary medical chemotherapy regimes are given continually from a small portable pump. One drug, often 5-FU, is given via a Hickman line, a soft, pliable tube inserted through the chest wall and tunnelled into the subclavian vein (Figure 10.9). This line allows easy venous access for blood sampling but also ensures that prolonged (usually six months) administration of chemotherapy does not damage peripheral veins.

The woman will have been taught how to care for her Hickman line by the hospital team responsible for her chemotherapy treatment. General practice and community staff back-up is essential to continue this support. Infection of the exit site of the Hickman line is fairly common and this should be recognized quickly and treated with antibiotics. Prompt action will prevent further ascending infection and possible septicaemia.

The wound site must be dressed regularly either by the woman herself, her practice nurse or a community nurse. The stitches should be removed from the incision site 7–10 days after the line has been inserted and from the exit site 3–4 weeks after insertion. This allows time for the woman's body to form scar tissue around the

cuff of Hickman line and therefore to anchor the line within the subclavian vein. Providing the site has completely healed the woman can continue many of her physical activities such as playing golf or tennis. She can lightly shower over the Hickman exit site but must not get the pump wet. Blockages of the Hickman line can occur and the pump occasionally malfunctions. The woman should have written instructions about what to do and contact numbers of the hospital team caring for her should this occur.

It can be quite disturbing for a woman to have a Hickman line protruding from the skin of her chest. In addition, this type of drug regime usually includes an anthracycline and platinum-based drug which for most women will mean some side-effects and hair loss. However, if appropriate support and careful explanation are given, and the treatment works at shrinking the tumour, most women cope very well (Smith and Powles, 1991)

Nursing care during chemotherapy

Side-effects from the chemotherapy are related to the types of drugs given and are usually limited to the parts of the body that have actively dividing cells (Goodman, 1989).

Hair loss or alopecia. Because most adjuvant breast chemotherapy regimes tend to be hair-sparing, complete hair loss does not often occur unless a strong anthracycline is included in the regime. Hair thinning is fairly common though and this can be devastating for the woman who has already lost part of or all of her breast. She is struggling to maintain her self-esteem and body image anyway so hair loss can take on an even greater significance. Support and practical advice can be invaluable to the woman at this time. Information on hair care, use of scarves and hats and how to obtain a National Health wig, if required, can ease the woman's distress and should be arranged before chemotherapy is started. Hair usually starts to regrow 4–6 weeks after chemotherapy has finished and can be softer and curlier than before.

Scalp cooling, by applying ice packs, cold caps or other methods to supercool the scalp can help to maintain the hair. By reducing the temperature of the scalp the blood supply to the hair follicles is depleted, thus depriving the hair follicle of the chemotherapy. The scalp cooling is usually left on the head for 20 minutes after the chemotherapy has been given, by which time the level of the circulating chemotherapy has dropped sufficiently to not have an effect on the hair. Scalp cooling does not always work but should be tried for any woman receiving an anthracycline as a bolus dose (Tierney, 1987; Judson, 1993)

Sore eyes. Antifolate and anthracycline chemotherapy often affect the conjunctiva of the eyes, causing stickiness and sometimes a dry soreness. Folinic acid given as an oral tablet can reduce the effects of an antifolate and the use of artificial tears can provide some comfort (Goodman, 1989).

Sore mouth. The mucous membrane of the mouth normally replaces itself quickly and is readily affected by chemotherapy. The woman should be advised to use a softer toothbrush to prevent unnecessary scratching of the mouth. Mouth hygiene should be encouraged and fluid input should be at least 2–2.5 litres per day. Any dental work should be completed before treatment starts or just before the next course of treatment when the blood count has recovered. Any fungal infections should be treated with nystatin or amphotericin. The woman may develop herpes simplex which must be treated promptly with Zovirax. Methotrexate often causes mucositis. This can be largely prevented by the administration of folinic acid 15 mg tablets for six doses at 24 hours post-chemotherapy.

Mouth washes containing a local anaesthetic such as Difflam may be soothing if mouth ulcers develop. A chlorhexidine-based mouth wash may be appropriate if there is evidence of oral infection. The woman's diet should be well-balanced, containing high proportions of vitamins and proteins to promote healing.

Nausea and vomiting. Because the body recognizes the chemotherapy as a toxic substance and because of increased gastric acidity, nausea and vomiting may occur. The woman is usually given anti-emetic tablets to take whilst at home but these may not be sufficient or appropriate. The woman should be encouraged to report her experiences of nausea prior to her next treatment so adjustments can be made to her anti-emetic control as appropriate. Anti-emetics which are 5-HT$_3$ antagonists can significantly reduce nausea and should be prescribed as appropriate. Because the side-effects of chemotherapy can be so traumatic, some women begin to associate attending the department with feeling sick. This anticipatory nausea can be treated prophylactically with conventional anti-emetics and sometimes anxiolytics may be useful. Women will receive their chemotherapy as an outpatient and will then be encouraged to continue in their normal routine. It is essential that care and support for symptoms should be shared and continued by their GP and practice nurse.

Nausea as caused by chemotherapy can also be eased by taking small, frequent meals and by eating bland food. Prolonged nausea can severely affect quality of life and considerable efforts should be made to reduce this unfortunate side-effect.

Nausea can also be eased by taking a prescribed antacid, drinking flat or fizzy drinks such as soda water, coke or lemonade, drinking ginger tea, or eating dry biscuits.

Lowered blood count. The bone marrow is constantly developing the cells that make up blood, i.e. white cells (neutrophils), red cells and platelets. The numbers of these circulating cells are reduced by chemotherapy. Depending on the chemotherapy given, the number of blood cells will reach a trough or nadir usually 8–12 days after the treatment has been administered. The numbers of white cells and platelets will start to recover after this point and should be at an acceptable level before the next treatment is given. The woman should be advised to contact her GP or the oncology clinic if she experiences bleeding gums or a tendency to bruise, the symptoms of a low platelet count. Infection, feverish chills and a high temperature could indicate a lowered white cell count and the woman must be aware of the significance of such symptoms. If the chemotherapy is particularly strong, blood levels will be taken at the predicted nadir and prophylactic antibiotics given if the white cell count is particularly low, i.e. below 2.0 $\times$ 10^9 per litre. For women receiving adjuvant chemotherapy a lowered white cell count is short and recovery is predictable (Judson, 1993).

Diarrhoea. This can be caused by chemotherapy damaging the gastrointestinal mucosa. Anti-diarrhoeal agents may be effective. If the problem becomes prolonged, management may require the use of parenteral nutrition in addition to fluid replacement. This would be unlikely with most chemotherapy regimes for breast cancer and would, of course, mean admission to hospital.

Lethargy. This insidious tiredness which is not eased by sleep affects most women who receive chemotherapy and increases towards the end of the usual six months of treatment. Some women manage to continue with their working lives perhaps with more flexible working hours whilst others require considerable rest and could not possibly work. No predictions should be made about how a woman might feel. The woman should be supported through this time and be reassured that her 'lethargy' is a normal response to the treatment although excessive tiredness could be an indication that the woman is not coping with her treatment or diagnosis and this needs to be addressed. She should be allowed to rest when tired, and family and friends should be involved to help them to understand this side-effect of chemotherapy.

Hormone therapy

The effectiveness of endocrine manipulation on breast cancers has long been known. Many newly diagnosed breast cancers and about one-third of metastatic breast cancers are responsive to hormone manipulation. The primary hormones involved are oestrogen and progesterone. Hormones are steroids which can be involved in stimulating tumour cell proliferation. They can affect tumour cells by interacting with the relevant hormone receptor within the cell's stroma and nucleus. The number of receptors can be measured by histopathologists once some breast cancer tissue has been removed from the tumour. The presence of oestrogen and progesterone receptors, ER and PR respectively, usually correlates with the clinical behaviour of the disease. The more oestrogen receptors the more likely the woman's breast disease will respond to hormone therapy. There are several types of hormone therapy; the most widely used in the first instance is the drug tamoxifen.

Tamoxifen

Tamoxifen is a steroid antagonist which acts by inhibiting the action of hormones on their target tissues. Tamoxifen has evolved from being a treatment for advanced metastatic disease, to being an effective adjuvant and primary therapy, and is now part of a national trial as a chemo-preventative agent for asymptomatic women with a high risk of breast cancer (Powles *et al.*, 1989). The tamoxifen tablet is taken daily at a dose of 20 mg and it is recommended that the drug is taken at a similar time each day. Side-effects include transient nausea, increased vaginal secretions, and hot flushes associated with an induced menopause (Jones, 1992). Unusual vaginal bleeding should be reported to the GP and investigated if it persists. There is no consensus for how long the drug should be taken but it is usual that the drug is prescribed for at least five years (Harris *et al.*, 1993).

Tumour regression can occur when a hormone drug is stopped, although six weeks should elapse before another hormone therapy is tried.

Progestogens

Medroxyprogesterone acetate (MPA) is similar to the hormone progesterone, and is designed to inhibit the circulating levels of oestrogen and block progesterone receptors. The drug is taken daily in tablet form. The particular side-effects of this drug can include acne, fluid retention, an irregular menstrual cycle and changes in libido. It is often given to post-menopausal women as a second-line treatment for metastatic disease.

Aromatase inhibitors

Aminoglutethimide. This drug is often used as a third-line hormone therapy for women who have already received tamoxifen and typically a progestogen. It has an antitumour activity in disseminated breast cancer similar to a surgical adrenalectomy. It works by blocking the conversion of androgens (produced by the adrenal glands) to oestrogens in the peripheral tissues. The tablets used to be given with hydrocortisone because one of the side-effects of aminoglutethimide is that it inhibits normal glucocorticoid production (the body's normal steroid hormones), although this does not occur at the lower daily dose of 250 mg. Other side-effects include transient lethargy, nausea, and muscle cramps. If these side-effects continue then the drug will be stopped. Some patients develop a widespread macular rash which generally disappears spontaneously and rarely requires cessation of treatment.

4-Hydroxyandrostenedione. This also works by blocking the conversion of androgens to oestrogens. The drug is given by intramuscular injection every two weeks, and there can be local reactions to the drug.

Ovarian ablation

In pre-menopausal women the ovaries are the main source of circulating oestrogen. Three methods are used to reduce the amounts of this circulating hormone. The ovaries

♦ can be removed surgically,

♦ have their function permanently ablated by radiotherapy, or

♦ can be suppressed by chemical means.

A chemical way of suppressing the ovaries is the administration of a luteinizing hormone-releasing hormone (LHRH) agonist. There are several LHRH analogues in use at the moment and these include goserelin (e.g Zoladex) leuprorelin (e.g. Prostap) and buserelin (e.g. Subrefact). Both goserelin and leuprorelin are administered as a depot injection into the abdominal wall on a monthly basis. Sometimes local anaesthetic is used to make the procedure more comfortable. The drug is then slowly released over the next month.

The advantage of a chemical castration is that once the drug is stopped the effect will be reversed, which is especially pertinent to women who wish to try for a family later if their treatment is successful. These LHRH antagonists can be used as adjuvant therapy and also for the treatment of advanced disease.

Nursing care

All hormone treatments work by blocking or manipulating the normal hormone levels and so can cause many symptoms associated with the menopause. These can include hot flushes, vaginal dryness, tiredness, weight gain, and night sweats. Clonidine has been given with limited effect to reduce some of these symptoms. Vitamin supplements such as evening primrose oil and vitamin B_{12} can also offer some relief. Menopausal symptoms need to be given as much credence as those caused by other treatments for breast cancer. The woman should be told what to expect and be allowed to discuss her feelings about such symptoms. The prospect of an early menopause can be yet another assault on a woman's body image and sexuality. Infertility can be a distressing side-effect for the woman who was planning a late pregnancy or for someone who has had problems conceiving. However, some younger women continue to menstruate whilst taking tamoxifen (Nolvadex), albeit irregularly and contraceptive advice should be given.

Radiotherapy

Radiotherapy is the delivery of high-energy ionizing radiation which destroys the cancer cells' ability to grow and multiply. Most radiotherapy departments use a linear accelerator or cobalt machine to deliver this high energy.

Radiotherapy can be used in three main situations for the treatment of breast cancer:

♦ As an addition to surgery

♦ As a primary treatment for a large invasive tumour

♦ For recurrent disease at the original site or for systemic metastatic disease, particularly bone or brain metastases.

As an addition to surgery

The usual schedule for external beam radiation therapy given as an adjunct to surgery is between 3 and 6 weeks. The treatment is given every week day with weekends off. It takes 10–15 minutes to set up the treatment machine for the individual patient, and then only 2–3 minutes for each 'fraction' to be given. The radiotherapist takes care to avoid delicate structures such as the lungs and heart. In order to align the radiotherapy machine markings are drawn on the skin and a small tattoo is usually made with Indian ink to ensure that the treatment is accurately reproduced every day. The woman should be warned about the permanency of these marks during the course of radiotherapy and the small tattoo will always remain. Following a wide local excision typical radiotherapy involves treatment to the whole breast followed by a 'boost' to the bed of the tumour. Women who undergo a mastectomy would not necessarily have radiotherapy, unless their tumour was poorly differentiated, was classified as a T3 (or greater) tumour, or had involved axillary lymph nodes.

Brachytherapy. Some radiotherapy centres use radioactive implants to give follow-up radiotherapy treatment. Under anaesthetic between 4 and 25 wide-gauge hollow needles are passed through the breast tissue to where the tumour was excised. Iridium-192 wire, a radioactive source, is then inserted into the tubes and secured firmly at each end. The wires stay in long enough to deliver the required dose of radiation, usually 2–5 days. The woman is nursed in a single lead-lined room to protect other patients, and also the nursing and medical staff from excessive radiation exposure.

Nursing care

Some women have a marked radiation reaction on the treated area, with skin eythema, soreness, swelling of the breast and rarely moist desquamation or breakdown of the skin. Topical applications are to be avoided unless necessary and then only hydrocortisone 1% ointment is the treatment of choice. Moist desquamation may mean that radiotherapy is stopped until the skin recovers. Even without a marked skin reaction, general advice about skin care will be given by the local treatment centre. There may be several reasons for

---

Box 10.5 Advice to give on skin care following radiotherapy

♦ Wear cotton or natural material next to the skin

♦ Do not use perfumed soaps or deodorants on the areas being treated

♦ Wash the area with water only and pat dry with a soft towel

♦ Do not wash off the markings

♦ If talc has to be used, baby powder is the best option.

---

variation in skin reactions to radiotherapy, including differences in intrinsic sensitivity (Turesson and Thames, 1989; Burnet *et al.*, 1992). General advice on skin care should be given (Box 10.5).

Some physical support needs to be given to the treated breast but a conventional bra may not be suitable. Cotton vests, 'crop tops' and sports bras can all give gentle support to the treated breast and will be better than an ill-fitting nylon bra (Oliver, 1988). It must be stressed that only the area being treated will be affected by the radiotherapy.

Some women find radiotherapy a depressing experience. Some of this is due to tiredness which can continue for up to seven weeks after the radiotherapy finishes (Graydon, 1994). Women can find the daily travelling to the radiotherapy centre quite a strain. Support at home with provision of home help and childcare as appropriate can be vital to ensure that the woman receives her full treatment. Involvement of the GP, practice and community nurses will also facilitate this treatment.

Side-effects from breast radiotherapy are purely local and it must be stressed that nausea and hair loss do not occur. The skin may darken further, changing a breast that has already had shape-altering surgery. Long-term effects may include the fibrosis of small blood vessels, causing even further discoloration.

Primary radiotherapy for a large invasive tumour

Women with large lesions which are inoperable by virtue of tumour extent or because of their general health can be managed with radiotherapy. Most radiotherapists will treat the whole breast and axilla, and the supraclavicular fossa. Intensive radiotherapy such as this can cause long-term side-effects such as fibrosis of the breast and lymphoedema (see section on lymphoedema). The prognosis for such women is particularly poor but the short-term benefits of local control are thought to outweigh the morbidity of the long-term effects.

The role of radiotherapy in metastatic disease will be discussed later in this chapter (see page 251)

Psychological care

For the woman with newly diagnosed breast cancer her whole world can appear to be falling apart. She may well feel relatively fit and healthy but will have to face up to treatment for a disease which will at some point alter her body shape, make her feel unwell, and will not carry a certainty of cure.

There can be a great disparity between what we as health professionals think the woman wishes to know or is experiencing and what she actually feels about her diagnosis. Becoming a recipient of care takes control away from the woman and this lack of control is one factor that can lead to psychological morbidity (Morris, 1983). Other factors that can predispose to psychological morbidity include:

♦ Lack of social support

♦ Not having a regular partner

♦ A change in body shape, especially if the woman's breasts were an important part of her self-image

♦ The physical effects of having treatment

♦ Doubts about her future.

Much can be done to recognize, ameliorate or prevent this psychological morbidity, starting from the time the woman is diagnosed with cancer. Morris *et al.* (1977) observed that newly diagnosed women with breast cancer display five different ways of coping with their diagnosis:

1 *Denial* The woman actively rejects her diagnosis. She 'blocks' any information given about her disease and cannot actively be involved with decisions about her treatment.
2 *Fighting spirit* The woman has the ability to display a hopeful, questioning attitude to her disease. She appears to want to make the best of what has happened.

3 *Stoical acceptance* Such women acknowledge their diagnosis but do not enquire any further about details. These women seem to carry on with their life without much concern for their illness.
4 *Anxious/depressed acceptance* Such women react to knowledge of their diagnosis with excessive anxiety or depression. They ask for large amounts of information but this information does not reassure them.
5 *Helpless/hopelessness* These women are completely overcome by their diagnosis. Their lives are disrupted by their anxieties so they can no longer function effectively.

It is not unusual for women who have been given their diagnosis to display one or more of these behaviours. As nurses caring for such women it is important to recognize these coping strategies and to suggest therapeutic intervention when appropriate. It is not within the remit of this chapter to teach counselling skills but rather to highlight the need for the skills of health care professionals who have formal counselling experience.

The breast care nurse, nurse counsellor, psychologist and specialist counsellor can all contribute to a woman's psychological care and their help should be offered as appropriate. But why is psychological care so important for the woman with breast cancer? In the late 1970s Maguire, a clinical psychologist, started to study women who were diagnosed and treated for breast cancer. He carried out several studies looking at the psychological morbidity of such women. One study concluded that as many as 25% of the women who had undergone a mastectomy needed psychological support for anxiety and depression (Maguire *et al.*, 1978).

Physically, psychologically, socially and financially, it makes sense to reduce or prevent the woman's psychological morbidity. This allows the woman to re-establish herself as a functioning member of society by returning to work and/or caring for her family more quickly, as well as freeing up other care agencies (Maguire *et al.*, 1982). A further controlled study carried out by Maguire and his colleagues showed that when women had the services of a specialist breast care nurse their physical and social recovery following mastectomy improved (Maguire *et al.*, 1983).

Work by Fallowfield questioned the concept that it was just the disfiguring surgery that caused psychological problems, and suggested that having breast cancer, with all its implications, was also a contributing factor. She concluded that specialist support should be available to all women who undergo treatment for breast cancer and not just those who undergo mastectomy (Fallowfield *et al.*, 1986). Watson and her colleagues suggested from their studies that a nurse specialist might offer more effective support if counselling were to begin as soon as the woman was diagnosed, and that counselling could follow a general framework for all women (Watson *et al.*, 1988). Their suggested framework concentrated on three different areas:

♦ Emotional support and facilitation of adjustment

♦ Information about the woman's physical state

♦ Practical advice on prostheses.

Emotional support and facilitation of adjustment

To strengthen a woman's coping mechanisms she should be encouraged to ask for support. The spouse, family and friends can give practical help and emotional support although this would involve permission from the woman herself, since not all women want their family and friends involved. Using the helpline numbers, support groups, the GP, practice nurses, community nurses, Macmillan and Marie Curie nurses (if appropriate) and the breast care nurse can reinforce the woman's support network. This support should help the woman regain some control over her life.

Information about her physical state

Most women need to understand something about their treatment. Gauging how much they want to know is difficult and requires skill. Because there is so much to know about breast cancer, and some of it is quite complex, time and sensitivity must be employed when explaining details. When first diagnosed, the woman will not be able to take in most of what she is hearing. The shock of being diagnosed as having breast cancer will be all that most women can immediately absorb. The role of the nursing team, including the breast care nurse, in reiterating what the women has already been told is crucial in helping her to come to terms with her diagnosis.

Treatment may not only be new to the woman but she may also be asked if she wishes to take part in a medical trial. Perhaps surprisingly, this does not appear to cause excessive stress. Providing the information given is adequate, women who allow themselves to be randomized do not suffer from any greater psychological, sexual or social problems from those treated outside a clinical trial (Fallowfield *et al.*, 1990). Later research by Fallowfield showed that the woman's need for choice is less important than her need for clear and accurate information (Fallowfield *et al.*, 1994).

Practical advice on prostheses

The restoration of a woman's external body image is linked with her ability to cope and adjust to her breast cancer (Denton and Baum, 1983). Helping to restore the woman's shape by giving advice on the right bras to wear, the fitting of the initial cumfie (soft breast form) and the fitting of the more permanent prosthesis can help the woman's return to normality. Advice on other clothing and swimwear can also facilitate recovery and the Breast Cancer Care association (formally the Breast Care and Mastectomy Association) can be very helpful.

A list of some of the many help agencies that can be contacted by the nurses caring for the woman, or the woman herself, to help her psychological adjustment is included in the list of Resources on page 255.

Female sexuality

A very important aspect of psychological care to consider when caring for the woman with breast cancer is her sexuality. Body image and sexual function are represented as a central, intellectual component of the way the woman feels about herself. Derogatis (1986) wrote that a positive body image is essential to effective sexual functioning. The self-esteem and therefore sexuality of the woman can be severely threatened by the loss or disfigurement of the breast and changes in her body as a whole. If the woman already feels insecure about herself and her body image prior to treatment for breast cancer, the problem can be amplified into a serious psychological disorder (Derogatis, 1986).

Although sex is an important aspect of life for most women, for some their sexuality is a central part of their life, and for these women the effects of treatment for breast cancer can be devastating. Baldwin (1990) writes that society's view of the perfect woman is constantly presented through the media as usually tall, thin and with two perfectly formed breasts. The breast is a symbol of many things about a woman:

♦ A symbol of womanhood

♦ A symbol of motherhood

♦ A symbol of sexuality.

For a woman who has undergone treatment for breast cancer which is disfiguring, the difference between the reality and the 'ideal' can be a cause of great stress (Baldwin, 1990). Sexuality is much more than the sexual act; it is about the quality of the human being. Individuals with a positive self-concept respect themselves and consider themselves worth while in a sexual sense, whilst those with a negative self-concept are often not satisfied with themselves sexually. A woman being treated for breast cancer may feel she is no longer sexually attractive even when her partner is trying to tell her otherwise. She may fear rejection by her partner and may withdraw from a physical and close relationship. Her partner in turn may view this as a sign that she no longer wishes a physical relationship, and so misunderstanding can be perpetuated.

Many research papers look at the sexual effects of losing a breast and there is sometimes a misconception that if a woman has breast conservation her psychological trauma will be less. However, work by Rutherford, who studied women undergoing a lumpectomy, highlighted the physical changes that occur. These include deformity, which may be substantial, thickening of skin and subcutaneous tissue, enlarged and pronounced pores, changes in breast contour, erythema and pain over the scar (Rutherford, 1988). Apart from the visual changes, the sensitivity of the breast can diminish because of radiotherapy or surgery.

Chemotherapy can cause fatigue, malaise, depression, alopecia, and amenorrhoea, the last of which is yet another assault on the woman's sexuality. A husband or partner can experience as much distress as the woman herself over the course of her treatment. Their feelings need to be taken into account and provision should be made for them to express their concerns.

Sexuality as an issue is rarely explored by nurses. Better education and more openness might encourage discussion and allow the woman to work through this very important issue. Women who tend to cope better with changes in their sexuality are those who have been able to resolve past life crises. Good sexual functioning prior to the illness tends to predict a return to a satisfactory sexual adjustment (Derogatis, 1986). The nature and quality of the woman's relationship with her primary partner and the size and nature of her support network are also important when re-affirming personal value and contributing to psychological adjustment. A woman's sexuality and her body image are about herself and the way she relates to the outside world. Such an important area of care should not be ignored by health care professionals when looking after the woman with breast cancer.

Metastatic disease

Breast cancer can spread to the bones, lungs, liver, brain, and almost any other soft tissue. Recurrence is sometimes detected by the woman herself, with the development of pain, another lump, breathlessness or feeling unwell. It may also be detected at routine follow-up visits. Investigations for metastatic disease include routine blood tests, X-rays, liver and bone scans, and perhaps the use of computerized tomography (CT) or nuclear magnetic resonance imaging (MRI) to determine the nature and extent of the metastatic disease.

The aims of management of metastatic disease are firstly to palliate symptoms and secondly to reduce the tempo of the disease. There is no longer an expectation of cure. The timing of recurrence in relation to first presentation and the site of relapse may predict the survival of the woman. Those women who have hormone-sensitive tumours and who have had a long interval between diagnosis and relapse are likely to do better than women who develop secondaries, especially in visceral sites, shortly after initial treatment (Leonard *et al.*, 1994). Some women, particularly post-menopausal patients with bone disease, may survive for many years with metastatic disease. The treatments for metastatic breast cancer are the same modalities as for primary disease.

Radiotherapy

Radiotherapy has a very large part to play in the palliation of metastatic disease. Painful bone disease is the most common manifestation of metastatic disease, and this can be treated very effectively with radiotherapy. Radiotherapy may also give considerable relief from disease in other organs, e.g. the brain, with a minimum of side-effects. Treatment may require several fractions of radiotherapy, but bony metastases in particular often respond well to a single treatment.

Hormone treatment

As described previously, there are a variety of hormone drugs available. Overall, the likely response rate for the first hormone treatment is about 30%. If the woman has disease which has responded to first-line hormone treatment, then it is more likely that a second line of hormone treatment will be effective. With each successive hormone treatment the probability of response diminishes.

Chemotherapy

Chemotherapy given for advanced disease has a response rate of between 40 and 60%, with a median relapse rate of 6–10 months (Leonard *et al.*, 1994). When treating the woman with chemotherapy the intent should be symptom control without paying the price of excessive toxicity. The drug regimes used in metastatic disease are similar to combinations used for adjuvant therapy. Multi-agent combinations including anthracyclines have the highest response rates, but also the highest toxicity. The choice of regime will depend on many factors.

Currently there is considerable work looking at the effectiveness of new drugs, e.g. taxol, and new combinations of existing drugs. High-dose chemotherapy has been used, mostly in the US, with promising results, but more studies are required to compare this treatment with conventional drug regimes. Careful symptom control is of paramount importance when women with metastatic disease are receiving such therapy (see main section on chemotherapy, page 240).

Pain

Pain can be controlled with effective analgesia as well as by treatment of the underlying disease with either chemotherapy or radiotherapy. Pain itself can be a complex problem with many components making up the subjective experience. In a woman who has chronic pain, fear, despair, anger and anxiety can all influence what she is experiencing. When caring for such a woman an accurate measurement of the site and severity of the pain is important to understand her experience and to measure the effectiveness of any interventions. The objective of pain control should be that the woman is pain-free at night, at rest and on movement.

Pharmaceutical intervention will start with mild analgesia, e.g. paracetamol (1 g 4 hourly) or soluble aspirin (300–600 mg 4 hourly). If the pain does not respond to this, a weak opioid analgesia will be tried, e.g. dihydrocodiene or coproxamol (Distalgesic), a dextropropoxyphene/paracetamol combination. If a stronger analgesia is needed then the opioid morphine is the drug of choice. Dose requirements may start at 5–10 mg 4 hourly but can be increased to 2–3 g 4 hourly, although there is no upper limit if the patient is experiencing pain. Measurement of the woman's pain is important so that drug dosage can be titrated against it.

Morphine can be administered as an elixir or tablet every four hours or as a slow release tablet (MST) every 12 hours. Any increase in the opioid dose should not be fully assessed until 24 hours has passed (Hanks and Mansi, 1988). Constipation is very likely to be a problem if the patient is receiving an opioid drug and regular aperients should be prescribed as well as giving advice about taking plenty of fluid, eating fresh fruit and vegetables and other fibre-containing foods.

Co-analgesics can be used with great effect to control pain and should be used with every category of analgesia. Non-steroidal anti-inflammatory agents can relieve bony pain or pain related to nerve compression. The use of steroids in advanced disease can also have a beneficial effect by relieving inflammation and by giving the woman a feeling of well-being. Bone pain can be significantly helped with the use of APD (pamidronate) which, when administered 2–3 weekly at a dose of 30–90 mg intravenously inhibits bone resorption when there is infiltration of the bone by breast cancer. Carbamazepine and amitriptyline can be useful for nerve pain. The use of anxiolytics such as diazepam can reduce the psychological component of the pain as well as helping with muscle spasm.

Non-drug measures for pain relief can include the use of massage, hot and cold packs, transcutaneous nerve stimulation and relaxation therapy. In an effort to relieve pain these are often more acceptable to the woman than taking more medication. By providing pain relief with non-interventionist measures the woman can feel more in control of her situation. More detail about these methods of pain relief can be found in the references in Hanks and Mansi, 1988.

Liver metastases

Liver metastases carry a grave prognosis. Chemotherapy is normally required, though care must be taken with the selection of drugs and dosages if there is significant impairment of liver function.

Lung metastases

Lung metastases can occur and typically present with shortness of breath. Management involves excluding other causes of breathlessness, including benign causes such as pulmonary embolus or tuberculosis, and other malignant causes such as pleural effusion. Treatment of pulmonary metastases has to be systemic, either with chemotherapy or hormone manipulation. The prognosis is generally poor.

Pleural effusions

Many women with metastatic disease develop a pleural effusion. This collection of fluid in the pleural cavity is caused by deposits of cancer cells, and has the effect of compressing the lung. The woman usually presents with shortness of breath and possibly pain on inspiration. The usual care is to insert a catheter into the intercostal space, drain the fluid off slowly and then to instil an irritant to adhere the pleural membranes together. Many different agents have been used but intrapleural bleomycin or tetracycline, plus a local anaesthetic, are most popular. Surgical intervention by a partial thoracotomy is sometimes used to drain off fluid and to instil an adhesive substance and in a fit woman this can be a very effective way of preventing reaccumulation of the fluid (Smith and Powles, 1991).

Pericardial effusion

Rarely, fluid can collect in the pericardium because of tumour infiltration. Diagnosis of this can be confirmed by ultrasound and, if tamponade is present, then drainage must be carried out quickly. If fluid collects again quickly a permanent 'window' can be surgically created in the pericardium for the long-term drainage of the effusion.

Malignant ascites

This is a rare site of secondary disease in women who have breast cancer. Deposits that develop between the peritoneum of the abdomen can cause fluid to accumulate in the peritoneal cavity. The fluid collection can be large in volume and cause discomfort, and breathlessness if pressing on the diaphragm. Drainage or paracentesis is carried out by inserting an indwelling catheter. The peritoneal fluid should drain at a rate of around 1 litre per four hours for 24 hours and then be allowed to drain freely. Treatments can be given intraperitoneally but these have not proved to be useful. Systemic therapy as for other sites of metastatic disease is more likely to be the treatment of choice. If the ascites becomes recurrent, a shunt may be inserted which drains fluid from the peritoneal cavity into the right subclavian vein or superior vena cava (Le Veen *et al.*, as cited by Smith and Powles, 1991).

Hypercalcaemia

This is a frequent complication of breast cancer and is caused by increased osteoclastic bone destruction releasing calcium into the bloodstream. Higher than normal calcium levels in the woman's bloodstream may make her feel thirsty, nauseous, disorientated, dehydrated and polyuric, and sometimes may make her have an altered conscious state. These symptoms are usually reversible if the condition is diagnosed and treated quickly. Hydrating the woman with i.v. 0.9% saline usually helps, but with the addition of specific agents to help to stabilize the bone, the calcium level can be kept within normal limits for longer. The most likely group of drugs to be used are the bisphosphonates which are very efficient at inhibiting the osteoclastic bone resorption. Pamidronate sodium (APD), at a dose of 30–90 mg is often used for this purpose. Other agents used include calcitonin, corticosteroids and mithramycin (Hanks and Mansi, 1988).

Brain metastases

Presentation may occur in a number of ways. These include symptoms of raised intracranial pressure, namely headache, vomiting, dizziness, visual disturbance and impaired intellectual function; neurological deficits specific to the site of disease, such as weakness or loss of balance; or less commonly fits.

The initial treatment would be the administration of steroids and then whole-brain irradiation. For single brain lesions in a woman who has no other evidence of disease, surgical intervention, or higher dose radiotherapy, can be offered. Radiotherapy treatment will be given with steroid cover to reduce excessive brain swelling. The woman may experience the side-effects of steroid use, which include weight gain, water retention, proximal myopathy, susceptibility to infection and possible steroid-induced diabetes.

Spinal cord compression

Metastatic deposits of disease within the vertebrae or dura can cause spinal cord compression. A woman developing spinal cord compression can have symptoms of leg or arm weakness, sphincter disturbance, and sensory changes. If any of these symptoms develop the woman should be referred to her oncologist as an emergency. Treatment starts immediately, with dexamethasone 4 mg q.d.s. and emergency radiotherapy. Less commonly, surgical decompression is used. The better the patient's neurological status when treatment begins, the better the long-term outlook. This condition can be extremely frightening for the woman as she is in danger of becoming paralysed.

Carcinomatous meningitis

Metastatic involvement of the meninges can cause headache, confusion, diplopia, cranial nerve palsies and impaired sensation. The clinical diagnosis is usually confirmed with a lumbar puncture, although cancer cells are not necessarily found in the CSF. The prognosis is poor, but treatment can be whole-brain radiotherapy or chemotherapy, particularly using intrathecal methotrexate.

The future

Because there is a strong correlation between drug dose and tumour response, the more chemotherapy that can be tolerated by the body the more cancer cells will be killed. When treating breast cancer patients doctors are attempting to increase the dose of chemotherapy to the limits of what the body can tolerate in terms of toxicity. To give such high doses doctors have to support the healthy body tissue as much as possible. Bone marrow, which produces blood cells, is very sensitive to chemotherapy and can be protected by administering colony-stimulating growth factors such as granulocyte colony-stimulating factor (GCSF). By promoting the growth of white cells the woman's immune system can be bombarded with high, but reasonably safe levels of chemotherapy. Prophylactic antibiotics can also be given to prevent infection. Symptom control is of paramount importance as this type of treatment can cause fairly marked side-effects.

Bone marrow preservation and transplantation after high-dose chemotherapy is being pioneered in the US. By giving back the woman her own bone marrow or that of another close match the woman can regenerate her immune system after the chemotherapy has killed off most growing cells including any malignant cells (Ghalie et al., 1994).

Nursing care during this type of treatment is intensive. The woman is likely to experience hair loss, nausea and vomiting and extreme lethargy. She may have to be barrier nursed until the bone marrow starts to regenerate. The woman will be an inpatient for a long time and, despite the intensive support a high proportion of these women will suffer from neutropaenic (lowered white cell count) sepsis (infection) (Ayash et al., 1994).

Doctors now understand that cancer (abnormal cell growth) can be caused by faults in individual's genes. By 'marking' the defective gene or genes, doctors may be able to detect residual cancer cells after surgery or chemotherapy has been given (Sikora, 1994). Other possible methods of destroying cancer cells includes their infection with controlled viruses so that the immune system of the body recognizes and destroys these cancer cells.

Some breast cancer cells produce high levels of the growth factor called c-*erb*B2 which stimulates cell growth. It is also known as an oncogene. Research is ongoing which will attempt to downregulate (reduce) this growth factor and thus prevent further proliferation of the cancer cell.

The use of molecular therapy in the treatment of cancer is still in its infancy and is due to the recent advances in molecular biology. The ethics of such treatment, i.e. gene manipulation, must be considered carefully. Such treatment will take many years to perfect and much more research needs to be undertaken before molecular therapy will take its place alongside the more conventional therapies.

Conclusion

Teamwork is an important factor in breast screening and caring for women with breast disorders. As we do not live in an ideal world treatment is often fragmented between hospital, screening unit and home, proving emotionally traumatic for the woman and her family. The research and advances being made into the diagnosis and treatment of breast disorders means that guidelines are constantly changing, requiring all health care professionals to keep up to date. The informed nurse can provide support and information, but most importantly can provide continuity of care for the woman undergoing treatment for a breast problem.

Resources

BACUP (British Association for Cancer United Patients)
3 Bath Place, Rivington Street, London EC2A 3JR
Cancer Information Service 0171 613 2121
Cancer Information Service freeline 0800 181199
Cancer Counselling Service 0171 696 9000
Cancer nurses provide information and emotional support by phone or letter. Booklets on cancer care are available. A one-to-one counselling service is also available.

Breast Cancer Care
Kiln House, 210 New Kings Road, London SW6 4NZ

Helplines: London 0171 867 1103; Glasgow 0141 353 1050; Edinburgh 0131 221 0407; Nationwide freeline 0500 245345.
Offers help, information and support to women who have breast cancer or other breast-related problems. Services include free leaflets, a prosthesis-fitting service and one-to-one emotional support from volunteers who have themselves experienced breast cancer.

British Association for Counselling (BAC)
1 Regent Place, Rugby CV21 2PJ
Tel. 01788 578328

British Lymphology Interest Group (BLIG)
Administrative Centre, Sir Michael Sobel House, Churchill Hospital, Oxford OX3 7LJ
Tel. 01865 225890

Cancer Link
17 Britannia Street, London WC1X 9JN
Information line 0171 833 2451; Asian language line 0171 713 7867; Scotland 0131 228 5557
Free, confidential emotional support and information in all aspects of cancer care. Resource to over 500 cancer self-help groups.

Lymphoedema Support Network
Tel. 0171 727 6973

Macmillan Services Development Department
Cancer Relief Macmillan Fund
15–19 Britten Street, London SW3 3TZ
Tel. 0171 352 7811

RAGE
Wellington House, Dixter Road, Northiam, East Sussex TN31 5LB
Support group for women who have undergone some axillary treatment and have suffered damage to their arm function.

Rigby Peller Corsetry Specialists
2 Hans Road, Knightsbridge, London SW3 1RX
Tel. 0171 589 9293;
22A Conduit Street, London W1R 9TB
Tel. 0171 491 2200
Able to advise women who need larger bras or have special requirements, for example after mastectomy.

Royal Marsden NHS Trust
203 Fulham Road, London SW3 6JJ
Tel. 0171 352 8171
Information leaflets on breast cancer and aspects of breast cancer treatments.

Women's Health
52 Featherstone Street, London EC1Y 8RT
Tel. 0171 251 6580

Women's Health Concern (WHC)
PO Box 1629, London SW15 2ZL
Tel. 0181 780 3007

Women's National Cancer Control Campaign
Suna House, 128–130 Curtain Road, London
EC2 3AR
Tel. 0171 729 4688

Further reading

BAUM, M., SAUNDERS, C. and MEREDITH, S. (1994) *Breast Cancer: A Guide for Every Woman.* Oxford: Oxford University Press.

DEVITA, S.R., HELLMAN, S. and ROSENBERG, S.A. (eds) (1993) *Cancer Principles and Practice of Oncology*, 4th edn. Philadelphia: J.B. Lippincott.

DIXON, M. and SAINSBURY, R. (1993) *Diseases of the Breast.* Edinburgh: Churchill Livingstone.

FALLOWFIELD, L. and CLARK, A. (1991) *Breast Cancer. The Experience of Illness Series.* London: Tavistock/Routledge.

SMITH, I.E. AND POWLES, T.J. (1991) *Medical Management of Breast Cancer.* London: Martin Dunitz.

WELLS, R. and TSCHUDIN, V. (1994) *Wells' Supportive Therapies in Healthcare.* London: Baillière Tindall.

References

AYASH, L.J., ELIAS, A. and WHEELER, C. (1994) Double dose intensive chemotherapy with autologous marrow and peripheral blood progenitor cell support for metastatic breast cancer: a feasibility study. *Journal of Clinical Oncology* 12: 37–44.

BADWE, R.A. (1993) Timing of surgery during the menstrual cycle for operable breast cancer. *Cancer Topics* 9(4): 42–43.

BALDWIN, E. (1990) Sexuality and breast cancer. *Midwife, Health Visitor and Community Nurse* 26 (10).

BCTCS of UKCCCR (1990) Breast Cancer Trials Coordinating Sub Committee of the United Kingdom. UK Coordinating Committee on Cancer Research. Cancer Research Campaign.

BURNET, N.G., NYMAN, J., TURESSON, I. *et al.* (1992) Improving radiotherapy cure rates by predicting normal tissue tolerance from *in vitro* cellular radiation sensitivity. *Lancet* **339**: 1570–71.

CHAMBERLAIN, J. (1993) Epidemiology. Chapter 13 in *Textbook of Mammography*. pp. 318–22.

CHILVERS, C.E.D., McPHERSON, K. PETO, J., PIKE, M.C. and VESSEY, M.P. (1993) Breast feeding and risk of breast cancer in young women. *British Medical Journal* **307:** 17–20.

CRC (1991) *Fact Sheet 6.1: Breast Cancer.* London: Cancer Research Campaign.

DENTON, S. and BAUM, M. (1983) Psychological aspects of breast cancer. In Margolese, R. (ed.) *Breast Care.* Edinburgh: Churchill Livingstone.

DEROGATIS, L. (1986) The unique impact of breast and gynaecologic cancers on body image and sexuality in women– a reassessment. In Vaeth, R. (ed.) *Body Image, Self Image and Sexuality in Cancer Patients*, 2nd edn. Basel: Karger.

DHSS (Department of Health and Social Security) (1986) *The Forrest Report.* London: HMSO.

DiSAIA, P.J. (1993) Hormone replacement in patients with breast cancer. *Cancer Supplement* **71**(4): 1490–98.

EBCTCG (Early Breast Cancer Triallists Collaborative Group) (1992) Systemic treatment of early breast cancer by hormonal, cytotoxic, or immune therapy. *Lancet* **339**(8784): 1–15, 71–85.

FALLOWFIELD, L.J., BAUM, M. and MAGUIRE, G.P. (1986) Effect of breast conservation on psychological morbidity associated with diagnosis and treatment of early breast cancer. *British Medical Journal* 293: 1331–34.

FALLOWFIELD, L.J., HALL, A., MAGUIRE, G.P. and BAUM, M. (1990) Psychological outcomes of different treatment policies in women with early breast cancer outside a clinical trial. *British Medical Journal* 301: 575–80.

FALLOWFIELD, L.J., HALL, A., MAGUIRE, G.P., BAUM, M. and A'HERN, R.P.A. (1994) Psychological effects of being offered choice of surgery for breast cancer. *British Medical Journal* 309: 448–551.

FOWBLE, B., GOODMAN, L.R., GLICK, J.H. and ROSATO, E.F. (1991) *Breast Cancer Treatment– A Comprehensive Guide to Management.* St Louis: Mosby.

GAZET, J.C., RAINSBURY, R., FORD, M., POWLES, T. and COOMBES, R. (1985) Survey of treatment of primary breast cancer in Great Britain. *British Medical Journal* 290: 1793–95.

GHALIE, R., RICHMAN, C.M., SOLOMON, S. *et al.* (1994) Treatment of metastatic breast cancer with a split course, high-dose chemotherapy regimen and autologous bone marrow transplantation. *Journal of Clinical Oncology* 12: 342–46.

GOODMAN, M. (1989) Managing the side effects of chemotherapy. *Seminars in Oncology Nursing* 5(2): Suppl. 1: 29–52.

GRAYDON, J.E. (1994) Women with breast cancer: their quality of life following a course of radiation therapy. *Journal of Advanced Nursing* 19: 617–22.

HAAGENSON, C.D. (1986) *Diseases of the Breast*, 3rd edn. Philadelphia: W.B. Saunders.

HANKS, G.W. and MANSI, J. (1988) The management of symptoms in advanced cancer: Experience in a hospital-based continuing care unit. *Journal of the Society of Medicine* 81: 341–44.

HARRIS, J., MORROW, M. and BONNADONNA G.

(1993) In DeVita, S.F. Hellman, S. and Rosenberg, S.A. (eds) *Cancer: Principles and Practice of Oncology*, 4th edn. Philadelphia: J.B. Lippincott.

IARC (1988) *Monographs on the Evaluation of Carcinogenic Risks to Humans: Alcohol Drinking.* IARC Scientific Publication 44. Lyon: International Agency for Research on Cancer, p. 387.

JONES, A.L. (1992) Hormonal treatment in post-menopausal breast cancer. In *Therapy Express– Advances in Therapy.* Brussels: CIBA-GEIGY Pharmaceuticals, pp. 591–94.

JUDSON, I.R. (1993) Toxicology of chemotherapeutic agents. In Andrews, P. and Sanger, G. (eds) *Emesis in Anticancer Therapy.* London: Chapman & Hall.

KALACHE, A. (1990) Risk factors for breast cancer, with special reference to developing countries. Chapter 5 in *Health Policy and Planning* pp. 1–22.

KISSIN, M., QUERCI DELLA ROVERE, G., EASTON, D. and WESTBURY, G. (1986) Risk of lymphoedema following the treatment of breast cancer. *British Journal of Surgery* **73**: 580–84.

LEONARD, R.C.F., RODGER, A. and DIXON, J.N. (1994) Metastatic breast cancer. ABC of breast diseases. *British Medical Journal* **309**: 1501–4.

McKINNA, J.A. (1983) Chapter 2 in *Diagnosis of Breast Disease.* p. 42.

McPHERSON, K., STEEL, C.M. and DIXON, J.M. (1994) Breast cancer – epidemiology, risk factors and genetics. ABC of breast diseases. *British Medical Journal* **309**: 1003–6.

MAGUIRE, G.P., LEE, E.G., BEVINGTON, D.J. *et al.* (1978) Psychiatric problems in the first year after mastectomy. *British Medical Journal* **1**: 963–65.

MAGUIRE, G.P., PENTOL, A., ALLEN, D. *et al.* (1982) Cost of counselling women who undergo mastectomy. *British Medical Journal* **284**: 1933–35.

MAGUIRE, G.P., BROOKE, M., TAIT, A. *et al.* (1983) The effect of counselling on physical disability and social recovery after mastectomy. *Clinical Oncology* **9**: 319–24.

MANSEL, R.E. (1994) Breast pain. *British Medical Journal* **309**: 866–68.

MANSI, J.L., SMITH, I.E., WALSH, G. *et al.* (1989) Primary medical therapy for operable breast cancer. *European Journal of Cancer and Clinical Oncology* **25**(11): 1623–27.

MORRIS, J., ROYLE, G.T. and TAYLOR, I. (1989) Changes in the surgical management of early breast cancer in England. *Journal of the Royal Society of Medicine* **82**: 12–15.

MORRIS, T. (1983) Psychosocial aspects of breast cancer: a review. *European Journal of Cancer and Clinical Oncology* **19**(12): 1725–33.

MORRIS, T., GREER, H. and WHITE, P. (1977) Psychosocial and social adjustment to mastectomy– a 2-year follow-up study. *Cancer* **40**: 2381–87.

NHSBSP (1993) *Guidelines for Cytology Procedures and Reporting in Breast Cancer Screening*, No. 22, p. 12.

OLIVER, G. (1988) Radiotherapy. Chapter 5 in Tschudin, V. (ed.) *Nursing the Patient with Cancer.* Hemel Hempstead: Prentice Hall.

PAGE, D.L. STEEL, C.M. and DIXON, J.M. (1995) Carcinoma in situ and patients at high risk of breast cancer.

ABC of breast disease. *British Journal of Medicine* **310**: 39–42.

PARKIN, D.M., SRJEINSWAARD, J. and MUIR, C.S. (1984) Estimates of the worldwide frequency of twelve major cancers. *Bulletin of the World Health Organization* **62**: 162–63.

POWLES, T.J., HARDY, J.R., ASHLEY, S.E. *et al.* (1989) A pilot trial to evaluate the acute toxicity and feasibility of tamoxifen for prevention of breast cancer. *British Journal of Cancer* **60**: 126–31.

RICHARDS, M.A. (1991) Systemic treatment of breast cancer. *Journal of the Royal Society of Health* August: 141–45.

RUTHERFORD, D. (1988) Assessing psychosexual needs of women experiencing lumpectomy. *Cancer Nursing* **11**(4): 244–49.

SAINSBURY, J.R.C., ANDERSON, T.J., MORGAN, D.A.L. and DIXON, J.N. (1994) Breast cancer. ABC of breast diseases. *British Medical Journal* **309**: 1150–53.

SIKORA, K. (1994) Genes, dreams and cancer. *British Medical Journal* **308**: 1217–21.

SMITH, I.E. and POWLES, T.J. (1991) *Medical Management of Breast Cancer.* London: Martin Dunitz.

SOLOMON, J. (1986) The good news about breast reconstruction. *Registered Nurse* November: 47–54.

THORNTON, H. (1993) A sacrifice for others? *Professional Nurse* **8**(6): 402–4

TIERNEY, A.J. (1987) Preventing chemotherapy induced alopecia in cancer patients. Is scalp cooling worthwhile? *Journal of Advanced Nursing* **12**: 303–10.

TUCKER, A.K. (1993) Introduction. In Tucker, A.K. (ed) *Textbook of Mammography.* Edinburgh: Churchill Livingstone pp. 2–3.

TURESSON, I. and Thames, H. (1989) Repair capacity and kinetics of human skin during fractionated radiotherapy: erythema, desquamation and telangiectasia after three and five years follow-up. *Radiotherapy and Oncology* **15**: 169–88.

UICC (1987) *TNM Classification of Malignant Tumours*, 4th edn. Berlin: Springer-Verlag.

UK National Case-Control Study Group (1989) Oral contraceptive use and breast cancer risk in young women. *Lancet* **1**: 973–82

VERONESI, U., SALVADORI, O., LUINI, A. *et al.* (1990) Conservative treatment of early breast cancer. Long-term results of 1232 cases treated by quadrantectomy and radiotherapy. *Annals of Surgery* **211**: 250–59.

WARD, D.J. (1987) Breast reconstruction. *Hospital Update* September: 725–34.

WATSON, J.D., SAINSBURY, J.R.C. and DIXON, J.M. (1995) Breast reconstruction after surgery. ABC of breast diseases. *British Journal of Medicine* **310**: 117–121.

WATSON, M., DENTON, S., BAUM, M. and GREER, S. (1988) Counselling breast cancer patients: a specialist nurse service. *Counselling and Psychology Quarterly* **1**(1): 23–32.

WILSON, R.G., HART, A. and DAWES, P.J.D.K. (1988) Mastectomy or conservation: the patient's choice. *British Medical Journal* **297**: 1167–69.

YEOWELL, M. (1993) Chapter 3 In Tucker, A.K. (ed) *Textbook of Mammography.* Edinburgh: Churchill Livingstone pp. 28–54.

11: Cervical screening and abnormalities

Vicky Padbury

OBJECTIVES

After reading this chapter you will understand:

♦ how to inform and update on the NHS Cervical Screening Programme

♦ the nature of abnormalities of the cervix

♦ the ethics of cervical screening

♦ the relevant anatomy and physiology of the cervix and associated structures and organs

♦ what is entailed in the treatment and management of cervical abnormalities

♦ how to take a cervical smear.

Introduction

Cervical screening has suffered, like no other screening procedure, from considerable adverse publicity in the UK in recent years. This has been due to various factors including:

♦ inadequately trained professionals taking cervical smears;

♦ failures in communicating results;

♦ misreading at laboratory level of the samples sent for cyto-analysis.

There is much the appropriately trained nurse can do to help counter this unfortunate situation. The majority of cervical screening takes place in the primary care setting, in GP surgeries (Table 11.1) and it has been shown (Atkin *et al.*, 1993) that 75% of practice nurses are undertaking the role of cervical smear-taker.

It is worth reminding nurses that as health professionals we are all accountable for our own actions, and therefore should not take on any tasks that we do not feel competent to undertake, but should seek out further training. The UKCC documents *Code of Professional Conduct* and *The Scope of Professional Practice* (UKCC, 1992) are useful to refer to.

The NHS Cervical Screening Programme (NHSCSP)

Organized screening programmes have been in operation in parts of Europe and North America for over 30 years. The Nordic countries – Denmark, Finland, Iceland and Sweden – started screening in the 1960s with highly organized programmes, achieving almost complete coverage of

Table 11.1 *Percentage of smears examined by source of smear, England, 1991/2*

SOURCE	PERCENTAGE
General practice	77.6%
Community clinic	8.2%
GUM clinic	2.5%
NHS hospital	9.7%
Other	1.4%

Source: DOH, *Cervical Cytology*, England (1991/2), 1993. Reproduced with permission of Cancer Research Campaign, 1994

their target populations. We should remember that these countries are very small and effective screening is therefore easier.

Britain has been screening since 1964, although initially in an *ad-hoc*, uncoordinated way. Recently more efficient organization, computerization and government initiatives have made screening more effective. An Intercollegiate Working Party was set up in 1987 and they made recommendations for effective screening. Following Department of Health guidelines the District Health Authorities (DHAs) established computerized call/recall systems, and in 1988 organized cervical screening really started in England and Wales.

In the Department of Health Guidelines (DOH, 1988a) updated in 1993 (DOH 1993) the main points were:

♦ The provision of clear policy guidelines recommending five yearly cervical smear tests for women aged between 20 and 65.

♦ Introduction of a computerized call and recall scheme based at Family Practitioner Committees as the Family Health Service Authorities (FHSAs) were then called.

♦ The production of professional guidelines through the medium of an Intercollegiate Report (1987).

♦ The introduction of a number of policy initiatives designed to improve the quality of the service.

♦ Clear guidelines on fail-safe systems and identification of one person as being responsible for the coordination of the fail-safe system.

♦ Introduction of an external laboratory quality

assurance system, funded by Regional Health Authorities (RHAs).

♦ The requirement that RHAs should organize, or provide training for those people reading cervical smear tests.

♦ The nomination of an individual who could be held to account for the 'organization and effectiveness of cervical cancer screening' (NCN, 1991a).

The National Coordinating Network (NCN) of the NHSCSP

Following the publication of Guidelines HC(88)1 (DOH, 1988a) a number of people representing five main interest groups: women, research workers, service providers, policy-makers and professional organizations, was convened to see what could be done to improve the management of cervical screening in the United Kingdom. This group met for three years with the aim of promoting the exchange of good ideas for quality improvement. The DOH was fully involved in this work and negotiations with the Department resulted in resources being made available to support and develop the work of what became the National Coordinating Network (NCN, 1991b).

The NCN continues to assist those running the cervical screening programme and is a source of updating and useful information. They liaise and coordinate between laboratory and Family Health Service Authority (FHSA) and produce authoritative guidelines and initiatives such as their LINKS newsletter.

To complete the picture of the history of our cervical screening programme, two more events need mentioning.

The first event was the 1990 GP's Contract which brought in target payments as incentives to GPs to screen 50% (lower payment) and 80% (higher payment) of their target population of women (aged 20–65 years) every five years (Table 11.2). This initiative has been very successful and has led to a marked increased in cervical screening activity, but may have raised some problems:

♦ Not all 20-year-olds and onwards will be sexually active, some will be inappropriately screened.

♦ If a GP has a highly mobile practice population

Table 11.2 *Percentage of GPs reaching screening targets, England*

YEAR	% GPs REACHING		
	80% target	50% target	Neither
April 1990	53	32	15
October 1990	67	24	9
October 1991	72	20	8
October 1993	83	14	3

→ introduction of target payments

it may be difficult to reach targets, therefore cervical screening might become a low priority within the practice.

♦ Coercive tactics have been reported to encourage women to have their smear test at their GP's surgery.

This creates a conflict, in that it goes against the spirit of enabling women to make informed choices about whether or not they wish to be screened and where they wish to go for screening (Austoker and McPherson, 1992).

The second event was the publication in July 1992 of the Department of Health's *Health of the Nation* document (DOH, 1992). In this document the DOH set targets for the reduction of preventable disease to improve the health of the nation. Cancers are the second most common cause of death (25%) in England. In the *Health of the Nation* document, four cancers (breast, cervical, lung and skin) were targeted for action. With cervical cancer the aim is to reduce the number of women with newly detected invasive cervical cancer by at least 20% by the year 2000.

The figures we have so far (in 1996) are for the year of 1993 when deaths from cervical cancer in England and Wales were 1369 women (O.N.S. Report, 1996). This figure shows a continued reduction in mortality from the disease. Evidence of improved coverage up to 1993 is shown in Table 11.3. The latest figures on coverage (NCN, 1996)

♦ show that over 85% of women in the screening age range have had a smear in the preceding 5 years.

Never before have health professionals, purchasers, providers and RHAs been given such a challenge. The *Health of the Nation* document has given an impetus to the cervical screening programme to carry on the good work of the 1988 reforms.

Screening in itself can cause stress and anxiety. It should be remembered that we are dealing with a seemingly healthy population and if a smear has to be repeated for any reason at all it can be the source of much worry. The belief by some women that the test will be 'painful, embarrassing or unpleasant' is a strong reason for non-attendance (Gillam, 1991). The principles of screening for disease are outlined in Box 11.1. You will see as we go through this chapter how well cervical screening fits in with most of these principles.

Table 11.3 *Percentage coverage in the target age range, England 1988/9–1992/3*

YEAR	% COVERAGE[a]
1988/89	43
1989/90	62
1990/91	74
1991/92	80
1992/93	83

Source: DOH, *Cervical Cytology*, England, 1988/89–1992/93. Reproduced with permission of Cancer Research Campaign, 1994
[a] percentage of women in the target age range (20–64 years) screened in the last 5.5 years of the given year.

Scenario

Gwyneth, a 58-year-old woman, had been called by the FHSA computer for her first smear ever. The *practice nurse realized that she would have to explain everything carefully to Gwyneth who looked very nervous and said even though she'd given birth to two children, having a smear had always sounded horrific. She had called the test the 'cancer smear'. The practice nurse thought that this was a good area to start giving information and explained that the test was in fact looking for very early changes in the cells from the cervix, that if left undetected*

Box 11.1   The principles of screening
The *Principles and Practice of Screening for Disease* was a Public Health Paper formulated in 1968 for the World Health Organization by Wilson and Junger and seems just as appropriate three decades later when we are considering cervical screening. The basic principles are as follows:

♦ The condition should pose an important health problem

♦ The natural history of the disease should be well-understood

♦ There should be a recognizable early stage

♦ Early treatment should be more beneficial than at a later stage

♦ There should be a suitable test

♦ The test should be acceptable to the population

♦ There should be adequate facilities for the diagnosis and treatment of abnormalities detected

♦ For disease of insidious onset, screening should be repeated at intervals determined by the natural history of the disease

♦ The chance of physical or psychological harm must be less than the benefits

♦ Cost of screening should be balanced against the benefits it provides.

and untreated might over a period of years change to cancer. This, along with giving Gwyneth more up-to-date information and spending some time showing her the equipment, helped to make the situation less formidable.

When the nurse took the cervical smear there was some contact bleeding. She informed Gwyneth of this and said that the laboratory might not be able to get such a good look at the cells that they want to see, and in that case they would most likely request a repeat of the smear.

She was 'not to panic' therefore if she was called back to the surgery. All this was understood by the patient who went home much better informed than when she had arrived, and because the nurse had spent time explaining things to her, Gwyneth was less likely to worry if called back for a repeat smear.

What is cervical screening looking for?

Cervical screening is undertaken to detect very early changes in cells from the cervix which, if left untreated, could lead to squamous cell carcinoma. In other words, cervical screening is a way of interrupting the natural history of the disease at an earlier and more treatable stage.

Other abnormalities may be picked up coincidentally by the cervical smear and these will be discussed later in the chapter.

The cervical smear test or the 'Pap' smear

We have the Greek scientist and humanitarian George N. Papanicolaou (1883–1962) to thank for the modern smear test. He began scientific work in Monaco in the field of oceanography and physiology, but moved to New York in 1913 where he joined the department of pathology at Cornell Medical College. Here he demonstrated changes in vaginal epithelium at different phases of the menstrual cycle, and developed a cytological test for malignant change in the squamous epithelial tissue of the cervix uteri.

It took many years for his research to be recognized, but his test for the early detection of cervical cancer has been widely used since the late 1940s and is known as the 'Pap' smear test. ('Smear' refers to the action of smearing the cells within the mucus onto the glass slide.) It is said (Barker, 1987) that Papanicolaou used his wife as a volunteer to obtain cervical cells. He used a pipette to draw fluid from the posterior fornix of the vagina in which can be found cervical cells (as cells from the cervix exfoliate like any other epithelial covering).

While we no longer use this pipette method to obtain the sample of mucus, the principles of the test remain the same.

Epidemiology of cervical cancer (Cancer Research Campaign, 1994)

Cervical cancer rates vary greatly throughout the world. In developing countries cervical cancer is the commonest female cancer. Of the estimated 460 000 new cases occurring annually in the world, 77% are in developing countries. Taking the world as a whole, cervical cancer is the second commonest female cancer after breast cancer.

Incidence and mortality rates in the UK are amongst the highest in Europe. The UK has the second highest incidence rate (in the European Community) after Denmark and one of the highest death rates. In 1992 1860 women died from cervical cancer in the UK. The trend over the past 20 years shows a substantial decrease in mortality rates (Figure 11.1), from 88 in 1972 to 63 per million population in 1992, but little change in incidence rates. Prior to 1988 two-thirds of the women found to have invasive carcinoma of the cervix had never had a smear test.

The natural history of cervical cancer

The majority of cancer of the cervix is squamous cell carcinoma; adenocarcinomas are rare (5–12%) and originate deep within the glands of the endocervical canal. It is not common to diagnose adenocarcinoma from a cervical smear and its origins are not thought to be associated with sexual activity. When we hear of celibate women dying

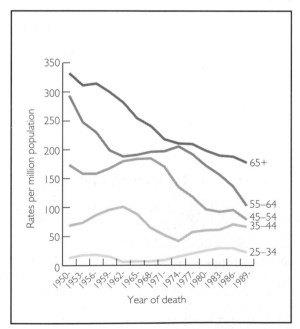

Figure 11.1 *Death rates for cancer of the cervix, England and Wales, 1950–91. (Reproduced with permission from Cancer Research Campaign* Factsheets. Cancer of the Cervix Uteri, *1994)*

from cervical cancer, it is most likely to be adenocarcinoma.

Squamous cell carcinoma

Epidemiological evidence has linked squamous cell carcinoma with sexual habits. One of the first people to take an epidemiological approach to cancer was a doctor called Domenico Rigoni-Stern who was born in 1810 in Italy. He graduated as a medical doctor and surgeon from the University of Padua in 1834 and published numerous papers during the 1830s and 1840s on the incidence and mortality of various cancers. In 1842 he published his most notable study of '*Statistical data relative to the disease of cancer*' (Scotto and Bailar, 1969). In this study he noted the higher frequency of breast cancer among unmarried women and nuns, relative to married or widowed women. He also found that uterine cancer (data did not distinguish between uterine cervix and uterine corpus, but it is thought that most of the uterine cancer was probably primary in the cervix), was not common in unmarried women and was very rare in nuns. This finding was later confirmed by Gagnon (1950) in a study of nuns in Quebec, Canada.

Singer and Szarewski (1988) commented in their book that the wives of Colombian businessmen from social class 1 had a high incidence of the disease. The wives were usually faithful to their husbands but it was found that the husbands were accustomed to regularly visiting prostitutes.

In the 1960s attention turned to the role of the male in the incidence of cervical cancer. It was found that wives of men whose first wives had died from cervical cancer were more likely to develop the disease; wives of husbands with penile cancer (Smith *et al.*, 1979) were also found to have a high incidence. These studies led to the concept of the 'high-risk' male, a category which can include men who work away from home and consequently have greater opportunity to have more than one sexual partner.

In general the disease is more common in women of lower socio-economic groups (Figure 11.2). There may be many co-factors within this, such as smoking habits (Simons *et al.*, 1993) and early age of sexual intercourse, leading to the likelihood of having more than one partner in a lifetime and increased probability of having more pregnancies.

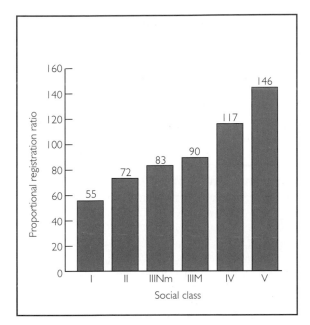

Figure 11.2 *Cancer of the cervix uteri: proportional registration ratios by social class, England and Wales, 1984. (Reproduced with permission from Cancer Research Campaign* Factsheets, *1994,* Cancer of the cervix uteri*)*

The sexually transmitted agent that is strongly linked with cervical cancer is the human papillomavirus (HPV) (Eluf-Neto *et al.*, 1994), and is also known as wart virus. There are over 40 different kinds of wart virus, identified by the type of DNA they contain. The association with cervical cancer is verified by the fact that around 90% of women with cervical cancer have antibodies to HPV in blood samples, while antibodies to HPV have also been found in about 95% of people who have genital warts.

When a group of women without genital warts or cervical cancer or pre-cancerous changes was studied, virtually none had antibodies to HPV. With all this evidence, Singer and Szarewski (1988) concluded that the wart virus is a major cause of cervical cancer.

Unfortunately, the high-risk viruses thought to be associated with cervical cancer – HPV 16, 18, 31 and 33 – cannot be specifically identified from a cervical smear test alone. When a cell is invaded by a wart virus, characteristic changes can be seen under the cytologist's microscope (the nucleus gives the appearance of having a halo round it).

The cells invaded are called koilocytes. To distinguish which HPV was present, the DNA would need to be examined.

Risk factors associated with cervical cancer

Sexual behaviour

It is recognized that certain areas of sexual behaviour are associated with increased risk of cervical cancer. These include the following:

♦ *Age at first sexual intercourse* The 'transformation zone' (see pages 266 and 267) is very evident and active in puberty making it would more susceptible to possible carcinogens such as HPV.

♦ *Number of sexual partners* Because HPV is transmitted through sexual activity, the numbers of sexual partners of both the women and her partner are risk factors.

♦ *Number of pregnancies* During pregnancy the transformation zone is very evident and active and therefore more vulnerable to sexually transmitted agents. Pregnancy also suppresses the immune system.

Within these risk factors associated with sexual behaviour run the previously discussed risk factors of smoking and socio-economic group (see page 262).

Suppression of the immune system

A weakened immune system would make the cervix more susceptible to the disease if the following risk factors were also present:

♦ *Smoking over 20 cigarettes per day* Barton *et al.* (1988) showed that nicotine found in high concentrations in the cervical cells of smokers damages the cells' immune response (Langerhans cells), making them more susceptible to forms of infections such as wart virus. Women who smoke have over ten times the normal risk of developing cervical cancer.

♦ *Acquired immune deficiency syndrome* (AIDS).

◆ *Treatments for cancer* – chemotherapy.

◆ *Post-transplant treatment* to prevent rejection of the new organ.

Method of contraception

The combined oral contraceptive pill has been implicated in cervical cancer, possibly due to the oestrogen in the pill making the ectropion (see Colour plate 3) on the cervix more extensive, therefore offering a larger area where metaplasia can be more vulnerable to HPV.

The connection with pill use is inconclusive and studies continue. We do know that the pill used correctly offers up to 99% protection from pregnancy and that pregnancy itself is a risk factor for cervical cancer.

The co-factor could be that pill users are less likely to use barrier methods in addition to their pill. The message that health professionals should give to clients is that the pill will protect from pregnancy and the use of condoms will protect from HIV, STDs and cervical abnormalities. The use of both is known as the double dutch method.

Alternative sexual practices

So far we have been discussing risks associated with penetrative sexual intercourse. Not all women are in a heterosexual relationship, and lesbian relationships need to be considered. A lesbian coming for a cervical smear should have sexual intercourse and her own sexual activities discussed in a sensitive manner. Knowing that the high risk agent is wart virus, sexual practices should be addressed, to decide whether the woman is at risk and whether a smear is relevant. If the cervical smear is decided against then there are many other well-woman checks that can be undertaken, e.g. breast awareness, and health advice given on other topics such as diet, smoking, etc.

Anatomy and physiology

Uterus

The uterus is a hollow, pear-shaped muscular organ situated in the pelvic cavity between the bladder and the rectum. In 80% of women it is anteverted (tilted forward) and anteflexed (curved forward on itself) from the level of the internal os (Figures 11.3 and 11.4).

The body or corpus of the uterus is 5 cm long, with the neck or cervix uteri 2.5 cm long; the lower part of the cervix protrudes at approximately 90° into the upper part of the vagina. Because the cervix protrudes into the high vagina it forms a space around it, which is divided into four fornices:

◆ The anterior space or fornix between the cervix and bladder

◆ The posterior space or fornix between the cervix and the rectum,

◆ The right and left (or lateral) fornices, taken up

Figure 11.3 *The pelvic organs in sagittal section.*

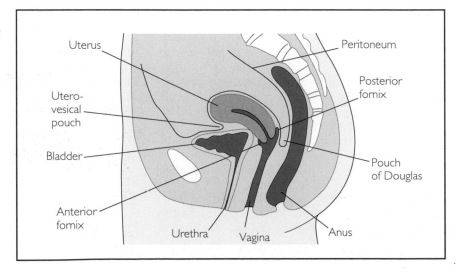

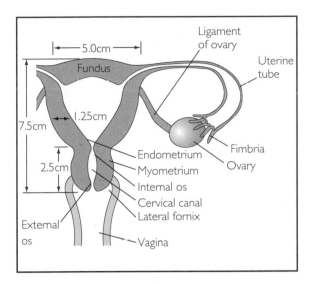

Figure 11.4 *The uterus and left Fallopian tube and ovary.*

by the ovaries and Fallopian tubes. These are called the right and left adnexae.

The inner layer of the body of the uterus is lined with endometrial cells which are constantly changing in thickness and vascularity according to the phases of the menstrual cycle. The superficial layers are shed during menstruation and evidence of them can be found up to days 10–12 of the next menstrual cycle if cervical mucus is examined under the microscope. This underlines the need to put the first day of the last menstrual period on the laboratory form. If there are endometrial cells present and your patient is more than 10–12 days into her menstrual cycle the laboratory may ask for a repeat smear (your patient may have an endometrial tumour).

The importance of informing the laboratory of an intrauterine contraceptive device being *in situ* is also associated with endometrial cells being present later in the cycle (Hopwood, 1995).

The cervix

The outer part of the cervix, the ectocervix, is covered by thick multilayered stratified (meaning horizontal sheets) squamous epithelium. In healthy women in their reproductive years, this consists of up to 20 layers of cells which arise at the basement membrane and mature in an orderly

way, gaining increased amounts of cytoplasm as they approach the surface of the epithelial covering. The blood vessels and glands are contained in the basement membrane under the tough squamous epithelium, giving the ectocervix a dusky pink sheen, which can be a helpful guide to you when endeavouring to locate the cervix during smear taking. It is quite different from the darker pink epithelium of the vaginal walls.

Under the microscope, the surface of the ectocervix is not smooth but rather like the coastline on a map, irregular with many folds. Sometimes these folds become blocked with mucus. When this happens they look like little cysts on the surface of the cervix and are called retention cysts or Nabothian follicles (see Colour plate 2).

Looking at the cervix from the vagina it could be likened to a Victoria plum in shape and size, with the 'stalk' at the cervical hole or os. The cervical os is the opening into the cervical canal. The endocervical canal is lined by epithelium only one cell thick, arranged in columns called columnar epithelium (Figure 11.5). Within these cells are found deep branching glands called compound racemose glands, which secrete alkaline mucus. It is within these glands that the uncommon adenocarcinoma can arise.

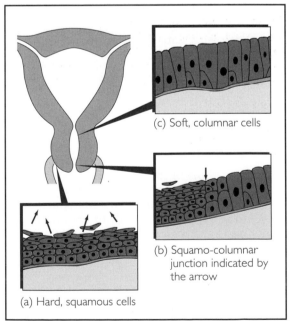

Figure 11.5
Squamo-columnar junction of the Cervix.

Separating the endocervical canal from the cavity of the uterus is the internal cervical os, which has a strong muscle surrounding it. This is important for maintaining a pregnancy.

The cervix is a very dynamic organ and changes throughout the different phases of a woman's life. It is under the influence of ovarian and pituitary hormones which are very active at puberty and during pregnancy. These start to decline during the climacteric and cease completely after the menopause. An experienced smear taker could probably guess the approximate age of a woman by just looking at her cervix.

The squamo-columnar junction (SCJ)

The point at which the squamous cells of the ectocervix meet the columnar cells of the endocervix is known as the squamo-columnar junction (SCJ). Depending on the age and hormonal state of the woman this junction could be in the lower third of the endocervical canal or out on the ectocervix (Box 11.2). See Colour plate 1.

Box 11.2 Factors that decide the position of the squamo-columnar junction

♦ Individual endogenous hormones during adolescence, puberty, the reproductive years and the climacteric/menopause.

♦ Extra exogenous hormones in the form of the oral contraceptive pill and hormone replacement therapy.

Within the confines of the alkaline endocervical canal the delicate columnar cells are protected from the acid pH of the vagina and also from the natural friction of the penis pushing against the cervix during sexual intercourse. It is a natural process for the columnar cells to migrate downwards on to the ectocervix, moving the SCJ to a new position. Ectropion, or ectopy, is the appearance of a red area of columnar epithelium around the cervical os by this process (Hopwood, 1990). This is a normal physiological state and the term 'erosion' formerly used should be avoided as it is liable to conjure the impression of something 'wearing away' (see Colour plate 3).

Scenario

The nurse was clearing up her room after a busy afternoon in the surgery undertaking 'well-woman' checks which included taking cervical smears. The phone rang. On the line was a very tearful patient, Sharon, a 25-year-old woman, who had seen the nurse for a smear that afternoon. The nurse had commented when taking the smear that there was an 'erosion' present on her cervix. Sharon, not wanting to seem ignorant, did not ask for more information, but on arriving home had looked up 'erosion' in the dictionary and was distraught to see it connected with 'wearing away'. The nurse was able to reassure her and admitted to using a term that is no longer in common use and instead talked of an ectopy which now made sense to Sharon. This was a salutory lesson to the nurse to be more careful and sensitive when offering information to patients.

Transformation zone or transitional zone

The migrated columnar cells at the squamo-columnar junction on the ectocervix will start to break down in the acid environment of the vagina. Squamous cells begin to grow from beneath the columnar epithelium and gradually replace it. This normal replacement of one type of cell by another is called squamous metaplasia and where it takes place is called the transformation or transitional zone (Figure 11.6).

The squamo-columnar junction and the transformation zone are the most common sites where pre-cancerous changes originate (Chomet and Chomet, 1989) due to these areas being active and vulnerable. It is imperative that the smear-taker understands this concept in order to take the best possible smears.

The nurse's role as a smear-taker

It is important for you, the smear-taker, to be up to date and well informed regarding all aspects of cervical cytology and this in turn will allow you to give your patient advice and information prior to her smear being taken.

Your attitude is very important. Not only is it

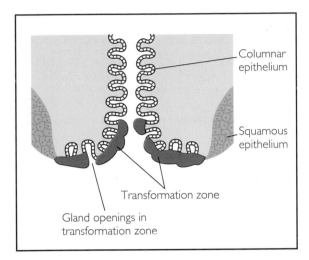

Figure 11.6 *Transformation zone. The surface of the everted columnar epithelium gradually changes to squamous epithelium. This altered area, consisting of metaplastic squamous epithelium, is known as the transformation zone. In post-menopausal women there is a reduction in size of the cervix. The squamo-columnar junction and part of the transformation zone come to lie in the endocervix.*

desirable to have someone who is sensitive to the patient's fears, feelings and possible misgivings about having a smear taken, but also someone who is comfortable with undertaking this most intimate of examinations. It is a presumption that all nurses feel able to undertake the role of smear-taker. Nurses may have problems with their own sexuality, which is not necessarily associated with the 'older' or 'younger' nurse. It may not be until the nurse starts learning how to take smears, that she realizes she has such a problem that she may have subconsciously denied or hidden until this time.

Scenario

An instructing nurse was discussing smear taking with her new family planning student. She had been aware of a distinct feeling of discomfort and embarrassment while observing the student taking a smear. The feeling certainly was not coming from the patient who was a very relaxed and chatty woman who, knowing it was a training session for the student was doing all she could to help the situation. When the instructing nurse enquired of the student how she felt she had done, the nurse became quite emotional and said that she had found it a most embarrassing situation to be in, and that if smear taking was an essential part of the course she wondered if she should continue.

After sitting down together and discussing the matter it transpired that the nurse had an unconsumated marriage of four years, and up to then had not admitted this to anyone. The instructing nurse was able to put the student in touch with a local psychosexual counsellor. The nurse did not continue with the course but hoped to do so when she had sorted out her own problems.

As a smear-taker, you will not only have to be quite happy with your own sexuality, but also be able to discuss any problems or anxieties that your patient may reveal at this most sensitive and intimate of times (Tunnadine, 1970).

It is not expected that you will have all the answers to whatever a patient reveals, but very often just the fact that the woman has voiced some concern or anxiety to you can be of enormous benefit to her, even though you may have said very little, apart from listening.

Training to become a smear-taker

Ideally all nurses who take cervical smears should have undertaken an appropriate course. Various courses are available:

♦ The ENB N28 Women's Health Screening Course

♦ The ENB 901 Family Planning in Society Course

♦ The ENB AO8 Advanced Family Planning Course

♦ The Marie Curie Cancer Screening for Practice Nurse Course (similar courses are available in Scotland, Wales and Northern Ireland).

Smear taking should not be task-orientated. A sound knowledge of relevant anatomy and physiology, the natural history of the disease, associated risk factors, abnormalities and possible treatment would not only be a distinct advantage to you but also to your patients, to whom you can give up-to-date information and advice.

It is quite common for many of the more popular courses to be oversubscribed. There can be problems getting funding to attend courses and it is not always easy to get time away from work. 'In-house' training from doctors and experienced nurses may be the only alternative, and can be excellent for practical sessions, but the knowledge gained from a reputable course is invaluable.

Information for women before the smear

Before attending for a cervical smear, women should be provided with information about how to prepare for the procedure. This could be in the form of a leaflet given out in your practice or clinic, or details given over the telephone when patients make their appointments, or added to a letter that you routinely send to your patients, inviting them to attend for a smear. The information should include the following recommendations:

♦ Ideally you smear should be taken half-way between your periods

♦ Avoid having a bath on the day of your smear, a shower or stand-up wash would be better.

♦ For about 48 hours before your smear use a condom or abstain from sexual intercourse.

♦ If you have recently used a vaginal pessary for treating an infection such as thrush, allow yourself to have a period before your next smear, to make sure all traces of the pessary have gone.

♦ If you are using an oestrogen cream, do not apply on the day of your smear.

This useful information is based on common sense and will enable you to obtain the best possible smear for cytological analysis. Remember these are ideals, and few women can manage all of them. The most important is that she is not too near the time of her period.

Taking a cervical smear

A smear test should be taken in such a way as to provide an adequate sample for assessment with the minimum of distress or discomfort to the client.

The client should be fully informed of the reason for the procedure and the implications for her future health and well-being.

Environment

Privacy is an essential prerequisite when a smear is taken. Ideally the room should also:

♦ Be warm

♦ Have a screen around the examination couch

♦ Have a good adjustable lamp

♦ Have a trolley or work-surface next to the couch

♦ Have a sink with hot and cold water supply.

The examination should be performed without interruptions.

Equipment

The following equipment will be needed:

♦ An autoclave which is regularly serviced and complies with current guidelines (DOH, 1988b, 1994) if instruments are sterilized within the clinic

♦ Vaginal speculae (assorted sizes)

♦ Cytology slides with frosted ends and a sharp pencil

♦ Fixative containing alcohol and carbo wax (dropper or spray)

♦ Assorted spatulae and cervical brushes currently recommended

♦ Swabs for culture

♦ Latex examination gloves

♦ KY lubricating jelly

♦ Smear request forms and boxes for transporting slides

♦ Disposable paper roll for the couch.

Interview and completion of the smear form

It is very important to record a menstrual/obstetric/contraceptive history in the patient's notes as these are relevant to cervical cytology.

This is also a good opportunity for the patient to air any anxieties or recent problems she may have had. Key questions are listed in Box 11.3.

Box 11.3 Key questions to ask prior to taking a smear

♦ Do you understand the purpose of this test?

♦ Do you have any bleeding after sexual intercourse (post-coital)?

♦ Are you currently using a method of contraception?

♦ Do you have any intermenstrual bleeding (if the patient is using oral contraception this may be the reason)?

♦ Do you have any pain during or after sexual intercourse (dyspareunia)?

♦ Do you have painful or heavy periods? (This would be important if the pattern and severity had altered without any changes in circumstances or lifestyle.)

♦ Have you noticed any difference in your vaginal discharge?

With the appropriate range of questions you will have formed a full picture of the woman's menstrual and sexual health. Relevant information should be recorded in her notes. It is very important to allow the patient to know what is being recorded, and to check that she does not object to you writing an item down that she may have disclosed which is of a sensitive or confidential nature.

Useful reading is the UKCC's *Standards for Records and Record Keeping* (UKCC, 1993).

Filling in the laboratory request form

This may seem rather a mundane item to discuss, but in today's world of computers, where every patient is recorded by name, address and date of birth, it is vital for the correct information to be clearly entered on the laboratory form. If the name is spelt incorrectly then the computer does not accept the information. Using the NHS number, if available, will help to verify information given. A checklist is given in Box 11.4.

The glass smear slide

It is a good idea at this point to write in pencil the name and date of birth of the patient on the frosted

---

Box 11.4 Checklist for filling in the laboratory request form

♦ Patient's name (correctly spelt) and maiden name if appropriate

♦ Address with postcode

♦ Date of birth

♦ NHS number if known. It can be found on the invitation letter if the FHSA has requested the test

♦ Today's date

♦ The first day of the last menstrual period, or bleed if using oral contraception or hormone replacement therapy (see page 265 for relevance of this)

♦ Date of the last smear

♦ Contraceptive type: Oral contraceptive with name; HRT type with name. State if intrauterine device (IUD) is present

♦ Referral source (GP/HA clinic or other)

♦ Call/recall; previous abnormal; clinical reason; – signify which

♦ If early recall state last test result or if known give the slide serial number from the previous laboratory form.

---

end of the glass slide, at the same time ensuring (by wiping with a tissue) that the slide is free from dust and grease.

Women who do not need smears

Now that women are sent a request for a smear by age alone, it will mean that many women who do not need smears at the present time are sent for. Austoker and McPherson (1992) state that 'all women aged 20–64 who are or ever have been sexually active should be screened'.

During the interview with the patient you should be able to carefully and sensitively find out if the woman is or ever has been sexually active. This could be by way of asking 'are you using any contraception at the moment'. If the answer is 'no' it may mean that she is celibate, trying to become pregnant or that she or her partner is sterilized. If this is not the case then the conversation could continue: 'if you don't mind me asking, are you sexually active?'. It may be necessary to be even more explicit, 'sexual activity' does not have to include sexual intercourse.

With care and sensitivity you can ascertain the need or not for a smear at that time. It is worth mentioning to the woman that if circumstances change and she becomes sexually active then she can return for a smear. The FHSA should be informed by writing only 'not applicable at this time' and they will recall her at a suitable interval, depending on the local policy.

Many nurses have been in the embarrassing position of having prepared a woman for a smear, only to get to the point of looking at her vaginal opening (introitus) to then have doubts as to whether she has ever been sexually active. Unfortunately, the woman has also had to go through the ordeal of very nearly having a procedure undertaken that is not appropriate.

It need not be a wasted journey for the woman if she finds she does not need a smear as such activities as teaching breast self-awareness (see page 226) and offering information on other well-woman issues may be of great value and interest.

Women who have had a hysterectomy for benign reasons do not need smears. A hysterectomy undertaken for pre-cancer/cancer is different and the woman would have vault smears at intervals according to the present guidelines (Austoker and McPherson, 1992).

A woman who has had a subtotal hysterectomy (for whatever reason) with the cervix remaining will still need to have cervical smears according to the present guidelines and local policy.

Taking the smear

Prior to starting the procedure, run through a checklist of preparations (Box 11.5).

Warm (or cool) the speculum under running water to reach body temperature. If necessary, lightly smear the sides but not the end of the speculum with a water-based lubricant, usually the warm water is sufficient. Inspect the vulva, looking for any sore areas, genital warts or unusual skin textures or colours. A gentle one-finger examination to locate the cervix can be helpful but care should be taken that the immediate area surrounding the os is not touched roughly. Pass the speculum into the vagina gently, with due regard to the

---

Box 11.5 Checklist prior to taking a smear

♦ Does the patient need to empty her bladder?

♦ Is all the equipment needed on a trolley/work-surface as close as possible to the examination couch?

♦ Have you asked permission of the patient to take the smear?

♦ Is the patient in a comfortable position on the couch with underwear removed?

♦ Have you offered the patient a cover if she has not got a petticoat on?

---

woman's reaction. Locate and visualize the cervix, making sure the cervical os is well in view. It is only after the os has been seen that the appropriate spatula can be chosen.

Note the position of the squamo-columnar junction to ensure that the transformation zone is sampled. Insert the spatula well into the cervical os and rotate it twice (using pencil pressure) through 360°. A cervical brush may be used (if the os is very tight) but first the blunt end of a spatula should be rotated around the ectocervix, then the brush inserted for sampling the endocervix. Due to the horizontal position of the bristles there is no need to twist the brush through 360°, introducing it gently into the cervical canal and twisting through only about 45° is sufficient to sample the endocervical canal without causing too much discomfort and bleeding.

A plastic Cervex brush if used has the advantage of sampling both the endo-and ectocervix at the same time. Care should be taken, as the Cervex brush should only be rotated clockwise (Waddell, 1994) through five turns. In a study by Szarewski et al. (1993) it was found that the quality of the sample obtained was very often due to the experience of the smear-taker more than the type of spatula used (Figure 11.7).

Quickly transfer the cells from the spatula on to the slide, using two lengthways strokes, spreading the specimen evenly. If a cervical brush is used, the specimen should be applied using a rolling action. Once the cells are removed from the cervix they are dying and must be preserved without delay. Whichever fixative is used it must be applied immediately, gently flooding the slide, and left to dry horizontally for at least 10–15 minutes. The

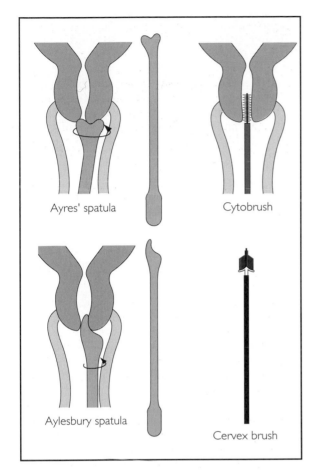

Ayres' spatula

Cytobrush

Aylesbury spatula

Cervex brush

Figure 11.7 *Cervical spatulae and their position within the external os. The Ayres' spatula and the cytobrush are designed to be used together (first the spatula and then the brush), whereas the Aylesbury spatula and the Cervex brush sample both endo-and ectocervix and can be used alone. (Redrawn with permission from Szarewski, A.* A Woman's Guide to the Cervical Smear Test. *London: Optima, 1994.)*

more experienced smear-taker will remove the speculum at the same time as the sample is taken, having a receptacle at hand to drop the used speculum into. Nurses new to the procedure may find it better to leave the speculum in position until the specimen is fixed. Leaving the speculum in the vagina also has the advantage of you being able to have a second look at the cervix and to note its condition and any bleeding that might have occurred on contact.

A bacterial swab could be taken after the smear if there is a heavy or unusual discharge; if the cervix looks sore or if the patient has commented on symptoms arising from her vaginal discharge.

Gently remove the speculum, making sure that it is clear of the cervix before allowing the blades to start closing.

Bimanual examination of the pelvis

Bimanual pelvic examination need not be undertaken as a routine procedure on an asymptomatic woman. However, if the patient has any of the following symptoms a bimanual examination of the pelvis should be done (RCN, 1995):

♦ Very painful and/or heavy periods

♦ Intermenstrual bleeding

♦ Urinary symptoms

♦ Abdominal swelling

♦ Lower abdominal pain or discomfort

♦ Pain on sexual intercourse

♦ Post coital bleeding.

If you are not trained to undertake this, it is advisable to ask for assistance from a relevantly trained nurse or a doctor. If this is not possible, discuss with the patient whether she could return at her convenience to complete the check.

If she has none of the symptoms mentioned, a simple check for cervical excitation could be performed:

♦ Ask the patient's permission to examine her.

♦ Apply KY jelly to the index and third finger of the examining hand.

♦ Gently insert one finger into the vagina, followed by the second finger.

♦ The idea is to gently hold the end of the cervix between the tips of the two fingers and move the cervix slightly from side to side (laterally).

♦ This should not cause any sudden pain or discomfort to the patient.

♦ If this is painful, it could be due to pelvic inflammatory disease (PID) (see page 407), a pregnancy outside of the uterus (ectopic) (see page 409), a deep-seated carcinoma or ovarian cysts.

♦ Ask for a second opinion from an experienced nurse or doctor while keeping your patient informed of what is happening.

Completing the laboratory request form

The clinical observations of the cervix should now be recorded on the laboratory request form. It is not up to you to diagnose what has been observed on the cervix. It is much easier to describe exactly what is seen: 'red cervix, bled on contact', 'large ectropion-like area seen', 'greenish vaginal discharge at os'. The cyto-screener has only a few cells in front of him or her to base a diagnosis on, therefore the more you can describe what is seen on the cervix at the time the better. It is important for you to sign your own name and possibly print it underneath. This allows for audit of smear results either by the laboratory or your self.

Problems inserting the vaginal speculum

At all times you should be sensitive to the woman's reactions, particularly as you are about to insert the speculum into the vagina. Many things could happen:

◆ The patient clamps her thighs together and says 'I can't go through with this'. You then have to put the speculum down and gently ask the woman what is on her mind and would she like to talk about it. This may reveal anything from abuse, rape, a previous miscarriage or termination of pregnancy, depression, a previous experience of a painful gynaecological examination – in fact the list is endless. The condition when a woman cannot allow a speculum (or a penis) to enter her vagina is called vaginismus (Valins, 1988) (see page 47 for more details).

The smear would have to wait until the woman felt able to cope with the procedure whilst also receiving help from other professionals.

◆ The opening to the vagina (introitus) looks small and when a fingertip is put into the entrance to the vagina an intact hymen is present. The woman has not had sexual intercourse (virgo intacta). You should explain that women who have never had sexual intercourse do not need smears, but if her circumstances change, she should return for a smear about one year after she becomes sexually active.

◆ When the outer folds of the vagina (labia majora) are parted the inner folds (labia minora) look unusual, the whole area looks as though it has been surgically treated, the introitus may be very small, even tiny, scar tissue may be obvious. If these signs are present in a woman from the east, north-eastern or west parts of Africa, or some parts of the Middle East or South-East Asia, it may well be that she has undergone female genital mutilation (Box 11.6)

> **Box 11.6** Female genital mutilation
> This is a collective term used for different degrees of mutilation of the female external genitals (Royal College of Nursing, 1994). As more refugees from Africa arrive in the UK, so more nurses working in primary care will come across women who have been genitally mutilated.
>
> The procedure is illegal in Britain under the Prohibition of Female Circumcision Act 1985, though parents determined to have it carried out may take their children abroad.
>
> It has no benefits to the woman and can cause problems such as painful intercourse (dyspareunia), no orgasms (as the clitoris is removed) and urinary and menstrual problems. Often the first time the mutilation is observed is during pregnancy. Problems commonly occur during labour. There are no easy answers to this problem, but when found, you should be sensitive, non-judgemental and supportive to the woman. It may be impossible to take a smear without surgical intervention. (See also page 105).

◆ Women who have had a Caesarean section may have tight vaginal muscles which have never been stretched by the head of the baby in the birth canal. The inserting of the speculum can be quite uncomfortable. You should try to pick a speculum that is not too big; it is useful to have a good assortment of sizes and lengths of vaginal speculae available.

◆ Peri-menopausal and post-menopausal women often present with drying and thinning of the vaginal epithelium. Again, a smaller speculum should be chosen and the use of KY jelly (sparingly smeared) on the blades of the speculum will make the procedure more comfortable, as described in the Report of the Intercollegiate Working Party (RCOG, RCP, RCGP, FCM, 1987).

Doubts when the cervix is visualized

If the cervix is covered with thick mucus, do not clean it. The cells that might be abnormal may be in the mucus which you have cleaned off. Take a first sweep of the cervix with the spatula, immediately followed by a second sweep with another spatula, spread them side by side on the slide, fixing without delay. On the laboratory form explain: 'left side of slide – first sweep of cervix; right side of slide – second sweep of cervix'. If the laboratory does not object, two slides could be sent marked '1st' and '2nd'.

If there is a mucus plug in the cervical os, this can be carefully lifted off without disturbing the cervical mucus with the tip of an Aylesbury spatula and discarded. If this plug of mucus were to get on to the slide it would make a very poor smear for the cyto-screener to look at.

If the cervix bleeds on the first sweep round with the spatula, do not make a second sweep. Spread the specimen immediately and fix and record the bleeding on the laboratory request form.

If the cervix looks sore and very red, take a high vaginal swab and a swab for chlamydia after the smear is taken, and add a comment to the laboratory request form. The patient should be told of the difference between cytology and bacteriology.

If there is a wide transformation zone on the ectocervix, take a first sweep with an Aylesbury spatula within the cervical os, and a second sweep with the blunt end of the spatula to sample the wide transformation zone. Spread the specimens side by side on the one slide and fix immediately.

A cervical polyp, which is an overgrowth of epithelial tissue (of varying sizes) often on a stalk and looking a little like a grape, may be seen (See Colour Plate 4). Polyps are rarely associated with malignancy, but it is felt they are worth a referral to the gynaecological outpatients for removal. There is a chance that the polyp may originate from the endometrium (on a long stalk), therefore on removal profuse bleeding might occur. Record on the laboratory form what you have seen ('polyp-type structure'), explain to your patient, and follow your policy for referral.

If the cervix looks unusual in any way it is appropriate to get a second opinion from a practitioner. It is quite acceptable for a patient to be referred for further investigations and colposcopy on the look of the cervix alone.

Pelvic inflammatory disease (PID)

If PID is suspected then an endocervical swab needs to be taken. The type of sampling equipment used varies from clinic to clinic. If there are no facilities for taking endocervical swabs, then the procedure should not be attempted; your patient should be referred to a clinic of genito-urinary medicine (GUM) where the appropriate equipment is available.

A swab result returned as negative might still mean that *Chlamydia* is present if this has not been tested for. *Chlamydia* left undetected and untreated could lead to salpingitis and pelvic inflammatory disease with the high risk of future fertility problems.

Common faults when trying to locate the cervix

You can never judge by outward appearances (height, weight) exactly where and in what position your patient's cervix will be. The 'one-finger' examination (page 270) will be a good guide as to the position and angle of the cervix.

Incorrect position of the speculum

You have inserted the speculum into the vagina, open up the blades and all you can see is a space surrounded by the vaginal walls. Often this is because you are in the posterior fornix.

Solution. Gently ease the speculum towards you while watching carefully to see if the cervix drops into view; it is useful to ask your patient to cough. When having to manoeuvre your speculum while it is in the vagina, great care should be taken not to cause pain or discomfort. A useful tip is to hold the lower or posterior part of the speculum with your thumb and index finger and apply slight pressure which moves the speculum slightly.

Good idea. When inserting the speculum, open it up slightly when about half of it is inside the vagina; you may be surprised to see the cervix coming into view sooner than you would have thought. If it is seen, continue introducing the closed speculum towards the observed position of the cervix.

Acute position of the cervix (1)

The cervix is pointing into the anterior wall of the vagina, due to a retroverted uterus. You cannot encompass the cervix with your speculum.

Solution. Ask your client to half-sit-up resting on her elbows (if possible), keeping her informed of why you are asking her to do this, or ask her to put her hands underneath her buttocks to raise her pelvis.

Acute position of the cervix (2)

The cervix is pointing into the posterior wall of the vagina, due to a very anteverted uterus. You cannot encompass the cervix with your speculum.

Solution. Ask your client to press down with her hands over her lower abdomen (retro-pubic area) or ask her to bring her knees up against her abdomen holding them with her arms. Either of these solutions could help flip the cervix forward, allowing you to locate it with your speculum.

If these fail, ask her to get into the left-lateral position where, by inserting the speculum into the vagina from the back the cervix should be able to be viewed. This may seem awkward but when you have viewed a difficult cervix once this way, you will find it to be a useful alternative.

Prolapsed vaginal walls obscuring the view of the cervix

This is a common problem. You insert the speculum and can only see the lateral walls of the vagina fall into your field of view.

Solution. Instead of turning the speculum through 90° (just after you have inserted the tip into the introitus) keep the speculum in the position of having the blades remain in the lateral position, then continue introducing the speculum further into the vagina. The walls will be against the blades and unable to collapse. This method can only be used if the space or area around your client's inner thighs allows.

Alternatively, use a latex condom or the finger of a latex glove with the closed end cut off and 'sheath' the speculum with this. Either method will hold back the vaginal walls.

A very deep (posterior) cervix

Solution. Use a Winterton speculum, which has extra long blades, or ask your client to press over her lower abdomen, or come-up into the semi-sitting position, either of which may push the uterus down a little, allowing you to visualize and encompass the cervix.

It is important for you to remember the very delicate structures that your speculum may be pressed closely against:

♦ The clitoris

♦ The labia minora

♦ The labia majora – remember pubic hairs can easily be snagged in the screws of the speculum.

It is essential to keep checking that your speculum is not pressing on or pinching any of these structures.

It is also important to keep your client informed of what is happening during the examination and why you are asking her to do a certain thing. Reassure her that she is not abnormal and that each person has slight variations within their body which makes your job more 'interesting'.

A good standard to follow is to treat all your clients the way you would like to be treated yourself. As you progress and see more and more cervices, you will begin to realize that there are indeed many different shapes and sizes of them, ranging from small flat, to long pointed ones.

It is an essential part of your job as a smear-taker to inform your client of how and when she will receive her results and what action to take if no results appear. The National Coordinating Network document *Improving the Quality of the National Health Service Cervical Screening Programme* (NCN, 1994) sets standards for the maximum waiting time for smear results to be sent out as 'not be more than one month'.

Finally, remember to offer advice and interpretation of smear results, should your client need to contact you.

Completing your responsibilities

Before the cytology slides are put into their transport boxes, having had time to dry for at least 15 minutes, check that there is a correctly completed laboratory form for each slide, and that names and dates of birth correspond. Do not let individual slides come into contact with each other and do not overfill the transport box so that the last slide is touching the side of the box. It may adhere to the box and be overlooked at the laboratory, or the specimen may be spoiled. Remember that if a slide is broken or is badly named or sent without its laboratory form it could mean your client having to return for a repeat smear which is both worrying and inconvenient for her.

The responsibilities of the smear-taker are outlined clearly in the Royal College of Nursing *Guidelines For Good Practice* (RCN, 1994).

The opportunistic smear

You should seize the chance of doing the 'opportunistic' smear when it presents itself, even if the woman has consulted you on an entirely different subject, as you may never see this patient again.

It is on such occasions when you have a patient with you and you have been trying to encourage her to have a smear, or she may have had a slightly abnormal result previously, that, regardless of the fact that she may even be menstruating at this time, it is thought best to take the smear than not have one at all. A blood-stained slide is easier to read by the cytologist if it is spread thinly.

It will always be up to the individual to decide whether or not to take up the offer of a smear test and it is important not to become coercive or judgemental, but to offer all the known facts regarding screening and abnormalities of the cervix which will allow your patient to make an informed decision.

You should discourage people from calling it the 'cancer smear' or 'cancer test' and try to dispel myths and misinformation surrounding the test. Elkind *et al.* (1989) explain how many women thought the test was inappropriate to them.

Any woman who presents with the following symptoms may need a smear earlier than the local recommended guidelines:

♦ Blood-stained vaginal discharge

♦ Intermenstrual bleeding

♦ Post-coital bleeding

♦ Post-menopausal bleeding.

Obstacles and dangers

Beware of the woman who always seems to have a 'period' so that she 'cannot have a smear today'. The 'period' that always gets in the way of a smear being taken could be due to some underlying pathology, or it might be that she is using her 'period' as an excuse for a smear not to be performed. You may be well advised to take a smear at this time whether she is menstruating or not again with your client's permission.

Sometimes our clients are not as knowledgeable as we sometimes presume. The difference between a bacterial swab and a cervical smear can be confusing for them to understand.

You may have a new client with you, whose notes have not arrived from her previous doctor. On enquiring about her last smear test she says that she had one some time ago and that the result was negative. Hopefully her medical records will appear soon to verify this, but there is always the chance that she could have had only a swab taken and that her last smear was not negative and that she is overdue for the needed repeat.

Hopefully with the continued linking up of different computers in the primary health care setting this will become a problem of the past. Good practice is to check if you are in any doubt at all, regarding past smear history. This could be done simply by contacting the previous surgery, the notes may still be there, or contacting the Family Health Service Authority concerned.

The postnatal smear

Before the setting up of the call/recall system in 1988, opportunistic smears were taken at the six-week postnatal check. Many doctors and nurses are mistakenly continuing this practice. A smear should only be taken if it is due under the local guidelines, or if the woman has any symptoms that suggest the need for an early smear. If the smear is due, ideally it should be postponed until at least ten weeks postnatally if you feel your patient will return.

Often smears taken at six weeks have to be

repeated due to 'postnatal changes' 'inflammatory', or 'atrophic' changes and may cause needless anxiety.

Smear results and classifications

Waddell (1994) states that an 'adequate smear is one which is suitable for the purpose for which it was obtained', therefore it follows that an inadequate smear is unsuitable for the purpose for which it was obtained.

Inadequate smears

Inadequate smears may be due to insufficient or unsuitable material being present. This could be due to various causes:

♦ Transformation zone not sampled sufficiently.

♦ Excessive lubricant used.

♦ Atrophic cervix. This can be due to low oestrogen levels not allowing exfoliation of cervical cells.

♦ Cytolysis. This is the normal process of cell disintegration due to the high glycogen content in the cells during the second half of the menstrual cycle. Excessive cytolysis may render the smear unsuitable. If a repeat is requested the smear should be taken before ovulation, when the glycogen content is less.

♦ Poor spreading of cervical mucus on the slide.

♦ Inadequate fixation Was the fixative shaken before use? Is the fixative out of date? Did you check to see that all the mucus was covered on the slide? Was the slide flooded too much, pushing off the cells? Was the slide allowed to stand for at least 15 minutes to dry before putting it in the transport box?

♦ The smear consists mainly of blood, pus or inflammatory exudate.

If your laboratory sends back a smear result reported as 'inadequate' they will usually write details of why it is classified as such. If you have any doubts or concerns about the result, it is a good idea to get to know your laboratory staff who are usually more than happy to give you advice and information. More liaison between smear-takers and cyto-screeners allows for the free flowing of information which is useful to everyone concerned.

Additional findings on smears

The cervical smear, though taken primarily to look for pre-cancer changes, may also identify specific infections present.

Anaerobes or anaerobic bacteria

Organisms such as bacteria or fungi which can live without oxygen may be found in the moist airless genital tract.

Gardnerella vaginalis

This is a bacterium normally found in the vagina but only causes problems if its numbers increase. The smear result may say 'Clue cells present' which indicates the presence of *Gardnerella*. Clue cells are ordinary epithelial cells to which these bacteria become attached (see page 295).

Candida albicans/*monilia/thrush*

This is another quite innocent vaginal infection which often shows up on a smear and can give rise to 'many polymorphs or neutrophils obscuring' the cells on the slide. You should be guided by the laboratory's suggested action; if they are not happy with the sample, an early recall will be suggested.

Trichomonas vaginalis

This is a protozoan and is sexually transmitted, giving a frothy, fishy smelling discharge with severe vaginal itching. The presence of *Trichomonas* makes cervical smears very difficult to read, often mimicking pre-cancer in the cervical cells. Your client and her partner should be treated with antibiotics. The laboratory will ask for a repeat smear after treatment. A *Trichomonas* infection can give the cervix the appearance of looking strawberry like. (See Colour plate 5.)

Herpes simplex virus (HSV)

This can be identified on a cervical smear, and would be indicated by multinucleated giant cells.

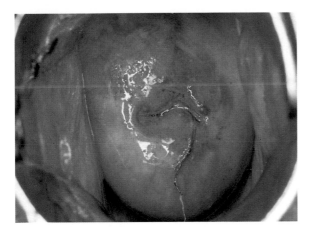

Plate 1 *Multiparous os showing a typical transformation zone and IUD threads. Reproduced with permission from Professor A. McLean, The Royal Free Hospital, London.*

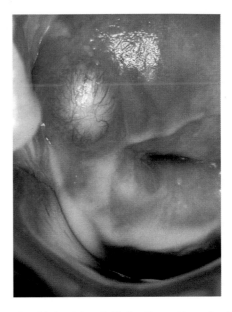

Plate 2 *Nabothian follicle. Reproduced with permission from Mr Peter Greenhouse, Ipswich Hospital, Ipswich.*

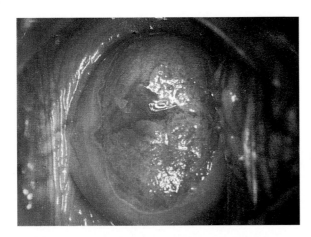

Plate 3 *Cervical ectropion. Reproduced with permission from Mr Peter Greenhouse, Ipswich Hospital, Ipswich.*

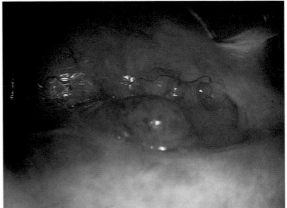

Plate 4 *Cervical polyp. Reproduced with permission from Professor A. McLean, The Royal Free Hospital, London.*

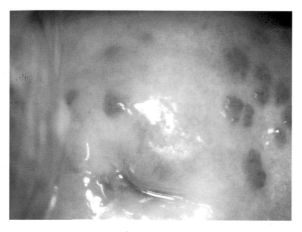

Plate 5 *'Strawberry' cervix. Characteristic of infection with Trichomonas vaginalis. Reproduced with permission from Professor A. McLean, The Royal Free Hospital, London.*

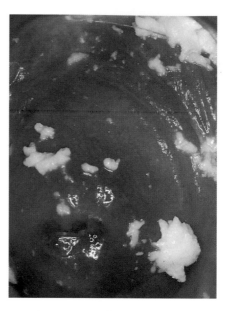

Plate 6 *Candidiasis. Characterized by a thick, white lumpy discharge adhering to the vaginal walls. Reproduced with permission from Mr Peter Greenhouse, Ipswich Hospital, Ipswich.*

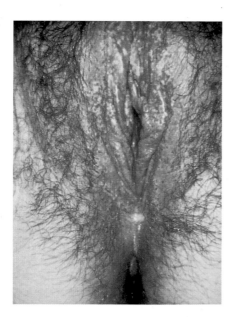

Plate 7 *Vulvovaginitis caused by candida. Reproduced with permission from J. Bingham (1984) Sexually Transmitted Diseases. London: Gower Medical Publishing.*

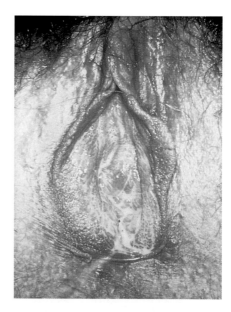

Plate 8 *Bacterial vaginosis. Characterized by a grey malodorus discharge at the vulva. Reproduced with permission from J. Bingham (1984) Sexually Transmitted Diseases. London: Gower Medical Publishing.*

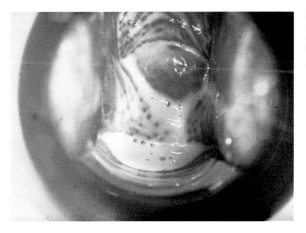

Plate 9 *Trichomonas vaginalis. Characterized by a frothy greenish-yellow discharge exuding from the vaginal wall. Reproduced with permission from J. Bingham (1984)* Sexually Transmitted Diseases. *London: Gower Medical Publishing.*

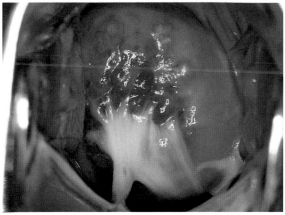

Plate 10 *Purulent cervicitis associated with gonorrhoea and chlamydia. Reproduced with permission from Mr Peter Greenhouse, Ipswich Hospital, Ipswich.*

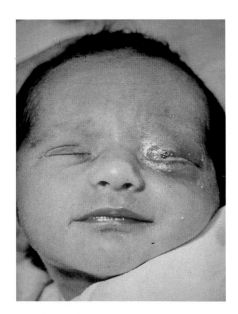

Plate 11 *Ophthalmia neonatorum with gonorrhoea. Symptoms appear within 2–5 days of delivery. Reproduced with permission from J. Bingham (1984)* Sexually Transmitted Diseases. *London: Gower Medical Publishing.*

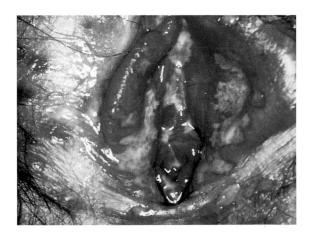

Plate 12 *Herpes lesion on labia majora and labia minora associated with vulval oedema. Reproduced with permission from J. Bingham (1984)* Sexually Transmitted Diseases. *London: Gower Medical Publishing.*

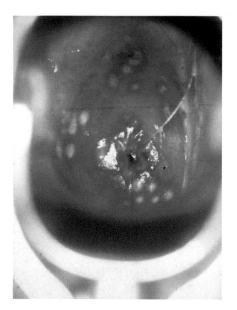

Plate 13 *Herpetic lesions on the cervix.
Reproduced with permission from J. Bingham
(1984)* Sexually Transmitted Diseases. *London:
Gower Medical Publishing.*

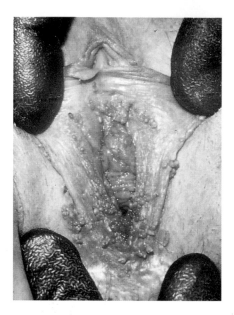

Plate 14 *Vulvo-vaginal warts extending down
into the perineum. Reproduced with permission
from J. Bingham (1984)* Sexually Transmitted
Diseases. *London: Gower Medical Publishing.*

Gonorrhoea and Chlamydia

These cannot be diagnosed from a cervical smear, but there can be intracellular detail that may suggest to the cyto-screener that one or the other is a possibility. The cytologist would suggest further bacterial investigations to be undertaken.

Actinomyces-type organisms

These are bacteria which live normally in the mouth and intestines. In women who have an intrauterine device (IUD) *in situ* this bacterium can often colonize around the IUD and its threads, and show up on the cervical sample. Treatment of this will depend on whether the woman has any symptoms and on local clinic guidelines (see also page 206).

Human papillomavirus (HPV) / koilocytosis

This is a very common result. There is no treatment for it. It is not the same as having warts and this distinction is very important. HPV appearing alone on a smear result does not mean a referral for colposcopy is needed. However, an early recall may be recommended as the link between HPV and early pre-cancer changes is strong (see page 263) (Downey and Barin, 1994).

Great care should be taken when discussing a result of HPV, as your client may wonder (particularly if she is in a stable, long-term relationship) how she came to have the virus. You should emphasize the fact that the natural history of HPV is fairly obscure, that it is very common and can lie dormant for many years before it is seen in cervical cells.

The types (according to the DNA in the cell) of HPV associated with pre-cancer changes are HPV 16, HPV 18, HPV 31 and HPV 33. These do not show up as genital warts in either women or men and there is no way of knowing if a man has it on his penis.

To confuse things further, the genital warts that are visible are HPV 6 and HPV 11 and are not thought to be important as far as cervical cancer is concerned.

Your client may ask why men do not get penile cancer if they have HPV (albeit invisible). The answer lies in the difference between the soft vulnerable area of transformation zone on the cervix, compared to the tough squamous cells of the penis.

'Inflammatory smear' or 'inflammatory changes'

These changes can be caused by a background infection. If there is a suspicion of an undiagnosed infection, a referral for full bacterial/viral screening should be suggested. There can be many simple explanations for an inflammatory smear, such as one taken near to menstruation, but repeated inflammatory changes or severe inflammatory changes may need a referral for colposcopy as they can be implicated in advanced cancer.

Borderline changes

This term is used to describe a cellular appearance that cannot definitely be described as normal. They are usually severe inflammatory changes on the borderline with mild dyskariosis.

The classification of inflammatory and borderline smears is very subjective, that is to say it depends on the particular cytologist who is looking at the cervical cells as to which classification is given.

Cytology and histology

It is important to understand the difference between cytology and histology and to keep these distinctions in mind, as many people confuse cytological with histological terms.

Cytology

Cytology is the study of individual cells, focusing on the size and shape of the nucleus within the cytoplasm, giving due regard to the general shape of the cell itself. This screening is undertaken on cervical smears that you send to the laboratory, by cytologists.

The outer layer of the cervix (ectocervix) is covered by thick, stratified squamous epithelium of up to 20 layers of cells in healthy women in their reproductive years. The cells arise at the basement membrane and mature in an orderly way, gaining increasing amounts of cytoplasm as they approach the surface of the epithelium.

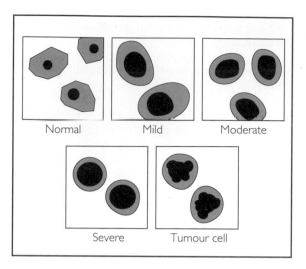

Figure 11.8 *Dyskariotic changes in the cell*

They appear in the cervival smear as parabasal, intermediate and superficial squamous cells. If cell division at the basement membrane is defective, abnormal nuclei are formed, these are *dyskariotic* cells (dys means 'bad' or 'abnormal' and karyon means 'kernal' or 'nucleus', i.e. bad nucleus). The cytologist looking at the cervical cells can identify changes in the squamous cells which, in a high proportion of women, if left untreated might become cancer.

There are three grades of abnormality between a normal cell and a tumour cell which the cytologist can recognize (Figure 11.8):

♦ Mild dyskariosis

♦ Moderate dyskariosis

♦ Severe dyskariosis.

Histology

Histology is the study of a portion (or biopsy) of epithelium from the cervix, looked at under the microscope. This kind of sample could only be obtained at colposcopy.

Just as dyskariosis is a cytological term describing the abnormal nucleus, *dysplasia* is a histological term describing the abnormal architecture of the epithelium (dys means 'bad' and plasia means 'change', i.e. bad change).

Looking at a sample of cervical epithelium under the microscope, the histologist can see how far through the layers of squamous cells, the dyskariotic cells have progressed.

Cervical intraepithelial neoplasia (CIN)

Cervical intraepithelial neoplasia (CIN) means 'new change in the outer layer of the cervix'. There are three levels of CIN recognized (Figure 11.9):

♦ *CIN I* occurs if just the outer third of the epithelium is abnormal (mildly dyskariotic cells appear in the smear) and the epithelium is said to show **mild dysplasia**. CIN I may resolve without any intervention but more frequent smears

Figure 11.9 *The CIN grading system.*

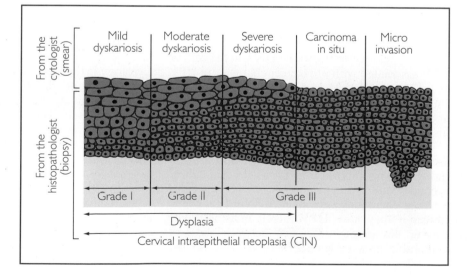

may be necessary for a period of time depending on local policy.

♦ *CIN II* occurs if a half to two-thirds of the epithelium is involved (moderate dyskariotic cells appear in the smear) and the epithelium is said to show **moderate dysplasia.**

♦ *CIN III* occurs if the full thickness of the epithelium is involved, with complete architectural chaos between the basement membrane and the surface of the epithelium (severely dyskariotic cells appear in the smear) and the epithelium is said to show **severe dysplasia**. This is also called **carcinoma** *in situ.* This CIN III is still 'skin deep', being confined by the basement membrane.

CIN I, II and III are histological findings, but many cytologists in a bid to give as much information as possible on the smear result will say 'moderate dyskariosis suggestive of CIN II', meaning that they are predicting that if a biopsy was taken the result would probably be CIN II.

Microinvasion

If the basement membrane has been breached by the abnormal cancer cells for a distance of 2 or 3 mm then microinvasion is said to have occurred. This is the first sign that the abnormal cells on the surface of the cervix are becoming malignant and starting to invade the cervix.

Invasive tumour

If the depth of invasion reaches 5 mm, involvement of the lymphatic channels and blood vessels becomes likely. At this stage your patient would no longer be asymptomatic but may present with a blood-stained vaginal discharge, intermenstrual bleeding, post-coital bleeding or unexpected bleeding post-menopausally.

On examination of the cervix the tumour may appear as a bleeding ulcer.

If left to invade further, the tumour may spread down the vagina, up into the uterus and out on to the ligaments on the side of the cervix and uterus (which holds the uterus in place). The tumour may invade forward into the bladder causing haematuria, or it may invade backwards into the rectum causing blood in the stools.

The patient may well have sought advice earlier with a low, dull, dragging backache.

Invasive cervical cancer is staged as described by Barker (1987):

Ib   The cancer is confined to the cervix and uterus

IIa The cancer has encroached on to the top of the vagina

IIb The cancer has invaded the tissue around the cervix (parametrium)

III There is extensive involvement of the vagina and/or invasion out to the bones of the side wall of the pelvis

IV   The cancer has invaded beyond the pelvis and/or adjacent organs such as the bladder or rectum.

The nurses role in giving results

The cytology laboratory will report the result of the smear and recommend the timing for future recall or if treatment or referral is necessary. We all should comply with this and if we are in doubt or have a query should contact the laboratory direct. There are mechanisms that come into play when a smear result needs a referral to a colposcopy clinic. The National Coordinating Network document *Guidelines on Failsafe Actions* (NCN, 1992) explains this well. If you are the nurse who took the cervical smear and your client has come to trust your approach, attitude and knowledge, then she may well come to you for clarification, reassurance or further information on her result and to know more about what happens next or just to talk to someone.

It is important for you to share with your client all the information written on the smear report, ideally reading the report together. This will only prove difficult if you are not sure of the facts.

We should be willing to act as advocates for our clients, and not fall into the trap of slightly altering the facts so that we feel more comfortable with the information we are giving.

Scenario

The nurse had worked hard in encouraging Mary to have a long-overdue smear. They had got to know one another from Mary's visits to the surgery with each of her four children over a period of years. Now aged 46, Mary

had a bit more time for herself and had come into the surgery for a 'check-up'. She had heard from a friend that she could come and have her blood pressure checked, and be given advice on diet. She said that she would love to try and stop smoking.

When the subject of having a cervical smear arose the nurse was aware of a feeling of apprehension in Mary and managed to give reassuring information and advice about the improved cervical screening service. Mary said she would make an appointment to see the nurse at one of the weekly well-woman sessions that the nurse ran.

A few days later the nurse was pleased to see Mary at the surgery. She had come to have her well-woman check. Mary was visibly relieved when everything was over. The nurse felt very pleased for having encouraged her patient to have the smear taken. One week later the nurse was shocked to see the smear result returned early as 'severe dyskariosis suggestive of CIN III. Invasion cannot be ruled out, requires urgent referral'. The nurse immediately felt as though she had just opened the proverbial 'can of worms'. She contacted Mary herself, as she had been the only person involved with the smear taking and consequent results.

The nurse explained exactly what all the terminology meant on the report which she saw was helpful to Mary. The most worrying thing for Mary was the next step – where, when and what would happen. The nurse told Mary all about the appointment, for colposcopy that had been arranged, that it was an outpatient appointment, and what to expect there.

The colposcopy clinic sent Mary a leaflet of explanation before her visit which she discussed with the nurse. Mary came to see the nurse after she had been to the colposcopy clinic, where she had undergone investigations and treatment. Thankfully the cancer had not been invasive, but CIN III. Mary had been very aware that the nurse was actually feeling 'guilty' for being the one who had found the abnormality and reassured her that she was so thankful to have had the smear taken when she did. Mary admitted that she had been worried over the fact that she was very overdue in having a repeat smear and in a subconscious way was hoping that someone would talk her into having the test.

Mary thanked the nurse for all her help.

Colposcopy

'Colpos' means bay, hollow or in this case, vagina; 'oscopy' means to inspect. Therefore, colposcopy means inspection of the vagina (to enable viewing of the cervix).

Colposcopy referrals are usually seen on an outpatient basis. Many colposcopy clinics nowadays send out patient information leaflets giving details of what will happen at their consultation with clarification of some of the abnormalities that are being investigated with the colposcope (Box 11.7). This certainly helps to make the referral to a colposcopy clinic less of an ordeal due to fear of the unknown.

Box 11.7 Useful information sent out by colposcopy clinics prior to a first consultation

♦ You should cancel your appointment if you are likely to be menstruating.

♦ Bring a friend with you.

♦ Arrange to have some time off work in case you have any treatment at your appointment; minor abnormalities may be dealt with the same day.

♦ If you are pregnant you can still have colposcopy, but if you require treatment this may be deferred until after the birth of your baby.

♦ Wear loose clothing, ideally in two halves, as you will be asked to remove your underwear.

♦ It will be useful for you to know the first day of your last menstrual period.

♦ Write down any questions that you would like to discuss.

The colposcope

The colposcope is a binocular microscope which allows the whole cervix to be viewed in detail (Figure 11.10); it allows for magnification of up to ten times life size (Barker, 1987). It can be used not only for inspection of the vagina and cervix but also of the vulva and anus. It has been used in Germany since the 1920s, but achieved widespread use in Britain from the 1960s onwards.

The patient can feel very frightened and alone,

Figure 11.10
Colposcopy.

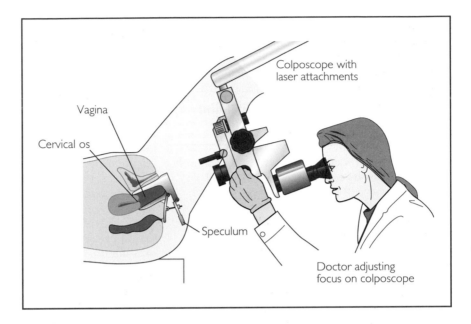

Colposcope with
laser attachments

Vagina

Cervical os

Speculum

Doctor adjusting
focus on colposcope

even though there is always a nurse present at colposcopy who will be able to give the patient reassurance and act as the 'vocal local' (Hopwood, 1990). Nowadays there may be the opportunity for the patient to see what is actually happening at the 'business end' of the couch on a television screen (via a video camera which is fixed to the colposcope). Some women may find this even more frightening, whilst others find it reassuring or even fascinating to watch the procedure. It is important to be sensitive to the woman's feelings regarding this.

The procedure as far as the patient is concerned should be very similar to that of having a smear taken, apart from the fact she is on a special couch with her legs in a lithotomy position. A vaginal speculum is inserted and the colposcope is placed near to the vaginal opening. It is important for you to tell your patient that the rather complicated looking colposcope does not go into the vagina.

The examination

Once the colposcope is in place, various procedures can be carried out. These include the following:

♦ A repeat cervical smear may be taken.

♦ The cervix may be swabbed gently with saline to remove any excessive discharge.

♦ The colposcopist will note any polyps, retention cysts, ulcers or warts.

♦ Dilute acetic acid is applied to the cervix to show up any protein-rich 'active' areas which will show up as extra white or 'acetowhite'. The degree of acetowhite change gives an indication of the likely severity of the underlying CIN, though the abnormality may not be the same throughout the affected area.

♦ Lugol's iodine (1 part iodine, 2 parts potassium iodine, 97 parts distilled water) may be applied next. This is known as Schiller's test and is useful in delineating the extent of an abnormal area. The iodine reacts with glycogen (normally present in healthy, mature squamous cells), staining healthy areas dark brown. 'Active' areas produce less glycogen and so do not stain so darkly.

♦ If the upper limit of the squamo-columnar junction cannot be visualized then the extent of the lesion will not be known, it could extend much higher up in the endocervical canal. In such a case local treatment at a colposcopy examination could not be carried out.

♦ One or more colposcopically directed 'punch' biopsies may be taken from what appear to be the most severely affected areas. A local anaesthetic will be introduced into the cervix using a dental syringe with a very fine needle. Adrenaline may be added to the lignocaine to minimize bleeding.

Treatment of cervical intraepithelial neoplasia

Treatment of CIN can be achieved by local ablative therapy or by excision.

Local ablative therapy

Laser treatment

The laser beam is directed under colposcopic control and boils the water in the cells, vaporizing the tissue. The lesion is destroyed to a depth of approximately 1 cm. Sufficient depth is important as abnormalities often extend deep into the endocervical glands. The ablation should also extend beyond the margin of the lesion. The advantages and disadvantages are listed in Box 11.8.

Box 11.8 Advantages and disadvantages of laser treatment

Advantages

♦ Laser treatment is flexible, not only cervical but vaginal lesions can be treated.

♦ The laser may also be used to take a cone biopsy for diagnostic purposes and as treatment.

♦ The squamo-columnar junction remains accessible after treatment.

♦ It does not affect childbearing.

Disadvantages

♦ It may be uncomfortable and painful.

♦ It uses an expensive piece of equipment.

♦ The machine and extractor for smoke and vapour are noisy and can alarm people.

♦ If an intrauterine device (IUD) is *in situ* it is difficult to avoid destroying the thread that protrudes from the cervical os. Therefore the IUD is usually removed before the procedure, a new one being fitted straight away afterwards.

Cold coagulation

This is, in fact, not cold, but is not as hot as diathermy or laser. Probes are used depending on the contour of the area to be treated. They are heated electrically and are applied to the cervix for up to 30 seconds. This method has mainly been superceded by loop excision.

Cryocautery

This destroys the abnormal cells by freezing them via a cryoprobe which is applied to the cervix, through which a high-pressure gas such as nitrous oxide or carbon dioxide is released. This method has mainly been replaced by loop excision, but is still used for cervical ectopy (see page 266), an entirely physiological (normal) state which can sometimes cause excessive vaginal discharge or post-coital bleeding. Cryocautery is often used in this condition to 'seal' the affected area.

Excisional treatment

Diathermy – 'hot' loop excision

LLETZ (Large Loop Excision of Transformation Zone) has become an increasingly popular method of treatment for CIN and could be used for routine management of CIN or reserved as a quick and acceptable outpatient alternative to other cone biopsy techniques.

There are different designs and sizes of loop which can be used to excise the abnormal tissue. The advantages and disadvantages are listed in Box 11.9.

After treatment some clinics insert a 'pack' of antibiotic or antiseptic cream into the vagina. There will be a blood-stained vaginal discharge which may last for a few days. The patient should be advised to contact the clinic or her own doctor if she is concerned about this. She should also be advised to avoid sexual intercourse for about 4–6 weeks to allow the cervix to heal. Internal tampons should also be avoided for the first menstrual period after treatment.

Each colposcopy clinic may have a slightly different procedure for follow-up checks. There should be liaison between the clinic and the patient's own family doctor so that she does not

Box 11.9 Advantages and disadvantages of LLETZ

Advantages

♦ Cheaper than laser machine

♦ No noise or smell

♦ Can reduce the need for a biopsy and therefore a second visit for treatment

♦ Provides an interpretable specimen for histology with evidence that all the affected area has been removed.

Disadvantages

♦ May be uncomfortable and painful

♦ Can cause excessive bleeding

♦ There is a possibility of overtreatment of minor abnormalities

♦ Can require a general anaesthetic for treating extensive areas

♦ If a deep cone is taken there could be implications for future childbearing.

slip through the net. When repeat smear-taking recommences the timing of these will be governed by local guidelines and the cytologist's report.

Surgical cone biopsy

On the whole, the need for this operation has been superceded by LLETZ, but it should be noted that if a very deep cone is taken it is usually carried out under general anaesthetic.

The indications for conization are:

♦ The upper limit of the lesion cannot be visualized

♦ Microinvasion is suspected from colposcopy

♦ Previous unsuccessful local ablative treatment

♦ Where there is wide divergence between cytology and histology reports.

A cone biopsy that is very deep can lead to two problems:

(1) The external cervical os may become very tight after treatment, which can result in painful menstruation.

(2) The internal cervical os may become damaged by treatment, weakening the muscle fibres. The internal os is responsible for keeping a pregnancy in the uterus, and after the 12th week of pregnancy an incompetent cervix might cause the pregnancy to miscarry.

If this problem is suspected, the treatment would be to have a stitch (like a purse string) inserted into the cervix, this is called a Shirodkar suture. It is removed once the patient has reached 38 weeks of her pregnancy and she then goes into labour normally.

With the advent of LLETZ problems of cervical incompetence are not as common as they were.

Psychological and psychosexual problems

Following treatment for abnormalities of the cervix, psychological or psychosexual problems may occur for either the patient or her sexual partner. There may be time for discussion and counselling at the colposcopy clinic, but this is not always possible or ideal.

You may well be the person that your patient would like to come and talk to about her anxieties after her treatment. You may feel as though you are not equipped to help, but you will soon find that one of the most important things about helping your patient is to be there and listen to her.

If you feel there is a need for more counselling than you can give your patient, be prepared to refer her to a local psychosexual counsellor.

Hysterectomy

A hysterectomy is indicated by:

♦ Recurrent abnormal smears and/or colposcopic appearance despite repeated local ablative therapy or conization

♦ A request for sterilization in the presence of severe or recurrent dysplasia

♦ Associated gynaecological problems such as menorrhagia or fibroids.

Invasive disease

If invasive disease has been diagnosed, the patient will be treated surgically and (depending on the stage of the disease) by radiotherapy or chemotherapy.

Wertheim's hysterectomy is the removal of the uterus and the upper third of the vagina with lymph node clearance. The ovaries may be removed if the woman is approaching the menopause or is post-menopausal.

Innovative methods of screening for the future

Cervicography

Cervicography is the taking of a photograph of the cervix after 5% acetic acid is applied. The cervicograms obtained are projected on a screen, thus obtaining a magnification and resolution that compares to that at colposcopy. These can be interpreted by a colposcopist in much less time than it would take to perform a colposcopic examination. Szarewski *et al.* (1991) describe the use of cervicography in a primary screening service.

The Polarprobe

The Polarprobe prototype is a computerized diagnostic instrument specifically developed to detect pre-cancers and cancer of the uterine cervix. Studies in England are at present being carried out at the Whittington Hospital, London by Professor Albert Singer and his team, and have been described by Coppleson *et al.* (1994).

Human papillomavirus (HPV) testing

The polymerase chain reaction (PCR) is a process by which the DNA of human papillomavirus is amplified to ascertain which type of HPV is present on the cervix. Recent research has demonstrated that the addition of HPV testing can substantially increase the detection rate of high-grade CIN. It may also be important in preventing the increasing proportion of invasive cancers among women with apparently adequate screening histories. More

large randomized trials need to be done before it can be recommended for routine screening (Cuzick *et al.*, 1995).

Conclusion – the way forward

This chapter started on an optimistic note with good news regarding the National Health Service Cervical Screening Programme being 'up and running' and increasingly doing very well. The chapter nears its end on a rather sad note, discussing the treatment for invasive cervical carcinoma. As the smear-taker, you can do your very best to make sure that the cervical screening programme reaches all women who need (and want) to have a cervical smear.

In becoming a competent, sensitive smear-taker you will not only be helping to spread the positive news about the programme but also be helping to discover this disease in its early, very treatable stages.

Resources

Videos

British Society for Clinical Cytology
Video and booklet: *Taking Cervical Smears*, 1989, to be updated. For further information, contact Dr K. Randall, Red Tree House, Pine Glade, Keston Park, Orpington, Kent BR6 8NT.

University of Newcastle upon Tyne Medical School
Video: *Cervical Smears – A training video for doctors and nurses*, 1995. The Audio Visual Centre, The Medical School, Framlington Place, University of Newcastle, Newcastle upon Tyne NE2 4HH.
Tel. 0191 222 6633

Useful addresses

Action on Smoking and Health (ASH)
109 Gloucester Place, London W1H 3PH
Tel. 0171 935 3529

BACUP (British Association of Cancer United Patients)
3 Bath Place, Rivington Street, London EC2A 3JR
Tel. 0800 181199

Cancer Research Campaign Primary Care Education Group
65 Banbury Road, Oxford OX2 6PE

Imperial Cancer Research Fund
Lincolns Inn Fields, PO Box 123, London WC2A 3PX

National Co-ordinating Network of the NHS
Cervical Screening Programme, Julietta Patnick (National Co-ordinator), Fulwood House, Old Fulwood Road, Sheffield S10 3TH
Tel. 01142 82357

Women's Health Concern
PO Box 1629, London SW15 2ZL
Tel. 0181 780 3007

Women's National Cancer Control Campaign
Suna House, 128 Curtain Road, London EC2 3AR
Tel. 0171 729 4688

Further reading

BRITISH SOCIETY FOR CLINICAL CYTOLOGY (1989) *Taking Cervical Smears* (video and booklet).

HASLETT, S. (1994) *Having a Cervical Smear.* Beaconsfield, Bucks: Beaconsfield.

HASLETT, S. and JENNINGS, M. (1992) *Hysterectomy and Vaginal Repair*, 3rd edn. Beaconsfield, Bucks: Beaconsfield.

NATIONAL COORDINATING NETWORK (1994) *Report of the First Five Years of the NHS Cervical Screening Programme.* London: NCN.

NATIONAL COORDINATING NETWORK of the NHS Cervical Screening Programme. *Links* magazine.

PARKER, S. (1994) *Medico-Legal Aspects of Screening for Cancer in Women for the Practice Nurse.* London: Medical Defence Union.

QUILLIAM, S. (1992) *Positive Smear*, 2nd edn. London: Letts & Co.

ROYAL COLLEGE OF NURSING (1994) *Female Genital Mutilation.* London: RCN.

SZAREWSKI, A. (1994) *A Woman's Guide to the Cervical Smear Test.* London: Optima.

References

ATKIN, K., LUNT, N., PARKER, G. and HIRST, M. (1993) *A National Census of Practice Nurses.* Report. York University.

AUSTOKER, J. and McPHERSON, A. (1992) *Cervical Screening*, 2nd edn. Oxford: Oxford University Press.

BARKER, G.H. (1987) *Your Smear Test.* London: Adamson.

BARTON, S.E., MADDOX, P.H., JENKINS, D., EDWARDS, R., CUZICK, J. and SINGER, A. (1988) Effects of cigarette smoking on cervical epithelial immunity. *Lancet* **11:** 652.

CRC (1994) Factsheets. London: Cancer Research Campaign.

CANCER STATISTICS REGISTRATIONS (1988) England and Wales Series MBI No. 17. London: HMSO.

CHOMET, J. and CHOMET, J. (1989) *Cervical Cancer.* London: Grapevine/Thorson Publishing.

COPPLESON, M., REID, B.L., SKLADNEV, V.N. and DALRYMPLE, J.C. An electronic approach to the detection of pre-cancer and cancer of the uterine cervix: a preliminary evaluation of the Polarprobe. *International Journal of Gynaecological Cancer* **4:** 79.

CUZICK, J., SZAREWSKI, A., TERRY, G. *et al.* (1995) Human papillomavirus testing in primary cervical screening. *Lancet* **345:** 1533–36.

DOH (Department of Health) (1992) *The Health of the Nation.* London: DOH.

DOH (1988a) HC(88)1 now superseded by HSG (93) 41. London: DOH.

DOH (1988b) *Decontamination of Instruments and Appliances used in the Vagina*, EL 88 MB 210. London: DOH.

DOH (1994) *Instruments and Appliances used in the Vagina and Cervix: Recommended Methods for Decontamination.* 'Safety Action Bulletin' SAB(94)22, June. London: DOH.

DOWNEY, G.P. and BAVIN, P.J. (1994) Relation between human papillomavirus type and potential for progression of minor grade cervical disease. *Lancet* **344:** 432–35.

ELKIND, A.K., HARAN, D., EARDLEY, A. and SPENCER, B. (1989) 'Well you can come in but I'm not having it'. *Health Visitor* **62:** 20.

ELUF-NETO, J., BOOTH, M., MUÑOZ, N. BOSCH, F.X., MEIJER, C.J.L.M. and WALBOOMERS, J.M.M. (1994) Human papilloma virus and invasive cervical cancer in Brazil. *British Journal of Cancer* **69:** 114.

GAGNON, F. (1950) Contributions to the study of the etiology and prevention of cervical cancer. *Journal of Obstetrics and Gynaecology* **60:** 516–22:

GILLAM, S.J. (1991) Understanding the uptake of cervical cancer screening. *British Journal of General Practice* **41:** 510.

HOPWOOD, J. (1990) *Background to Colposcopy and Treatment of the Cervix.* Burgess Hill: Schering Healthcare.

HOPWOOD, J. (1995) *Background to Cervical Cytology Reports*, 3rd edn. Burgess Hill: Schering Healthcare.

NCN (1991a) National Co-ordinating Network of the NHS Cervical Screening Programme – The First Annual Report. London: NCN.

NCN (1991b) *Links Magazine* no. 5, January.

NCN (1992) *The NCN Guidelines on Failsafe Actions.* London: NCN.

NCN (1994) *Improving the Quality of the NHS Cervical Screening Programme.* London: NCN.

NCN (1996) *Links Newsletter*, no 16, March. Office for National Statistics (1996) *Population and Health Monitor*, April.

RCN (Royal College of Nursing) (1994) *Cervical Screening Guidelines for Good Practice.* London: RCN.

RCN (1994) *Female Genital Mutilation.* London: RCN.

RCN (1995) *Bimanual Pelvic Examination – Guidance for Nurses.* London: RCN.

RCOG, RCP, RCGP, FCM (Royal College of Obstetricians and Gynaecologists; Royal College of Pathologists; Royal College of General Practioners; Faculty of Community Medicine) (1987) *Report of the Intercollegiate Working Party on Cervical Cytology Screening.*

SCOTTO, J. and BAILAR, J.C. III (1969) Domenico Rigoni-Stern and medical statistics (a nineteenth century approach to cancer research). *Journal of the History of Medicine and Allied Sciences* **24:** 65–75.

SIMONS, A.M. PHILLIPS, D.H. and COLEMAN, D.V. (1993) Damage to DNA in cervical epithelium related to smoking tobacco. *British Medical Journal* **306:** 1444–48.

SINGER, A. and SZAREWSKI, A. (1988) *Cervical Smear Test.* London: Optima.

SMITH, P.G. *et al.* (1979) Mortality of wives of men dying with cancer of the penis. *British Journal of Cancer* **41:** 422.

SOUTH WEST THAMES REGIONAL HEALTH AUTHORITY (1992) *A Framework for Better Health.* Annual Report of the Director of Public Health.

SZAREWSKI, A., CURRAN, G., EDWARDS, R. *et al.* (1993) Comparison of four cytologic sampling techniques in a large family planning centre. *International Academy of Cytology* **37:** 457.

SZAREWSKI, A., CUZICK, J., EDWARDS, R., BUTLER, B. and SINGER A. (1991) The use of cervicography in a primary screening environment. *British Journal of Obstetrics and Gynaecology* **98:** 313.

TUNNADINE, P. (1970) *Contraception and Sexual Life.* London: Tavistock.

UKCC (United Kingdom Central Council) (1993) *Standards for Records and Record Keeping.* London: UKCC.

UKCC (1992) *The UKCC Code of Professional Conduct* and *The UKCC The Scope of Professional Practice.* London: UKCC

VALINS, L. (1988) *Vaginismus.* Bath: Ashgrove Press.

WADDELL, C. (1994) Update in cytology with a focus on smear adequacy. *Journal of the National Association of Family Planning Nurses* **27:** 43–48.

WILSON, J.M.C. and JUNGNER, O.G.H. (1968) *Principles and Practice of Screening for Disease*; The World Health Organization. A report; Paper 34. Geneva: WHO.

12: Sexual health and sexually acquired infection

Jim Nash ◆

OBJECTIVES

After reading this chapter you will understand:

◆ the importance of sexual health and sexual health promotion

◆ some causes of vaginal discharge and genital ulceration

◆ the basic features of sexually transmitted diseases, with particular reference to women

◆ issues for women with HIV and AIDS

◆ the difficult emotional and practical problems that sexually transmitted diseases can have on a woman's life and interpersonal relationship

◆ nursing issues in promoting sexual health.

Introduction

In your professional role as a nurse, whether in general practice, family planning clinics, gynae outpatients or genito-urinary medicine (GUM) clinics, you will encounter women who are anxious about their sexuality, sexual health and particularly their vaginal discharge. It is within the context of the GUM clinic that sexual health, vaginal discharge and sexually acquired infection in women will be discussed in this chapter, but the philosophies of GUM can be easily be adapted to your own clinical settings.

Vaginal discharge should never be trivialized or dismissed. When a pathological discharge is apparent it can be both psychologically and physically very distressing and can profoundly undermine a woman's sense of well-being. Consideration of this fact and sensitivity from nursing staff will make a visit to the sexual health clinic far less of an ordeal.

Historical perspective

Within the past few years the type of service provision provided for patients attending GUM clinics has changed rapidly as a sort of Darwinian cross-fertilization of ideas of care has taken place. The core service of GUM is still to diagnose, treat, manage and maintain effective epidemiological control of sexually transmitted diseases whilst also increasing the range of sexual health services available to clients. Such facilities include family planning services, psychological and counselling services and sexual health promotion. Other aspects of service provision include cervical cytology and colposcopy and specialist clinics provided for patients who are positive for human immuno-deficiency virus (HIV) or who have developed acquired immune deficiency syndrome (AIDS).

Today's sexual health service is underpinned by a strong research portfolio. The provision of primary health services looks likely to expand even further in the future within genito-urinary medicine and this more enlightened attitude is to be welcomed. Sadly, such an enlightened attitude has not always been the case and part of your professional role should be to challenge vigorously discrimination of any type that your clients may experience when using the sexual health service.

Davenport-Hines (1990) discussed that the historical aspects of sexually transmitted disease (STD) are closely woven into the fabric of society and individuals who suffered from such diseases often experienced hysteria, hypocrisy and social condemnation. The history of STDs reflects the changing values and belief systems both in the individual and in society.

In 1916 the Venereal Disease Regulations defined only three venereal diseases: syphilis, gonorrhoea and chancroid, and clinics were established to diagnose and treat these conditions. In 1917 the Venereal Diseases Act protected patients' rights to obtain free treatment and to have a confidential, open-access medical service. These early clinics were under the auspices of the local authorities and were incorporated into the National Health Service in 1948. There are at present 230 GUM clinics in the United Kingdom.

In the pre-antibiotic era, these designated STDs were often difficult to treat. Syphilis in particular had bequeathed an historical legacy of high levels of morbidity and mortality. Drugs used to treat the conditions were often toxic, but with the introduction of penicillin in 1943 the 'therapeutic situation was revolutionised' (Oriel, 1978). Classic venereal diseases such as syphilis and gonorrhoea could now be cured. A gradual change in the public perception of STDs also began to take place as a reduction in guilt, fear and anxiety occurred. By the 1950s, however, the second generation of STDs was beginning to increase rapidly. Such infections were caused by bacteria like *Chlamydia trachomatis, Ureaplasma urealyticum, Gardnerella vaginalis* and by viruses such as herpesvirus hominis, hepatitis B virus and the human papillomavirus (Catterall, 1983). An increased incidence of non-specific genital infection was also seen in both sexes. Catterall also points out that serious complications from some of these infections were beginning to be seen in women, e.g. pelvic inflammatory disease (PID), with the attendant risk of infertility, ectopic pregnancy and chronic relapsing salpingitis, together with the added problem of damage to the unborn baby or infection during the perinatal period.

Since the original classification of venereal diseases the category of STD-producing pathogens has extended the nomenclature considerably. The term 'venereal disease' has now fallen into disuse as it is a pejorative description and does not adequately describe the new service direction towards sexual health.

All GUM clinics are responsible for making statistical returns to the Department of Health on the number of cases seen each year categorized by diagnosis and sex. This is a standard public health measure. The *Health of the Nation* document (DOH, 1992) gave additional impetus to the campaign for improved sexual health by setting a target to reduce the incidence of gonorrhoea by 20% by the end of 1995. Gonorrhoea was chosen, even though it is less commonly diagnosed today, as it is seen to be a marker for other sexually transmitted diseases.

The World Health Organization in a recent study estimated that at least 333 million new cases of *curable* STDs occurred in the world in 1995. These STDs, which are not only curable but also preventable, and their complications rank in the top ten causes of healthy days lost by adults in the urban areas of the developing world and therefore have a large socio-economic impact on financial planning. According to the World Bank, 'provision of treatment for curable STDs represents one of the most cost effective interventions to improve health in the world' (WHO, 1995). This is of particular concern and relevance due to the links between STDs and HIV. Many of these curable STDs cause genital lesions and inflammation and there is strong evidence to suggest that these greatly increase the sexual transmission of HIV.

The changes in GUM cannot be divorced from the wider social changes that have occurred in the UK, including the greater freedom of sexual expression, improved standards of living, easier access to safe effective contraception, the use of recreational drugs, the rise of an articulate and informed women's movement and gay movement and the shift in the political and sexual arena. Sexual health is an idea which has been forced on to the social agenda by the arrival of HIV and AIDS, and should recognize individual needs and sexual diversity.

Consent and confidentiality

The ethical perspectives of informed consent and confidentiality in GUM are of paramount importance. Every patient has the right to determine what is done to them. Patient consent is implied from their presentation at the clinic and request for help. The amount of information a patient receives should enable them to make a reasonable and informed decision about what is to happen to them. This respect for the patient's integrity and autonomy is crucial to the wider epidemiological management of STDs. A relationship of trust and confidence should be established by all levels of clinic staff, regardless of age, sex and race.

If a client is diagnosed as having an STD, the tracing of sexual contacts, also known as partner notification, needs to be undertaken. The health adviser working within GUM and who interviews the client in private, needs the client's full cooperation to motivate them to persuade their sexual contacts to attend the clinic to exclude the risk of infection. The health adviser is able to acknowledge that telling a partner is not easy, particularly when the woman may be feeling hurt, angry, frightened or even guilty. There is no right or wrong way to tell a partner but the health adviser will be able to give advice and recommend different approaches to the discussion, or even suggest leaving an appropriate leaflet around in order to get the conversation started.

If the client is unable to do this or is too embarrassed, the health adviser then needs to undertake this responsibility personally, whilst maintaining the anonymity and preserving strict confidentiality for the client. Such a task requires tact, dedication and diplomacy. The wider role of the health adviser within GUM is now well accepted and established and includes counselling, health education, health promotion and discussion of safe sex and safer sex (see Chapters 2 and 9).

The idea that clients attending GUM clinics are sexually irresponsible, feckless and indifferent to the welfare of others is a myth. The majority of clients will make a considerable effort to contact sexual partners and encourage them to attend GUM clinics to seek treatment. For this to happen they need a clear idea of why it is necessary, and also absolute confidence that respect will be given to the confidential nature of their disclosures.

Informed consent has been reinforced by the complex legal, financial and personal issues clients must consider when thinking about having the HIV antibody test. Within GUM a balance has to be maintained between the rights of the individual, versus the responsibility to society, a balance that is often tricky and can on occasion create tension.

With the advent of HIV and AIDS, Austoker (1988) remarked that there were 'calls for dramatic, legally enforceable, coercive measures such as segregation and confinement of those identified as having AIDS'. Compulsion has been tried before in the field of STDs and has either been counterproductive or has failed. For example, in 1942 local authorities were granted powers to treat patients compulsorily and to notify details of them and their contacts to central government. These regulations (known as Defence Regulations 33B) resulted in large numbers of doctors failing to implement them as they constituted a major breach of patient confidentiality. As a consequence these controversial Defence Regulations were repealed in 1947.

Confidentiality is not an absolute concept and may be broken in a limited number of circumstances: with a patient's consent, by due legal process, or if on balance the doctor's duty to society outweighs their responsibility to the individual. However this is rare in practice. Robertson *et al.* (1989) illustrate the issue of consent and confidentiality with examples of case law in STD and conclude that 'compulsory measures are inappropriate' but persuasion, voluntary compliance and the knowledge that respect for patient confidentiality will prevail is more effective.

Taking a sexual history

'A sexual history alerts the nurse to possible infections that will need to be screened during the physical assessment' (Andrist, 1988) and will also help to inform the nurse of the woman's sexual health education requirements. Taking a sexual history takes time, practice and expertise and may create problems for the inexperienced health care professional, particularly if they are ill at ease not only with discussing sexual matters but also with their own sexuality. Box 12.1 outlines the areas that need to be looked at in order to gain the maximum knowledge about your client's sexual history so that you can help her effectively.

Box 12.1 Points to remember when taking a sexual history

♦ Ensure the woman understands why taking a sexual history is necessary and recognize that the issues involved are both personal and sensitive.

♦ Recognize your own feelings in relation to discussing sex with a client. Try to acknowledge your own embarrassment, attitudes and your own belief and value systems which may have an influence on the nature of the interaction between you and your client.

♦ Do not be reluctant to use street language if appropriate to the context of the interview, particularly if that is more comfortable for your client.

♦ Listen attentively to what the woman is saying and particularly note any non-verbal communication.

♦ Be purposeful in your questions but do not make assumptions or apply sexual stereotypes. Adopt a non-judgemental attitude, particularly in relation to lifestyle or sexual orientation, and concentrate instead on sexual activity. Refer to all partners as partners and not by gender.

♦ Always work within your professional boundaries and within the framework of the law.

♦ Protect the patient's right to confidentiality.

Specific questions that should be asked include:

♦ What is the nature of the present problem? Has the client a past history of STDs and if so what was the nature of the previous problem?

♦ What type of recent sexual activity has occurred and what sites were used for sex (vaginal, anal or oral)? This will indicate the areas to be examined and the type of specimens to be taken.

♦ Has the woman been overseas recently and did sexual intercourse occur abroad?

♦ Has there been any recent partner change, or has there been multiple contacts? Is the partner experiencing any symptoms?

♦ What, if any, method of contraception is used?

♦ What is her level of alcohol consumption?

♦ Does she take any drugs? What is the type and frequency of the drug and the method of administration?

♦ What was the date of her last menstrual period and the date of her last cervical smear? Is there any dyspareunia? An obstetric history is also relevant.

♦ How old was she when she had her first sexual experience? This is relevant as the younger a woman is at first intercourse the more at risk she is of cervical dysplasia. Sometimes you might not get an accurate answer to this question, but the answer that your client feels she should be telling you and feels more comfortable with herself.

Additional information should also include anything that the woman considers important to her present problem, including any rash, arthralgia or abdominal pain.

In order to take a satisfactory sexual history it is important to be aware of the barriers that can make effective communication between you and your client more difficult. These could include:

♦ *Gender*   A patient may have difficulty talking to someone of the opposite sex.

♦ *Culture*   Women from some ethnic minorities may have problems discussing sexual topics. The interview needs to be culturally sensitive and the information obtained will inevitably depend on the woman's education, religion and length of residence in this country. If there are language problems, additional care needs to be taken with confidentiality if a third party is used to act as an interpreter.

♦ *Age*   The young adult years are the time of highest sexual activity but you should remember that sexual activity continues throughout life and well into the third age. Preconceived notions that older people do not engage in active sex should be avoided and your recognition of the older individual's life experiences is important.

Bor and Watts (1993) state that 'patients are willing to answer questions about their intimate sexual behaviour and lifestyle provided that they do not feel judged or ridiculed'. A woman must be given time, space and a private place to discuss her sexual history and you should always try to provide her with a rationale for your questions.

When taking a sexual history you must also discuss and offer advice on safe sex (see Chapter 9) and health education advice on lifestyle issues (see Chapter 2). This is an extremely important part of the health promotion work within GUM by any health professional dealing with sexual health.

Vaginal discharge

The vagina is lined with stratified squamous epithelium which is covered by a surface film of transudate moisture. This, in conjunction with the normal vaginal flora (containing both aerobic and anaerobic bacteria) keeps the vagina moist and constitutes part of the vagina's non-specific defence mechanism against infection. 'The vagina secretes a carbohydrate which the bacteria feed on, producing lactic acid in the process. This makes vaginal secretions acidic and thus hostile to many fungi, bacteria and viruses' (Gamlin, 1988). Doderlein's bacilli (a normal inhabitant of the vagina) are responsible for converting this vaginal carbohydrate (glycogen) into lactic acid. The Doderlein's bacilli also help maintain the normal environment of the vagina, they compete for nutrition and produce anti-fungal properties. This mechanism also helps to maintain the normal vaginal acidity at pH 4.5, which keeps the vagina clear of pathogens which cannot survive in the environment. This delicate balance may be upset if the bacilli are killed by a course of antibiotics intended for a systemic infection elsewhere in the body.

Vaginal discharge to some degree, is normal in all women and does not necessarily indicate a pathological condition. Occasionally there will be a variation in the amount or colour of this normal discharge due to a number of different causes:

♦ The menstrual cycle – there will be an increase of clear mucus just prior to ovulation which is often described as looking like the white of an egg (spinnbarkeit mucus).

♦ Pregnancy

♦ Method of contraception – the contraceptive pill gives rise to a thicker discharge whilst spermicides when recently used make the vaginal discharge thinner.

♦ Sexual arousal

♦ Stress.

A normal physiological discharge should not cause an offensive odour, irritation or soreness. When a woman complains of a vaginal discharge that is different from normal and causing her a problem, care needs to be taken that assumptions are not made that she is automatically suffering from a sexually transmitted disease (STD).

A pathological discharge can be either infectious or non-infectious in origin. Whatever the cause of the discharge, however, the symptom is a very subjective one with the 'normal' discharge being a very arbitrary concept for individual women. Serious STD infection in women is often unapparent or asymptomatic and, as Adler (1990) states, 'symptoms in women are a poor guide to the exact nature of the condition.'

'Neither the patient's symptoms nor a subjective description of the colour and quantity of the discharge are of much value in reaching an accurate diagnosis' (Adler, 1990). The potential problems that also need to be considered are: (a) whether the cause of the vaginal discharge is due to more than one single cause; and (b) what the risk index is for sexual spread of an STD like hepatitis A and B and possibly C, syphilis and HIV infection.

Many of the organisms attributed to be responsible for producing vaginal discharge, e.g. *Candida albicans*, *Gardnerella vaginalis*, *Ureaplasma urealyticum* and *Mycobacterium hominis* have been isolated from healthy women who are asymptomatic and not complaining of a particular problem. The development of signs and symptoms of vaginal discharge is discussed by Masfari *et al.* (1986), who suggest that a quantitative change occurs in the polymicrobial balance of the vaginal flora. A corresponding change to both the number and the yield of organisms may influence the vaginal environment which then allows some organisms to become pathogenic.

Many women are frequently embarrassed about their vaginal discharge and although they recognize the need for medical advice will wash themselves thoroughly or douche before going to the doctor. Unfortunately this may not only make diagnosis and treatment more difficult as the symptoms will be masked, but it also may exacerbate the condition due to the alteration of the vaginal pH.

Common causes of vaginal discharge are listed in Box 12.2. Other possible causes of vaginal discharge include the cytomegalovirus which has been isolated from semen, the cervix and saliva. Enteric pathogens and B haemolytic streptococci have also been implicated as a cause of vaginitis and cervicitis.

Box 12.2   Causes of vaginal discharge

Pathological discharge (infective)

♦ *Candida albicans*

♦ Bacterial vaginosis

♦ *Trichomonas vaginalis*

♦ *Chlamydia trachomatis*

♦ *Neisseria gonorrhoea*

♦ Genital ulceration, e.g. herpes

Non-infective

♦ Cervical ectopy

♦ Cervical polyp

♦ Cervical neoplasm

♦ Retained products (e.g. tampon, post-abortion)

♦ Trauma

♦ Atrophic vaginitis

♦ Allergic reactions (e.g. douches)

The differences in the reproductive tract and the respective anatomical structure between men and women accounts for the greater risk of complications of STDs in females. In men a urethral discharge is usually confined to the anterior urethra and symptoms of a discharge are recognized early. In women the pattern of infection is considerably more variable, often silent, and several sites may be infected, including the cervix, urethra and rectum. Robertson *et al.* (1989) point out that with gonorrhoea in men 85–90% will develop an obvious urethral discharge. However, in 75–85% of women a discharge is not apparent or they are asymptomatic.

An abnormal vaginal discharge is a common presenting complaint of women attending their doctor or GUM clinics. Frequently the discharge is accompanied by other symptoms, e.g. vaginal soreness or irritation, unpleasant odour, dyspareunia and bleeding. Sometimes women will also complain of 'cystitis', which may be an external dysuria due to vulval soreness or due to a urinary tract infection. Frequently women may attend a GP practice complaining of a vaginal discharge when they are actually needing help with another problem, e.g. contraception, pregnancy or a psychosexual problem.

The standard management of a woman attending a GUM clinic complaining of vaginal discharge needs careful and considerate explanation at all stages. After a routine general and sexual history has been taken, the woman will undergo a general examination, a bimanual pelvic examination and a detailed genital examination.

♦ A vaginal speculum will be inserted and specimens for both microscopy and cultures will be taken from the lateral vaginal wall, the posterior fornix, cervix and urethra (and occasionally the rectum).

♦ A smear for cytology will be taken if required.

♦ All glands adjacent to the genital area will be checked.

♦ A serological test for syphilis will be taken as part of the routine care – this should be repeated after three months as the incubation period for syphilis is very variable.

♦ A routine urinalysis is also performed.

♦ Screening for hepatitis B or an HIV antibody test following pre-test counselling may be performed if required.

A good light source should be available for the routine examination. A hand lens is of particular value when trying to identify very small warts, infestations and in assisting to distinguish dermatological conditions of the vulva from STDs.

Physically, it takes longer to examine a woman,

and the examination is far more detailed. Specimen taking needs to be particularly accurate with sufficient material taken to inoculate cultures. Differential diagnosis can often be difficult to establish. The clinical picture may be made more complex if the woman is also experiencing a urinary tract infection.

Non-infective causes of vaginal discharge

Cervical ectopy

An ectopy occurs when the columnar epithelium which lines the cervical canal replaces some of the stratified squamous epithelium which covers the exterior of the cervix. It is a very common condition, particularly if the woman is taking the contraceptive pill, and usually causes no problems. Occasionally the ectopy may cause a mucoid discharge which may be blood-stained if cervicitis is present. The ectopy is treated by cryocautery (see page 282).

Cervical polyp

Many women with cervical polyps are asymptomatic but they can cause a blood-stained vaginal discharge. Surgical removal is necessary.

Cervical neoplasm

Irregular bleeding (particularly post-coital) is the most common first symptom of a cervical neoplasm and there may be a watery discharge which is often offensive.

Retained products

Postnatal or post-abortion. Retained products of conception can cause bleeding and an offensive vaginal discharge, particularly if there is an accompanying infection. Treatment is with antibiotics and an evacuation of the retained products of conception (ERPC).

Retained tampon. A retained tampon, or part of a tampon that has broken off, will very quickly give rise to a characteristically offensive discharge. This will settle on removal but occasionally antibiotics may be required if the tampon has been present for any length of time.

Atrophic vaginitis

Atrophic vaginitis is a common problem in postmenopausal women, the majority of whom are asymptomatic. However, some women are more susceptible and complain of vaginal and vulval soreness, dyspareunia, occasional spotting and a blood-stained discharge. After careful inspection of the vagina to exclude malignancy, the treatment is with systemic oestrogen or topical oestrogens in the form of creams, pessaries, tablets or a silastic ring. Initially topical oestrogen is poorly absorbed by the atrophic vaginal mucosa so should be continued for a minimum of 4–6 weeks.

Pathological discharge

Vulvovaginal candidiasis

Vulvovaginal candidiasis or yeast infection (commonly known as thrush or monilia) is one of the most common causes of vaginal discharge throughout the world. *Candida* species may be present as blastospores in up to 20% of asymptomatic women (Sobel, 1990) or as germinated yeasts which have successfully adhered to vaginal epithelial cells in women with symptoms. Candidiasis is not considered to be sexually transmitted, although Sobel noted 'penile colonization with candida is present in approximately 20% of male partners of women with recurrent vaginal candidiasis'. Some specialists believe that *Candida* may be a normal commensal in the vagina and it only becomes pathogenic when the vaginal environment becomes altered.

There are three yeasts that are commonly found in the vagina of asymptomatic women (Thin, 1982)

♦ *Candida albicans*   81%

♦ *Torulopsis glabrata* (now called *Candida glabrata*)   16%

♦ Other *Candida* species   3%

The incubation period remains undetermined because it is difficult to establish at what precise moment the yeast begins to colonize the vagina.

Predisposing factors and clinical manifestations of candidiasis are listed in Boxes 12.3 and 12.4. Symptoms of candidiasis may be exacerbated a few days before the onset of menstruation and the soreness and excoriation may extend down to the peri-anal region.

Box 12.3   Predisposing factors for candidiasis

♦ Pregnancy

♦ Oral contraceptive pill (particularly those with a high oestrogen content)

♦ Diabetes mellitus

♦ Broad-spectrum antibiotics

♦ Steroid and immunosuppressive drugs

♦ HIV infection (when cell-mediated immunity is damaged)

♦ Tight restrictive clothing and nylon underwear, resulting in poor ventilation to the genital area.

♦ Trauma to the vaginal mucosa (chemical irritants, douching).

Box 12.4   Clinical manifestations of candidiasis (see Colour plates 6 and 7)

♦ Acute pruritus

♦ Vaginal discharge (which may range from watery to homogeneously thick and commonly described as looking like cottage cheese)

♦ Vulval erythema and burning

♦ Vaginal soreness and irritation

♦ Dyspareunia

♦ External dysuria

♦ Odour (is often minimal and non-offensive)

♦ Fissuring and oedema (may occur).

Diagnosis

A high vaginal swab should be taken and microscopic examination by Gram stain or by wet mount preparation will usually demonstrate Gram-positive bacilli and yeast cells, mycelia and spores. A urine test should be done to check for sugar and protein as diabetic women are particularly prone to candidiasis. The vaginal pH is normal. No serological test is available to diagnose vulvovaginal candidiasis.

Treatment

A variety of preparations are now available to treat vulvovaginal candidiasis and the treatment regime will depend on whether the episode is a primary attack or a recurrent and difficult to treat genital candidiasis. No treatment is recommended for asymptomatic women.

A single episode.   The following regimes are recommended to treat a single attack of candidiasis:

♦ Clotrimazole 500 mg pessary at night and 1% cream applied topically twice daily for up to 14 days.

♦ Clotrimazole 200 mg pessary for three nights and 1% cream applied topically twice daily for up to 14 days.

♦ Clotrimazole 10% cream applied stat (or with hydrocortisone 1% cream – French, 1995).

♦ Fluconazole 150 mg stat oral dose.

♦ Econazole nitrate 150 mg pessary and 1% cream.

Recurrent and relapsing candidiasis.   The picture here is more complicated, and women you encounter in your clinical practice with recurrent candidiasis should all be referred to GUM as this condition can cause considerable distress and is often difficult to treat. You should be able to reassure the woman that ultimately her condition is manageable. Treatment regimes may combine topical and oral therapy, involve the use of intermittent prophylaxis, and include the treatment of the partner.

The important aspect of the care of this group of women is the psychological support they need as recurrent problems can eventually put stress on a relationship as intercourse tends to be avoided due to discomfort and pain. Women will often self-medicate without medical advice and they should be advised against this.

In pregnant women local therapy should be used as systemic therapy is contraindicated. There is no indication for routine screening of pregnant women for candidiasis.

Advice and follow-up

There are many useful patient information leaflets (particularly from the Health Education Authority) about candidiasis which you should have available and can give to your patients to back up any verbal advice you offer. This advice could include the following:

♦ Avoid the use of douching as this may alter the acid/alkaline balance of the vagina therefore encouraging yeasts to multiply.

♦ Use baths to give relief from local discomfort but do not wash the genital area too frequently and avoid bubble baths, disinfectants such as Dettol, strongly perfumed soaps and vaginal deodorants.

♦ Change to a non-biological washing powder.

♦ Avoid tights, nylon underwear, tight jeans, etc. and wear loose clothing with a high proportion of non-synthetic fibres.

♦ Use pads and panty liners rather than tampons.

♦ Take care with genital and anal hygiene (wiping from 'front to back') to avoid autoinoculation from the bowel of *Candida* species.

♦ Apply live natural yoghurt to the vulva if an attack is not too severe.

♦ If antibiotics usually give rise to candidiasis, then ask for prophylactic *Candida* treatment at the same time.

♦ Avoid intercourse until all symptoms have disappeared as this will naturally encourage local cellular repair.

If the episode of candidiasis is an isolated attack then follow-up is usually not necessary.

For women who experience recurrent vulvovaginal candidiasis, a routine follow-up is recommended. Adler (1990) suggests male contacts should be seen 'firstly, if they have symptoms and secondly, if the woman is having repeated recurrences. The man should be thoroughly investigated as was his female partner, to make sure that he has no concurrent sexually transmitted disease, since this is likely to predispose to candidal infection'. Vaginal recurrence of candidiasis may occur because a small number of organisms may persist and escape detection and re-emerge at another time. The need to ensure that clients comply with the full length of treatment is crucial in order to avoid a recurrent attack.

Bacterial vaginosis (non-specific vaginitis)

Bacterial vaginosis (sometimes called gardnerella) is a common cause of vaginal discharge among women of childbearing age. The epidemiology of bacterial vaginosis reveals that the highest group of women experiencing the problem are seen at GUM clinics. Hillier and Holmes (1990) ask 'is bacterial vaginosis sexually transmitted?' The evidence is conflicting as bacterial vaginosis microorganisms have been isolated in studies from male partners of some women, and bacterial vaginosis is more common in sexually active women. However its presence has also been demonstrated in the absence of sexual activity. Ison (1993) states that 'bacterial vaginosis occurs when the vaginal ecology is altered.' Ison then describes the condition as 'sexually associated' which is not the same as sexually transmitted. Prostatic fluid is known to exacerbate the condition.

Bacterial vaginosis is a complex condition which results in a shift in the ecological balance of the vaginal flora. The lactobacilli protecting the vagina are substantially reduced in number and replaced by a mixed bacterial flora consisting of *Gardnerella vaginalis* and anaerobes like *Mycoplasma hominis*, *Bacteroides* and *Mobiluncus* species. Why this change occurs is unknown, and because the pathogenesis of bacterial vaginosis is poorly understood, the incubation period is unknown.

However, it is known that bacterial vaginosis can occur in the presence of another STD pathogen such as *Trichomonas vaginalis*, *Neisseria gonorrhoea* and *Chlamydia trachomatis*, and Ison (1993) notes that 'there is a strong association with the presence of an intrauterine device for contraception'.

The clinical manifestations are listed in Box 12.5.

Diagnosis

Bacterial vaginosis is primarily a diagnosis of exclusion. Other sexually transmitted pathogens

> **Box 12.5** Clinical manifestations of bacterial vaginosis (see Colour plate 8)
>
> ♦ Discharge – a malodorous vaginal discharge which is often described as watery with a fishy or cheesy odour, and is frequently worse after sexual intercourse or at the time of a period. Occasionally there is an increase in the amount of discharge or a change of colour (grey or yellow).
>
> ♦ Abdominal discomfort (may be experienced)
>
> ♦ Pruritus
>
> ♦ Dysuria.
>
> There is little or no inflammation of the vaginal epithelium and no vulval erythema, oedema or fissuring present, unless a coexisting pathogen is also causing additional pathology.

need to be eliminated first as a possible cause of the pathology. The vaginal discharge is characteristic and may be viewed on the labia and fourchette prior to internal examination.

A Gram-stained slide is considered the definitive diagnostic test and shows the replacement of normal vaginal flora with mixed flora and the presence of 'clue cells'. Clue cells are epithelial cells which are readily identified under the microscope as their margins are crowded and they are often obscured by bacteria sticking to them. The vaginal pH is raised between 4.7 and 7.0.

The amine test is carried out when a drop of vaginal discharge is placed on a slide and mixed with a drop of 10% potassium hydroxide. If the test is positive there will be a transient release of a characteristic ammonia-like smell. This test is also known as the 'whiff test' for obvious reasons.

A vaginal culture for bacterial vaginosis is of limited value as mixed bacterial flora can be isolated in asymptomatic women.

Treatment

The current treatment with a satisfactory therapeutic success is oral metronidazole 2 g given stat. For patients with recurrent bacterial vaginosis then metronidazole 400 mg should be given twice daily for five days. Patients should be advised to avoid alcohol as this can produce a disulfiram-like reaction with nausea, flushing, headache and sweating. Extra care should also be taken if women are also taking anticoagulants, as the prothrombin time may be prolonged. Metronidazole is contraindicated in the first trimester of pregnancy because of its possible teratogenic risks.

Alternatively clindamycin 2% cream used intravaginally with an applicator at night for seven nights can be given.

There is no evidence that treating the male partners of women diagnosed of having bacterial vaginosis has any therapeutic value. Contact tracing is not indicated as it is not a sexually transmitted disease and is usually self-limiting. The release of prostatic fluid by the male during intercourse may compromise the normal bacterial flora of the vagina by promoting the release of amines. The use of condoms is recommended.

Easmon (1993) observes that bacterial vaginosis 'is perceived as a mild medical problem' but warns that there is evidence to suggest that the condition may predispose to post-operative infection after a hysterectomy, to postpartum endometritis after childbirth, and to premature rupture of the membranes and pre-term delivery in the pregnant woman. Easmon also feels that bacterial vaginosis is underdiagnosed in the primary care setting for a variety of reasons. This could be due to a shortage of consultation time, a 'basic reluctance to undertake vaginal examination' and the lack of a chaperon. Easmon recommends that practice nurses should learn more about bacterial vaginosis in order to improve the sexual health of their clients and to facilitate better management of the problem in primary care.

Bacterial vaginosis along with vaginal candidiasis are not sexually transmitted diseases although women may experience similar anxieties, distress and discomfort as women who do present at a GUM clinic with an STD. It is important that you listen to your clients' worries and discuss them thoroughly rather than dismiss them as trivial. Good communication between you and your client is vital because if the conditions are not clearly understood they can cause additional stress for the woman within her sexual relationship.

Trichomoniasis

Trichomoniasis is a sexually transmitted infection caused by a flagellated protozoan called *Trichomonas vaginalis*. In women the organism is usually isolated from the posterior vaginal fornix, where it attaches itself to areas of vaginal squamous epithelium. Columnar epithelium seems to demonstrate resistance to *Trichomonas vaginalis*; however, the cervix is involved in the inflammatory response. *Trichomonas vaginalis* may also be present in the urethra, bladder, Skene's ducts and Bartholin's ducts. Perinatal transmission is the main method of non-venereal spread. Up to 40% of women with trichomoniasis attending GUM clinics may have gonorrhoea (Mohanty, 1990).

Trichomonas vaginalis is ovoid in shape and can be observed down the microscope making a jerky swaying motion. Movement is provided by four free anterior flagella and an undulating membrane. *Trichomonas* reproduce by binary fission and feed by phagocytosis. Two other trichomonads can be found in humans: *Trichomonas tenex*, which is found in the mouth and has been associated with gingivitis, and *Pentatrichomonas hominis*, which is isolated from the large intestine and is associated with acute diarrhoeal problems. All three species are thought to be site-specific.

The incubation period is thought to be between one and four weeks. The reason for such a variable length of time for a woman to produce symptoms will depend on her susceptibility and reactivity.

The clinical manifestations are listed in Box 12.6, although the woman may well be asymptomatic and any clinical features present are variable.

Box 12.6   Clinical manifestations of trichomoniasis (see Colour plate 9)

♦ Vaginal discharge is most frequently described as profuse, yellow to green in colour, offensive in odour and frothy in appearance.

♦ Vaginal pruritus and vulval soreness and erythema may be present although are not common.

♦ Dyspareunia

♦ Dysuria (often with urinary frequency)

♦ Colpitis macularis (small punctate haemorrhages of the cervix may be present, giving the cervix a characteristic 'strawberry' appearance, see Colour plate 5).

Diagnosis

Trichomoniasis can be diagnosed by microscopy when a wet mount slide (with a coverslip) is viewed under the microscope. The flagella can be seen making a characteristic whiplash motion. The undulating membrane can also be seen pulsating. There are an increased number of polymorphonuclear neutrophils present as part of the acute inflammatory response. The infection can also be diagnosed using Feinberg Whittington culture or Amies transport medium. No serological test is available. The vaginal pH is raised to 5.5. The amine test may also be positive.

Treatment

The treatment of choice is metronidazole 2 g given stat to the client and to her sexual partner and the same advice outlined on page 296 given.

All male partners need to be seen, examined and treated. Mohanty (1990) remarked that 'ninety per cent of male contacts of women with trichomonas are asymptomatic'. To isolate the organism in men is notoriously difficult and they should be treated epidemiologically in the absence of a definitive diagnosis if the female contact is positive. A follow-up test of cure is recommended for both partners.

For recurrent *Trichomonas* infections it is important to check that the partner has been correctly treated and to consider the possibility of reinfection. If the condition is more obstinate, then metronidazole 400 mg twice daily may be prescribed for five days. Abstinence from sexual intercourse is essential until a cure has been established.

Chlamydial infection

Infection by *Chlamydia trachomatis* can be difficult to diagnose in women and may easily escape detection. The organism infects the columnar or transitional epithelium of the urethra, endocervix, and may spread to the endometrium, Fallopian tubes, peritoneal cavity and rectum, producing inflammation, ulceration and scarring. At least a third of women with *C. trachomatis* will have signs of local infection.

Chlamydia trachomatis is the commonest cause of pelvic inflammatory disease (PID) and there is now accumulating evidence of a major role of *C. trachomatis* in the pathogenesis of infertility (Teare, 1986). Studies from America show that 30–50% of women with laparoscopically diagnosed pelvic inflammatory disease are infected with *C. trachomatis.*

Chlamydia trachomatis is often difficult to detect and this can pose problems for women due to the long-term consequences of untreated infection, i.e. pelvic inflammatory disease, chronic pelvic pain, infertility and an increased risk of ectopic pregnancy. It can also cause ophthalmia neonatorum in infants born to infected mothers.

Some of the predisposing factors for *C. trachomatis* in asymptomatic women have been discussed by Romanowski (1993). It is noted that chlamydial infection is more common in:

♦ sexually active women under 25 years of age;

♦ women who do not use contraception, or those who use a non-barrier method of contraception;

♦ women who have had two or more sexual partners in the last year; and

♦ GUM clinic attenders having a partner with non-specific urethritis or gonorrhoea.

Chlamydia trachomatis is an obligate intracellular parasite and depends on the host cell to provide it with its energy source and other nutrients. The organism has a unique growth cycle that depends on attachment and penetration of the host cell using an enhanced phagocytic process. Being an intracellular body, *C. trachomatis* is best isolated from cell scrapings rather than from discharge from the infected site.

The incubation period is 7–21 days as confirmed from male urethral infection.

The women may be asymptomatic and may harbour the organism for a considerable length of time with few or no symptoms to suggest infection. Alternatively women may present with pelvic inflammatory disease (see also page 407).

Some of the clinical manifestations are listed in Box 12.7.

Diagnosis

All new patients attending a GUM clinic or old patients re-attending with a new problem will have a routine chlamydia test done as part of the screening process. New tests to detect *Chlamydia trachomatis* are being developed but diagnostic tests vary locally according to the local laboratory policy. With current tests there is a small possibility of a false positive or a false negative result.

Box 12.7 Clinical manifestations of chlamydial infection which may be present (see Colour plate 10)

♦ Mucopurulent vaginal discharge

♦ Hypertrophic ectopy of the cervix, which becomes oedematous, congested and bleeds easily

♦ Urethritis

♦ Bartholinitis

♦ Endometritis

♦ Salpingitis (which may present as in the Fitz–Hugh Curtis syndrome where the chlamydial infection has spread to the liver capsule causing right upper quadrant abdominal pain or shoulder pain).

Usually, a swab is used to detect chlamydial antigen, which is measured by enzyme-linked immunosorbent assay (ELISA). A chlamydial cell culture will be done if the woman then produces an equivocal result, is pregnant or has been the victim of a sexual assault.

All female contacts of men with non-specific urethritis will routinely have an endocervical chlamydial test. Serological tests for chlamydial antibodies are available but their use is of limited value (Goh and Forster, 1993).

Testing for *Chlamydia* prior to a termination of pregnancy or an IUD insertion is now routine in many units so that effective treatment can be commenced if necessary before the invasive procedure is carried out.

Treatment

Several antimicrobials have proved to be effective in the treatment of *Chlamydia.* Doxycycline 100 mg twice daily for seven days or erythromycin stearate 500 mg twice daily for 14 days are the main drugs of choice. No follow-up test of cure is usually done except in the case of pregnant women when a repeat culture is performed. All women should be seen a week after treatment to check treatment has been complied with and tolerated, and no further exposure has occurred. It is ideal if both individuals can be treated concurrently and they should be advised to avoid sexual intercourse until the course of treatment is complete. All patients found to be *Chlamydia* positive need to see a health adviser for contact tracing of current and/or recent sexual partners.

Women who are contacts of men diagnosed as having non-specific urethritis are treated for *Chlamydia* irrespective of whether the organism is isolated from them or not. Very often women who have *Chlamydia* at the time a cervical smear is taken may find the result shows 'inflammatory changes'. Full bacterial and viral screening should be performed and the smear repeated when the cervical inflammation has been treated. *Chlamydia* is often a co-infection when another STD (notably gonorrhoea) is present causing a vaginal discharge, or when a mucopurulent cervicitis is diagnosed with a non-specific cause.

Gonorrhoea

Gonorrhoea is one of the oldest STDs and reference is made to the condition in the Old Testament. Hippocrates is often credited with being the first person to describe the condition. In England, by the Middle Ages, the disease was well-documented. The historical epidemiology of gonorrhoea is linked to changes in sexual behaviour and the recent fall in the incidence of gonorrhoea is probably a result of 'safer sex techniques' (Adler, 1990).

In approximately 70% of women gonorrhoea is asymptomatic. Symptoms when they are present are often associated with a concurrent infection such as *Chlamydia* in 20–40% of cases or *Trichomonas vaginalis* in 20% of cases.

The cause of gonorrhoea is an organism called *Neisseria gonorrhoea*. It was discovered by Albert Neisser, after whom it is named. *Neisseria gonorrhoea* is a Gram-negative diplococcus that is non-motile and non-spore-forming and characteristically grows in pairs. Serotyping of the gonococci has demonstrated at least 70 different strains.

Gonococci attach to cellular membranes of columnar and immature squamous epithelium causing substantial mucosal cell damage in a very short time. Submucosal invasion is accompanied by a heavy polymorphonuclear leucocyte response. In women the primary site for the gonococci to grow is the endocervix, where the pH is neutral. Auto-inoculation may result in infection of the Skene's glands, Bartholin's ducts and colonization of the urethra and rectum.

The incubation period in men for urethral gonorrhoea is 3–7 days. For women the incubation period is more variable but in women who are symptomatic it is approximately 10 days.

The woman may be asymptomatic or may present with pelvic inflammatory disease as for *Chlamydia trachomatis*. Symptomatic women may present with any of the manifestations listed in Box 12.8.

Box 12.8 Clinical manifestations of gonorrhoea (see Colour plate 10)

♦ Mucopurulent vaginal discharge

♦ Cervicitis

♦ Intermenstrual uterine bleeding

♦ Menorrhagia (can be severe)

♦ Erythema and oedema of the cervix (may bleed on contact with a swab)

♦ Dysuria.

Diagnosis

A Gram-stain slide is taken to identify the Gram-negative intracellular diplococci. A wet-mount slide is also done to exclude a co-infection with *Trichomonas vaginalis*. Swabs are taken from the cervix and urethra and cultured on blood agar plates or transported in Stuart's medium. Taking cultures from women is essential as up to 50% of cases of gonorrhoea will be missed in women if the Gram-stain slide is relied on alone. Women who are known contacts of partners with gonorrhoea or those who complain of rectal discomfort will also have a rectal culture done.

Blood tests are available to detect antibodies to *N. gonorrhoea*; however, they are not sufficiently sensitive or specific to be used in uncomplicated gonorrhoea.

Treatment

In uncomplicated cervical, urethral and rectal gonorrhoea the usual treatment of choice is amoxycillin 3 g stat and probenicid 1 g stat orally. Patients allergic to penicillin can be given ciprofloxacin 500 mg stat. Ciprofloxacin should not be used for pregnant women, adolescents or in patients with a history of convulsions. For penicillin-resistant strains of *N. gonorrhoea* or if the woman is pregnant, then spectinomycin 2 g intramuscularly can be used. Mohanty (1989) explains that the reason for giving a single-dose treatment 'is based on the high default rate of follow-up examination for a test of cure'.

French (1995) indicated that patients diagnosed with cervical and urethral gonorrhoea should also be treated with a course of doxycycline 100 mg twice daily for seven days in case of concomitant chlamydial infection. Routine screening for *Chlamydia* and other infections will be taken as part of the diagnostic procedure.

All patients with *N. gonorrhoea* are referred to the health adviser for contact tracing and advised to abstain from sexual intercourse until a follow-up test of cure has been done. Gonorrhoea can have serious sequelae if untreated. In the short term, complications like salpingitis, Bartholin's gland abscess and pelvic inflammatory disease may ensue. Disseminated gonococcal infections can lead to septic arthritis and longer term there is an increased risk of chronic pelvic pain, ectopic pregnancy and infertility. If a pregnant woman develops gonorrhoea, Godley (1993) reports a risk of intrauterine growth retardation, premature membrane rupture, chorioamnionitis and postpartum sepsis. There is the additional risk of ophthalmia neonatorum in the neonate (see Colour plate 11).

Genital ulceration

Most genital ulceration in young adults is likely to be infectious, whilst in the older woman the possibility of neoplastic disease has to be considered. The average age for developing vulval carcinoma is 60 years (Hall, 1993). When discussing genital ulceration the history taking from the patient needs to be particularly detailed and it is important to find out if the woman has recently had sexual intercourse abroad. This is for two reasons: first, because it may be necessary to consider a tropical STD, and secondly, genital ulceration is a co-factor throughout the world implicated in the spread of HIV infection.

Other important questions to ask a patient about genital ulceration are:

♦ When was the last episode of sexual intercourse?

♦ Is the ulcer painful or painless?

♦ Is it a single ulcer or multiple?

♦ Is it the first attack or is it recurrent in nature?

♦ Has she taken any drugs recently? This could indicate Stevens–Johnson syndrome (a drug reaction causing genital ulceration usually associated with tetracyclines).

♦ Is there a history of any allergies?

♦ Is the area itchy and is there any excoriation present?

Common causes of genital ulceration are listed in Box 12.9.

Box 12.9 Causes of genital ulceration

Infective

♦ Genital herpes

♦ Syphilis

♦ Tropical STDs
  - chancroid
  - lymphogranuloma venereum
  - granuloma inguinale

♦ Pyogenic infection

♦ Scabies and infestations

♦ Candidiasis (severe)

♦ Condylomata acuminata (genital warts – these do not usually ulcerate but if ulceration occurs it is often as a result of treatment, with the added risk of a secondary infection because of local tissue damage).

Non-infective

♦ Trauma

♦ Drug eruptions

♦ Carcinoma

♦ Behçet's disease

♦ Paget's disease

♦ Crohn's disease

♦ Dermatitis artefacta.

Genital herpes

Genital herpes is endemic to all population groups. Mindel and Adler (1984), in a review of genital herpes, say attendance at GUM clinics for the condition showed a 58% increase between 1976 and 1981. The notable feature of the herpesvirus is its ability to remain latent in the host and then to reactivate periodically. At present there is no cure for herpes. The morbidity of the condition is of particular concern as genital herpes tends to affect the woman's personal relationships due to its chronic nature. Breslin (1988) points out that 'emphasising that the disease is not curable is non productive'. When talking to women with herpes you should listen carefully to all their concerns and encourage them as far as possible to try to gain psychological control of the virus.

Several viruses are classified as herpesviruses. They are herpes simplex virus 1 and 2 (HSV-1 and HSV-2), varicella-zoster virus, Epstein–Barr virus, cytomegalovirus and human herpesvirus 6. HSV-2 resides in the sacral ganglia causing genital lesions, whilst HSV-1 resides in the trigeminal ganglia and is principally associated with facial lesions. The increase in oral–genital sex means that HSV-1 can cause genital herpes.

Some population prevalence studies of HSV-2 have demonstrated an antibody level 25% higher than those who present with clinical disease. Large numbers of individuals are asymptomatic, whilst others have a very mild symptomatic infection which is often not reported.

Active HSV-2 infection has an incubation period of 2–20 days. HSV-2 is a sexually transmitted disease and auto-inoculation from one site to another is feasible. HSV-2 has been demonstrated to be more virulent than HSV-1. Non-venereal spread of HSV-2 to the neonate can occur intrapartum and postpartum.

Clinical manifestations

First attack. The first attack of herpes is usually the most severe, with a prolonged period of viral shedding. The woman may have a systemic illness with fever, malaise, myalgias, headache, genital irritation, vaginal discharge, inguinal tenderness and lymphadenopathy. The lesions in a primary herpes episode of the genital area in women are frequently located on the vulva, vagina, perineum and may also occur on the thighs or buttocks (see Colour plates 12 and 13 . Breslin (1988) noted that 'HSV cervicitis can be found in over 80% of women with initial genital disease'.

The lesions begin as erythematous papules which then develop into vesicles. The vesicles then rupture and leave ulcerative lesions; some of the ulcers coalesce, producing larger areas of ulceration. The ulcers then crust over and re-epithelialization takes place, usually without leaving a scar. The severity and duration of a first attack varies enormously. Some women find the lesions heal within a week, whilst in others the duration may be as long as 3–6 weeks. The median duration for viral shedding from the onset of the lesions is generally agreed to be approximately 12 days.

Complications of a primary herpes infection include dysuria, retention of urine, constipation due to pain on defecation, aseptic meningitis and transverse myelitis. The local symptoms can cause considerable psychological distress.

Recurrent herpes infection. Recurrent attacks of genital herpes are usually much milder and shorter in duration than the primary attack. This is partly due to the fact that women have established good levels of neutralizing antibodies to the virus. The recurrence rate for genital herpes will depend on a number of factors including immunological reactions in the host, age, race, site of inoculation, past exposure and genetic background. Lesions in recurrent attacks of herpes often occur at the initial infection site in small clusters and rupture within 48 hours. Viral shedding is for a much shorter period (about five days) and re-epithelialization takes place on average within ten days. The constitutional symptoms associated with the primary attack are absent.

Mindel and Adler (1984) note that 50% of patients experience 'prodromal symptoms' prior to an attack which the woman, if warned, will learn to recognize. These prodromal symptoms may consist of a mild tingling sensation at the respective site and shooting pain to the buttock, leg or hip. There may also be mood alterations and the woman may become more irritable, tearful and easily upset. You can educate your client to recognize this prodrome, which will help her to manage the condition and encourage her to feel that she is more in control of the virus.

Diagnosis

Diagnosis of HSV-2 is made by taking a culture for viral isolation. The ideal specimen is obtained from a fluid-filled vesicle by rupturing the vesicle with a sterile needle. The fluid is collected on a sterile swab and transferred to a viral transport medium. In the laboratory the specimen is inoculated into a living cell maintained at body temperature to observe its growth and confirm diagnosis.

Treatment

As with all other STDs, treatment should aim at promoting comfort, promoting healing, preventing secondary infection and decreasing transmission of the disease. The main treatment is oral acyclovir 200 mg five times daily for five days. Treatment should begin as early as possible in an attack. You should try to choose an appropriate moment to point out to your clients that acyclovir is not a cure for herpes and the drug acts by suppressing viral replication. Saline bathing of the ulcerated area produces some relief of the discomfort. Mild analgesia is recommended for pain relief.

Acyclovir is not recommended for infrequent recurrent episodes. It is an acyclic nucleoside analogue and acts by inhibiting the viral DNA polymerase. The use of acyclovir as a prophylaxis against recurrent herpes appears to be limited but women who experience more than six attacks a year may qualify for oral acyclovir suppressive therapy as a means of controlling the virus. However, a number of women are unhappy taking suppressive therapy as it is a constant reminder to them of their condition.

All women should see the health adviser for both contact tracing, and education and counselling about the condition. Sexual intercourse should be avoided until the lesions have completely re-epithelialized.

Pregnant women who have previously suffered from herpes often express concern about the risk to their unborn baby. Corey (1990) points out that 'the vast majority of pregnant women with recurrent genital herpes deliver normal infants'. What is vital is that the woman informs her midwife and obstetrician of the fact that she has previously had the virus, as herpes in pregnancy and herpes of the neonate are complex and require an individual approach to care. The woman should be kept fully informed and encouraged to share in the decision-making process regarding delivery of her baby. If a woman has active lesions at the time of delivery then it is recommended that a Caesarian section should be performed (Corey, 1990; Godley, 1993).

Godley (1993) points out that the results of routine viral cultures from the lower genital tract are of no predictive value in women who have asymptomatic viral shedding at the time of delivery and additionally a culture result takes an average of a week to be confirmed – frequently too late to be of value. Routine screening of pregnant women for genital herpes is not recommended.

The psychological aspects of genital herpes

Breslin (1988) describes women as having a sense of shock, anger, isolation and loneliness on being made aware of the diagnosis of genital herpes. Initially the anger tends to be directed to the person thought to have given them the infection but is then frequently aimed at the medical profession for having diagnosed the condition and then not being able to provide a cure. Anxieties arise about relationships, childbirth and cancer. There is an increased incidence of psychiatric morbidity and depressive illness and self-destructive feelings can be experienced. Breslin's comments have been validated and confirmed by Carney et al. (1994) who found the psychological impact of the first episode of genital herpes had a 'profound effect on patients'. If there were no recurrences of the condition then the woman's psychological state improved. However, if there was a recurrence the level of anxiety remained as high as for the primary attack.

The link of genital herpes with cervical cancer still remains unproven and tenuous but annual cervical cytology is recommended – consequently giving the woman yet another reminder of the long-term effects of genital herpes.

Nurses therefore need to give positive assurances that the condition is manageable. Helping women to manage the disease means helping them to identify stress factors which may contribute to a recurrence. These may include:

♦ hormonal changes, e.g. ovulation;

♦ local heat from tight clothing or from prolonged exposure to sunlight;

♦ emotional distress and life-changing events; or

♦ stress, lack of sleep, overwork and not taking sufficient time for emotional and physical repair and an opportunity to get things into perspective.

In your clinical practice you should remember that listening to a woman's fears and anxieties about herpes can act as a major catharsis for her. This listening in itself may be enough to help, as many women feel isolated and unwilling to discuss the condition with others from whom they would normally draw support. Additionally it will give you an idea whether the patient would benefit from psychological assistance or from joining a support group.

Syphilis

Syphilis has been described as a social model for HIV and AIDS and has been called 'one of the most fascinating diseases of humans' (Sparling, 1990). It is impossible to do justice to the complexities of the condition of syphilis in an introductory chapter such as this on sexually transmitted diseases.

The origins of syphilis have been lost in time but from 1495 the disease begins to be recorded, and has since been extensively written about by poets, novelists, dramatists and social historians as well as medical researchers. Looking back over history, syphilis was pandemic causing high levels of morbidity and mortality and was originally a disease of greater virulence than the type of presentation seen today.

Syphilis is divided into four stages: primary, secondary, latency and tertiary. It is a rare condition in the UK today, but worldwide the disease still causes significant problems and you should be aware of this in patients who present with symptoms who have been overseas. Any patient presenting with genital ulceration needs to be screened for syphilis as part of the diagnosis of exclusion.

The causative organism of syphilis is *Treponema pallidum*, which is classified as a spirochaete. It is one of a group of diseases referred to as the treponematoses, which includes yaws and pinta. These latter two conditions are described as 'variants of syphilis' and are acquired by non-venereal spread, usually in childhood (Arya *et al.*, 1980). Syphilis is acquired by sexual contact, except for congenital syphilis when the unborn infant acquires the condition by transplacental transmission from the infected mother.

The incubation period for primary syphilis is nine days to three months. The median duration is three weeks. The reason for the varied incubation time is related to the amount of the *T. pallidum* inoculum. *Treponema pallidum* cannot enter the body through intact skin but will enter through small abrasions that occur in the mucous membrane during sexual intercourse. 'When a concentration of approximately 10 million organism per gram of tissue is reached, clinical lesions appear' (Tillman, 1991).

Clinical manifestations

Primary syphilis. The primary stage is characterized by the appearance at the site of inoculation of a primary chancre (sore). The chancre is usually a painless ulcer that has a punched in centre and indurated edge. There may be some oedema to adjacent tissue, and lymph glands local to the chancre site may be slightly enlarged. In women the common sites for the chancre are the vulva, labia, vagina and in 25% of cases the cervix. If untreated, the chancre heals spontaneously in a few weeks.

Secondary syphilis. The characteristic lesions of secondary syphilis usually occur 4–12 weeks after the appearance of the primary chancre. By this stage the disease has become systemic and the patient may present with malaise, headache, fever and a bilateral symmetrical rash. The rash occurs on the trunk, face, legs, arms and diagnostically on the soles of the feet and palms of the hands. Other lesions referred to by Adler (1990) include the appearance of condylomata lata (wart-like papules occurring on the labia and anus). These condylomata can be very infectious and are often a prime site for isolating the *T. pallidum*. The secondary stage of syphilis has a duration of approximately two years. It is important to realize that the stages of syphilis are very fluid and there is no clear demarcation line. Once the secondary stage subsides the patient enters the latent stage.

Latent syphilis. This is usually characterized as a period absent of any clinical manifestations of disease although the serology would be positive. The patient may remain in the latent stage of syphilis for as little as two years or for as long as 40 years.

Tertiary syphilis. This is now a very rare condition and can be divided into three presenting categories: gummatous, cardiovascular and neurosyphilis. The two classic conditions of neurosyphilis are tabes dorsalis and general paralysis of the insane. It is not always appreciated by health care practitioners today that these conditions would have been extremely common in this country before the advent of penicillin and called for considerable nursing expertise. Today treatment for syphilis, at any stage of the disease, is successful.

Congenital syphilis. This is more accurately known as transplacental syphilis and can still be a problem in some parts of the developing world. A dramatic decline has taken place in the UK partly due to the serological screening of pregnant women.

Diagnosis

In the primary stage a dark ground microscopy is done on the primary chancre to identify the *T. pallidum*. The serology may be negative at this stage but is positive within ten days of the primary chancre appearing. Serological testing for syphilis began in 1906 when Wasserman first described the serological reaction.

Treatment

The main treatment of choice for primary and secondary syphilis is procaine penicillin 600 000 units intramuscularly daily for ten days and 500 mg probenicid twice daily for ten days. Alternative therapies include erythromycin 500 mg four times a day for 15 days or doxycycline 100 mg twice daily for 15 days. For latent and tertiary syphilis the treatment regime is increased both in dosage and length. Clients must be warned that it is essential to complete the medical treatment in order to stop asymptomatic disease progression.

All clients with syphilis need to be seen by the health adviser for contact tracing and must abstain from sexual intercourse until two follow-up blood tests have been performed.

In dealing with women from other cultures you should remember that woman testing positive for syphilis should not be classified automatically as suffering from syphilis as serological tests cannot distinguish between syphilis and non-venereal treponematoses like yaws, pinta and bejel.

Condylomata acuminata (genital warts)

Genital warts have been described as far back as classical times. Lucas (1988) discusses the fact that the Roman physician Celsus documented genital warts in the year AD 25. The possible link between cervical cancer and genital warts was first discussed in oncology literature in the 1840s.

For clients, both male and female, genital warts are a distressing problem as not only do they look aesthetically upsetting on the external genitalia but women may also have heard of the possible link with cervical cancer and be anxious for their future. Genital ulceration may result from treatment of the warts, particularly when women self-treat, mistakenly thinking that a more aggressive application of the caustic agent will clear them up faster. This is not the case as the warts often remain and the patient is left with chemical burns.

Genital warts are caused by the human papillomavirus (HPV). 'Seventy three genotypes of HPV have been identified so far, of which more than 30 types can affect the genital tract' (Bowman, 1994). Papillomaviruses are classified according to their natural supporting host. HPV are DNA viruses, meaning that they carry all their genetic information in a single strand of DNA. HPV tend to be site-specific in infectivity, but auto-inoculation from one site to another does occur.

Genital warts can be associated with many strains of HPV, however most are caused by types HPV 6 and HPV 11 which are more often associated with benign warts or mild dysplasia. Cervical intraepithelial neoplasia (CIN) has been linked particularly to HPV 16 and 18 and is present in over 80% of invasive squamous carcinomas of the cervix, vulva and penis. The severity of the cervical dysplasia appears to be linked to the HPV type.

The incubation period for HPV is very variable and can be anywhere between three weeks and nine months. Schneider (1993) states that 'sexual transmission is the main pathway for genital HPV's, however, vertical, peripartal [during pregnancy and childbirth] and oral transmission are also possible'. HPV enter through breaks in the skin and mucous membrane. Genital warts are described as hyperproliferative benign epithelial neoplasms, they are self-limiting tumours which may spontaneously regress. They are often exacerbated in pregnancy, old age and in immunosuppressed patients.

Clinical manifestations and predisposing factors

Genital warts are the third most common STD in the UK. Clinical and subclinical warts can be present anywhere from the cervix to the anus. In women the most common sites are the introitus, labia minora and elsewhere on the vulva. They are also seen on the perineum (see Colour plate 14). Tinkle (1990) describes clinical genital warts as 'flesh coloured verrucous lesions' that tend to occur on warm, moist areas of the genitalia. Oral lesions may occur, probably due to oro-genital sexual practices.

Several co-factors have been associated with HPV which may promote its progression including:

♦ The early onset of sexual activity

♦ Smoking (tobacco metabolites have been found in the cervical mucus)

♦ Other STDs – particularly *Chlamydia*, *Trichomonas* and herpes simplex

♦ Multiple sexual partners

♦ Poor genital hygiene

♦ Hormonal changes

♦ Poor nutrition.

Lucas (1988) has argued that any additional inflammation, irritation or erosion will help to promote the integration of the virus into the cell. Women with cervical or vaginal clinical warts may experience bleeding, itching and a vaginal discharge following sexual intercourse.

Diagnosis

In clinical practice a diagnosis of clinical warts is made on their appearance. Any suspect or atypical growth will be biopsied to exclude a differential diagnosis such as carcinoma. The diagnosis of subclinical HPV might follow a cervical smear when the cytology report notes that koilocytes are identified, or during a colposcopy. The cervical transformation zone is particularly important as this is the area where columnar epithelium undergoes a process of metaplasia, developing into squamous epithelium. This area of cellular change at the cervix is thought to make it more vulnerable to viral infection and to neoplastic change. Only 20% of women with genital warts will demonstrate clinical HPV of the cervix (Tinkle, 1990).

Other diagnostic methods discussed by Tinkle include the use of DNA hybridization studies that employ molecular biological techniques to identify the particular HPV genotype, and immunoperoxidase studies directed at identification of HPV antigens. Both of these tests are not yet standard, being expensive and difficult to obtain.

Treatment

The main treatment for genital warts is the topical application of 25% or 10% podophyllin to vaginal, vulval and anal warts. The resin is applied two to three times a week and must be washed off within 4–6 hours. Surrounding skin should be protected with Vaseline beforehand. A strict and accurate record should be kept of the number of treatments and the condition of the skin at each treatment. Treatment regimes for genital warts are often very protracted and should be reviewed every two weeks. If treatment is not effective then alternative forms of treatment should be considered.

Cryotherapy, electrocautery, carbon dioxide laser, liquid nitrogen and treatment with trichloroacetic acid may be attempted. Some women with extensive genital warts which have failed to respond to other forms of treatment may eventually consider surgical excision.

Women may be able to self-treat with podophyllotoxin twice daily for three days but will need clear written instructions and warnings about overenthusiastic self-treatment. Podophyllin and podophyllotoxin are contraindicated in pregnant women as they are toxic to the fetus.

Internal rectal warts can take longer to clear, partly because the most caustic agents cannot be used in this area. The treatment of cervical warts is aimed at obliterating the lesions by freezing techniques, laser and surgical procedures. Treatment to the cervix can often result in an increase in vaginal discharge which women need warning about. This discharge tends to be self-limiting as the treated area heals.

Condom usage is recommended all the time genital warts are present. All sexual partners should be seen and screened for warts even if these are not obviously apparent as 60% of sexual partners will acquire warts. When a woman presents with warts for the first time a routine screen for other STDs is done, and the anal canal should be checked with a proctoscope if peri-anal warts are seen. Even if there are no visible warts, weak acetic acid may be applied to suspect areas and minor warts would then be highlighted. If a cervical cytology smear has not been performed in the past 12 months then this should also be done.

All these treatments for clinical HPV are time-consuming, socially disruptive and often profoundly uncomfortable. Recurrences of clinical warts are common so women are asked to return as soon as they notice any new condylomata so that treatment can be started quickly before they become too extensive.

Infestations

The main infestations seen in GUM clinics are the crab louse and scabies. Infestations of the genital area produce an intense itching which in turn may become secondarily infected. The woman may present with excoriation to the external genitalia resembling genital ulceration. Infestations are distressing and care needs to be taken in explaining treatment to the patient who also should be warned that purchasing additional proprietary products and overtreating the infestation can result in dermatitis.

Contact tracing of sexual partners is required. All women should have a routine STD screen as infestations are the result of sexual contact.

Lice

Three species of lice infest humans. Transmission of *Pediculosis pubis* is by intimate physical contact, usually sexual intercourse.

The nit of the crab louse is oval shaped and opaline to look at. The eggs usually hatch in 5–10 days, once they are incubated by the host's body heat. The nits are secured to the base of the pubic hair by a cement-like substance. The louse is parasitic and feeds on human blood for its nourishment.

Diagnosis is usually made on the woman's

symptoms and treatment is with malathion 0.5% applied to the pubic and other affected areas and washed off after 12 hours.

Scabies

Infestation with *Sarcoptes scabiei* results in severe itching in 2–6 weeks. The adult female burrows into the horny layer of skin and deposits 2–3 eggs a day. These eggs develop into an adult in about ten days. Transmission is by close contact and it is usually sexually transmitted.

Diagnosis is made on the symptoms and the itching is worse at night when the body is warm. Burrows may be present and these can be opened using a sterile needle and the scabies mite observed under low-power light microscopy.

Treatment is with malathion 0.5% applied to all body surfaces except the face and washed off after 24 hours. Clothing and bed linen need laundering or dry cleaning and no other precautions are necessary.

Human immunodeficiency virus (HIV) infection and acquired immune deficiency syndrome (AIDS) in women

---

The literature on HIV and AIDS has become very extensive since the condition was first recognized in 1981. Today nurses face complacency to the topic both from within the profession and from the wider society. This chapter can only briefly look at ongoing issues that concern women, but further information can be obtained from the books, support groups and helplines which are listed at the end of this chapter. In order to gain an accurate picture of the impact of HIV and AIDS in women it is important to bear in mind not only the national but also the global perspective of the disease.

The number of HIV and AIDS cases that were projected for the UK early on in the epidemic has not occurred. There are many reasons for this. First, the statistical estimates of numbers possibly infected were inaccurate. Secondly, it can be argued that the rapid response by GUM clinics to provide information and counselling to the general public did much to raise public awareness of the disease. Thirdly, the excellent work done by the many voluntary organizations such as the Terence Higgins Trust (THT) moved the debate into the political and social arena. They alerted the public consciousness to the potential threat of HIV and AIDS and broke down traditional ideas about sexuality and sexual practice.

The idea that HIV and AIDS was a 'gay man's disease' however took hold and this has disadvantaged women so that even now, over a decade into the infection, women still have a low index of suspicion that they are at risk or could be infected (Glenn *et al.*, 1991). A decade ago less than 10% of people with AIDS were women but by the end of 1994 women represented 40% of all new AIDS cases – a rapid fourfold increase. By the year 2000 the World Health Organization estimate that four million women will have died of AIDS.

The global epidemiology of HIV and AIDS provides a sharper perspective of how the infection is having an impact on women and their children. Worldwide it is estimated that vaginal intercourse accounts for 60–70% of all HIV infection (Johnson, 1992) and WHO estimates that 7–8 million women of childbearing age have been infected with HIV – a figure that is expected to double by the end of the century. Leading authorities in the field of HIV and AIDS are almost in universal accord that if the pandemic spread is to be controlled then empowerment of women in relationships is vital and Blakey (1991) discusses how such strategies for reaching and empowering women can be achieved.

Empowerment is discussed in nursing in a very loose way and you should remember that it is a very sophisticated concept and takes considerable time for women to implement. A woman does not wake up one morning and say 'I think I will be empowered today'. Empowerment means fundamentally altering cognitive and behavioural patterns that have occurred and been instilled over years of socialization, which have produced thinking and behavioural patterns in women that are comfortable for her, and which have never previously been questioned. For many women, but particularly those from an ethnic minority, the concept of empowerment is an alien one and feminists argue that the empowerment of women when it does occur is on male terms. All of this does not mean that empowerment should not take place but you need to keep in mind that the change in attitude for some women may be difficult to understand and achieve. The whole concept of empowerment is complex and necessitates considerably more thought than merely teaching a woman to be responsible by carrying condoms in her handbag. Women need to learn to make informed choices to improve the quality of their lives.

Other issues that put women at a disadvantage include the socio-economic obstacles at both the microeconomic and macroeconomic level. Horton (1995) states a need for investigators and policy-makers to address the complexity of HIV disease in women, and mentions that contributory factors like 'domestic violence, substance abuse, prison detention, mental illness, poverty and limited access to care all impinge on women at risk of HIV'. The sexual and economic subordination of women has certainly fuelled the HIV and AIDS pandemic.

For many women who are HIV positive their history reveals very few sexual partners. Flanigan and Carpenter (1994), discussing HIV infection through heterosexual transmission in the Rhode Island study, found that 70% of positive women had been in a stable relationship with a single partner for at least two years, and that their median number of sexual partners over the previous ten-year period had been three. The route of transmission of the virus to women is overwhelmingly through heterosexual intercourse.

Women are often much sicker by the time they arrive under the care of the physician because of the perception that they are at low risk. Evidence is now accumulating which demonstrates that there are positive advantages for women who manage to reach medical care earlier as early medical intervention can limit some of the problems that could occur. HIV-positive women are at greater risk of cervical dysplasia and cancer associated with HPV and should therefore have annual cervical smears. There is an increased risk of vaginal candidiasis, particularly as the CD4 (white lymphocyte) count falls, genital ulcerative disease, cervicitis, salpingitis and pelvic inflammatory disease (Baker, 1995) and all these can be carefully monitored with early medical support.

Women will need contraceptive information and advice on what is best for them. Condoms (both male and female) play an important part in the strategy to prevent the transmission of sexually transmitted diseases including HIV as they are the most effective method of preventing transmission. Other barrier methods, e.g. the diaphragm or cervical cap, may reduce transmission to a lesser extent. The role of spermicides is uncertain. Oral contraceptive use has been implicated in some circumstances to be immunosuppressive, but Howe *et al.* (1994) says the risk of oral contraception contributing to the increased transmission of HIV remains 'controversial'. The use of the intra-uterine contraceptive device is contraindicated in HIV-positive women, as for women with other STDs, because the risk of infection is increased and also the risk of HIV transmission may be increased.

Studies with HIV-positive homosexual men have indicated that if a patient receives good primary care facilities whilst HIV positive and fit, this then extrapolates through into a longer period before developing an AIDS diagnosis and correspondingly a longer life expectancy. Women, as well as men, need to benefit from these advantages.

The science of HIV infection is constantly changing and new technology like the polymerase chain reaction (PCR) is being used which is capable of measuring a patient's viral load in conjunction with the CD4 count. Such advances are altering the care and management of the disease. A new generation of antiretroviral drugs also look set to change the treatment modalities in patient care.

Sound advice to patients, in conjunction with good dental, podiatry, nutritional and psychological care have made a marked improvement to patient well-being. The coordination of these services within the nursing of this client group is complex. All health care professionals need to give consideration to the additional support patients, their partners and their families need. It is undoubtably a considerable strain on all involved having their life medicalized, monitored and subject to continuous assessment. HIV infection consequently can trigger responses of depression, grief and anger (Silebi, 1995).

HIV testing in pregnant women is generally offered on an 'opt-out' basis, i.e. the woman can decline to be tested. Women who test HIV positive require ongoing assessment, education and counselling and aggressive early intervention for any infection. They also need strategies to assist them to maintain their good health. The problems of HIV infection in pregnant women have been looked at in detail by Mok (1992). Vertical transmission may occur intrauterine, intrapartum and postpartum. The European Collaborative Study (1991) established the vertical transmission rate at 12.9% but the relative risk for each stage has not been quantified. In a healthy HIV-positive woman there is no reason why the pregnancy should not progress normally to term. The case management of a pregnant woman will be more detailed because of her HIV status and care will need to be coordinated between the woman's obstetrician, the GUM physician and the multidisciplinary team. Invasive techniques such as amniocentesis, umbilical cord blood sampling and fetal scalp electrodes are contraindicated, as is breastfeeding, in order to reduce the risk of infection to the unborn infant or neonate.

The possible benefits of antiretroviral drug use in pregnant women in reducing the vertical transmission rate of HIV has been demonstrated by Connor *et al.* (1994) and means that pregnant women will have additional difficult decisions to make. The ethical problem is crystallized by Bayer (1994) when he states: 'in view of the remaining uncertainties about the long term consequences of zidovudine treatment during pregnancy for both mother and her offspring, the principal of consent to both screening and treatment is even more relevant'.

Both men and women with HIV share many worries and health concerns but women have many additional anxieties. Women have to confront gynaecological HIV-related clinical manifestations, contraceptive concerns, the worry of vertical transmission in pregnancy and the future care of any children she may already have.

The whole perspective of HIV infection in women is markedly very different from men and you should be aware of these differences in your planning and implementation of nursing care. You also need to be aware and sensitive to your own feelings, beliefs and attitudes towards women who are HIV positive or have AIDS. If you are uncomfortable about treating and talking to such women then you have a professional responsibility to refer on to other colleagues. However, if your attitude is empathetic, understanding, caring and helpful then your client, her partner and her family will be able to benefit from your skills.

Nursing issues in sexual health

Over the past decade the National Health Service has undergone significant change. Government initiatives such as the *Health of the Nation* document (DOH, 1992) and the Patients' Charter, combined with local management policies have all been designed to improve patient care, meet local population needs and have instigated changes for the benefits of patients.

These changes have increased the work of the general practitioner and have inevitably resulted in a corresponding reconfiguration of the work of the practice nurse. Traditionally doctors used to examine patients and were responsible for taking a medical and sexual history but this fixed role is becoming more flexible. Increasingly nurses and health advisers are becoming responsible for health promotion and counselling patients in relation to safer sex, harm minimization and sexual health. More nurse-led clinics are being established, which means that taking a history from patients is becoming part of the nurse's role. Both Andrist (1988) and Bor and Watts (1993) discuss this issue in relation to defining what the woman's actual and potential problems are in relation to her sexual health needs.

The general principles of nursing care remain the same, but the context in which that care is delivered during the last decade has changed. There has been the development of outreach work to cover schools, sex industry workers, drug users and the homeless. GUM clinics now have extended opening hours with longer appointments for consultation, examination and investigations. Patients who are HIV positive have regular check-ups and access to counselling which is particularly important for those who have progressed on to an AIDS diagnosis. Additionally there has been the development of improved shared care with GPs.

Woolley (1993) thinks there is a role for practice nurses to promote sexual health, particularly when the context of the nurse–patient interaction is appropriate to the issue, e.g. when the woman attends for contraceptive advice or for cervical cytology. Woolley also suggests that 'well-adolescent' clinics could be run from the general practice setting. The use of specific clinics with specific targets, directed at a particular population group are by definition a better way of reaching the heterogeneous groups of women in society whose needs are very different in each group.

In all clinical settings, information leaflets should be available about how to prevent STDs. These leaflets (some excellent ones are available from the Health Education Authority) should clearly explain safe sex, the use of barrier methods of contraception, the risks of multiple partners or a partner with multiple partners, how to tell a partner and where to go for appropriate help.

The psychological response to STDs is another issue that nurses need to consider. A sexually transmitted disease damages an individual's self-concept and lowers self-esteem, resulting in anxiety, impaired social interactions, hopelessness, depression and a feeling of isolation. Most women will recover a sense of equilibrium in due course and self-worth should be restored without recourse to psychological support. However, for a few, the consequences of a sexually acquired infection can be continued shock, pain and unresolved latent anger, hostility and aggression. This may disturb future relationships with feelings of mistrust and sexual dysfunction. When dealing with such women in your clinical practice you should remember to let them express their anger and let them cry and validate their feelings. Assisting the woman to articulate her unhappiness can then lead to helping her develop effective coping skills.

Whittaker (1993), looking at the experience of female nurses and female patients in GUM, found that nurses gained job satisfaction from relationships with their patients and demonstrated skill in utilizing short amounts of time with patients to establish a rapport. This 'supportive and talking work' as Whittaker calls it often went unrecorded. It is not the amount of time that the nurse spends with the client that is important but the way that the time is used for educating and discussing with the woman the issues that concern her sexual health. The time is also used in counselling, assisting the woman with problem-solving, decision-making and allowing her time to reflect on her feelings. The female patients in the study confirmed the importance of the nurse's role in explaining issues and giving support, i.e. quality of advice not quantity of time.

Whittaker (1993) confirmed in her study what researchers have previously identified: that both female clients and female nurses had strong negative feelings towards the internal examination – a finding which contradicts the acquiescent behaviour of both groups in the examination room. For women the lithotomy position in itself is disempowering and she will need a clear explanation from supportive staff of what is happening to her and why it is necessary. Interestingly, nurses working within GUM tend to undervalue the chaperoning role, whilst the client values the nurse chaperon to both explain, validate and legitimize what occurs during the internal examination procedure. In your clinical practice you should try and remember these two important points raised by Whittaker and be caring, supportive, nonjudgemental and sensitive to your client's anxieties and needs.

In your dealings with clients from both sexes you should consider and reflect on the way men have little knowledge and have frequently been excluded from appreciating the woman's sexual health perspective. Educating both male and female clients about their sexual drive, sexual response time, sexual performance anxieties and sexual techniques, as well as sexual health promotion needs in the opposite sex will help to reduce the division and misunderstanding between them. A woman's sexual health will improve immeasurably if men are taught to value it. Recent research has shown men are equally ill-informed about their own health care needs and suggests much remedial work needs to be done in this area of health promotion as well.

STDs are more difficult to detect in women than in men and the risk of chronic sequelae remains much higher. Demographically the women most at risk of contracting an STD are young women, ethnic minority women and socially and economically disadvantaged women. Women attending GUM clinics often use a pseudonym and will also give a fictitious address. If this is done the responsibility rests with the client to ensure that she returns for her test results and this should be carefully explained to her. If a culture result comes back as positive there is no way the health adviser could contact the woman. Information is never released to a third party, including the woman's GP, without the woman's express consent.

Munday (1990) surveyed 300 patients in GUM and found the majority did not want the results of their consultation sent to their general practitioner without their consent. However 71% of women agreed to their GP being informed of their cervical cytology result – perhaps this was due to the fact that having a smear test is seen as being more 'normal' and does not carry a social stigma. Munday's studies looking at consumers' views have demonstrated just one of the ways GUM

nursing can change by recognizing and responding to clients needs.

The use of clinical audit in GUM as Mercey (1992) has discussed is to 'improve standards driven by honest admission that our service is rarely perfect'. Clinical audit in GUM tends to be multidisciplinary and is able to define more accurately what nurses do in their clinical practice and the contribution they make to the sexual health service. Information that is given to women needs to be consistent with regard to universal precautions, safer sex practice and clinic policies and procedures. Lack of information, conflicting information and inconsistency between staff were some of the aspects of the service found to be most irksome to female patients in Whittaker's study (1993) of clients' views. Obviously these should be avoided in order to improve care.

Conclusion

Sexual health is a concept that means different things to different people. In your nursing role you should aim to have a holistic approach to sexual health which encompasses health promotion advice, recognizes varying sexual behaviour, understands that disease interferes with sexual function, and most importantly accepts that psychological factors impair and inhibit sexual functioning and relationships. In short, sexual health may be considered the physical and emotional state of well-being that enables women to enjoy and act on their sexual feelings (Boston Women's Health Book Collective, 1985).

Nurses, whether in primary care or in hospital departments and clinics, have an important role in maintaining the sexual health of women. You should be able to assess and identify sexual concerns and problems and be able to intervene effectively in order to help your clients. The key to successful and practical management of STDs lies in the accurate diagnosis and appropriate treatment for the condition both within general practice and within GUM so that a rapid solution can be found to the client's problem.

Sexually transmitted diseases pose a serious threat not only to women's sexual health but also to the general health and well-being of millions of women worldwide. The problem of STDs has still not been tackled adequately on a global scale and until this is done, numbers worldwide will continue to increase. The education about and adoption of safer sex practices and the increasing availability of condoms have a vital part to play in reducing rates of STDs. With good STD services and active AIDS prevention programmes it is hoped to limit the spread of HIV.

Resources

AVERT (AIDS Education and Research Trust)
11–13 Denne Parade, Horsham, West Sussex RH12 IJD
Tel. 01403 210202

BHAN (Black HIV/AIDS Network)
111 Devonport Road, London W12 8PB
Tel. 0181 749 2828
Counselling in Hindi, Urdu, Gujerati, Punjabi and Kiswahili. Counselling can also be arranged in other Middle Eastern and Far Eastern languages.

Blackliners
Unit 46, Eurolink Business Centre, 49 Effra Road, London SW2 1BZ
or
100 Shepherdess Walk, London N1 7JM
Tel. 0171 738 7468 (Administration); 0171 738 5274 (Helpline)
Support for African, Caribbean and Asian people.

Body Positive
51b Philbeach Gardens, London SW5 9EB
Tel. 0171 835 1045 (Office); 0171 373 9124 (Helpline)
Body Positive provides support, counselling and advice for people who are HIV positive, also will provide details of Body Positive groups and services nationwide.

Department of Health
Head of Communicable Diseases Branch, Wellington House, 133–155 Waterloo Road, London SE1 8UG
Tel. 0171 972 4020
Responsible for integrating HIV and AIDS into the mainstream of health care and health promotion. Publish leaflets offering occupational guidance to health care professionals.

Health Education Authority
Hamilton House, Mabledon Place, London WC1 9TX
Tel. 0171 383 3833

Provide a wide range of publications for professionals. Leaflets and posters can be ordered from local Health Promotion Units and a complete publications catalogue and ordering service is available from the HEA.

International Planned Parenthood Federation (IPPF)
Sexual Health Project, PO Box 759, Inner Circle, Regent's Park, London NW1 4NS
Tel. 0171 487 7933
Promotes sexuality awareness and sexual health among the family planning associations who form the IPPF.

London Lighthouse
111–117 Lancaster Road, London W11 1QT
Tel. 0171 792 1200
Centre for people affected by HIV and AIDS, including support groups and residential care.

National AIDS Helpline (all Freephone)
0800 567 123 (24 hours)
0800 555 777 for free copies of leaflets
0800 521 361 minicom for hearing impaired (10 am–10 pm)
0800 282 445 Bengali, Gujerati, Hindi, Punjabi, Urdu and English (Tues 6–10 pm)
0800 282 446 Cantonese and English (Tues 6–10 pm)
0800 282 447 Arabic and English (Weds 6–10 pm)

Positively Women
5 Sebastian Street, London EC1V 0HE
Tel. 0171 490 5501 (Office); 0171 490 2327 (Helpline)
Provides a range of free and confidential counselling and support services for women with HIV and AIDS.

Scottish AIDS Monitor
26 Aderson Place, Edinburgh EH6 5NP
Tel. 0131 555 4850
Scottish AIDS Monitor also provides a full range of advice, information and support services.

Terence Higgins Trust
52–54 Grays Inn Road, London WC1X 8JU
Tel. 0171 831 0330; 0171 242 1010 (Helpline); 0171 405 2381 (Legal line) (Mon and Weds 7–9 pm)
Practical support, help, counselling and advice for people with or people concerned about AIDS.

The Herpes Association
41 North Road, London N7 9DP

Tel. 0171 609 9061
Offers support to herpes sufferers and provides information sheets.

The Women's Group
PO Box 201, Manchester M60 1PU
Tel. 0161 839 4340
Support group for HIV-positive women in the northwest of England.

Further reading

For nurses

BARTER, G., BARTON, S. and GAZZARD, B. (1993) *HIV and AIDS – Your Questions Answered*. Edinburgh: Churchill Livingstone.

CSONKA, G.W. and OATES, J.K. (eds) (1990) *A Textbook of Genitourinary Medicine*. London: Baillière Tindall.

CURTIS, H., HOOLAGHAN, T. and JEWITT, C. (eds) (1995) *Sexual Health Promotion in General Practice*. Oxford and New York: Radcliffe Medical Press.

EDGE, V. and MILLER, M. (1994) *Women's Health Care*. Mosby's Clinical Nursing Series. St Louis: Mosby.

ILETT, R. (1993) *Women and HIV/AIDS: a bibliography*. Glasgow Women's Library.

PRATT, R. (1995) *HIV and AIDS. A Strategy for Nursing Care*, 4th edn. London: Edward Arnold

For clients

BRODMAN, M., THACKER, J. and KRANZ, R. (1993) *Straight Talk About . . . Sexually Transmitted Diseases*. Facts on File. New York: Facts on File Inc.

KNOX, H. (1995) *SEXPlained . . . The uncensored guide to sexual health*. London: Knox Publishing.

MAIN, J., MOYLE, G., PETERS, B. and COKER, R. (eds) (1995) *What We Should All Know About HIV and AIDS*. London: Mediscript.

NORTHRUP, C. (1995) *Women's Bodies Women's Wisdom*. London: Piatkus.

PHILLIPS, A. and RAKUSEN, J. (1989) *The New Our Bodies, Ourselves, A Health Book by Women and For Women*. Harmondsworth: Penguin.

RICHARDSON, D. (1989) *Women and the AIDS Crisis*. London: Pandora Press.

References

ADLER, M.W. (1990) *ABC of Sexually Transmitted Diseases*, 2nd edn. British Medical Journal

ANDRIST, L.C. (1988) Taking a sexual history and educating clients about safer sex. *Nursing Clinics of North America* 23(4): 959–73.

ARYA, O.P., OSOBA, A.O. and BENNETT, F.J. (1980) *Tropical Venereology*. Edinburgh: Churchill Livingstone.

AUSTOKER, J. (1988) AIDS and homosexuality in Britain: a historical perspective. In Adler, M.W. (ed.) *Diseases in the Homosexual Male*. Berlin: Springer-Verlag, pp. 185–97.

BAKER, D.A. (1995) Management of the female HIV-infected patient. *AIDS Patient Care* April: 78–81.

BAYER, R. (1994) Ethical challenges posed by zidovudine treatment to reduce vertical transmission of HIV. *New England Journal of Medicine* 331(18): 1223–25.

BLAKEY, V. (1991) Promoting sexual health: strategies for reaching and empowering women. In Curtis, H. (ed.) *Promoting Sexual Health*. London: Health Education Authority, pp. 87–95.

BOR, R. and WATTS, M. (1993) Talking to patients about sexual matters. *British Journal of Nursing* 2(13): 657–61.

BOSTON WOMEN'S HEALTH BOOK COLLECTIVE (1985) *The New Our Bodies, Ourselves*. New York: Simon & Schuster.

BOWMAN, C. (1994) Perspectives on HPV. *British Journal of Sexual Medicine* May/June: 24–25.

BRESLIN, E. (1988) Genital herpes simplex. *Nursing Clinics of North America* 23(4): 907–15.

CARNEY, O., ROSS, E., BUNKER, C., IKKOS, G. and MINDEL, A. (1994) A prospective study of the psychological impact on patients with a first episode of genital herpes. *Genitourinary Medicine* 70: 40–45.

CATTERALL, R.D. (1983) The British service for patients with sexually transmitted diseases. *Health Trends* 15: 82–85.

CONNOR, E.M., SPERLING, R.S. GELGER, R. *et al.* (1994) Reduction of maternal–infant transmission of human immunodeficiency virus type I with zidovudine treatment. *New England Journal of Medicine* 331(18): 1174–79.

COREY, L. (1990) Genital herpes. In Holmes, K.K., Mardh, P.A., Sparling, P.F. *et al.* (eds) *Sexually Transmitted Diseases*. New York: McGraw-Hill.

DAVERNPORT-HINES, R. (1990) *Sex, Death and Punishment*. London: Fontana Press.

DOH (Department of Health) (1992) *The Health of the Nation*. London: HMSO.

EASMON, C.S.F. (1993) *The Diagnosis and Management of Bacterial Vaginosis*. London: Royal Society of Medicine.

EUROPEAN COLLABORATIVE STUDY (1991) Children born to women with HIV-1 infection: natural history and risk of transmission. *Lancet* 337: 253–58.

FLANIGAN, T.P. and CARPENTER, C.C.J. (1994) HIV infection in women: review and recommendations. In Daniels, V.G. (ed.) *The AIDS Letter* no. 40 London: Royal Society of Medicine.

FRENCH, P. (1995) The Clinic Guide (Unpublished). Mortimer Market Centre, Mortimer Market (off Capper Street), London WC1E 6AU.

GAMLIN, L. (1988) The human immune system. *New Scientist*, 10 March.

GLENN, P.S.F., NANCE-SPRONSON, L.E. McCARTNEY, M. and YESALIS, C.E. (1991) Attitudes toward AIDS among a low-risk group of women. *Journal of Obstetric and Gynecological Neonate Nursing* 20(5): 398–405.

GODLEY, M.J. (1993) The management of sexually transmitted diseases in pregnancy. *Medicine International* 21(3): 74–81.

GOH, B.T. and FORSTER, G.E. (1993) Sexually transmitted diseases in children: chlamydial oculo-genital infection. *Genitourinary Medicine* 69: 213–21.

HALL, J. (1993) Management of genital ulceration in general practice. *British Journal of Sexual Medicine*, May/June.

HILLIER, S. and HOLMES, K.K. (1990) Bacterial vaginosis. In Holmes, K.K., Mardh, P.A., Sparling, P.F. *et al.* (eds) *Sexually Transmitted Diseases*. New York: McGraw-Hill.

HORTON, R. (1995) Women as women with HIV. *Lancet* **345**: 531–32.

HOWE, J.E., MINKOFF, H.L. and DUERR, A.C. (1994) Contraceptives and HIV. *AIDS* 8(7): 861–67.

ISON, C.A. (1993) The aetiology of bacterial vaginosis. In Easmon, C.S.F. (ed.) *The Diagnosis and Management of Bacterial Vaginosis*. London: Royal Society of Medicine.

JOHNSON, A.M. (1992) Epidemiology of HIV infection in women. *Baillière's Clinical Obstetrics and Gynaecology* **6** (1).

LARSEN, S.A., HUNTER, E.F. and CREIGHTON, E.T. (1990) Syphilis. In Holmes, K.K., Mardh, P.A. Sparling, P.F. *et al.* (eds) *Sexually Transmitted Diseases*. New York: McGraw-Hill.

LUCAS, V.A. (1998) Human papillomavirus infection: a potentially carcinogenic sexually transmitted disease (condylomata acuminata, genital warts). *Nursing Clinics of North America* 23(4): 917–31.

LURIE, P., HINTON, P. and LOWE, R. A. (1995) Socioeconomic obstacles to HIV prevention and treatment in developing countries: the roles of the International Monetary Fund and the World Bank. *AIDS* 9(6): 539–44.

MASFARI, A.N., DUERDEN, B.I. and KINGHORN, G. R. (1986) Quantitative studies of vaginal bacteria. *Genitourinary Medicine* **62**: 256–63.

MERCEY, D. (1992) Clinical audit in genitourinary medicine 'Why, Who, What, How and When?' *Genitourinary Medicine* **68**: 205–6.

MINDEL, A. and ADLER, M.W. (1984) *Genital Herpes, A Review*. Aldershot: Gower Medical Publishing.

MOHANTY, K.C. (1989) Gonorrhoea. *British Journal of Sexual Medicine* May: 206–7.

MOHANTY, K.C. (1990) Trichomoniasis. *British Journal of Sexual Medicine* July: 210–12.

MOK, J.Y.O. (1992) Vertical transmission. *Baillière's Clinical Obstetrics and Gynaecology* 6(1): 85–99.

MUNDAY, P.E. (1990) Genitourinary medicine services; consumers' views. *Genitourinary Medicine* 66: 108–11.

ORIEL, J. D. (1978) Genitourinary medicine? *British Journal of Venereal Diseases* **54**: 291–94.

ROBERTSON, D. H. H., McMILLAN, A. and YOUNG, H. (1989) *Clinical Practice in Sexually Transmitted Diseases*. Edinburgh: Churchill Livingstone.

ROMANOWSKI, B. (1993) Sexually transmitted diseases in women: symptoms and examination. *Medicine International* 21(3): 82–86.

SCHNEIDER, A. (1993) Pathogenesis of genital HPV infection. *Genitourinary Medicine* **69**: 165–73.

SILEBI, M.I. (1995) Case management of the perinatal patient with HIV infection. *AIDS Patient Care* April: 82–84.

SOBEL, J.D. (1990) Vulvovaginal candidiasis. In Holmes, K.K., Mardh, P.A., Sparling, P.F. *et al.*, (eds) *Sexually Transmitted Diseases*. New York: McGraw-Hill.

SPARLING, P.F. (1990) Biology of *Neisseria gonorrhoeae*. In Holmes, K.K., Mardh, P.A., Sparling, P.F. *et al.*, (eds) *Sexually Transmitted Diseases*. New York: McGraw-Hill.

TEARE, E.L. (1986) How to . . . diagnose and treat chlamydial infections. *British Journal of Sexual Medicine* January: 20–22.

THIN, R.N. (1982) *Lecture Notes on Sexually Transmitted Diseases*. Oxford: Blackwell Scientific.

TILLMAN, J. (1991) Syphilis an old disease, a contemporary perinatal problem. *Journal of Obstetric and Gynecological Neonate Nursing* 21(3): 209–13.

TINKLE, M.B. (1990) Genital human papillomavirus infection a growing health risk. *Journal of Obstetric and Gynecological Neonate Nursing* 19(6): 501–7.

WHITTAKER, D. (1993) 'In The Room' – Invisible Work and Hidden Experiences of Women Nurses and Women Patients in a Genito-Urinary Medicine Clinic: An Exploratory Study (Unpublished). Mortimer Market Centre, Mortimer Market (off Capper Street), London WC1E 6AU.

WHO (1995) Sexually transmitted diseases: three hundred and thirty-three million new curable cases in 1995. Press Release WHO/64. Geneva: World Health Organization.

WOOLLEY, P. (1993) Promoting sexual health in general practice. *British Journal of Sexual Medicine* November/December: 4–5.

13: Premenstrual syndrome
Gilly Andrews

OBJECTIVES

After reading this chapter you will understand:

♦ some of the theories about the possible causes of PMS

♦ the variety of symptoms and the devastating effect that severe PMS can have on a woman's life

♦ how to recognize and help to diagnose when a woman is suffering from PMS rather than a psychiatric problem

♦ how to advise a PMS sufferer to help herself to overcome the problem

♦ the different treatment options available for severe PMS.

Introduction

Premenstrual syndrome (PMS) is a topical and controversial issue, with increasing interest in the subject both in medical journals and in women's magazines, which frequently have articles debating and explaining this complex topic. Yet in spite of all this many doctors still refuse to believe that PMS exists and it can be extremely difficult for some women to find understanding and supportive advice for a problem that she feels is ruining her life – not only her personal and social relationships but also in her work environment.

Too often sufferers will hear negative comments such as: 'It is all part of being a woman'. 'It's that time of the month again – ignore it and you will feel better in a few days' time' or 'Pull yourself together'. Such remarks and lack of advice and understanding only serve to isolate women even further in their misery and despair – many feel that they have a real psychiatric illness and are terrified that they 'are going mad'. Even worse, some women will have been given the wrong treatment which can be more harmful than no treatment at all.

Attitudes towards PMS are slowly changing as women take an active and positive role in trying to understand health issues which affect their life. This chapter will give you an insight into this bewildering and occasionally frightening disorder so that you will be able to help and counsel female clients who ask for your advice.

Historical perspective

Premenstrual syndrome is frequently thought of as a twentieth-century disorder that the modern woman has 'invented' in order to provide a convenient excuse for occasions when she does not live up to her own lifestyle expectations. However, Hippocrates in 460 BC observed that 'women are subjected to intermittent "agitations" and as a result the "agitated" blood finds its way from the head to the uterus whence it is expelled'. He also noticed that 'shivering, lassitude and heaviness of the head denote the onset of menstruation' (Chadwick and Mann, 1950). The fact that this correlation of psychological symptoms with menstruation was observed and written about two and a half thousand years ago contradicts the suggestion that premenstrual syndrome is a disease of the twentieth century.

Nevertheless, it was not until 1931 that the term 'premenstrual tension' was used when Frank published a description of a small group of women who had symptoms of tension, depression, headaches and weight gain for 7–10 days before menstruation. Greene and Dalton in 1953 first used the term 'premenstrual syndrome' when they recognized and wrote about the wide range of symptoms which may occur with the menstrual cycle. Premenstrual syndrome (PMS) is the term which is now more generally accepted.

Over four decades later, despite considerable scientific and medical research, we are little further forward in understanding the disorder. There is confusion and disagreement in the medical profession over the definition of PMS, its causes, the diagnostic criteria and the best methods of treatment. The American Psychiatric Society (APA) says that PMS is a psychiatric disorder and have renamed it 'late luteal phase dysphoric disorder'. It is hardly surprising, therefore, that women who suffer from premenstrual syndrome often find it extremely difficult to obtain information, advice and help for their symptoms when doctors cannot agree amongst themselves.

Definition

The World Health Organization does not recognize premenstrual syndrome as an illness and consequently there is no WHO definition. Reading through medical and nursing journals you will come across numerous definitions which can only add to your confusion in trying to understand the disorder. The diverse nature of PMS symptoms necessitates a definition broad enough to cover the variability of symptoms which will also vary from cycle to cycle in individual women in their severity, timing and duration.

A logical definition of PMS by Magos and Studd (1984) is 'distressing physical, psychological and behavioural symptoms not caused by organic disease which regularly recur during the same phase of the ovarian (or menstrual) cycle, and which significantly regress or disappear during the remainder of the cycle'. It is the repetitive cyclical nature, not the type of symptoms, which is important to the definition and diagnosis of premenstrual syndrome. More recently, Reid (1991) has in addition stressed that the severity of symptoms is important. Many women suffer premenstrual symptoms but in most cases they are mild. It is only a minority of women whose symptoms are of such extreme severity to interfere with function, and it is only this latter group who should be said to suffer from PMS.

Some researchers have tried to classify PMS into different subgroups (Abraham, 1980) but these 'subtypes' are often arbitrary and women report their own unique combinations of symptoms.

Menstruation itself is not necessarily a prerequisite of the diagnosis, as cyclical symptoms may continue to occur following hysterectomy if the ovaries have been conserved (Backstrom *et al.*, 1981). This condition would be better termed 'ovarian cycle syndrome' and women who suffer from it may not realize what their problem is, as they have no outwardly visible signs (i.e. menstruation) which would signal a relief of their distressing symptoms. Consequently they often suffer many months and even years of cyclical symptoms following a hysterectomy without realizing that their problem is identical with premenstrual syndrome. Once diagnosed, the treatment of these women is very straightforward.

Incidence

Although PMS has been described as 'one of the world's commonest diseases' the true prevalence is difficult to assess. This is mainly due to the wide differences in the definition and diagnostic criteria.

Up to 90% of women are aware of some body changes or symptoms during the fourth week of their menstrual cycle, which forewarn them of the imminent start of their period. These changes are mild and may only consist of a slight increase in breast tenderness. True PMS is said to affect approximately 40% of women, with about 5–10% so severely incapacitated that it dominates their life during this phase of the cycle (Reid and Yen, 1981). This means that a GP with an average

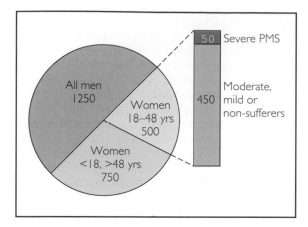

Figure 13.1 *Approximately 50 women in a practice list of 2500 may have severe pre-menstrual syndrome.*

number of 2500 patients might expect between 25 and 50 women to have severe PMS (Figure 13.1).

PMS is no respecter of class. Although Snowden and Christian (1984) in a WHO global study of patterns and perception of menstruation suggest that PMS is a phenomenon of Western 'civilized' society, other studies have found PMS to be just as prevalent in Third World countries when its existence is specifically sought out (Shershah *et al.*, 1991). Age, parity, race, socio-economic groups and familial predisposition are thought likely to have distinct effects on the incidence of PMS but studies show conflicting results.

A young person's attitude to her periods develops from those who first introduced her to menstruation, e.g. her mother or her teacher. If their outlook viewed menstruation in a negative way and if a young woman has been told since childhood that PMS exists and has experienced these problems at first hand with her mother, then the daughter will expect that time of the month to be dreadful. It is a self-fulfilling prophesy.

Nowadays the average age for puberty is 12 years, and for the menopause 51 years. An average woman may thus expect to have over 450 menstrual cycles in her life, with only short breaks for pregnancy and breastfeeding. If she is adversely affected during the premenstrual phase of her cycle, even for only two or three days a month, it can be seen that PMS can create a significant problem throughout her life.

Changes in social structure during the twentieth century and contemporary lifestyle expecta-

tions means that the modern woman, who is frequently trying to juggle the varied demands of a job, alongside those of being a wife, lover, mother and carer, is no longer prepared to tolerate symptoms which result in her feeling less than at her best. Attitudes differ though and an ardent feminist has said 'you can't have equality and PMS!'

Symptoms and effects

The symptoms of PMS are less frequent during the early reproductive years, tend to become progressively worse with age and then merge with similar climacteric symptoms as the menopause approaches. Symptoms are frequently said to start after stopping the oral contraceptive pill or following a pregnancy. The severity of the symptoms may fluctuate from cycle to cycle but the type of symptoms will usually remain constant.

The symptoms of premenstrual syndrome are numerous – over 150 different symptoms have been recorded in research literature (Moos, 1969). Unfortunately PMS symptoms are so diverse and are also symptoms of other disorders, which can be experienced by both men and postmenopausal women, that this can often lead to difficulties when trying to make a diagnosis.

Magos and Studd in 1985 wrote about the effects of the menstrual cycle on medical disorders and noted that the severity of symptoms of over 160 medical conditions fluctuated with the menstrual cycle. You might find it helpful to enquire whether any of your female patients with pre-existing medical conditions such as asthma, epilepsy, migraine, rheumatoid arthritis and herpes find that these conditions worsen during the premenstrual phase of their cycle and then be able to give advice and reassure them of the cyclical nature of their symptoms.

PMS symptoms are numerous and diverse and almost any system of the body can be affected. Symptoms are often broadly classified into three categories and women may often have a mixture of symptoms from each group:

♦ Physical

♦ Psychological

♦ Behavioural.

Physical symptoms

Typical physical symptoms are listed in Box 13.1. The common symptoms of bloating, fluid retention and mastalgia cause the uncomfortable *sensation* of weight gain, but the majority of women show no demonstrable premenstrual weight increase. Interestingly some PMS sufferers clearly experience an altered perception of body image premenstrually, which may at least partially explain this (Faratian *et al.*, 1984). There is possibly a redistribution of body fluids rather than fluid retention which could account for these differences. Such symptoms cause considerable distress to many PMS sufferers who often have to wear looser, more comfortable clothes and a larger and more supportive bra. One woman describes her wardrobe as her 'normal clothes' and her 'fat clothes'. Wald *et al.* (1981) showed that gastrointestinal transit time is significantly increased during the luteal phase of the cycle when there is an increase in progesterone levels which inhibit the smooth muscle of the gut. This will then give rise to constipation, gaseous distension and the sensation of being bloated.

Box 13.1 Typical physical symptoms of PMS

♦ Breast tenderness and swelling

♦ Abdominal bloating

♦ Peripheral oedema

♦ Headaches and migraine

♦ Hot flushes

♦ Dizziness

♦ Palpitations

♦ Visual disturbances

♦ Pelvic discomfort

♦ Altered bowel habits

♦ Appetite changes or cravings

♦ Nausea

♦ Acne or skin blemishes

♦ Reduced coordination.

The impression of putting on weight premenstrually is in itself very depressing and the effect can be devastating for those who are on a diet. Many women experience cravings for certain types of food in the few days before their period. These cravings may be for unusual, highly savoury meals but, more frequently are for sweet, high-carbohydrate snacks such as bread, cakes, chocolate and fizzy drinks. Women who are normally vigilant about their diet and weight often find their willpower will suddenly desert them and can munch through one or two bars of chocolate. Whether these are genuine cravings or whether women eat because they are feeling miserable and food is a great comforter is a point that is difficult to determine. As a result of their extra eating and cravings they consequently feel more bloated and fat and this makes them even more miserable – a vicious circle!

Scenario

Jenny, a fitness instructor, who is normally conscientious to the point of being fastidious about her diet, found her willpower deserted her in her premenstrual week and she craved highly flavoured crisps and salted nuts. These salty foods then made her want to drink plenty of fluids and she then felt bloated, obese and miserable. She would then push herself even harder during her exercise classes to try and offset the effects of her cravings – making her feel even more guilty and miserable.

Some PMS sufferers complain of headaches during the premenstrual phase of their cycle. These headaches can vary from mild diffuse pain to a classic migraine associated with nausea, vomiting, visual disturbances and a blinding unilateral headache. Headaches and migraine are unpredictable in whether they respond to treatment and how long they last. You should advise all women who present with headaches as part of their PMS problems to take appropriate analgesia at the first symptoms so that an ordinary headache does not develop into a full-blown migraine.

Clumsiness and lack of coordination can increase premenstrually and some women drop and break crockery, cut themselves on knives, burn themselves whilst cooking and continually bump into furniture. It is tempting to assume that these women are normally clumsy, uncoordinated and accident-prone throughout the month but this is not the case. Perhaps this clumsiness is caused by a lack of concentration when women feel edgy and tense premenstrually? Women who play a lot of sports find their coordination and concentration is lacking, and they frequently get angry and aggressive both towards themselves and their opponents.

Psychological symptoms

Many women find the psychological manifestations of premenstrual syndrome the hardest group of symptoms to tolerate as they often feel totally out of control, and are completely bewildered by their own behaviour. Colleagues, friends and relatives offer kindness and understanding for physical problems such as headaches and breast tenderness but rarely give sympathy and support for symptoms of depression, mood swings, irritability and tension.

The most common psychological symptoms are listed in Box 13.2.

Box 13.2 Common psychological symptoms of PMS

♦ Tension

♦ Irritability

♦ Depression

♦ Mood swings

♦ Anxiety

♦ Restlessness

♦ Lethargy

♦ Lack of libido

♦ Lack of concentration.

Women or their partners will frequently complain of a 'Jekyll and Hyde' personality. A woman who is normally even-tempered and calm may find that some small and trivial incident can completely upset her equilibrium and she can rapidly lose her temper and become bad tempered and aggressive. This is frequently followed by feelings of guilt and tearfulness at her own unreasonable behaviour and occasionally she might even develop suicidal ideas.

Scenario

Alice and John came to a specialist PMS clinic together for the first time. This was the third appointment that Alice had been sent as she had failed to attend on two previous occasions. Alice explained that she missed these appointments as they had coincided with times when she was not premenstrual and she was feeling very positive about herself and felt in control of her PMS. This third clinic appointment was also at such a time but John insisted that both he and Alice should attend as he was finding it very difficult to cope with Alice who suffered violent mood swings and he occasionally feared for the safety of their six-year-old twins. Twice in the past week he had come home from work and found the children on their own. On one occasion the children were left alone in the kitchen with a broken glass all over the floor which Alice had dropped when they had been naughty. The second time he had arrived home to find that Alice felt that she could not cope any longer with the boys and had just walked out, leaving them to cope on their own for over two hours.

John was very keen to relate how dreadful the situation was becoming and how important it was for Alice to get some expert help. He was anxious that as this third clinic appointment coincided yet again with a postmenstrual phase that Alice would not explain how desperate the situation was at home. Alice was treated with oestrogen therapy and within three months was virtually back to a more even-tempered disposition. John later said that if she had not received treatment when she did, that he could see that their marriage was in imminent danger of breaking up. John, needless to say, was delighted with the result.

Eighteen months later John again attended the clinic with Alice – she had forgotten how bad she had been with her premenstrual mood swings and was intending to see how she could manage without treatment. John was very keen for her to continue as he really feared for the safety of the twins and for the future of their marriage if she reverted back to her aggressive mood swings.

Leather *et al.* (1993a) in a study of 100 women found that PMS influenced most daily activities but the greatest effect was felt in the home.

Table 13.1 *Effect of PMS on lifestyle in 100 women with PMS*

	Not applicable	Number affected	Severely affected (%)
WORK PERFORMANCE	14	80	27.5
WORK RELATIONSHIPS	23	70	22.1
HOUSEHOLD CHORES	1	97	45.5
RELATIONSHIP WITH PARTNER	6	93	82.8
RELATIONSHIP WITH CHILDREN	22	77	61.0
SOCIAL RELATIONSHIPS	2	94	41.5

Relationships with their partner were severely affected in 82% of PMS sufferers, and 61% said their relationships with their children were also severely affected. Fortunately, women seem more able to control their mood swings and anger at work with only 22% saying that their work relationships were severely affected (Table 13.1).

Clare (1983) found that women presenting with premenstrual syndrome are more likely to complain of intrapersonal conflicts and marital disharmony, and that they also have high anxiety levels. Laws (1985) suggests that women focus on the complaints of premenstrual syndrome instead of acknowledging and dealing with existing problems such as stressful relationships or adverse circumstances. Therefore in dealing with women who claim to have PMS it is important for you to distinguish between those who have genuine PMS and those who are just 'complaining' and unhappy about their stressful situations.

It is also important to distinguish women who have premenstrual syndrome from those with a psychiatric disorder whose symptoms are not related to the ovarian endocrine cycle. Failure to make these two distinctions can lead to inappropriate and ineffective treatment. However, women with depression or underlying psychiatric disorders will often experience a premenstrual exacerbation of their symptoms (Halbreich *et al.*, 1983) which can be severe enough to warrant admission to a psychiatric hospital.

Behavioural symptoms

A wide range of behavioural changes are reported to increase during the premenstrual phase. These include agoraphobia, absenteeism from work, loss of concentration and work performance and avoidance of social activities (Moos, 1969). Accidents, alcoholic binges, criminal behaviour (Dalton, 1961), suicide attempts and psychiatric admissions (Glass *et al.*, 1971) all seem to occur more frequently during the premenstrual phase.

PMS and its behavioural symptoms have occasionally been used as a defence in criminal proceedings. This obviously has important legal implications since although many of these prosecutions may be for minor offences, the issue has occasionally been raised during trials for murder or manslaughter. In the absence of agreement within the medical profession as to a definition of PMS, it is difficult for the legal profession to know how to proceed on this.

It is your professional duty to try and ensure that a genuine sufferer from premenstrual syndrome receives the help and treatment she needs rather than a criminal record. You also have to ensure that the plea of PMS is not abused by those who do not suffer from the problem.

Scenario

Lesley, a 44-year-old housewife, had been seeing her doctor for the past two years complaining of increasing premenstrual symptoms. Her doctor had tried Lesley on a variety of tranquillizers and antidepressants but basically told her 'it was a woman's lot'. Lesley felt her premenstrual behaviour was becoming increasingly out of control and after a particularly tearful session with her GP she was eventually referred to a specialist PMS clinic. Unfortunately the week before her first appointment she stole a pair of woollen gloves from a department store, an item she clearly did

not need as it was the middle of summer and she had plenty of money in her purse. The store had a policy of prosecuting shoplifters and Lesley wondered if the clinic would write a letter to the court confirming that she suffered from PMS and was premenstrual when the crime was committed.

Positive symptoms

PMS is not necessarily all about distressing symptoms and bad news. Logue and Moos (1988) found that between 5 and 15% of women actually feel better during the premenstrual phase of the cycle. They reported an increase in well-being, energy and confidence. Libido is also said to improve during this phase as testosterone levels rise premenstrually.

Scenario

 Jane, a 28-year-old advertising executive, found that she was at her most dynamic and resourceful in the week leading up to her period. She would find a tremendous surge of energy and enthusiasm, often clearing her desk of all the paperwork that had been accumulating over the past three weeks. She got her best creative ideas for work during this phase and due to an increased libido and sex drive her relationship with her partner was also at its best.

Causes of PMS

Numerous theories have been put forward to explain why PMS occurs (Box 13.3) but as yet, the precise cause remains unknown despite extensive research. Psychological, endocrine, social, environmental and dietary theories have been widely investigated and extensively reviewed in the medical literature (O'Brien, 1987; Sampson, 1989) but none of these hypotheses have been proved to be solely relevant.

Progesterone deficiency has been the most fashionable theory for many years, but there is no evidence of such a deficiency, or that it causes PMS. Studies demonstrate contradictory and varying levels of progesterone between patients

Box 13.3   Possible causes of PMS
♦ Psychological
♦ Progesterone deficiency
♦ Oestrogen/progesterone imbalance
♦ Sodium and water retention
♦ Prostaglandin deficiency/excess
♦ Prolactin excess
♦ Vitamin B_6 deficiency
♦ Trace element deficiency
♦ Hypoglycaemia
♦ Thyroid abnormality
♦ Serotonin deficiency.

and controls (Backstrom and Carstensen, 1974; O'Brien *et al.*, 1980). This is hardly surprising since the secretion of progesterone is pulsatile and occasional blood sampling will fail to detect the subtle differences that were thought to exist.

Recent research has indicated that a central neurotransmitter abnormality is suggested by reduced platelet uptake of serotonin and reduced peripheral blood serotonin levels in PMS sufferers during the luteal phase of the cycle (Menkes *et al.*, 1992; Sundblad *et al.*, 1992).

The symptomatology of PMS in many women bears a close resemblance to that of depression. This has led to the theory that PMS is a form of cyclical depression which has become 'entrained' to the menstrual cycle. That is, the hormonal changes themselves do not cause PMS, but merely act as a cue for an independently cycling primary depressive disorder (Schmidt *et al.*, 1991).

The best information that we have at present is that there is an obvious link between PMS and cyclical ovarian activity (Studd, 1979) as symptoms only occur between puberty and the menopause. They disappear during anovulatory cycles and pregnancy, yet persist after hysterectomy if the ovaries have been conserved (Backstrom *et al.*, 1981). If ovarian function is completely suppressed by gonadotrophin-releasing hormone analogues or by bilateral oophorectomy then PMS symptoms will disappear. This does not mean that the primary abnormality is in the ovaries – it could lie anywhere in the hypothalamo-pituitary-ovarian (HPO) axis or in the higher centres that influence this HPO axis. This association with ovarian function is not in conflict with a central neurotransmitter theory of the cause of PMS, as there is increasing evidence that ovarian hormones can influence neurotransmitter function (Guicheney *et al.*, 1988).

Considerable research has been conducted and numerous papers written on all the above hypotheses but there is no real evidence that any of them explains the true cause of PMS. Although researchers have been keen to find one particular reason for PMS it is more probable that there are several factors and PMS is probably a combination of physiological, psychological and social factors that interact with life events.

Diagnosis

Correct diagnosis is essential for the successful treatment of PMS. Unfortunately, there are no universally agreed objective diagnostic criteria for PMS and no biological markers, such as blood tests, which can be used to confirm a diagnosis. Many 'informed' women have read that PMS is caused by a hormone imbalance and so will often demand a 'hormone measurement test'. Such tests are useless in diagnosing premenstrual syndrome but can be more appropriately used in excluding other disorders which might be causing similar symptoms, e.g. anaemia, hypothyroidism, polycystic ovarian disease and the peri-menopause.

A full menstrual, contraceptive, gynaecological and obstetric history should be obtained. Women should be asked when they first noticed symptoms of PMS and if these symptoms were absent during pregnancy. The onset of PMS has often been linked to starting or stopping the contraceptive pill, the birth of a child or sterilization.

As mentioned earlier, symptoms can vary from cycle to cycle. It is important to find out what type of symptoms the woman is complaining of (both positive and negative), when these start in relation to the onset of menstruation and how quickly they resolve after bleeding has commenced. Some women might have minor symptoms for a day or two which they can easily cope with, whilst others have symptoms which start at ovulation and become progressively more severe during the next 14 days until menstruation starts. If they then also suffer from menorrhagia and dysmenorrhoea these women, unfortunately, do not have many 'good' days in a month.

The contribution of any underlying psychological disease and previous psychiatric history should also be taken into account – although in practice this can be difficult to determine. Many self-assessment questionnaires, visual analogue scales and menstrual diaries have been introduced in an attempt to make it easy for the woman and her doctor to assess whether she suffers from premenstrual syndrome (Box 13.4).

> **Box 13.4** Menstrual Distress Questionnaire
> The 'Menstrual Distress Questionnaire', developed by Moos in 1968 is widely used to assess symptoms on a daily basis. It consists of 47 symptoms divided into eight symptom clusters:
>
> ◆ Pain
>
> ◆ Concentration
>
> ◆ Behavioural change
>
> ◆ Autonomic reactions
>
> ◆ Water retention
>
> ◆ Negative effect
>
> ◆ Arousal
>
> ◆ Control
>
> The eighth 'control' group consists of six symptoms not normally associated with the menstrual cycle and is included to help to identify 'complainers'. Women are asked to complete the chart every evening for two or three cycles scoring their symptoms on a scale of 0–3 (0 = none, 1 = slightly, 2 = moderately, 3 = a lot). They are also asked to chart when they start and stop bleeding. An adaptation of this menstrual questionnaire is shown in Box 13.5.

When symptom assessment charts are analysed after two or three cycles it is readily apparent whether a woman is suffering from the cyclical symptoms of PMS, or perhaps has some other underlying physical or psychiatric disorder which is present throughout the month.

Management of PMS

Numerous approaches and treatments for PMS have been advocated since Frank first described premenstrual tension over six decades ago. The fact that so many treatments are available suggests

Box 13.5 Symptom assessment chart for use in the Menstrual Distress Questionnaire

Name: . . . .

Please complete every evening.

Describe how you felt during the day, scoring each symptom from 0–3: 0 = none; 1 = slight; 2 = moderate; 3 = a lot.

If applicable, indicate days of period with a 'p'.		Mon	Tue	Wed	Thu	Fri	Sat	Sun
Pain	Muscle stiffness							
	Stomach pains/cramps							
	Backache							
	Tiredness							
	General aches/pains							
Concentration	Difficulty sleeping							
	Forgetfulness							
	Confusion							
	Difficulty concentrating							
	Clumsiness							
	Accidents, e.g. cutting finger							
	Difficulty making decisions							
Behavioural Changes	Lowered work performance							
	Taking naps, staying in bed							
	Staying at home from work							
	Avoid social activities							
	Loss of efficiency							
Autonomic Reactions	Dizziness or faintness							
	Cold sweats							
	Feeling sick/vomiting							
	Hot flushes							
Water Retention	Weight gain							
	Skin disorders (spots, rash)							
	Painful or swollen breasts							
	Feeling swollen/bloated							
Negative Effect	Crying spells							
	Loneliness							
	Anxiety							
	Restlessness							
	Irritability							
	Mood swings							
	Depression							
	Tension							
Arousal	Feeling affectionate							
	Orderliness							
	Excitement							
	Feelings of well-being							
	Bursts of energy/activity							
Control	Feelings of suffocation							
	Chest pains							
	Ringing in the ears							
	Heart pounding							
	Numbness, tingling							

that the majority of them are ineffective, and confirms that researchers are no further forward in understanding the aetiology of PMS or the treatment of the condition. Harrison (1982) says it is the *woman* with PMS who should be treated rather than the PMS itself.

Hallman (1986) estimated that only 7.5% of women with PMS seek the advice of a doctor. This means that the vast majority of women will try many different approaches and self-help remedies in order to obtain help and relief from their cyclical symptoms.

All women can be helped by simple, straightforward discussion and counselling with advice regarding diet, stress avoidance and their general lifestyle. It is difficult to find an effective drug therapy for mild to moderate symptoms and thus the treatment for this grade of PMS is often unsatisfactory. It is a paradox that women who have severe PMS are easier to treat than those who suffer from mild to moderate PMS. This is because severe symptoms can have such a disruptive effect on women's lives that they are willing to try more active intervention by suppressing the ovarian cycle.

Whatever the method used to manage PMS, it is important to realize that the syndrome demonstrates a *high placebo response rate*. This rate has been reported to be as high as 94% (Magos *et al.*, 1986) although the generally agreed figure is nearer 50%. Some studies have shown that the placebo response has been more marked with psychological rather than physical symptoms but other studies disprove this. Why a placebo response is so high is uncertain – it may be due to the effect of counselling and having the problems validated and taken seriously that symptoms become better tolerated, together with a real desire to improve. Such placebo responses usually disappear within three months.

Reports of successful, but uncontrolled, treatments are consequently impossible to interpret and virtually meaningless. Drug trials which make no attempt to compare the effects of placebo should be ignored.

Self-help measures

Discussion

Discussion about the different symptoms that the woman is experiencing will help you to establish the severity of her problem. It is important for you to find out how long these symptoms last, how severe they are and whether they are relieved immediately by menstruation. In an ideal world we should also try to establish the woman's threshold of complaining and tolerance, and the degree of disruption that PMS has on her normal life. In practice, however, it can be very difficult to ascertain these facts.

As a nurse, you are often perceived by your patients as being more approachable than other health care professionals. Nurses are also seen as having more time to chat about a problem that might seem 'too trivial to bother the doctor with'. Discussion with a helpful and sympathetic nurse can be very therapeutic, especially for those women who have found other health care professionals not so understanding. If you can give the woman a greater understanding and knowledge about menstruation and premenstrual syndrome it will reduce her anxiety and hopefully lessen her symptoms. Once premenstrual problems have been voiced, you should encourage the woman to talk to others who may not have appreciated that there was a problem. These can include colleagues at work, friends, her partner and her family.

A sympathetic ear can be very comforting. Simple reassurance that she is 'not going mad' and that there is 'light at the end of the tunnel' can have an enormous psycho-therapeutic effect. Women frequently report that their worst fear is that they are 'going crazy' and that this fear is not being taken seriously. You should listen carefully to what they have to say, support them as women and confirm that their experiences are real and that other women also experience similar problems.

It can be helpful to find out why the woman is coming forward at this particular moment in time for help and advice. Has she experienced any major changes in her life during the past year which have tipped the balance, and made symptoms she was normally able to tolerate become unbearable? These problems can range from relationship difficulties, job changes, stresses with children or ageing parents to financial crises. Being able to talk to someone about these problems can be very therapeutic and you might well be able to refer the woman to local organizations for help. Some helpful suggestions you could make include:

♦ Belonging to a mother and baby group

♦ Relationship counselling

♦ Joining a local carers' group

♦ Referral to social services to see if extra financial support is available.

These suggestions, although they seem basic, might be all that is needed to tip the balance back again from seemingly unmanageable and distressing problems into tolerable but manageable difficulties.

Dietary changes

There is an abundance of conflicting advice that women are given about how to modify their diet to improve the symptoms of PMS. The best advice that you as a nurse can give to any woman, whether or not she suffers from PMS, is to eat well and healthily (see Chapter 2).

Recommendations that some women have found helpful include those listed in Box 13.6.

Your patients may find it helpful if you remind them not to expect an instant result from altering their diet. It can often take a few months for the beneficial effects to be felt both on their general health and on their PMS symptoms.

Self-help groups

Unfortunately there are few PMS self-help groups in the UK but advice about starting a local group can be obtained from the organizations and societies listed at the end of this chapter (see Resources, page 334). These societies also supply further advice about suitable books, leaflets and videos. It is important to read these books yourself before recommending them to PMS sufferers as the information might be very biased towards a particular method of treatment and not give a well-balanced overview of premenstrual syndrome.

In general practice it is sometimes more practicable for PMS support groups to be set up and run alongside other clinics and activities that involve women, e.g. family planning clinics and mother and baby clinics, rather than being a separate entity of their own.

Many PMS sufferers have their own small, unofficial self-help groups. Neighbours, friends and colleagues at work can all get together, have a moan and swap experiences and remedies that they have tried and found to be beneficial (or useless). It is hardly surprising that women get a lot of support

---

Box 13.6 Dietary recommendations to alleviate PMS

♦ *Reduce the intake of salt* Excess salt – whether added during cooking or at the table – can cause fluid retention, leading to feelings of bloatedness and mastalgia. Foods with a high salt content should also be restricted, e.g. cheese, preserved meats or fish, salted nuts, etc.

♦ *Reduce fluid intake* This advice is particularly suitable for women whose main symptoms include bloating and mastalgia.

♦ *Limit intake of caffeine* Restrict the amount of coffee, tea or cola. Caffeine can increase levels of anxiety and irritability. Many women find decaffeinated coffee or herbal teas are acceptable alternatives. Camomile tea is a great relaxant, peppermint tea helps with nausea and lime blossom tea settles mood swings.

♦ *Reduce dietary fat intake.*

♦ *Reduce intake of 'junk foods'* Eat as much fresh, unrefined food as possible. Have a varied diet containing a broad spectrum of nutrients.

♦ *Eat regularly* It is amazing how many women will skip meals or pick at their food at exactly the time of the month when they should be eating regularly and having a well-balanced diet.

♦ *Do not overeat* Some women have been advised to keep their blood sugar levels up (therefore avoiding the risk of hypoglycaemic-like symptoms of tiredness, irritability and headaches). Consequently they nibble at frequent intervals on sugary snacks and chocolate. This should be avoided as they will only end up fat and premenstrual rather than just premenstrual! If they feel the desire to nibble frequently then fresh fruits and vegetables should be substituted.

♦ *Limit intake of alcohol and tobacco* Women often use alcohol or tobacco for short-term relief of mood symptoms but both can lead to long-term problems.

---

and encouragement from others who can empathize with their problems, and it can also reveal a wealth of successful remedies and strategies for dealing with premenstrual syndrome.

Exercise and relaxation techniques

Any form of exercise is beneficial for women who have PMS and should certainly be encouraged. It is not certain why this should be so but exercise undoubtedly improves general health, well-being and self-esteem and may increase a woman's tolerance to premenstrual change, thus reducing the impact that premenstrual syndrome has on her life (Goodale *et al.*, 1990).

Walking, jogging, aerobics, swimming and yoga are all therapeutic and should be recommended. Some women find relief from their symptoms by using meditation, breathing exercises and relaxation techniques similar to those used in antenatal classes.

You should advise women who suffer from PMS that they should try to find some time every day in which they can be on their own and free from outside interruptions. In practice, unfortunately, this is often difficult when women are trying to juggle the varied demands of having a busy career with those of being a wife and mother. Reading, watching television, listening to music or even masturbating are all effective ways of relaxing. If none of these appeal then you can always advise going to a quiet place and screaming loudly, making a punch-bag out of pillows or cushions or anything else which might help!

Scenario

Sue, a normally calm mother, found that her main premenstrual problem was that she was becoming increasingly bad tempered and aggressive. She would shout at her children for trivial reasons, stamp around the house and slam doors in her fury. She eventually found an outlet for all this pent-up anger by realizing that if she made bread when she was premenstrual she could knead and pummel the dough very heavily, thereby calming her anger and filling her freezer with bread for the next few weeks!

Stress management

In general, advice about stress management can seem very simple and basic but it is surprising how few women have actually thought logically about how they can effectively manage their lives in order to help themselves. Many women benefit from simple advice and by making minor adjustments to their normal work schedule or family life if they are able to plan when they are likely to be suffering from PMS. Suggestions that you could make might include:

♦ Arrange appropriate childcare to give a 'break'

♦ Avoid having in-laws or guests to stay

♦ Avoid having friends to dinner

♦ Postpone driving tests

♦ Do not start a strict new diet

♦ Postpone a starting date for a new job.

Some women (and their families) have found it helpful if days that are likely to be stressful are marked on the family calendar. This means that both partners and children might be able to avoid discussing potentially difficult issues during these few days and hopefully avoid head-on clashes. This form of stress management, whilst being very successful, does unfortunately mean that PMS can effectively dominate the rest of the month as women constantly have to refer to the calendar to check where they are in their menstrual cycle.

Women who have demanding and stressful jobs often find that PMS can have a very debilitating effect on their working relationships and how they are perceived by their colleagues. They may be extremely efficient and competent for most of the month, but need only lose their temper once, or walk out of a meeting in tears and their credibility is immediately diminished. Potentially awkward meetings should be arranged, if possible, for times when she is not at her most vulnerable. If this cannot be managed then advice in relaxation techniques (see page 36), can certainly help the woman cope with the strains and responsibilities of her employment.

Alternative therapies

Many women have found relief from various 'alternative' or 'complementary' practitioners. These can include aromatherapists, reflexologists, herbalists, hypnotists, homeopaths and acupuncturists.

Aromatherapy can be really helpful in alleviating specific PMS symptoms. Use a couple of drops of oil in the bath, in massage oil or for inhalation (Box 13.7).

Box 13.7 Aromatherapy oils used to relieve PMS symptoms

♦ *Fatigue:* geranium, orange, lavender and mint.

♦ *Fluid retention:* eucalyptus, geranium and juniper.

♦ *Headaches:* camomile, lavender, rosemary and mint.

♦ *Tender breasts:* geranium.

♦ *Anger:* camomile, mint and ylang ylang.

♦ *Grumpiness:* rosewood.

♦ *Lethargy:* cypress, juniper, lemon, orange and rosemary.

♦ *Hypersensitivity:* mint.

Although there have been few controlled trials to show the beneficial effects of 'alternative' therapies on PMS, many women have found them extremely useful in reducing stress levels and helping them adapt to the strains of PMS and a busy lifestyle. Such therapists are generally only available privately but some do have sliding scales of fees for those who are unable to afford the full rate. It is useful to compile a list of locally recommended therapists which you could give to any women who might be interested. It might also be helpful to have a price list and a note of who has recommended them.

General advice

Women will appreciate any advice that you can give them (Box 13.8).

Nutritional supplements and non-hormonal drugs

If response to the above measures has not been satisfactory then treatment with pills may be tried. As a nurse, you might often find that you are consulted first for advice on any 'over-the-counter'

Box 13.8 General advice for women with PMS

♦ If your main symptom is abdominal bloating then don't try to squeeze into a garment that you usually wear, but to try some looser, more comfortable clothes with elasticated waistbands.

♦ If breast tenderness is a problem then wear a well-fitting, supportive bra.

♦ Don't arrange to go out and socialize when you don't feel like it, but stay in and read a book or watch a video.

♦ Get a good night's sleep.

♦ Some women find that sex is helpful as an orgasm is a powerful way of relieving tension (Masters and Johnson, 1966).

---

remedies that might help. The woman may not be visiting you ostensibly to discuss her PMS but will often ask for advice following a cervical smear or a contraceptive check.

You should remember that, as mentioned previously, any medication has a high placebo response and that if you can 'add in' some counselling as well then your patient may feel much better. Any improvement in symptoms, even if it is only a placebo response from non-prescription therapies, should be valued and the woman should be encouraged to continue with her treatment no matter how illogical the therapy seems, as it certainly will not be causing her any harm, unlike the side-effects that may occur from wrongly prescribed drugs for PMS.

Pyridoxine (vitamin B₆)

Pyridoxine appears to be the most widely used self-prescribed medication with up to 92% of women with PMS having tried it (Leather *et al.*, 1993a). It is widely available from chemists and health food shops. Trials of pyridoxine therapy give conflicting results with some studies showing it is no more effective than placebo (Stokes and Mendels, 1972) though others have shown it to have a therapeutic benefit (Williams *et al.*, 1985).

Pyridoxine is a co-factor in neurotransmitter synthesis and if benefits have been obtained it should be taken at a maximum dose of 100 mg daily throughout the cycle. At higher doses pyridoxine can cause peripheral neuropathy.

Multivitamin and mineral supplements

The best advice is for women to have a healthy, well-balanced diet with plenty of fresh food as discussed earlier. However, many women will supplement their dietary intake by taking extra nutritional treatments which are widely advertised and marketed as being able to treat PMS successfully.

Many types and varieties of multivitamin and mineral (mainly zinc and magnesium) supplements are available at chemists and health food shops. They differ enormously both in content and in price. The cheapest are of little use as they contain only small amounts of nutrients, whilst the most costly contain ingredients of doubtful relevance and are prohibitively expensive.

General advice that can be given is that extra vitamins and mineral preparations taken in moderation will not cause any harm. As they might have a placebo effect it may well be worth trying them for a three-month period to see if PMS symptoms improve.

Royal Jelly has also been reported by some women to be helpful in relieving the symptoms of PMS.

Evening primrose oil (EPO)

Evening primrose oil is a fashionable medicine. It is rich in an oil containing the essential fatty acid gamolenic acid, and has been strongly promoted in recent years as a cure for PMS. Gamolenic acid is thought to correct a disorder of E_1 prostaglandins which have many complicated functions within the body. Supplements of gamma-linolenic acid are believed to correct the theoretical disorder that exists between E_1 prostaglandins and essential fatty acids.

There are a bewildering number of new formulations of evening primrose oil being marketed at present which either combine EPO with marine oils, or with other sources of gamolenic acid such as borage seed oil and star flower oil. All these preparations are expensive and their value is doubtful. There are wide variations between the doses recommended by different manufacturers, ranging from 295 mg to 3000 mg daily.

Controlled studies using EPO for the treatment of premenstrual syndrome are lacking and their results are contradictory (Khoo et al., 1990). Little benefit seems to be gained from using evening primrose oil and the therapeutic efficacy of it has most likely been overstated. However, EPO certainly does not have any adverse side-effects, and women should be allowed to self-medicate to see if they have any relief from their symptoms.

Evening primrose oil has certainly proved to be effective in the treatment of cyclical mastalgia and benign breast disease (Pye et al., 1985) and is available on prescription for women suffering from these disorders.

Medical treatments

All the means of managing PMS symptoms that have so far been described are methods that the PMS sufferer can use and try on her own, or buy at a chemist or health food shop without a prescription. Women have usually investigated and tried many of these different treatment approaches and remedies to see if they can help and give relief to all or a few of their symptoms. If symptoms show no significant improvement then she may well consult her doctor for advice and help.

Nurses are well-placed in the medical setting to talk to the woman before she sees the doctor and can often offer valuable advice and support. Confirmation of the validity of her experiences and an understanding attitude will often be a great relief in itself.

Unfortunately, some doctors might only have a passing interest in premenstrual syndrome and not be able to give the support and help that is needed. They may be unsympathetic towards PMS sufferers and show little sensitivity in dealing with their problems. 'It is something women have to live with' and 'pull yourself together' are comments that sufferers hear all too frequently. It is important that the doctor conveys to the woman that PMS has a physical basis related to her hormones, that she is not going mad and that effective treatment is available. Such treatment has to take account of the needs and requirements of the individual woman, which differ according to her age, wishes for future pregnancy, the severity of her symptoms and her menstrual pattern.

Diuretics

Many women experience bloating and a feeling of weight gain, although, as mentioned earlier, very few have a demonstrable weight increase. The use of diuretics should be reserved for those who have an appreciable weight increase during the luteal phase of their cycle. If diuretics are prescribed then they should be taken on alternate days, although women then tend to increase the dosage and frequency if they get no immediate relief from their symptoms.

Care is needed in the prescribing of diuretics as electrolyte imbalances can occur if the course is extended, and continuous use can exacerbate fluid retention, consequently worsening the condition that it was meant to improve. This can be prevented to some extent by the use of an aldosterone agonist such as spironolactone which has shown to be effective for PMS symptoms of swelling and weight increase (O'Brien, 1987).

Prostaglandin inhibitors

Prostaglandin levels fluctuate throughout the cycle in response to the changing levels of oestradiol and progesterone. Prostaglandin inhibitors have many effects on the central nervous system including sedative and analgesic properties and they also reduce menorrhagia. In PMS where generalized aches and pains, headaches and fatigue are reported then mefenamic acid (250–500 mg three times a day) has been found to be more beneficial than placebo in a double-blind crossover study (Mira *et al.*, 1986).

If a woman suffers from premenstrual migraine, pelvic pain, dysmenorrhoea and menorrhagia then prostaglandin inhibitors may well be worth considering. Treatment should start from about day 16 of the cycle, and you should advise the woman that gastrointestinal side-effects can be reduced if the drug is taken with food.

Tranquillizers and antidepressants

PMS sufferers are all too frequently prescribed tranquillizers and antidepressants in the mistaken belief that they will alleviate the many psychological symptoms of PMS. While this would seem a logical treatment there is little evidence of any benefit except in the small group of women who also have an underlying psychological illness as well as premenstrual syndrome.

Modern antidepressants, however, which are serotonin re-uptake inhibitors such as fluoxetine (Prozac), appear to be an effective treatment for PMS and early studies have shown promising results (Menkes *et al.*, 1992). The relevant studies have included women suffering from irritability and depression, which is often exacerbated premenstrually, so it is possible that the disorder treated in these studies has really been a variant of depression rather than true premenstrual syndrome. Further trials of these drugs will be watched with interest.

Bromocriptine

Bromocriptine has been used to treat premenstrual breast tenderness but it has no effect on general premenstrual syndrome. It is a powerful drug and many women experience unpleasant side-effects and it is therefore not used widely these days.

Progestogens and progesterone

Despite no scientific evidence that progesterone deficiency is a cause of PMS, progestogens and progesterone continue to be among the most commonly used first-line treatments prescribed by doctors. This method of treatment has been strongly advocated and enthusiastically promoted by Dalton (1984) who has done a significant amount of writing on premenstrual syndrome, and has certainly increased awareness of the enormity of problems associated with PMS. However, her views on the treatment of PMS with progesterone must be considered controversial and unsubstantiated by controlled trials.

There is no evidence of a lack of progesterone during the luteal phase, and several randomized double-blind placebo-controlled trials show that progesterone therapy is no more effective than a placebo (Freeman *et al.*, 1990) so it remains hard to understand why this method of treatment is still so widely prescribed by doctors.

Research into the menopause has shown that cyclical progestogen (norethisterone 5 mg) given to prevent endometrial hyperplasia, causes symptoms that are very similar to those of premenstrual syndrome (Magos *et al.*, 1986), so it seems even more bizarre that women with PMS are given treatment that can worsen an existing condition which they were trying to avoid!

If progesterone has any place in premenstrual syndrome it is one of causation rather than therapy. However many women will request progesterone treatment (normally given as Cyclogest® suppositories) or oral progestogen (dydrogesterone is structurally similar to natural progesterone) as this method of treatment has been widely written about in women's magazines.

Suppression of the ovarian cycle

The most successful treatments for severe premenstrual symptoms are those that suppress ovulation and ablate the cyclical biochemical changes 'whatever they are' which cause PMS.

All methods that suppress the ovarian cycle need to be used in conjunction with sympathetic counselling and a supportive medical team. Discussion needs to be centred around future pregnancy plans as all these treatments will affect fertility in the short term.

Pregnancy itself will effectively treat PMS but this may not be a convenient or appropriate solution. Women should be advised that pregnancy is an option and will certainly 'cure' their PMS in the short term, but that symptoms will most likely return after delivery. Many women may then decide to 'speed up' their pregnancies and then seek effective treatment once their family is complete.

The following medical treatments all act by suppressing ovulation and are reversible.

Combined oral contraceptive pill

The combined oral contraceptive pill would seem to be the ideal treatment for PMS as it effectively suppresses ovulation and also gives contraceptive cover. Endocrine cyclicity remains, however, as hormones are only given for three weeks out of four, or in fluctuating doses with the biphasic and triphasic pills.

Surprisingly there have been no conclusive placebo-controlled studies to assess the effect of the combined oral contraceptive pill on premenstrual symptoms, and those studies which have been done show conflicting results. Moos in

1969 showed that the pill reduced the incidence and severity of premenstrual complaints, especially psychological symptoms, whilst Marriott and Faragher (1986) and others have been unable to demonstrate any beneficial effect.

The Pill though is a suitable first-line treatment option for a large percentage of women, particularly those who also require effective contraception. Women will experience the additional benefits of reduced dysmenorrhoea and menorrhagia. Symptoms may reappear during the pill-free week and if this is the case, it may be more logical to take the combined pill continuously for three months without any break between packets, followed by a seven-day break (tricycle regime). This will reduce the number of pill-free intervals and withdrawal bleeds with their associated symptoms per annum, but there is a small incidence of breakthrough bleeding, particularly in the first cycle.

The symptoms of a significant number of women appear to get worse whilst they are on the Pill. This is thought to be due to the side-effects of the progestogen element of the contraceptive pill (Cullberg, 1972). It is well worth changing to a different pill with a different progestogen content to see if this might help. Any change of pill should be tried for a minimum of three months before any conclusion can be made about the benefits or otherwise.

Scenario

Anna, a 19-year-old student, needed contraception. *Whilst taking a full history Anna mentioned to the nurse that she always felt moody and irritable for four or five days before her period, but had learned to cope with this so long as it did not occur just before exams. She was commenced on the combined oral contraceptive pill but returned three months later complaining of general moodiness and depression throughout the cycle which worsened during the pill-free week. Anna was given a pill with a different progestogen content which certainly improved her generalized depression but symptoms definitely returned when she did not take the pill for a week. It was decided to see if Anna would be symptom free if she avoided the pill-free week by taking three packets without a break.*

Anna returned at her next follow-up visit feeling pleased as she was having no cyclical symptoms and also had the added benefit of fewer episodes of bleeding.

The exact role and the effect of the combined oral contraceptive pill in the treatment of PMS are unresolved. There is a great need for proper prospective randomized placebo-controlled studies to look at this area and, in particular, the use of tricyclic regimes needs to be fully evaluated.

The progestogen-only pill and depot progestogens for contraception have not been carefully evaluated regarding premenstrual syndrome. Again, some women have reported a relief of symptoms, but others say their problems get much worse.

Danazol

Danazol is a synthetic steroid which has multiple effects on the pituitary–ovarian axis. Given continuously and in high doses (400 mg daily) danazol will suppress ovulation and menstruation. It has been shown to be beneficial for those women with severe mastalgia and other PMS symptoms (Halbreich *et al.*, 1991). However many women discontinue treatment at these doses as they experience androgenic side-effects which they find unacceptable, e.g. acne, hirsutism, bloating and weight gain (Watts *et al.*, 1987).

Danazol has been shown to be effective at reducing symptoms in some women at lower doses (Deeny *et al.*, 1991), thus avoiding the masculinizing side-effects. Studies (Sarno *et al.*, 1987) have also shown there is some benefit if danazol is taken only during the luteal phase.

Given over a long-term, danazol has a detrimental effect on lipids and regular monitoring needs to take place. It should not be given for more than six months.

Gonadotrophin-releasing hormone analogues

At high continuous doses, gonadotrophin-releasing hormone (GnRH) analogues suppress ovarian function completely, thereby causing a 'medical oophorectomy' and complete absence of cyclical and premenstrual symptoms. These drugs are usually given as subcutaneous injections (leuprorelin acetate) and implants (goserelin). They are also available as nasal sprays (buserelin) but these give less precise suppression of the ovarian cycle and symptoms may recur intermittently.

GnRH analogues have been shown to be more effective than placebo (Muse *et al.*, 1984) but the consequences of causing a medical oophorectomy limits their use to only six months. Long-term treatment cannot be justified because of the risks of osteoporosis and ischaemic heart disease associated with low oestradiol levels. Women tolerate the menopausal symptoms of hot flushes and night sweats if adequately counselled before therapy starts and in fact will often prefer these new symptoms to the cyclical tyranny of PMS.

Studies have been made to see if the skeleton and cardiovascular system can be protected by supplementing the treatment of GnRH analogues with conventional low-dose hormone replacement therapy ('add-back' therapy). The progestogens in such therapy may cause symptoms to recur to a degree in some women but others experience relief (Leather *et al.*, 1993b).

The use of GnRH analogues, even in the short term, is beneficial in a number of cases as it can convince the woman, her family and her colleagues at work that her symptoms are in fact caused by her ovarian cycle and not by an underlying personality or psychiatric disorder.

Scenario

Margaret, a solicitor in her early thirties, had been *in a stable relationship with Tony for over four years. The relationship had come under increasing strain when the responsibilities of Margaret's job took her overseas for short periods. Margaret had always complained of PMS and had some insight into the problem, but normally kept her symptoms at a manageable level using stress avoidance, exercise and relaxation techniques. She also took vitamin B$_6$, although she admitted that this most likely gave little benefit. The problems between Margaret and Tony increased over six months with Margaret becoming increasingly depressed, irritable and aggressive in the ten days before her period. Tony thought that Margaret was 'going mad' and threatened that unless she received psychiatric*

*help urgently he would leave her as he felt
completely unable to cope with her moods.*

*Fortunately Margaret's doctor referred her to a
specialist clinic where she was initially treated with
GnRH analogues. Margaret and Tony began to
notice a distinct improvement in her depression
and mood swings, in spite of experiencing
menopausal symptoms of hot flushes and night
sweats. Their relationship began to return to an
even keel, despite the increasing pressures of
Margaret's work. This six-month trial of treatment
with GnRH analogues was enough to convince
both Tony and Margaret that her problems were
related to her menstrual cycle and that she
certainly did not have an underlying psychiatric
problem.*

Oestrogen therapy

First-line therapy for severe premenstrual syndrome should be aimed at suppressing the ovarian cycle with the administration of oestrogens that are widely used in hormone replacement therapy (HRT) (see also Chapter 14). This oestrogen therapy needs to be in the form of subcutaneous implants or transdermal patches as oral HRT will not sufficiently suppress the ovarian cycle and thus symptoms may remain. This work has been pioneered by John Studd, consultant gynaecologist, at the Chelsea and Westminster Hospital, London.

Oestradiol implants and patches contain natural rather than synthetic oestrogens and their route of administration avoids the liver. They therefore do not adversely affect clotting factors and lipid metabolism. They do not have the same restrictions that apply to the contraceptive pill and can safely be given to women beyond the age of 50 years regardless of blood pressure, weight or smoking habits.

The use of these highly effective percutaneous oestrogen treatments for PMS is made more complicated in women with a uterus, by the need to take a cyclical progestogen. This is important in order to prevent endometrial hyperplasia (Sturdee *et al.*, 1978) but it does mean that some women develop mild PMS-like symptoms during this phase of treatment. These symptoms are usually less severe and less prolonged than their previous symptoms but if persistently troublesome the dose and duration of the progestogen may be reduced, or a different progestogen can be tried. It is im-

portant to warn women that these side-effects are particular properties of the progestogens given and are not symptoms of untreated PMS.

Oestradiol implants

The ovarian cycle can be suppressed by subcutaneous implants of oestradiol (Greenblatt *et al.*, 1977) and the benefits of this in treating PMS sufferers was demonstrated in a placebo-controlled study (Magos *et al.*, 1986). This study showed a superior response of active treatment against placebo for all of the Moos symptom clusters in the Menstrual Distress Questionnaire despite an initial placebo response of 94%.

Implants (100 mg decreasing to 75 mg and then to 50 mg as symptoms are controlled) are given at six-monthly intervals and many women find this method of administration convenient and cosmetically more pleasing than wearing oestradiol patches. Testosterone 100 mg can be added if there are problems of loss of libido, loss of energy and profound depression. As this is often the case with PMS sufferers combined oestradiol and testosterone implants are often the best initial treatment.

This therapy is usually well liked and tolerated by women, but it does require a degree of commitment because of the prolonged duration of action of the implants and the consequent need to continue with cyclical progestogens to prevent endometrial hyperplasia. This prolonged action may last for approximately two years after the last implant and makes implant treatment unsuitable for women who may be planning a pregnancy in the foreseeable future. It is ideal for women who have completed their families and for those who have worsening PMS symptoms when approaching the menopause.

Scenario

Claire, a 38-year-old divorced mother, had suffered from PMS for most of her life. Her *symptoms got progressively worse after the birth of her two daughters. Initially she put this deterioration down to the stresses of coping with two boisterous and demanding children, and the added financial anxieties of her husband's business. Claire's main problem was of aggression and violent mood swings – she even once threw the television out of the window during an argument over which programme to watch.*

The marriage eventually ended and Claire hoped that her PMS might improve as one stressful area in her life had gone. However the duration of her PMS symptoms gradually increased despite the fact that she had modified her diet, did regular exercise and had tried most 'over-the-counter' remedies. She eventually sought the advice of her doctor after she became violent towards her youngest daughter. The strength of her anger and aggression had really frightened Claire and had persuaded her that she urgently needed help.

Her doctor referred her to a gynaecologist with a particular interest in PMS who decided after discussion with Claire that she would benefit from an oestradiol implant. The improvement was dramatic – her family and friends could not believe the transformation that took place over the next few months – no more mood swings and anger. Claire returned for a repeat implant every six months for two years but then did not attend for a further ten months. On enquiry it transpired that Claire had felt so well and 'in control' of herself that she thought she no longer needed oestrogen therapy and could discontinue treatment. Unfortunately her symptoms were beginning to reappear as her ovarian cycle was not sufficiently suppressed and her new partner persuaded Claire to return for treatment.

Oestradiol patches

Oestradiol patches provide an attractive alternative to implants. High doses are needed initially (100–200 μg twice weekly) – which is a much larger dose than that used for the menopause.

Studies have shown that patches are more effective than placebo in relieving psychological, behavioural and physical symptoms of PMS by more than 50% (Watson *et al.*, 1989). Treatment should be started on the first day of a period and a progestogen such as Provera 5 mg should be taken from day 17 to 26 of the cycle for endometrial protection.

Some women experience transient breast tenderness and nausea when starting treatment but you should encourage them to continue with the patches as these symptoms will normally resolve by the second month. Oestrogen patches can have adhesion problems and may cause skin reactions in some women – you can give simple advice regarding daily rotation of the patch site and letting some of the alcohol evaporate from the 'reservoir' type of patch before placing it on the skin. The newer single-membrane patches (where the oestradiol is contained in the matrix of the adhesive rather than an alcohol reservoir) seem to stick better and cause less skin irritation. If problems are encountered with the progestogen phase of the treatment then it is always possible to alter the type of progestogen, the dosage or the duration.

It is clear that oestrogen therapy either as an implant or as patches is the only convincingly effective pharmacological treatment for severe PMS which is both well-tolerated by women and suitable for long-term use and should be the first-line therapy for severe PMS.

Surgery

The ultimate, if drastic, solution – as for so many gynaecological problems – may be hysterectomy and bilateral salpingo-oophorectomy followed by straightforward hormone replacement therapy. This HRT can be with oestrogen alone, as progestogen need not be added as endometrial protection would not be required. The ovaries must be removed at surgery in order to alleviate PMS symptoms, otherwise the ovarian cycle remains and will continue to give rise to cyclical problems.

Obviously surgery is reserved for those women who have severe PMS, or whose PMS is compounded by menstrual and gynaecological problems. In a recent study nearly 40% of women whose families were complete were prepared to consider such major surgery in order to be relieved of their cyclical symptoms (Leather *et al.*, 1993a). That such a substantial number of women are prepared to consider major surgery in an attempt to be free of the stresses of PMS confirms the inadequacies of current treatment options and the extent to which severe PMS can destroy women's professional and domestic lives.

A summary of different treatment approaches is shown in Figure 13.2.

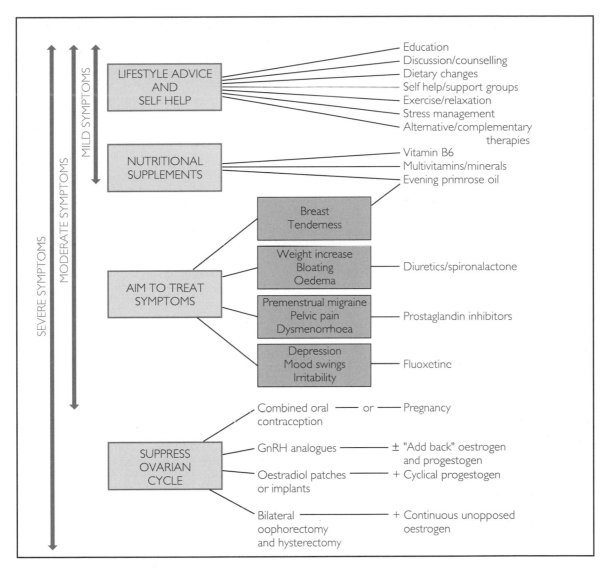

Figure 13.2 *Summary of treatment approaches to PMS.*

Conclusion

Pre-menstrual syndrome can affect up to 90% of women and includes a wide range of physical and emotional changes. The broad range of symptoms can vary from cycle to cycle in their severity, duration and their effect on women's lives. PMS unfortunately is not a straightforward problem as there is no recognized cause, and there is a wide range of management approaches and conflicting treatment options. It is important when women first

seek help and advice that they are able to discuss their problems with a sympathetic nurse who will be able to listen, counsel and support them through a variety of self-help approaches.

In severely affected women who have not been helped with these therapies then cycle suppression may be considered a suitable option. Women can also be referred to a small number of specialist PMS clinics which may be run by gynaecologists who have an interest in PMS and menopausal problems.

Resources

Menopause and PMS Trust
Chelsea & Westminster Hospital, Fulham Road, London SW10 9NH
Tel. 0181 746 8697

Women's Health
52 Featherstone Street, London EC1Y 8RT
Tel. 0171 251 6580

The Premenstrual Society (PREMSOC)
PO Box 429, Addlestone, Surrey KT15 1DZ
Tel. 01932 872560

PMS Help
PO Box 160, St Albans, Herts AL1 4UQ

National Association of Premenstrual Syndrome (NAPS)
P O Box 72, Sevenoaks, Kent TN13 1XQ
Tel. 01732 459378 (Office); 01732 741709 (Information line)

Women's Nutritional Advisory Service
PO Box 268, Lewes, East Sussex BN7 2QN
Tel. 01273 487366

Further reading

DAVIES, J. (1991) *Premenstrual Syndrome: Special Diet Cookbook*. London: Thorsons.
O'BRIEN, P.M.S. (1987) *Premenstrual Syndrome*. Oxford: Blackwell Scientific.
SHREEVE, C. (1992) *Premenstrual Syndrome*. London: Thorsons.
STEWART, M. (1994) *Beat PMS through Diet*. London: Vermilion.

References

ABRAHAM, G.E. (1980) Premenstrual tension. *Current Problems in Obstetrics and Gynecology* 3: 1–48.
BACKSTROM, T. and CARSTENSEN, H. (1974) Estrogen and progesterone in plasma in relation to premenstrual tension. *Journal of Steroid Biochemistry* 5: 257–60.
BACKSTROM, T., BOYLE, H. and BAIRD, D.T. (1981) Persistence of symptoms of premenstrual tension in hysterectomised women. *British Journal of Obstetrics and Gynaecology* 88: 530–36.
CHADWICK, J. and MANN, W.N. (1950) *The Medical Works of Hippocrates*. Oxford: Blackwell.
CLARE, A.W. (1983) Psychiatric and social aspects of premenstrual complaint. *Psychological Medicine Monograph Supplement* 4: 1–58.
CULLBERG, J. (1972) Mood changes and menstrual symptoms with different gestagen/estrogen combinations: a double-blind comparison with placebo. *Acta Psychiatrica Scandinavica (Suppl.)* 236: 1–86.
DALTON, K. (1961) Menstruation and crime. *British Medical Journal* 2: 1752.
DALTON, K. (1984) *Premenstrual Syndrome and Progesterone Therapy*, 2nd edn. London: William Heinemann Medical Books.
DEENY, M., HAWTHORN, R. and MCKAY HART, D. (1991) Low dose danazol treatment of the premenstrual syndrome. *Postgraduate Medical Journal* 67: 450–54.
FARATIAN, B., GASPAR, A., O'BRIEN, P.M.S., JOHNSON, I.R., FILSHIE, G.M. and PRESCOT, P. (1984) Premenstrual syndrome: weight, abdominal swelling, and perceived body image. *American Journal of Obstetric Gynecology* 150: 200–4.
FRANK, R.T. (1931) The hormonal causes of premenstrual tension. *Archives of Neurology and Psychiatry* 26: 1053–57.
FREEMAN, E., RICKETS, K., SANDHEIMER, S.J., and POLANSKY, M. (1990) Ineffectiveness of progesterone suppository treatment for premenstrual syndrome. *Journal of American Medical Association* 264: (3): 349–53.
GLASS, G.S., HENINGER, G.R., LANSKY, M. and TALAN, K. (1971) Psychiatric emergency related to the menstrual cycle. *American Journal of Psychiatry* 128: 705.
GOODALE, I.L., DOMAR, A.D. and BENSON, H., (1990) Alleviation of premenstrual syndrome symptoms with the relaxation response. *Obstetrics and Gynaecology* 75: 649–55.
GREENBLATT, R.B., ASCH, R.H., MAHESH, V.B. and BRIGNER, J.R. (1977) Implantation of pure crystalline pellets of estradiol for conception control. *American Journal of Obstetrics and Gynecology* 127: 520–24.
GREENE, R. and DALTON, K. (1953) The premenstrual syndrome. *British Medical Journal* I: 1007–14.
GUICHENEY, P., LEGER, D., BARRAT, J. *et al.*, (1988) Platelet serotonin content and plasma tryptophan in peri- and postmenopausal women: variations with plasma oestrogen levels and depressive symptoms. *European Journal of Clinical Investigation* 18: 297–304.
HALBREICH, U., ENDICOTT, J. and NEE, J. (1983) Premenstrual depressive changes. Value of differentiation. *Archives of General Psychiatry* 40: 535–42.
HALBREICH, U., ROJANSKY, N. and PALTER, S. (1991) Elimination of ovulation and menstrual cyclicity (with danazol) improves dysphoric premenstrual syndrome. *Fertility and Sterility* 56: 1066.
HALLMAN, J. (1986) The premenstrual syndrome – an equivalent of depression? *Acta Psychiatrica Scandinavica* 73: 403–11.
HARRISON, M., (1982) *Self-help for Premenstrual Syndrome*, revised edn. New York: Random House.
KHOO, S.K., MUNRO, C. and BATTISTUTTA, D. (1990) Evening primrose oil and treatment of premenstrual syndrome. *Medical Journal of Australia* 153: 189–92.
LAWS, S. (1985) Who needs PMT? A feminist approach to the politics of premenstrual tension. In Law, S., Hey, V. and Eagan, A. (eds) *Seeing Red. The Politics of Premenstrual Tension*. London: Hutchinson, pp. 16–64.
LEATHER, A.T., HOLLAND, E.F.N., ANDREWS,

G.D., and STUDD, J.W.W. (1993a) A study of the referral patterns and therapeutic experiences of 100 women attending a specialist premenstrual syndrome clinic. *Journal of the Royal Society of Medicine* **86** (4): 199–201.

LEATHER, A.T., STUDD, J.W.W., WATSON, N.R. and HOLLAND, E.F.N. (1993b) The prevention of bone loss in young women treated with GNRH analogues with 'add back' estrogen therapy. *Obstetrics and Gynecology* **81:** 104–7.

LOGUE, C.M., and MOOS, R.H. (1988) Positive peri-menstrual changes: towards a new perspective on the menstrual cycle. *Journal of Psychosomatic Research* **32:** 31–40.

MAGOS, A.L. and STUDD, J.W.W. (1984) The premenstrual syndrome. In Studd, J.W.W. (ed.) *Progress in Obstetrics and Gynaecology*, vol. 4. Edinburgh: Churchill Livingstone.

MAGOS, A.L. and STUDD, J.W.W. (1985) Effects of the menstrual cycle on medical disorders. *British Journal of Hospital Medicine* **33:** 68–77.

MAGOS, A., BRINCAT, M. and STUDD, J.W.W. (1986) Treatment of the premenstrual syndrome by subcutaneous oestradiol implants and cyclical norethisterone; placebo-controlled study. *British Medical Journal* **292:** 1629–33.

MARRIOTT, A. and FARAGHER, E.B. (1986) An assessment of psychological state associated with the menstrual cycle in users of oral contraceptives. *Journal of Psychosomatic Research* **30:** 41–47.

MASTERS, W.H. and JOHNSON, V.E. (1966) *Human Sexual Response*. Boston, MA: Little, Brown & Co.

MENKES, D.B., TAGHAVI, E., MASON, P.A., SPEARS, G.F.S. and HOWARD, R.C. (1992) Fluoxetine treatment of severe premenstrual syndrome. *British Medical Journal* **305:** 346–47.

MIRA, M., MCNEIL, D., FRASER, I.S., VIZZARD, J. and ABRAHAM, S. (1986) Mefenamic acid in the treatment of premenstrual syndrome. *Obstetrics and Gynaecology* **68:** 395–98.

MOOS, R.H. (1968) The development of a menstrual distress questionnaire. *Psychosomatic Medicine* **30:** 853–67.

MOOS, R.H. (1969) Typology of menstrual cycle symptoms. *American Journal of Obstetrics and Gynecology* **103:** 390–402.

MUSE, K.N., CETEL, N.S., FUTTERMAN, L.A. and YEN, S.C. (1984) The premenstrual syndrome effects of medical ovariectomy. *New England Journal of Medicine* **311:** 1345–49..

O'BRIEN, P.M.S. (1987) *Premenstrual Syndrome*. Oxford: Blackwell Scientific.

O'BRIEN, P.M.S., SELBY, C. and SYMONDS, E.M. (1980) Progesterone, fluid and electrolytes in premenstrual syndrome. *British Medical Journal* **ii:** 1161–63

PYE, J.K., MANSEL, R.E. and HUGHES, L.E. (1985) Clinical experience of drug treatments for mastalgia. *Lancet* **ii:** 373–77.

REID, R.L. and Yen, S.S.C. (1981) Premenstrual syndrome. *American Journal of Obstetrics and Gynecology* **139:** 85–104.

REID, R.L. (1991) Premenstrual syndrome. *Current Problems in Obstetrics and Gynecology and Fertility* **8:** 1–57.

SAMPSON, G.A. (1989) Premenstrual syndrome. *Baillière's Clinical Obstetrics and Gynaecology* **3:** 687–704.

SARNO, A.P., MILLER, E.J. JR. and LUNDBLAD, E.G. (1987) Premenstrual syndrome; beneficial effects of low-dose danazol. *Obstetrics and Gynecology* **70:** 33–36.

SCHMIDT, P.J., NIEMAN, L.K., GROVER, G.N., MULLER, K.L., MERRIAM, G.R. and RUBINOW, D.R. (1991) Lack of effect of induced menses on symptoms in women with premenstrual syndrome. *New England Journal of Medicine* **324:** 1174–79.

SHERSHAH, P.J., MORRISON, J.J. and JAFAROY, S. (1991) Prevalence of premenstrual syndrome in Pakistani women. *Journal of the Pakistan Medical Association* **41:** 101–3.

SNOWDEN, R. and CHRISTIAN, B. (1984) *Patterns and Perceptions of Menstruation*. New York: St Martins Press.

STOKES, J. and MENDELS, J. (1972) Pyridoxine and premenstrual tension. *Lancet* **i:** 1177–78.

STUDD, J.W.W. (1979) Premenstrual tension syndrome. *British Medical Journal* **277:** 410.

STURDEE, D.W., WADE EVANS, T., PATTERSON, M.E.L., THOM, M.H. and STUDD, J.W.W. (1978) Relations between bleeding pattern, endometrial histology and oestrogen treatment in post menopausal women. *British Medical Journal* **i:** 1571–77.

SUNDBLAD, C., MODIGH, K., ANDERSCH, B. and ERIKSSON, E. (1992) Clomipramine effectively reduces premenstrual and dysphoria: a placebo controlled trial. *Acta Psychiatrica Scandinavica* **85**(1): 39–47.

WALD, A., VAN THIEL, D.H., HOECHSTETTER, I. *et al.* (1981) Gastrointestinal transit: the effect on the menstrual cycle. *Gastroenterology* **80:** 1497–500.

WATSON, N.R., STUDD, J.W.W., SAVVAS, M., GARNET, T. and BABER, R.J. (1989) Treatment of severe premenstrual syndrome with oestradiol patches and cyclical norethisterone. *Lancet* **ii:** 730–32.

WATTS, J.F., BUTT, W.R. and LOGAN-EDWARDS, R. (1987) A clinical trial using danazol for the treatment of premenstrual tension. *British Journal of Obstetrics and Gynaecology* **94:** 30–34.

WILLIAMS, M.J., HARRIS, R.I. and DEAN, B.C. (1985) Controlled trial of pyridoxine in the premenstrual syndrome. *Journal of International Medical Research* **13:** 174–79.

14: The menopause
Kathy Abernethy ◆

OBJECTIVES

After reading this chapter you will understand:

◆ how the menopause occurs and the hormonal changes which occur

◆ the short-, intermediate and long-term effects of oestrogen deficiency

◆ hormone replacement therapy (HRT) and its uses, indications, contraindications and possible long-term risks

◆ how to counsel a woman before she starts HRT and how to effectively monitor HRT once treatment is established

◆ non-hormonal treatments for oestrogen deficiency symptoms

◆ factors, other than hormones, which influence a woman approaching the menopause.

A woman in the autumn of her life, deserves an Indian summer, rather than a winter of discontent.
(The Late Robert B. Greenblatt MD, formerly Professor of Endocrinology, Georgia, USA)

Introduction

All women who live long enough will experience the menopause. The menopause marks the end of fertility and the end of periods. Alongside this often comes acute menopausal symptoms and anxiety about long-term effects such as cardiovascular disease and osteoporosis. Emotionally, the menopause can signify a time of great change as women take the opportunity to make an assessment of life, perhaps having to adapt to a changing role in the family and in society, and also to come to terms with a changing body and changing expectations in life. Physical changes in her body, social and emotional changes in life and psychological changes in herself make the time of menopause one

of great turbulence and self-analysis for some women. The menopause is such an individual event, with its differing associated 'mid-life' problems, that how each women perceives and experiences this time of physical change, will vary enormously. Medicine will help some, counselling may be necessary for others and for others the time of menopause will slip by barely recognized.

This chapter aims to highlight the physical aspects of the menopause along with recognizing some of the non-physical effects and suggesting ways in which you can help women through this phase of their life in a positive way, using both medical and non-medical means.

Definitions

The 'menopause' is a term used to describe the final menstrual bleed in a woman's life. The term 'climacteric' covers the phase of time either side of the last bleed. It is during this climacteric phase that menopausal symptoms commonly occur. Both women and health professionals alike tend to use the term 'menopause' to describe the phase in a woman's life when fertility disappears and periods stop. The following terms are also used:

♦ *Pre-menopause* The time prior to periods stopping, usually before symptoms start.

♦ *Peri-menopause* The time around the menopause when bleeding can be irregular and symptoms may occur. Conception is still theoretically possible although cycles may be anovulatory.

♦ *Post-menopause* The time in a woman's life after periods have stopped for at least a year.

Age of menopause

In the UK, the average age at which periods stop is 51 years. This has remained constant for many years although general improvements in health care provision have resulted in a much greater life expectancy than was known by previous generations. Women now expect to live much longer after the menopause and it is partly for this reason that women themselves are thinking more about the long-term effects of oestrogen deficiency. Although 51 years is the average age of the menopause, it commonly occurs between the ages of 45 and 58 years and can occur much earlier in some women. A menopause which occurs earlier than age 40 years is described as a premature menopause and these women deserve special attention.

The age of menopause is affected by smoking which can bring this forward by 1–2 years. (Lindquist and Bengrsson, 1979).

The following factors do not seem to affect whether a woman has an early or late menopause:

♦ Race

♦ Use of oral contraception

♦ Number of pregnancies

♦ Age of menarche

♦ Socio-economic factors.

Some women experience a gradual stopping of periods over a couple of years whilst others will find that their periods stop suddenly. Others may see more frequent periods initially, gradually becoming less frequent. All of these patterns are normal.

In relation to types of menopause the following terms are used:

♦ *Natural/spontaneous* – periods stop of their own accord.

♦ *Surgical* – the ovaries are removed by surgery thus producing an instantaneous menopause.

♦ *Premature* – menopause occurs under the age of 40 years, for whatever reason.

♦ *Induced* – menopause is brought on by external factors such as chemotherapy or radiotherapy.

Hormonal changes at the menopause

During the peri-menopausal phase, oestradiol levels fall and levels of follicle stimulating hormone (FSH) and luteinizing hormone (LH) rise. However there is wide fluctuation in levels around the time of menopause. The rise in FSH is gradual and reaches a peak after the final bleed has occurred. The levels drop again about 10–20 years after the menopause (Chakravati *et al.*, 1976).

Prior to the menopause, oestradiol and oestrone are the principle oestrogens circulating in the body. They are produced mainly by the ovaries, with oestradiol the predominant hormone. Oestrone is also available through conversion of a hormone, androstenedione, which is secreted by the adrenal glands. After the menopause, levels of both oestradiol and oestrone drop markedly and oestrone becomes the dominant oestrogen.

Women themselves often believe that they need to have a blood test to measure hormone levels at the time of menopause. In practice, this is hardly ever useful or even necessary. Symptoms of the menopause do not correlate to actual oestrogen levels, with some women seemingly able to tolerate very low oestrogen levels with few symptoms, whilst others will experience profuse symptoms despite only a small change in oestrogen levels. We may consider measuring FSH levels, but these fluctuate widely around the time of the menopause and can be unreliable. A series of two or three measurements would be required for a diagnosis of the menopause and again would be of little value in predicting the need for hormone replacement therapy. FSH levels may be useful in a hysterecto-mized woman who is experiencing early symptoms of the climacteric. FSH levels are also used to diagnose a premature menopause when the medical implications are going to be greater than for the average age woman.

Premature menopause

Whilst it is common for the natural menopause to occur in the late forties or early fifties, some women experience the menopause much earlier. A menopause prior to age 40 years is described as premature. Long-term consequences for such women are even greater than with a so-called 'normal menopause', and many specialists would now agree that this group of women deserves special attention because of their additional physical needs. They also deserve special attention with regard to the psychological and emotional upsets which some women experience when undergoing an early menopause.

Causes of premature menopause

Surgery

If both ovaries are removed, the menopause occurs immediately. Symptoms can be quite severe even after a very short time. Hormone replacement therapy should be given not only to prevent symptoms but also to help protect against osteoporosis and cardiovascular disease. Hysterectomy alone (i.e. with conservation of one or both ovaries) has also been shown to bring forward the age of menopause in some women (Siddle *et al.*, 1987). Women should no longer be assured therefore that their remaining ovaries will necessarily carry on working until the normal age of menopause. Professionals must now listen more carefully to those women who may complain of menopausal symptoms soon after hysterectomy. FSH levels may be indicated in these women.

Scenario

Deborah is 42 years old. She had a hysterectomy with conservation of ovaries two years ago. Apart from her initial post-operative check she has not seen her doctor since. She now feels extraordinarily tired and often wakes at night feeling very hot. Eventually she sought medical advice. After checking her thyroid function was normal, the GP decided to do a series of FSH levels. He was surprised to discover they were in the post-menopausal range. Deborah started HRT and within a few weeks her symptoms were improved. Deborah is relieved that she is now getting the long-term oestrogen protection her body needs, as well as feeling so much better.

Natural

Occasionally the menopause occurs spontaneously at an unusually early age. This may be associated with chromosomal abnormalities or autoimmune diseases affecting the ovaries. Sometimes no cause is found for the early menopause. Typical menopausal symptoms may or may not be present, so careful investigations are needed. For women who are wanting children it is particularly important that a prompt diagnosis is made as implications with regard to their fertility are immense.

Iatrogenic

Iatrogenic early menopause, i.e. caused by outside influences, such as chemotherapy or radiotherapy, can be quite traumatic, especially when the woman has successfully faced malignant disease but has to come to terms with an early menopause as a result of her treatment.

Consequences of an early menopause

Menopausal symptoms

These are likely to be worse in a woman who experiences a sudden menopause, as a result of surgery, for example, than in those woman who experience a gradual ovarian failure (Chakravati *et al.*, 1977).

Cardiovascular disease

Early studies in the 1950s showed a higher incidence of heart disease in women with early menopause (Oliver and Boyd, 1959). More recently, the US Nurses Study demonstrated that the risk of myocardial infarction increased as the age of the menopause decreased and that bilateral oophorectomy under the age of 35 years incurred a sevenfold risk compared to pre-menopausal women (Rosenberg *et al.*, 1981). A later study showed that women who took oral hormone replacement therapy after oophorectomy had no increased risk in cardiovascular disease (Colditz *et al.*, 1987).

Osteoporosis

Premature menopause is associated with an earlier onset of osteoporosis. This is preventable by the use of hormone replacement therapy (Lindsay *et al.*, 1976).

Premature menopause and hormone replacement therapy

A woman with an early menopause needs special care with regard to HRT. She is likely to be taking it for many years so care must be taken to find a regime which suits her and gives acceptable hormonal replacement. The woman herself should be involved in a decision as to how she wants to take her HRT and every effort should be made to minimize side-effects. Younger women may need higher doses of oestrogen not only in order to feel well but also to maintain an adequate protection of the skeleton (Gangar and Key, 1993). The consequences of stopping treatment are potentially more damaging in women with premature menopause, so it is particularly important that they understand why the HRT is necessary and are given ample opportunity to express anxieties and ask questions about treatment.

Psychological effects of premature menopause

Experiencing an early menopause, whether natural or surgical, can cause emotional difficulty. Issues relating to sexuality in particular can become very important and for some women these issues can be difficult to handle. These may include:

♦ Loss of fertility

♦ Change in body image

♦ Feelings of loss of femininity

♦ Fear of ageing prematurely

♦ Feeling 'out of control' of their body

♦ Feeling that their body has 'let them down'.

It is helpful if such women are given the opportunity to discuss such issues openly. Some women value being able to talk within a group of other women who have also undergone early menopause. Young women often feel very isolated at the time of premature menopause and this is not helped by the fact that almost all literature on the subject of menopause is aimed at women in their fifties. Women undergoing planned surgery may have time for discussion within the gynaecology unit but those who undergo a natural early menopause are often left feeling angry, frightened and alone with no-one to turn to.

Scenario

Isobella is 34 years old. She has two children and had considered her family to be complete until she was diagnosed as experiencing an early menopause. Once confronted with the inevitability of having no more children, she had a constant desire for one more child, even though she knew it was not possible. She felt very bitter that this decision was taken from her. She did not tolerate HRT very well and was reluctant to take it. She was eventually seen by an experienced menopause counsellor who, over time, helped her to adjust to her new situation. As she came to terms with her infertility, she became more willing to try other HRT regimes and eventually found one which suited her.

Short- and intermediate-term effects of oestrogen deficiency

For many people, the most obvious symptom associated with the menopause is the hot flush. Almost all women and probably many men would be able to associate hot flushes with 'the change'. However, there are many other symptoms which can arise around the time of the menopause, some of which can be quite distressing, particularly if the woman herself does not realize that they may be related to her menopause.

Vasomotor symptoms

Approximately 75% of post-menopausal women do experience acute menopausal symptoms. Symptoms sometimes start before periods even become irregular and can continue for many years after the last bleed (Studd *et al.*, 1990). The average length of time that symptoms last is two years with 25% of women continuing to experience them for five years and 5% of women still experiencing them many years after the menopause (McKinlay and Jeffereys, 1974).

The hot flush

Women describe a flush as a feeling of intense heat, sometimes accompanied by sweating, starting in the chest area and rising through the neck and face. The frequency and length of flushes varies from woman to woman. Flushes which occur at night often result in profuse sweating, the so-called 'night sweat'. These can occur night after night for months or even years. The actual cause of the hot flush is not known although various theories have been suggested. Hormone levels cannot predict the onset of flushes and sweats and it seems that the fluctuation in oestrogen levels which occurs around the time of the menopause is more important than the actual physiological levels. Vasomotor symptoms respond extremely well to oestrogen therapy, which remains the treatment which has been most widely researched for this problem (Coope *et al.*, 1975). There is a strong placebo response with treatment for hot flushes so any study has to be carefully controlled if a true therapeutic effect is to be demonstrated.

If left untreated, vasomotor symptoms will eventually subside, leaving no long-term effects. The decision as to whether to treat them or not can only be taken by the woman herself according to her individual circumstances, a decision which will be based on how severe and unbearable her symptoms are.

Other treatments apaprt from oestrogen therapy which have been suggested to relieve hot flushes include:

♦ Vitamin E

♦ Clonidine

♦ Propanolol

♦ Oil of evening primrose.

Psychological symptoms

Many women complain of psychological upset at the time of the menopause but it is difficult to establish whether they are a true result of oestrogen deficiency or whether they are secondary factors related to other symptoms, such as flushes and sweats. Prolonged episodes of night sweats may lead to a very poor sleep pattern, which in turn results in poor concentration, poor memory, mood changes and even physical symptoms such as headaches and fatigue. This is described as the 'domino effect'.

Nevertheless, many studies have shown that minor psychological disturbances often precede the actual last bleed and seem to correlate with fluctuating oestrogen levels (Ballinger, 1975; Montgomery and Studd, 1991). These symptoms can include:

♦ Loss of confidence

♦ Depressed mood

♦ Fatigue

♦ Feelings of unworthiness

♦ Forgetfulness

♦ Difficulty in making decisions.

It should be remembered that many external factors will influence how a woman is feeling emotionally and psychologically around the time of the menopause and these should be taken into account when considering the effects of the menopause. These factors are discussed later in the chapter.

Women on hormone replacement therapy do describe a beneficial psychological effect (Campbell and Whitehead, 1977), but quite how the HRT works is unclear. Studies are difficult to perform objectively because of the strong placebo effect and because of the difficulty of allowing for all the external influences on psychological well-being.

Sexual function

Sexual function is another area where many influences, other than simply that of the menopause have an important role. Satisfaction within a relationship, emotional stability and psychological well-being will all help to contribute to a satisfactory sex life. Sexual activity involves both partners and we should not assume that a problem at mid-life is always due to the woman and her hormones. The male partner too, may be changing and male sexual dysfunction, such as impotence or loss of desire, may also contribute to a less than satisfactory sexual relationship. In the same way that we must not always blame the menopause for sexual disorders at the time of the menopause, we should not assume that HRT is always the answer.

Psychosexual counselling may be necessary even if oestrogen deficiency is playing an important role. Sexual difficulties which are likely to respond to HRT are:

♦ Lack of lubrication

♦ Loss of libido

♦ Dyspareunia.

The vaginal epithelium changes markedly after the menopause, resulting in the vaginal walls becoming thinner and less elastic. Vaginal secretions diminish and the vagina becomes more susceptible to infection because of the changing pH. This is known as atrophic vaginitis.

It is likely that simply relieving vaginal dryness and discomfort can break the cycle which is often seen, where a woman makes love but it is painful, so next time the desire is absent, leading to even less lubrication and therefore even more discomfort. If intercourse is expected to be painful, it occurs less and less frequently, resulting in further atrophy and consequently more discomfort. Oestrogen can help to break this cycle.

Some studies have shown that testosterone increases sexual desire and for some women this can be combined with their oestrogen therapy (Sherwin and Gelfland, 1985). Testosterone is given by implant and may be particularly useful for the hysterectomized woman. A trial of therapy may be necessary to see if the effects will be beneficial.

Bladder symptoms

Bladder symptoms worsen with age and are often assumed to be directly associated with the hormonal effects of the menopause. However no stud-ies have been able to directly relate menopausal status with specific urinary symptoms, although beneficial effects of oestrogen therapy have been shown (Hilton and Stanton, 1983). This beneficial effect may be due to collagen factors in the tissue around the urethra. It has been estimated that 50% of women attending a menopause clinic have urinary symptoms, such as stress incontinence, frequency of micturition, urgency, and nocturia (Cardozo, 1990). Whether these are a genuine response to oestrogen deficiency or are caused by other factors, they none the less need a sympathetic ear and helpful advice. A trial of oestrogen therapy may well be of benefit.

Box 14.1 Summary of typical oestrogen deficiency symptoms

Short term

♦ Flushes/sweats

♦ Psychological complaints

♦ Insomnia.

Intermediate

♦ Sexual difficulties

♦ Dyspareunia

♦ Vaginal atrophy

♦ Bladder symptoms.

Long term

♦ Osteoporosis

♦ Cardiovascular disease.

Long-term effects of oestrogen deficiency

Osteoporosis

More and more women are now becoming aware of the condition called osteoporosis, and the fact that it particularly affects women after the menopause. The National Osteoporosis Society, a national charity, has ensured that osteoporosis is much more fully understood now than in the past. The media has also covered the subject extensively, and many women are now presenting to their GPs expressing concern about the condition of their bones.

Osteoporosis is a condition in which bone mass per unit volume reduces to such an extent that fractures may occur, even following minimal trauma. This definition does not require a fracture to have occurred, but simply for the risk of fracture to be increased because of reduced bone mass. So some women are said to have osteoporosis even though they have not yet experienced a fracture.

Normal bone structure

Bone is a living part of the body, being constantly removed and renewed, with new bone being deposited on a continuous basis. Four main cells are found in bone, but the two most relevant to osteoporosis are the *osteoclasts*, which remove old bone, and *osteoblasts*, which replace it. In children and young adults, there is a net increase in bone density, resulting in skeletal growth. However, at around the age of 30–35 years, peak bone mass is achieved and less bone formation takes place. The bone becomes less dense as a result of greater bone destruction and less formation, resulting in a demineralization, leaving a less dense and consequently weaker bone structure (Figure 14.1)

This gradual thinning of the bone particularly affects trabecular bone, of which the long bones and vertebrae are mainly comprised. This trabec-

ular bone is surrounded by a hard cortical shell. Osteoporotic bones lose strength as they become less dense as a result of less bone formation. Therapies aimed at preventing osteoporosis aim either to increase bone formation (building) or to reduce bone resorption (destruction). Hormone replacement therapy is thought to work partly by preventing bone resorption, thus helping to restore the balance between bone resorption and formation.

Causes

Osteoporosis can be caused by various factors. Peak bone mass is achieved by early adult life and appears to be largely genetically predetermined, although lifestyle factors such as diet and exercise may be influential in promoting a healthy bone mass during skeletal development. Race is also an important factor, with Afro-Caribbean people having a greater bone mass than white people, who in turn have a greater bone mass than Asians (Ellerington and Stevenson, 1993).

Once peak bone mass is achieved, bone loss then occurs at varying rates throughout the rest of a person's life. Men lose bone density more slowly and also often achieve a greater peak bone mass in the first place, so are less at risk of osteoporosis. By far the greatest influence on the bone density of a woman is the menopause, after which bone density may be lost very rapidly. How much at risk of developing osteoporosis a woman is, will depend on how great a peak bone mass she achieves as a young adult, combined with how fast she subsequently loses bone density after the menopause. A woman who achieves a good peak bone mass, may subsequently lose bone rapidly, putting her at as much risk as the woman who has a lower peak bone mass, but after the menopause loses bone density more slowly. The initial 5–10 years after the menopause is the time when the greatest bone loss occurs, with a general slowing down of the rate some ten years or so after the menopause. Measures for preventing osteoporosis are therefore most effective in the first ten years after the menopause although benefit will still be achieved many years later (Nilas and Christiansen, 1988).

Although osteoporosis occurs most commonly in women after the menopause, it can also occur in both men and women as a result of the following contributory factors:

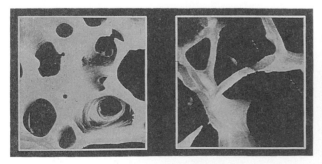

Figure 14.1 *Normal (left) and osteoporotic (right) bone. (Reproduced with permission from Dempster, D. et al., A simple method for correlative scanning electron microscopy of human iliac crest biopsies.* American Journal of Bone and Mineral Research **1**: *15–21.)*

◆ Corticosteroid therapy (above 75 mg prednisolone daily or equivalent on a regular basis)

◆ Hyperparathyroidism

◆ Cushing's syndrome

◆ Some malignant diseases

◆ Long-term immobilization

◆ Excessive exercise, such as with athletes or ballet dancers

◆ Chronic diseases, such as hepatic or renal failure

◆ Rheumatoid arthritis.

Risk factors

Various risk factors (Box 14.2) have been identified to try and predict women at risk of osteoporosis, but it has proved difficult to correlate these with actual incidence of osteoporosis in individual women. Some women seem to have all the risk factors and not develop osteoporosis, whilst others are not apparently at high risk yet develop the disease. At best such risk factors will only identify 30% of those people who will subsequently develop osteoporosis (Stevenson *et al.*, 1989).

Incidence

Osteoporotic fractures are extremely common. It is estimated that 40–50% of all women will experience a fracture related to osteoporosis during their lives (Ellerington and Stevenson, 1993). The three

> **Box 14.2**   Risk factors for osteoporosis
> ◆ Race
> ◆ Heredity
> ◆ Early menopause
> ◆ High alcohol intake
> ◆ Cigarette smoking
> ◆ Low body weight
> ◆ Nulliparity
> ◆ Episodes of amenorrhoea
> ◆ Sedentary lifestyle
> ◆ Secondary contributory factors.

most common sites for fracture as a result of osteoporosis are the wrist, the spine and the hip.

The wrist.   There are approximately 40 000 cases of Colles' fracture in the UK each year, with a dramatic rise in numbers among women over the age of 50. Men do not experience a rise in incidence such as occurs among women.

The spine.   Vertebral fractures occur when osteoporosis causes the vertebral bodies to collapse because of weakened bone mass. These fractures may occur without causing pain and only subsequently be shown by X-ray, or they may result in sudden, acute back pain requiring medical attention. Repeated vertebral fractures cause the so-called 'dowager's hump' (Figure 14.2) which typifies the image of an elderly lady and frightens so many younger ones..

Figure 14.2   *A woman with severe osteoporosis. (Reproduced with permission from slide set* A Woman's Guide to the Menopause, *produced by Wyeth Laboratories.)*

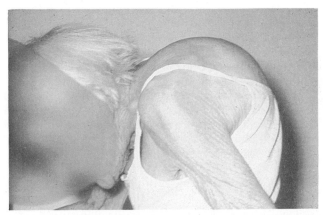

The hip.　Hip fractures are potentially very serious. Treatment of hip fractures is generally by surgery which carries the risks associated with general anaesthetic as well as risks from immobility in a generally frail and elderly person. Many elderly women who experience a hip fracture never regain their independence and have to rely on their family or society for help and support. About 20% of those who sustain a hip fracture will die within a year (Grimley-Evans *et al.*, 1979).

The incidence of hip fractures in the UK is high, with figures likely to rise as we experience an increasing elderly population. The cost to the NHS is enormous and the cost in terms of personal suffering, immeasurable (Hillard *et al.*, 1991).

Measuring bone density

Conventional X-rays are of little value in assessing osteoporosis because bone loss will only be evident when very severe. Obvious fractures will show up and past vertebral fractures which may have occurred without pain will also be evident. However as a means of predicting those at risk of osteoporosis and subsequent fracture, X-rays are seldom used.

The most usual way of currently assessing bone density is dual energy X-ray absorptiometry (DEXA). This measures bone density at various sites and is said to give an accurate result of bone density at the spine and hip. Fracture risk is directly related to bone density and even a single measurement at around the time of the menopause will give a good indication of future risk of fracture (Hui *et al.*, 1988). A further scan 12–18 months later will also help to assess the actual rate of bone loss over this period of time.

Measurements such as these are particularly helpful to the woman who would prefer not to take HRT but who would do so if there was evidence that she was likely to benefit. They also help to determine how long a woman may wish to stay on therapy, as a woman with more severe bone loss is more likely to remain on a treatment than one with only slight bone loss. Bone density measurements also help in assessing the effectiveness of a particular therapy, as repeat scans over a period of time will demonstrate the benefit of the therapy for an individual.

There are currently insufficient machines in the UK to make it feasible to offer this service to all women at the time of the menopause. Research is underway to assess whether bone density measurements may be used for screening a population as well as for individual diagnosis. If shown to be effective this would enable doctors to be more selective about targeting women who might need treatment and would enable women to be more sure that the treatment they were opting to take was really necessary. At present, we can only try to identify those women who we perceive to be most at risk, which particularly includes those women experiencing an early menopause or who have had long episodes of amenorrhoea earlier in life.

Other methods of measuring bone density include photon absorptiometry (single and dual) and quantitative computerized tomography (CAT) scans.

Calcium

Women sometimes believe that if they simply take extra calcium, they will prevent osteoporosis. Unfortunately this is too simplistic. Calcium, like all vitamins and minerals, is an essential part of a normal diet. If it is lacking during the years that the skeleton is forming, then the bones will suffer as a consequence. However, most people do get sufficient calcium in a modern Western diet. After the menopause, taking extra calcium alone will not stop osteoporosis. Women at the time of the menopause sometimes cut back on the calcium in their diet inadvertently whilst trying to diet, by reducing the amount of dairy products they eat. These women should be encouraged to maintain an adequate intake of calcium, either through dairy products or through other foods. Women on special diets for moral or religious reasons may not be getting sufficient calcium and supplements may be useful for these women.

Calcium may be useful as a treatment for established osteoporosis, particularly in an elderly person. Some regimes for established osteoporosis incorporate extra calcium, e.g. disodium etidronate (see page 359).

Hormone replacement therapy and osteoporosis

For the greatest benefit to the skeleton, HRT should be started soon after the menopause and continued for five years (Ettinger *et al.*, 1985). This is the phase when women lose bone density very rapidly and therefore conserving bone at this stage is most valuable in the long term. If HRT is started some years after the menopause the bone density will not be substantially reversed although further loss will be prevented. This may be sufficient for an individual to avoid a fracture and so is still considered of great value (Quigley *et al.*, 1987).

HRT has been shown to protect against fracture of the wrist, hip and spine. It has been estimated that five years' use of HRT reduces the risk of hip fracture by 50% (Melton, 1987). Women who experience an early menopause would need to continue HRT at least until the age of normal menopause (50 years) to sustain adequate protection. When HRT is stopped, bone loss is believed to continue at the same rate as if the menopause had just occurred (Christiansen *et al.*, 1981), thus the benefit of treatment is maintained for some years.

There is a minimum dose of oestrogen which is thought to be protective against bone loss for most women. However, a few women continue to lose bone on these doses. Only by performing regular bone density scans can we be sure that a dose is effective for an individual woman. It is not known why some women appear to need higher doses than others and it is impossible to predict who these women are. In practice this means that the majority of women receive a standard dose unless a bone scan indicates the need for a higher dose.

Exercise

It is known that long periods of immobilization lead to a decrease in bone density, however research has been unable to positively demonstrate whether taking extra exercise around the time of the menopause can increase bone mass on its own accord. Such studies would be difficult to conduct because of other influencing factors such as diet, drugs and lifestyle. It does seem evident, however, that weight-bearing exercises such as walking, running and dancing are of more benefit to the skeleton than swimming which is still of course an excellent exercise, particularly for the cardiovascular system (Stevenson *et al.*, 1990). Exercise also increases muscle tone, general fitness and agility, perhaps reducing the likelihood of a fall and consequent risk of fracture.

Excessive exercise such as that undertaken by athletes or ballet dancers reduces body weight to such an extent that periods may stop. This results in a loss of bone density pre-menopausally which will increase the risk of fracture later in life, particularly when combined with a later loss associated with the menopause (Drinkwater *et al.*, 1984).

Cardiovascular disease

Heart disease is the major cause of death in women aged over 50 years in the UK (OPCS, 1987). Heart disease has always been considered to be predominantly a male problem and it is true that until the age of 50 years it is men who are far more likely to suffer a heart attack or stroke. After this age, the incidence in women comes closer to that of men. This is considered to be partly due to a fall in oestradiol levels after the menopause, which appear to have a strong influence on various factors relating to heart disease (Colditz *et al.*, 1987). It is not clear which factors are most important, whether it is to do with changing lipids alone or whether other changes occur in blood vessels themselves as a result of oestrogen deficiency. It seems likely that the beneficial effects exerted by oestrogen therapy on cardiovascular protection are the result of a combination of direct effects on vessel walls, blood flow and lipid metabolism (Whitehead and Godfree, 1992).

Menopausal status

What is clear is that menopausal status and not simply age alone plays an important role in the incidence of cardiovascular disease in women. The Framingham Study in the USA showed that among a group of women in the same age band, the ones who had undergone menopause had a higher rate of cardiovascular disease than those women who had functioning ovaries. This was particularly so among the younger age groups, indicating that a premature menopause is a risk factor for future heart disease (Margolis *et al.*, 1974).

Other factors

Of course the menopause is not the only factor which will influence whether a woman gets cardiovascular disease. Lifestyle, medical and genetic factors all play an important role (Box 14.3).

Box 14.3 Risk factors for cardiovascular disease

Lifestyle

◆ Smoking

◆ Obesity

◆ Sedentary lifestyle

◆ High fat diet.

Medical

◆ Menopausal status

◆ Hypercholesterolaemia

◆ Family history of heart disease

◆ Hypertension

◆ Diabetes.

The role of hormone replacement therapy in preventing cardiovascular disease is very important and this should be emphasized when women seek advice about lifestyle and other changes. It can be all too easy to promote a healthy lifestyle and encourage the cessation of smoking in order to reduce heart disease and miss out on the advice about HRT unless a woman specifically asks.

The role of HRT in preventing cardiovascular disease

There is now a great deal of data relating to HRT and heart disease. Out of 31 published studies over 20 years, 25 have shown a reduced risk with oestrogen therapy, which in 12 of these studies showed a statistical significance. These have indicated a reduction in the rate of cardiovascular disease by at least 40% and of stroke by approximately 20% in users of oestrogen therapy (Smith and Studd, 1993).

Most of the studies were carried out using women taking oestrogen therapy on its own, usually conjugated equine oestrogen (Premarin). Initial concern was raised that the cardiovascular benefits seen with oestrogen-only therapy would not be maintained with the cyclical oestrogen plus progestogen regimes of HRT which are more commonly prescribed in the UK. However, further studies have demonstrated that when used in the low doses currently recommended in modern forms of HRT, the benefit is not lost (Hunt *et al.*, 1987). Further studies are underway to clarify this. Some progestogens may have an adverse lipid effect but as we have already seen, it is unlikely that the beneficial effect of HRT is solely due to lipid changes.

At present most women know that HRT will help acute menopausal symptoms and many are also aware of the beneficial effects to the skeleton. However fewer are aware of the very real benefits to the cardiovascular system and indeed many women believe HRT will be harmful to this system rather than of benefit. Greater education is necessary to ensure that women are learning of this benefit as well as all the others.

Alzheimer's disease

New research appears to indicate that HRT could lower the risk or slow the progression of Alzheimer's disease in some women. There is an urgent need for larger and longer trials before the treatment of this disease can be claimed an additional benefit of HRT (Paganini-Hill, 1996).

Hormone replacement therapy

Hormone replacement therapy (HRT) has become a hot issue for discussion among women in their fifties. 'Should I or shouldn't I take it?', 'Do I need it?', 'Will it harm rather than help?' These and other questions are very important to women as they go through their menopause. The decision to take HRT is a personal one for most women, with conflicting advice often being offered by doctors, nurses, friends and the media. Women need more information in order to be able to make an informed choice for themselves. It is estimated that around 75% of post-menopausal women will experience acute menopause symptoms, yet only about 10–20% will receive HRT. Even fewer will continue the treatment beyond the first few months. As a health professional you must give accurate information to women so that they can make an informed choice for themselves.

Principles of HRT

HRT consists of the two female hormones: oestrogen and progestogen. In hysterectomized women, oestrogen is used on its own but women with a uterus are generally prescribed both oestrogen and progestogen in order to prevent the endometrial stimulation which has been associated with oestrogen-only therapy (Henderson, 1989).

Oestrogens used in HRT are natural rather than synthetic. Natural oestrogens, which include oestradiol, oestrone and oestriol, cause the level of oestrogen circulating in the bloodstream to be similar to normal pre-menopausal levels. Synthetic oestrogens such as those found in the oral contraceptive pill have a much more potent effect and are not used in modern forms of HRT. Conjugated equine oestrogens (e.g. Premarin, a common form of HRT) act in a similar way to human oestrogens and are considered to be 'natural' rather than synthetic.

In most current forms of HRT in the UK, oestrogen is given on a continuous basis, i.e. without a break. Progestogens can be given cyclically or continuously, although in the UK, cyclical progestogen has become normal practice.

As HRT develops we are likely to see more preparations with continuous progestogen used in an attempt to avoid the need for a monthly bleed by producing an atrophic endometrium. This 'period-free HRT' is an attractive option for *post-*menopausal women wanting to start HRT. Studies have shown irregular bleeding and spotting are common in the first few months but these usually settle. New preparations of continuous combined oestrogen and progestogen are being researched and are available. Tricyclical regimes are also available, where progestogen is administered once every three months. This could minimize the likelihood of progestogenic side effects and produce a withdrawal bleed only once every three months.

Routes of administration

HRT can be given in various forms, and for the majority of women the final decision should be influenced by a personal choice. A woman who has chosen her favoured route of receiving HRT is more likely to continue the therapy than the woman who has been persuaded to use a regime with which she does not feel comfortable. HRT can be given in the following ways:

- ♦ Oral
- ♦ Transdermal
- ♦ Implants
- ♦ Vaginal creams/pessaries.

The main difference between the oral and non-oral routes of HRT is the avoidance of the gastrointestinal tract in non-oral routes and the subsequent 'first-pass effect' on the liver. Tablets also result in a greater change of oestradiol to oestrone, changing the ratio from that which is normally found in a pre-menopausal woman. Variation in circulating oestrogen levels between women is common as rates of absorption vary from individual to individual.

First-pass effect

The so-called 'first-pass effect' means that the liver receives a bolus of oestrogen after each dose, rather than a steady release. It results in metabolism of much of the oestrogen into a less active form. This means that a higher dose is necessary in order to achieve similar therapeutic effects to non-oral routes. This first pass will have an effect on various factors, including clotting and lipids. These effects are not all adverse and tablets have not been shown to result in any increase in hypertension or thrombotic disease (Whitehead and Godfree, 1992). Indeed, oestrogen given by any route will eventually pass through the liver and have similar effects. It is generally recommended that oral therapy should be avoided in women who are considered to be particularly susceptible to effects in the liver, such as those with hypertension, hypertriglyceridaemia or a previous history of venous thrombosis (Whitehead and Godfree, 1992). Women who have previously experienced severe gastrointestinal upset, such as Crohn's disease, may also benefit from a non-oral route, because of possible absorption problems.

Tablets

Tablets are the commonest way of receiving HRT. They have been available longer than any

Box 14.4 Oral HRT: advantages and disadvantages.

Advantages

♦ Convenient to take for most people

♦ Familiar way of taking medication

♦ Available as oestrogen-only and combined preparations

♦ Relatively inexpensive

♦ Regimens can easily be tailored to an individual's needs.

Disadvantages

♦ Some women consider any tablets to be 'unnatural'

♦ Ratio of oestradiol to oestrone is altered

♦ Compliance can be poor if pills are forgotten

♦ First-pass effect on the liver

♦ Slight nausea in some women in early stages.

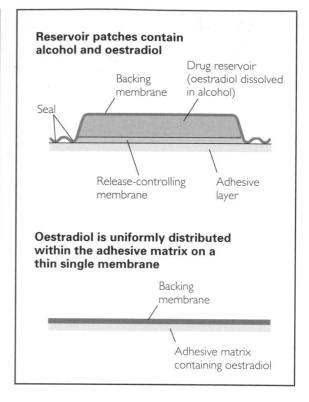

Reservoir patches contain alcohol and oestradiol

Seal
Backing membrane
Drug reservoir (oestradiol dissolved in alcohol)
Release-controlling membrane
Adhesive layer

Oestradiol is uniformly distributed within the adhesive matrix on a thin single membrane

Backing membrane
Adhesive matrix containing oestradiol

Figure 14.3 *Reservoir patches (top) contain alcohol and oestradiol. In matrix patches (below) the oestradiol is uniformly distributed within the adhesive matrix on a thin single membrane. (Reproduced courtesy of Janssen Cilag Ltd.)*

other form of HRT and much of the research into the long-term effects of HRT has been carried out using oral forms of therapy. They are available in different doses containing various natural oestrogens and in combination with a choice of progestogens. The advantages and disadvantages are listed in Box 14.4.

Transdermal

HRT can be given transdermally by either:

♦ patches or

♦ gel preparation.

Oestradiol patches deliver a constant dose of oestrogen over a 24-hour period. The patch is stuck to the abdomen or buttocks and changed once or twice weekly and is generally kept on during bathing and swimming. The first patch to be developed was the 'reservoir' patch, which consists of oestradiol dissolved in alcohol in a drug reservoir. An adhesive layer holds the patch in position on the skin whilst the alcohol carries the drug through the skin. The newer 'matrix' patches contain no alcohol and the oestradiol is contained in the matrix of the adhesive itself (Figure 14.3). These patches seem to stick better and for some women cause less skin irritation. Patches are available in

different doses and can be used in combination with progestogen, either orally or in a combined oestrogen/ progestogen patch.

The advantages and disadvantages of transdermal HRT patches are listed in Box 14.5.

HRT in the form of a gel is now available in the UK, after many years of use in France. It is recommended to be rubbed into the skin (upper arm and shoulders or alternatively the inner thighs) daily and it works in a similar way to patches. Women with a uterus must also take progestogen in order to prevent endometrial stimulation.

Implants

Oestradiol implants are small pellets containing oestrogen which are inserted under the skin of the abdomen or buttock through a small incision

> **Box 14.5** Transdermal HRT patches: advantages and disadvantages
>
> *Advantages*
>
> ♦ No need for tablets. A combined oestrogen/progestogen patch is available.
>
> ♦ Physiologically normal ratio of oestradiol to oestrone.
>
> ♦ Avoids first-pass effect on the liver.
>
> ♦ Perceived as more 'natural' by some women.
>
> *Disadvantages*
>
> ♦ Some women develop a skin irritation
>
> ♦ Degree of adhesion may vary between women
>
> ♦ Visual reminder to the women of her HRT
>
> ♦ Must remember to change the patch regularly.

(Figure 14.4). The oestrogen is released slowly over a period of months. They are available in varying doses: the higher the dose, usually the longer they last. Levels of oestrogen in the bloodstream tend to be higher than with other forms of HRT, but there is no evidence that this is damaging. Indeed some women seem to benefit from these higher levels. Implants can last a long time with great variation between individuals. The physiological effect of an implant can continue for up to two years and progestogen therapy may be necessary for that time if the women has a uterus. Rarely, a condition described as 'tachyphylaxis' has been observed, where women return for an implant at increasingly shorter intervals (Gangar *et al.*, 1989). Symptom control becomes poor even though oestrogen levels are high. So far there has been no evidence that this is harmful but some specialists consider it wise to try and offer lower doses less frequently until levels return to a more normal level. This may be difficult for a woman who has become used to high oestrogen levels.

The advantages and disadvantages of HRT implants are listed in Box 14.6 overleaf.

Vaginal treatments

Oestrogens administered directly to the vagina are useful for some women. They have a direct beneficial effect on atrophic vaginitis without the systemic effects of other routes. They are particularly useful for the older woman whose main complaint is of vaginal discomfort.

The oestrogens used in modern forms of vaginal preparations are oestriol and oestradiol. These are not absorbed systemically when administered at the recommended doses and therefore will not have an effect on vasomotor symptoms or confer benefit to the skeleton or heart. Preparations which comprise of creams, pessaries or vaginal tablets are recommended to be used 4–5 times a week for 2–3 weeks and then reduced to twice a week as a maintenance dose for two to three

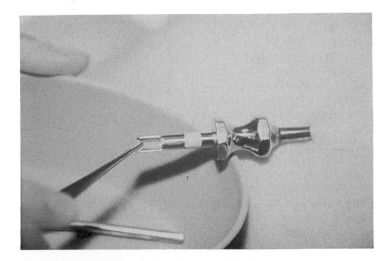

Figure 14.4 *Insertion of an oestradiol implant. (Reproduced courtesy of Organon Laboratories.)*

Box 14.6 HRT implants: advantages and disadvantages

Advantages

♦ Inserted two to three times a year and then nothing more to remember

♦ Compliance is ensured

♦ No first-pass effect

♦ Physiologically normal oestradiol to oestrone ratio

♦ Can be given alongside testosterone therapy

♦ Very convenient for women who do not need progestogen

♦ Cheap.

Disadvantages

♦ Has to be inserted by a medical practitioner

♦ Minor surgical procedure

♦ Prolonged action in some women

♦ 'Tachyphylaxis' in some women.

Box 14.7 Vaginal HRT treatments: advantages and disadvantages

Advantages

♦ No need for bleed

♦ Can be used alongside other HRT if necessary for women with severe urogenital symptoms

♦ Vaginal tablets very convenient to use

♦ Offers good relief of urogenital symptoms

♦ Vaginal ring offers more long-term relief with less intervention.

Disadvantages

♦ Some creams seem messy to use

♦ Older women may find an applicator or ring difficult to use

♦ Regulation of dose can be difficult.

months. Many women then repeat the course a few months later. A soft flexible ring containing oestradiol is also available and should be changed after three months. This has the advantage of being less intrusive on a woman's lifestyle and yet offers good relief of vaginal symptoms. It can be inserted either by a medical practitioner or, after instruction, by the woman herself.

Some women use oestrogen creams as a lubricant during sexual intercourse. This should be discouraged as oestrogen could be absorbed through the penile skin and cause adverse effects to the partner, although this is less likely with newer formulations (Di Raimondo *et al.*, 1980).

The advantages and disadvantages of vaginal HRT treatments are listed in Box 14.7.

Progestogens

Progestogen is added to oestrogen in order to offer protection to the endometrium. Studies have reported an increased risk of endometrial hyperplasia in users of oestrogen-only regimes and that these regimes have a prolonged effect on the endometrium even after treatment has stopped. The implication of this is that if women receive even a relatively short course of oestrogen-only therapy

they would theoretically need medical follow-up for several years after stopping treatment (Henderson, 1989).

This incidence of hyperplasia can be prevented by giving a cyclical progestogen alongside the oestrogen therapy (Box 14.8). The number of days that progestogen is taken is directly associated with the degree of protection offered (Paterson *et al.*, 1980). It is currently recommended that 10–13 days offers maximum protection and most HRT preparations work on this principle.

Box 14.8 Recommended daily doses of various progestogens in combination with oestrogen used in HRT

Norethisterone	0.7–2.5 mg (1 mg is most common)
Levonorgestrel	150 μg
Dydrogesterone	10/20 mg
Medroxyprogesterone acetate	5/10 mg

Progestogen only therapy. If a woman has severe vasomotor symptoms and is concerned about osteoporosis, but cannot or will not take oestrogen therapy, progestogen on its own may be useful. Doses necessary would be medroxyprogesterone acetate 10–20 mg or norethisterone 5–10 mg daily.

Bleeding. Approximately 80–90% of women who take a cyclical HRT regime will experience a monthly withdrawal bleed. You should counsel a woman that this bleed should be regular, lasting up to about six or seven days, but may be much shorter. It should not be painful or too heavy and should settle into a predictable pattern.

Breakthrough bleeding (i.e. unrelated to the progestogen) should not occur and repeated episodes need investigation. Occasional episodes may be due to:

♦ poor compliance – progestogen is missed;

♦ interaction with other drugs – such as antibiotics;

♦ gastrointestinal upset – progestogen is not absorbed; or

♦ stress.

Heavy prolonged bleeding may be caused by:

♦ poor compliance,

♦ fibroids,

♦ endometrial polyps,

♦ inadequate dose of progestogen, or

♦ endometrial hyperplasia.

Progestogen-releasing intrauterine system (IUS)

A T-shaped IUD containing levonorgestrel in a sleeve around the stem is now available and marketed in the UK under the name 'Mirena'. The insertion of this intrauterine system or IUS means there is a progestogenic effect directly on the endometrium with minimal systemic absorption. Potentially this has several advantages for the woman: cyclical progestogen is unnecessary as the endometrium is protected from hyperplasia by the steady release of levonorgestrel, progestogenic side-effects are minimized, reduced bleeding or amenorrhoea occurs in a substantial number of women and contraception would be provided for the peri-menopausal woman. Currently this product is only licensed in the UK for its contraceptive use, but studies in Finland have shown that the IUS offers a long term and convenient progestogen alternative when combined with oestradiol implants. The authors comment that women appreciated the simplicity of the method (no regular pill taking or patch changing) combined with the minimal bleeding and this increased the acceptability and convenience of HRT (Suhonen *et al.*, 1995.)

Tibolone

Tibolone is a therapy for relief of acute menopausal symptoms which is given continuously and theoretically does not produce a bleed. It has oestrogenic, progestogenic and androgenic properties and has been shown to be effective at reducing flushes, sweats, sleeplessness and in improving mood and libido in women (Benedek-Jaszmann, 1987). Irregular bleeding may occur in peri- menopausal women so it is only recommended for use in women who have had one year without periods. The majority of post-menopausal women on Tibolone will have amenorrhea, but any irregular bleeding on this therapy should be investigated (Sturdee, 1993). Long-term effects on the cardiovascular system are not yet known but it appears to have a beneficial effect on the skeleton (Hands, 1991).

Contraindications to hormone replacement therapy

In the past both health professionals and the lay public alike have been concerned about which women should not take HRT because of pre-existing medical conditions. Data based on research into the oral contraceptive pill have been wrongly applied to HRT and confusion has consequently arisen.

Absolute contraindications

Absolute contraindications are considered to be those medical conditions which will be worsened by the use of HRT. In these circumstances HRT use should be avoided, although occasionally women with such conditions seek the advice of a menopause specialist and may be prescribed HRT. This would be on an individual basis, however, and should not be taken as general guidelines.

Absolute contraindications to HRT are;

♦ Endometrial cancer

♦ Breast cancer

♦ Pregnancy

♦ Undiagnosed abnormal vaginal bleeding

♦ Severe, active liver disease.

Relative contraindications

In the past, some other conditions have been taken as contraindications but are no longer generally considered to be so. Some specialists would, however, recommend the use of the non-oral route as a preference for women with these conditions, because of the avoidance of the first-pass effect on the liver and subsequent lipid and clotting changes (Whitehead and Godfree, 1992). These conditions listed in Box 14.9, could be considered relative contraindications and referral to a specialist may be preferred. However it is important that women with these conditions are not led to believe that HRT would be out of the question.

Breast cancer and HRT

One of the greatest anxieties which is shared by both the lay public and health professionals is the possibility of increasing the risk of breast cancer in women taking HRT. Unfortunately, breast cancer is a common disease with hormonal factors being known to play an important role. The following are known risk factors for breast cancer:

♦ Early menarche

♦ Obesity (which is associated with higher levels of circulating oestrogen)

♦ Late first pregnancy

♦ Late menopause.

Breast cancer is naturally a very emotive issue and one which frightens many women. The idea of increasing the risk of developing cancer is unthinkable for many women even though the risk of developing other diseases, e.g. heart disease, may be greater without HRT. Women therefore look for reassurance that they will not get cancer and although the data about HRT is reassuring, especially in short- to medium-term use, it is impossible to give women the absolute reassurance they want. As more and more women are prescribed HRT it is inevitable that some will develop breast cancer and it will be very difficult to persuade these women that the HRT was unrelated.

The effect of HRT on breast cancer is not conclusive – a large number of studies have been carried out but little general agreement reached. In the last ten years some studies have shown a slight

---

Box 14.9 Medical conditions and HRT

♦ *Hypertension* Untreated hypertension should be treated prior to starting HRT but is not a contraindication.

♦ *Myocardial infarction or angina* One study has shown that the incidence of fatal MI in a woman with previous MI was 50% less in a group treated with HRT (Henderson *et al.*, 1986). Specialist advice is suggested.

♦ *Previous thrombosis* Previous thrombosis provoked by a known risk factor such as immobilization or surgery is not considered a contraindication, although non-oral therapy may be recommended. Clotting screens are recommended particularly in women who have had a previous unprovoked thrombosis or in women who experienced a thrombosis whilst pregnant or during use of the oral contraceptive pill. Abnormal clotting screen results would suggest that the woman be referred to a haematologist, (Whitehead and Godfree, 1992).

♦ *Varicose veins* Not a contraindication.

♦ *Heavy smoker* Not a contraindication and could be considered an indication in view of the increased risk of cardiovascular disease.

♦ *Diabetes* Glucose levels should be monitored in case insulin requirements change initially.

♦ *Gallstones* If a woman actually has gallstones HRT is usually avoided. Treated gallstones are not a problem.

♦ *Migraine* It is impossible to predict how migraine will respond to HRT. The only answer is for a woman to try it and monitor the migraines.

♦ *Otosclerosis* A condition of progressive deafness which has been shown to worsen in pregnancy. It has been suggested that HRT should be used with caution in case the changing oestrogen status worsens the condition, although referral to an ENT specialist may be helpful (Whitehead and Godfree, 1992).

---

increase in the risk of breast cancer with oestrogen use whilst others have not. Studies are difficult to conduct because of the necessary large numbers and also the need to allow for so many other influencing factors. Those women at an already high risk have in the past avoided use of HRT so are seldom included in the statistics (Bergkvist *et al.*, 1988).

If there is an increased risk of breast cancer with HRT it would appear to be with longer term use. A meta-analysis of many studies was conducted and showed no increase in the risk of breast cancer with up to five years use of HRT. Over ten years use has shown a slight increase in breast cancer risk (Steinberg *et al.*, 1991). The effect of 5–10 years' use is still unclear. However, if a woman develops breast cancer whilst on HRT, studies show that the mortality rate is lower, perhaps because the tumour will have been detected earlier or because the tumour is of a lower grade malignancy (Hunt *et al.*, 1987).

Preparing a woman for hormone replacement therapy

You should encourage women to make an informed choice about HRT, to decide for themselves whether or not to take it and how long they may take it for. Many doctors wait for a woman to ask for HRT rather than offering it to her and indeed some doctors appear only to prescribe for those women with unmanageable symptoms. Yet some women find accurate information about HRT difficult to find and making an informed choice can be very difficult for them. It is hardly surprising then to discover that only about 10% of post-menopausal women in the UK take HRT (Wilkes *et al.*, 1991) and that many start HRT only to stop it at a very early stage because of anxiety about side-effects. Of those women who stop treatment it is estimated that the vast majority do so without the knowledge of their family doctor (NOP, 1992). With the ever-increasing evidence that HRT is beneficial to both heart and bones it is essential that women at least consider taking it for more than just a few months.

Information

Women read about issues relating to menopause and HRT in the media. These articles are not always well-researched or accurate, yet women often believe them because they are in print. Some articles over-sensationalize HRT, making it out to be a modern wonder drug, whilst other articles emphasize only the negative aspects of HRT and encourage women to 'think natural' rather than trying HRT.

Women also receive information about HRT from sketchy medical consultations where time is short and the opportunity for discussion limited. It is therefore essential that you carefully consider how you can provide the necessary information for women so that they are better placed to make decisions for themselves. Some would suggest that all women attending for a medical consultation in their forties should be provided with information about the menopause so that they are prepared when the time comes. You could also consider the menopause to be a time in a woman's life, like pregnancy, where help and advice is essential but that ultimately the woman makes decisions for herself regarding the options open to her.

Ways of providing this information include:

◆ Leaflets/books/videos

◆ Group discussions

◆ Menopause information evenings

◆ Support groups

◆ Talks to local women's groups.

Scenario

One general practice decided to offer monthly information evenings on the subject of the menopause. Women were targeted with invitations through the age/sex register and offered a suitable date. The evenings were run jointly by the practice nurse and the health visitor. A video was shown which prompted discussion and questions of a general nature, and the opportunity was taken to discuss the benefits of HRT. Women were then encouraged to return for a personal consultation in order to discuss their own individual situation. They came to these consultations better informed and able to ask relevant questions because they had been to the information evening.

Unrealistic expectations

If you are able to, it is well worth evaluating with a woman about to start HRT what she is hoping it will do for her. Some women start HRT with hopelessly unrealistic ideas and, not surprisingly, are disappointed a few months later. You can assess which symptoms are most likely to be helped by HRT and warn her that some may take longer to improve than others. If she has the idea that HRT will make her look and feel 20 years younger, it is helpful to try and dispel this myth. Some women also expect HRT to repair broken relationships, restore sexual desires and generally perform miracles!

Side-effects

Women do worry about risks of HRT and unwanted side-effects (Box 14.10). It is therefore important that *you* raise these issues even before a woman starts HRT. You should have honest discussion about issues such as breast cancer, bleeding and other side-effects so that a woman starts treatment confident that she has received all the necessary advice. She will then start it with an open mind, prepared for early side-effects but willing to persevere. You should advise her as to when to expect her bleed and warn her that the first one is not necessarily an indication of how future bleeds will be. You should also warn her of early side-effects which are caused by the sudden rise in oestrogen levels when HRT is started. If you do not prepare women for these side-effects they may cause greater anxiety as women become concerned about underlying problems. For example, the woman with breast tenderness thinks the HRT is causing breast cancer, or the woman with leg cramps thinks she is getting a thrombosis. It is often these early side-effects which cause women to give up HRT after only a very short time.

Box 14.10 Understanding the side-effects of HRT

Breast tenderness
Nausea
Leg cramps
Headaches
} These are often oestrogen related and temporary

PMS-type symptoms
Fluid retention
Bleeding problems
} These are usually progestogen related

Scenario

Jill started HRT for relief of flushes. These disappeared rapidly but her breasts felt very sore and she experienced headaches for ten days out of the month. After a few weeks Jill decided the treatment was not worth the benefits and discontinued the HRT. She failed to keep her follow-up appointment. Her symptoms returned but she did not realize that the breast problem would probably have subsided and that the progestogen may have been the cause of the headaches and that this could be altered. The resulting flushes caused her to go without a good night's sleep for nearly two years.

Understanding her HRT

Many women are prescribed HRT without understanding what the treatment comprises of. Most HRT regimes are 'user-friendly' but women can still misunderstand the therapy and take it incorrectly. As with the contraceptive pill it is worth taking the time to explain the regime and reinforce how to take it. In the case of patches, it may be helpful to actually demonstrate them to some women. Women who are taking a combined oestrogen and progestogen therapy need to understand why the progestogen is important and necessary or they may be tempted to miss this part out, particularly if it is causing side-effects.

Scenario

Karen commenced on HRT for acute menopausal symptoms. She felt much better on it and her symptoms subsided. However she noticed that the extra tablets at the end of the packet caused her to feel bloated and generally less well. She decided to experiment and initially missed every other tablet and eventually missed them all. The bloated feeling disappeared yet her menopausal symptoms were still well-controlled. It was a further five months before she told her doctor what she had discovered and she was alarmed to realize that she had been potentially damaging the womb by taking unopposed *oestrogen. She had thought all the tablets in the treatment were simply to control her symptoms.*

Tailoring the dose

Women are often unaware that HRT is a whole spectrum of medications, doses and types of hormones. They may simply stop a treatment which is unsuitable thinking that they have 'given it a go' when in fact a different regime may be much more suitable. You need to encourage women to return with their complaints so that a different regime can at least be tried. This will sometimes mean moving away from the convenient packs of combined oestrogen and progestogen and prescribing the two hormones separately. It is particularly important that a woman on a 'tailored' dose understands when to take each component. Women on such regimes may find it easier to take the progestogen on a calendar month basis rather than on her own cyclical one, e.g. commencing the progestogen on the first day of every month.

Perseverance

You should prepare women for the fact that the first HRT regimen they try, may not be the one which is most suited to them. An open mind is necessary when starting HRT and a willingness to try different treatment variations. As a practitioner you also need to be open to the woman who wants to try different regimes until she finds the one which is most suitable for her.

Pre-treatment counselling

The secret to a woman's confidence in her HRT often lies in the information you offer her before she even starts it and in the way you deal with her anxieties once she is on therapy. Women want and deserve open and frank discussion before starting HRT with ample opportunity to ask questions.

Anxieties women have about HRT

Fear of cancer

The word 'hormone' can be off-putting for some women and cause them to have anxieties about how they will be affected if they take HRT. Education

and information is the answer to ensure that women fully understand both the risks and benefits of HRT. The issue of breast cancer must be discussed and not avoided and the need for progestogen in the non-hysterectomized woman must be stressed.

Risk of thrombosis

Some women (and some doctors!) are confused about the differences between the contraceptive pill and HRT. This leads to a belief that any risk associated with the Pill must also apply to HRT. They are often confused to be told at 35 years that they must stop the Pill because they smoke, only to be told at the age of 50 years that they should consider HRT because of the benefits to the cardiovascular system. Women who have had a previous thrombosis may have been led to believe that they should avoid HRT, despite current evidence to the contrary.

Fertility

Some women worry that if they resume a monthly bleed, then fertility will also return. An explanation about the mechanics of conception and of how HRT works will be helpful. Women should also be reminded that HRT is not contraceptive in its actions.

Side-effects

A careful explanation of common side-effects, e.g. nausea, leg aches and breast tenderness, is appreciated by most women, who would prefer to be forewarned and therefore prepared for any possible problems.

HRT is unnatural

Many people have the idea that if something is natural it must be good for you and if it is unnatural it must be harmful. Women look to those of previous generations for whom HRT was not available, and ask 'Why do I need it and they did not?', forgetting that life expectancy and the expected quality of life in old age has improved dramatically. You could argue that the menopause is a state of hormone deficiency and that by giving HRT you are simply replacing the hormones, but to discuss whether this is natural or not is not really helpful. Each woman should be encouraged to look at the facts herself and make her choice.

Bleeding

For many women, stopping the monthly periods is the only real advantage of the menopause. If a woman is to start HRT she should be prepared for the possibility of a monthly bleed, and be told when to expect it and how long it may last.

Monitoring and evaluation of HRT

When a woman starts any form of HRT, she wants to be sure that it is safe for her to do so and be confident that she will be adequately monitored whilst on therapy. The following baseline investigations are usually performed prior to a woman starting HRT:

♦ Height

♦ Weight

♦ Blood pressure

♦ Medical history

♦ Pelvic examination

♦ Breast examination.

These represent basic well-woman checks and ensure that there are no true contraindications to the use of HRT. Regular cervical smears and mammography should be recommended according to local policy for all women. These are not required more frequently because of HRT use.

Other investigations

Some women will require extra investigations because of a particular medical or family history. These should be assessed on an individual basis but may include the following:

♦ Thyroid function test

♦ Clotting screens

♦ Lipid profiles

♦ Mammography

♦ Follicle stimulating hormone levels

♦ Bone densitometry.

These tests may be clinically indicated prior to starting HRT but an abnormal result will not necessarily preclude the woman from taking HRT. Treatment for the relevant condition may be initiated, followed by HRT. Some of the results, e.g. low bone density, may give a stronger indication for using HRT than for not using it.

Ongoing evaluation

Initial evaluation is generally done after three months on HRT or after starting a new regime. Once established on a satisfactory treatment regime, follow-up visits can be 6–8 monthly. Assessments at follow-up visits will include:

♦ Weight

♦ Blood pressure

♦ Symptom assessment

♦ Assessment of side-effects

♦ Monitoring of bleeding

♦ Breast check.

Pelvic examination

Thorough pelvic examination should be performed prior to a woman starting HRT to exclude any obvious abnormalities. Once established on HRT they are generally performed three yearly along with cervical cytology, unless clinically indicated more frequently. Such indications may include:

♦ Abnormal bleeding pattern on HRT

♦ Presence of fibroids which require monitoring

♦ Presence of endometriosis

♦ Post-coital bleeding

♦ Pelvic pain.

Who should monitor?

As with many areas of medicine, preparing a woman for HRT and monitoring her whilst she takes it, has in the past been the responsibility of doctors, either general practitioners or consultants.

As nurses widen their roles, particularly in the community, it is becoming more common for women to turn to them for help and advice about well-woman and menopause-related issues. Nurses are already running health promotion clinics and advice and care at the time of the menopause could be incorporated into these. However you must ensure the following:

♦ Adequate training for the nurse

♦ Supervision and support from the GP

♦ Willingness to work as a team by both GP and nurse

♦ Consistency of information among team members.

Areas in which nurses are most likely to be involved are:

♦ History taking

♦ Information and explanations about HRT

♦ Answering specific enquiries, especially by telephone

♦ Organizing a clinic

♦ Providing literature and recommending books/videos

♦ Liasing with self-help groups

♦ Monitoring of women who are established on HRT.

It is important that you make it as easy as possible for women to ask questions once on HRT. Appointments may be busy but a Helpline will ensure that those women with anxieties are dealt with speedily and in time to prevent them simply stopping their HRT. This helpline may only need to be available for a couple of hours a week, but it is very useful for women to know that if they phone at a certain time on a certain day, they will receive adequate help. In the long term this will probably reduce the number of appointments needed as many minor issues can be easily dealt with over the telephone.

Non-hormonal treatments for oestrogen-deficiency symptoms

One of the commonest questions asked by women considering the use of hormone replacement therapy is, 'Is there an alternative?'. Those women who are advised against HRT for medical reasons seek other ways of relieving acute menopausal symptoms and protecting their bones and hearts. Other women see HRT only as a 'last resort' and would prefer to use anything but HRT to help symptoms. Some view taking HRT as failure to cope with life, believing that if they live a healthy, positive lifestyle, then they should not need it. However, women soon find that menopausal symptoms are non-discriminatory and even the woman with the healthiest lifestyle and strongest positive attitude may get unpleasant menopausal symptoms. The ability to cope with the symptoms may vary and some women will turn to HRT much sooner than others, whilst a few women will persevere with all sorts of other therapies before eventually turning to HRT.

There have been few studies to evaluate the success or otherwise of non-hormonal treatments, particularly the so-called alternative therapies which are becoming so widely talked about and tried by women. Reports are therefore often anecdotal rather than scientific and we can only suggest to women that they try them with an open mind. Menopausal symptoms have been demonstrated to have a strong placebo response to any treatment so a woman needs to try a therapy for quite a while to be sure of its long-term effectiveness. Some would argue that even a placebo effect is worthwhile if it improves quality of life for a while without being harmful. Some non-hormonal treatments are aimed more at assisting the woman to cope with her symptoms, rather than actually curing them. For many women this is sufficient to substantially improve quality of life.

Short-term symptom relief

Each symptom needs assessment individually and treatment offered accordingly. Clonidine may be offered for relief of hot flushes (Claydon *et al.*, 1974), vaginal lubricants for vaginal discomfort and sedatives for sleep problems. Obviously these do not treat the underlying oestrogen deficiency but may achieve good symptom control at least in the short term. Various vitamin complexes, such as vitamin B_6 and vitamin E, have been suggested for relief of some symptoms. Vitamin E, which is said to be useful for mood swings and breast tenderness, has also been shown to relieve hot flushes (McLaren, 1949). Oil of evening primrose is widely quoted as being useful for menopausal symptoms although scientific evidence is not conclusive. Other therapies which have been suggested for relief of menopausal symptoms are:

♦ Herbal remedies

♦ Acupuncture

♦ Aromatherapy

♦ Reflexology

♦ Shiatsu

♦ T'ai Chi

♦ Yoga.

Coping strategies

Some women discover ways of coping with their symptoms, particularly vasomotor symptoms, which enable them to continue a normal life. These include:

♦ wearing several layers of light clothing which can be easily removed;

♦ reducing caffeine/alcohol intake;

♦ showering frequently and avoiding hot baths;

♦ avoiding 'trigger' foods such as spices and curries;

♦ cutting down on smoking;

♦ opening plenty of windows;

♦ avoiding stressful situations where possible; and

♦ wearing a lightweight towelling dressing gown in bed to help absorb perspiration and reduce the need to change sheets so frequently.

Some women also find that relaxation techniques, stress management and counselling may help in coping with symptoms and also in coming to terms with this transitional life phase.

At the time of the menopause, many women take the opportunity to re-evaluate their lifestyle, perhaps making adjustments to their habits related to smoking, diet and exercise.

Whatever a woman does decide about taking hormone replacement therapy, it is important that she realizes that these 'natural' therapies may not be totally free from drawbacks themselves and that although her symptoms may improve, she should not assume that she is also benefiting her skeletal, cardiovascular and urogenital systems. Women need to understand that relief of symptoms alone is not the secret to successful menopause management.

Osteoporosis and cardiovascular disease

Women who take hormone replacement therapy for relief of acute symptoms, early in the climacteric, are also silently giving benefit to other body systems – the bones and the heart. Those women who do not get symptoms and so do not consider HRT are losing out on these benefits. Other factors which influence the rate of osteoporosis and heart disease should be considered if they decide against HRT. These include:

♦ *Exercise* This is beneficial to the whole body, leading to a general feeling of well-being and improved physical strength and suppleness. Beneficial to both the cardiovascular system and to the skeleton.

♦ *Diet* A good, varied diet is necessary to maintain a healthy body. Recommendations include low total fat intake, low sugar intake, low salt intake, increased fibre intake, good calcium intake. Calcium is an essential part of a balanced diet and women are particularly encouraged to think about this at the time of the menopause. Most women who take a healthy diet probably achieve a good calcium intake, but those women who have a restricted dairy intake may need supplements.

♦ *Lifestyle* Reducing alcohol intake and cutting back on smoking will help to promote good health. Cigarette smoking in particular is known to be harmful to the cardiovascular system and women who are serious about improving their health should stop smoking.

Other medications

Alternative drug therapies are available which may be suitable for those women who cannot take oestrogen therapy but who are concerned about osteoporosis.

♦ *Calcitonin* This is given as an injection although it is being developed as a nasal spray. It has some analgesic properties and is generally used for treatment not prevention of osteoporosis.

♦ *Bisphosphonates* This is a group of medications which works in a similar way to HRT on bone. Etidronate is used in conjunction with calcium supplements in a regime of 14 days of disodium etidronate and 76 days of calcium supplementation, it is licensed for treatment rather than prevention of osteoporosis so is more often used in the older woman. Newer bisphosphonates are likely to become available.

♦ *Progestogen alone* This cannot be described as 'non-hormonal' but is useful for those women who cannot take HRT for medical reasons (see page 350).

It is helpful to point out to women that whilst lifestyle changes are important they may not be of sufficient value to fully replace the benefits of HRT as we know them. A healthy lifestyle is always to be encouraged but we must ensure that we do not lead women to think that these alone are an effective alternative to HRT.

Other factors which influence a woman at the climacteric

The menopause is a time in a woman's life when her body undergoes immense physical change. The consequences can be long-lasting and can affect how she copes with other stresses which may arise at around the same time. It is all too easy to blame the menopause for every physical and emotional upset which occurs at around the age of fifty. This would be wrong but it is true that areas of a woman's life which she has always coped with successfully can suddenly become difficult to manage. Some women find life at the time of the menopause to be one of great change, whilst others find life continues as normal. Whether the physical effects of a changing body lead to the woman feeling less able to cope, or whether the emotional upsets appear to make physical symptoms worse, is unclear. Nevertheless, the woman, her problems and her hormones must be viewed together rather than in isolation from each other. Some women

will need treatments and therapies other than hormone replacement therapy in order to help them cope with some aspects of their lives. Some problems which arise around mid-life will be better treated by these other therapies than by simple HRT.

Changing body image

It is an unfair fact of life that society accepts the concept of a youthful figure as one to be constantly strived for. In the UK women spend large sums of money trying to keep slim, with no wrinkles and youthful looking hair. The cosmetics industry would have us believe that this is not only desirable but essential for the modern lifestyle. Both men and women need to accept that our bodies do change as we get older. Fat distribution changes, metabolic rate slows down and skin and hair may lose their youthful texture.

A change in how women view their body image is therefore required from women around mid-life if they are to come to terms with their changing bodies. This does not mean that women should resign themselves to being overweight and unattractive but they may need to make more effort to keep to the same weight. Extra exercise will be necessary to firm up sagging muscles and lifestyle changes become more pertinent at this time. The menopause occurs at a similar time to these other body changes and women tend to blame their hormones alone for all these changes.

Relationships

Mid-life can be a time when women re-evaluate the things that are important to them. Marriages which have become stale, relationships which are faltering, may be re-assessed and decisions made about the future. Women sometimes take the opportunity to discuss issues which have remained unspoken for many years. Relationships with children can become confrontational as teenagers become more rebellious and independent.

Failed dreams

Some women look upon the time of the menopause as a landmark in their lives and a time to evaluate their life. They may be disappointed that they have not achieved all that they had hoped for. Perhaps they did not succeed at work as they had expected. Maybe they did not have the longed-for children and the menopause has finally closed that door. Sometimes the disappointment may lie with their partner, the promotions which were never realized and the expectations which were not met.

Ageing parents

Some women expect the menopause to signify a time when they will be free of some of their previous responsibilities, particularly if children are getting older and more independent. It can therefore come as a shock to realize that their own parents, or those of their partner are becoming more dependent on them. Women may find themselves the unpaid carer, leading to feelings of frustration and sometimes resentment that their own freedom has been restricted.

'Empty nest'

The so-called 'empty nest syndrome' occurs in women who have dedicated their lives to the upbringing of their children to the exclusion of their own independence. When the children leave home it leaves a gap which is hard to fill. With more and more women having responsibilities both inside and outside the home, this phenomenon seems to be lessening. Indeed many women cannot wait for the last child to flee the nest!

Sexuality

Some women view the menopause as being the culmination of fertile years. The ability to bear children was a driving force behind sexual satisfaction and once fertility declines, new desires and expectations must be met. Women may feel less attractive and therefore consider themselves less desirable to their partner. For others, the freedom from the need for contraception can be a release and sexual relationships improve. For some, the stability of a longstanding relationship represents freedom for sexual expression, whilst for others it can lead to feelings of boredom and frustration. Physical symptoms of the menopause such as vag-

inal dryness may lead to sexual frustrations as women try to avoid painful and uncomfortable intercourse, as well as emotional upsets.

Fear of death

For some, the menopause may mark the beginning of old age. Fear of getting older and of death in particular, may influence how they feel. Attitudes to ageing vary from individual to individual and it is important that we consider this when discussing mid-life problems and the menopause. For some, the menopause prompts a sad realization that life is getting shorter and that old age, and ultimately death, are inevitable.

Work

In a society which values youth, it is easy for a woman to feel undervalued in the workplace despite her greater experience. Finding a job in her fifties is much more difficult than in younger years, even though she may be better qualified for the job than some younger applicants. Some women find that symptoms of the menopause cause them to give up a job because they feel less able to cope with difficult situations a decision they may then regret when their symptoms subside, only to discover that it is difficult to find work again.

Contraception at the peri-menopause

For many women, a real advantage of the menopause is that the fertile years are over and concerns about contraception can be forgotten. A freedom from these anxieties can lead to a renewed sexual enthusiasm and greater satisfaction within a relationship. Whilst one must appreciate that for some women, particularly the childless, this end of fertility marks a sad disappointment that children will not now be born, for others the relief that contraception can stop, can be just as great.

Yet some women do not realize the point at which fertility stops is very difficult to pinpoint and in theory, can only be done retrospectively. Fertility begins to decline during the late thirties continuing into the forties. Women may consider themselves infertile during the peri-menopausal phase when in fact they could still conceive. With the well-known physical risks attached to pregnancy in older women and the psychological trauma this can bring, it is particularly important that you counsel women appropriately about the ongoing need for contraception at this time.

The current Family Planning Association (FPA) recommendations are that contraception should continue in women over 50 years until they have not had a period for one year. Women under the age of 50 should continue using contraception for two years after their last period. The FPA recommendations are easily understood for those women who do not start HRT, but because HRT often causes bleeding to continue or to resume, the actual last period can be masked. This means that advising a woman when to stop contraception can at best, only be a guide. HRT cannot be considered to be contraceptive, so some women will need to consider a change of contraception at this time.

The Pill and HRT

If a woman is using the combined oral contraceptive pill then she is unlikely to notice menopausal symptoms as the levels of oestrogen in the pill will be controlling them. Regular bleeds are likely to continue and the last physiological period will be masked. Healthy, non smoking women, who are of normal weight and normotensive may continue using the combined pill providing that they are considered to be at a low risk of thrombosis and heart disease. In the light of recommendations from the Committee on Safety of Medicines (1995), it is particularly important that women are carefully assessed before continuing to use the combined pill. Women themselves must be informed of the small risk of thrombosis, when considering the risks and benefits (Mills *et al.*, 1996).

Those women who decide to come off the Pill will find either that their periods return, in which case they can follow the usual FPA guidelines and use contraception for a further one or two years after they stop, or that their periods have stopped. Measurement of FSH levels on two or three occasions over a six-month period can confirm that the menopause has occurred. Alternative contraception should be used whilst awaiting confirmation of FSH levels.

The progestogen-only pill

Use of the progestogen-only pill will not usually mask menopausal symptoms, although bleeding patterns may be unpredictable. Amenorrhoea should not be assumed to indicate that the menopause has occurred. Measurement of FSH levels on several occasions can help to give an indication of menopausal status. Occasionally the progestogen-only pill is prescribed alongside conventional HRT. Theoretically this should be contraceptive, but no studies have been carried out to confirm that the mini-pill continues its effect alongside exogenous oestrogen. Women who stop the progestogen-only pill and go straight on to HRT will not know when their last period occurs.

Depot progestogens

The main drawback of this method is its irreversibility and long-lasting effect. Menopausal symptoms can occur and if oestrogen therapy is required, irregular bleeding can result. In practice this method is rarely used by peri-menopausal women, particularly those wanting HRT.

Intrauterine devices and HRT

With modern IUDs, women can continue using them up until the time of the menopause. An IUD inserted from the age of 40 years onwards is unlikely to be replaced unless it causes problems, and can simply be removed after the menopause. One disadvantage is that if the IUD is left *in situ* for the recommended one or two years after the last bleed, it may be more difficult to remove than if a woman were still menstruating because of stenosis of the cervical os. A levonorgestrel releasing device is now available (see page 351) which is ideal for the perimenopausal woman.

Sterilization

Sterilization of one or other partner is a very secure way of preventing a pregnancy. It is unlikely, however, that a couple would choose this method at a time close to the menopause, because of the need for surgery. Sterilization at an earlier age will have no effect on the woman's subsequent menopause.

Natural methods of family planning

It is not recommended that women rely on natural methods of family planning around the time of the menopause. Irregular periods and changing vaginal and cervical mucus will make these methods very unreliable.

Barrier methods

Barrier methods, such as the condom, cap and spermicides, provide an effective method of contraception at the peri-menopause. They will not alter menstrual pattern and will not influence symptoms of the menopause. If a couple are already familiar with the use of a cap or condoms it is relatively easy to simply continue using them. It may be more difficult for those women who have not been used to barrier methods to start at this time. The decline in fertility leading up to the menopause means that those methods which might be considered unreliable in younger women, such as spermicides used alone will probably offer sufficient protection for this group of women. Barrier methods are easily stopped when contraception is no longer required.

The issue of contraception is one which must be discussed alongside advice about HRT. Some women think that HRT will act as a contraceptive and the consequences of such a belief could be disastrous for that individual. The question of when to stop using contraception is much more difficult to answer and will vary from woman to woman. If the actual date of the menopause is not known, only an arbitrary guess can be made as to when to stop contraception. To be on the safe side, some would say this should be to the age of 54 years.

Future developments

Nasal spray

A promising route for the future would seem to be a nasal spray of oestradiol which achieves plasma oestradiol levels sufficient to control menopausal symptoms. Research is underway to establish the doses required and to assess whether it also confers long term benefits.

Newer progestogens

It is likely that newer progestogens will be added to HRT in an attempt to minimize side effects and enhance cardiovascular benefit.

More 'period free' treatments

For many women, it is the thought of returning to regular withdrawal bleeds which makes HRT unacceptable. Products are available which offer a continuous oestrogen and progestogen in an attempt to achieve amenorrhoea. Others are likely to become available.

Testosterone patches

These are available for use in men. We may see them being developed as an adjunct to HRT for some women.

Combined single matrix oestrogen/progestogen patches

These would have the advantage of avoiding the need for tablets, whilst minimizing the risk of skin reactions.

Vaginal rings

Oestradiol and progestogen could be administered vaginally via a silastic hormone-releasing ring, making the use of patches or tablets unnecessary. Absorption through the vaginal mucosa would be sufficient for systemic effects to be achieved.

Conclusion

HRT is a rapidly changing field and you are likely to see many new products becoming available over the next few years. With a greater variety of regimes and products available, women are more likely to find a form of HRT which suits them, making it more convenient to use and therefore more beneficial in the long term. As more research is carried out and we learn more about the effects of oestrogen on the entire body, the whole field of HRT is likely to widen.

Resources

British Menopause Society
36 West Street, Marlow, Bucks SL7 2NB
Tel. 01628 890199

Institute of Psychosexual Medicine
11 Chandos Street, London W1M 9DE
Tel. 0171 580 0631

National Osteoporosis Society
PO Box 10, Radstock, Bath BA3 3YB
Tel. 01761 471771
Please enclose SAE.

Women's Health Concern
PO Box 1629, London W8 6AU
Tel. 0171 938 3932
Please enclose SAE.

Relate
Herbert Gray College, Little Church Street,
Rugby, Warwickshire CV21 3AP
Tel. 01788 573241

The Amarant Trust
11–13 Charterhouse Buildings, London EC1M
7AN
Please enclose large SAE.

Further reading

COOPER, W. (1988) *No Change*, 3rd revised edn.
London: Arrow Books.
NATIONAL OSTEOPOROSIS SOCIETY
(1993) *Menopause and Osteoporosis Manuals for
GPs and Practice Nurses.*
NICOL, R. (1993) *HRT – Your Guide to Making
an Informed Choice.* London: Vermillion.
SHEEHY, G. (1993) *The Silent Passage.* London:
Harper Collins.
STOPPARD, M. (1994) *Menopause.* London:
Dorling Kindersley.
WHITEHEAD, M. I. and GODFREE, V. (1992)
HRT – Your Questions Answered. Edinburgh:
Churchill Livingstone.

References

BALLINGER, C.B. (1975) Psychiatric morbidity and the menopause; screening of general population sample. *British Medical Journal* **3**: 344.

BENEDEK-JASZMANN, L.J. (1987) Long-term placebo controlled efficacy and safety study of ORG OD14 in climacteric women. *Maturitas* suppl. 1: 25.

BERGKVIST, L., PERSSON, I., ADAMI, H.O. *et al.* (1988) Risk factors for breast and endometrial cancer in a cohort of women treated with menopausal oestrogens. *International Journal of Epidemiology* **17**(4): 732.

CAMPBELL, S. and WHITEHEAD, M.I. (1977) Oestrogen therapy and the menopausal syndrome. *Clinical Obstetrics and Gynaecology* **4**: 31.

CARDOZO, L. (1990) Oestrogen deficiency and the bladder. In Drife, J.O. and Studd, J.W.W. (eds) *HRT and Osteoporosis.* London: Springer-Verlag, p. 57.

CHAKRAVATI, S., COLLINS W.P., FORECAST, J.D. *et al.* (1976) Hormonal profiles after the menopause. *British Medical Journal* **ii**: 784.

CHAKRAVATI, S., COLLINS, W.P., NEWTON, J.R. *et al.* (1977) Endocrine changes and symptomatology after oophorectomy in pre-menopausal women. *British Journal of Obstetrics and Gynaecology* **84**: 769.

CHRISTIANSEN, C., CHRISTIANSEN, M.S. and TRANSBOL, I. (1981) Bone mass in postmenopausal women after withdrawal of oestrogen/gestagen therapy. *Lancet* **i**: 459.

CLAYDON, J.R., BELL, J.W. and POLLARD, P. (1974) Menopausal flushing: double blind trial of a non-hormonal preparation. *British Medical Journal* **1**: 409.

COLDITZ, G.A., WILLETT, W.C., STAMPFER, M.J. *et al.* (1987) Menopause and the risk of coronary heart disease in women. *New England Journal of Medicine* **316**: 1105.

COMMITTEE ON SAFETY OF MEDICINES (1995) Combined oral contraception and thromboembolus (letter) CSM, London.

COOPE, J., THOMPSON, J.M. and POLLER, L. (1975) Effect of 'natural oestrogen' replacement therapy on menopausal symptoms and blood clotting. *British Medical Journal* **4**: 139.

DI RAIMONDO, C.V., ROACH, A.C. and MEADOR, C.K. (1980) Gynaecomastia from exposure to vaginal oestrogen cream. *New England Journal of Medicine* **302**: 1089.

DRINKWATER, B.L., NILSON, K., CHESHUNT, C.H. *et al.* (1984) Bone mineral content of amenorrheic and eumenorrheic athletes. *New England Journal of Medicine* **311**: 277.

ELLERINGTON, M.C. and STEVENSON, J.C. (1993) *Osteoporosis, Questions and Answers.* Kingston, UK: Merit Communications.

ETTINGER, B., GENANT, H.K. and CANN, C.E. (1985) Long term oestrogen replacement therapy prevents bone loss and fractures. *Annals of Internal Medicine* **102**: 319.

GANGAR, K., CUST, M. and WHITEHEAD, M. (1989) Symptoms of oestrogen deficiency associated with supraphysiological levels of plasma oestradiol concentrations in women with oestradiol implants. *British Medical Journal* **299**: 601.

GANGAR, K. and KEY, E. (1993) Individualising HRT. *Practitioner* **237** (1525): 358.

GRIMLEY-EVANS, J., PURDHAM, D. and WANDLESS, I. (1979) A prospective study of fractured proximal femur – incidence and outcome. *Public Health* **93**: 235.

HANDS, D. (1991) New product assessment – Tibolone. *Hospital Pharmacy Practice* November: 293.

HENDERSON, B.E. (1989) The cancer question: an overview of recent epidemiologic and retrospective data. *American Journal of Obstetrics and Gynecology* **161:** 1859.

HENDERSON, B.E., ROSS, R.K., PAGININI-HILL, A. and MACK, T.M. (1986) Estrogen use and cardiovascular disease. *American Journal of Obstetrics and Gynecology* **154:** 1181.

HILLARD, T.C., WHITCROFT, S., ELLERINGTON, M.C. *et al.* (1991) The long term risks and benefits of HRT. *Journal of Clinical Pharmacology and Therapeutics* **16:** 231.

HILTON, P. and STANTON, S.L. (1983) The use of intravaginal oestrogen creams in genuine stress incontinence. *British Journal of Obstetrics and Gynaecology* **90:** 940.

HUI, S.L., SLAMENDA, C.W. and JOHNSTONE, C.C. (1988) Age and bone mass as predictors of fracture in a prospective study. *Journal of Clinical Investigation* **81:** 1804.

HUNT, K., VESSEY, M., McPHERSON, K. *et al.* (1987) Long term surveillance of mortality and cancer in women receiving HRT. *British Journal of Obstetrics and Gynaecology* **94:** 620.

LINDSAY, R.L., HART, D.M., AITKEN, J.M. *et al.* (1976) Long term prevention of post menopausal osteoporosis by oestrogen. *Lancet* **i:** 1038.

LINDQUIST, O. and BENGRSSON, C. (1979) The effect of smoking on menopausal age. *Maturitas* **i:** 191.

McKINLAY, S.M. and JEFFEREYS, M. (1974) The menopausal syndrome. *British Journal of Preventative Medicine* **28:** 108.

McLAREN, H.C. (1949) Vitamin E in the menopause. *British Medical Journal* **2:** 1378.

MARGOLIS, J.R., FILLUM, R.F., FEINLAB, M. *et al.* (1974) Community surveillance for coronary heart disease: The Framingham Cardiovascular Disease Survey; methods and preliminary results. *American Journal of Epidemiology* **100:** 425.

MELTON, L.J. (1987) Postmenopausal bone loss and osteoporosis: epidemiological aspects. In Zichella, L., Whitehead, M.I. and Van Keep, P.A. (eds) *The Climacteric and Beyond*. Carnforth, UK: Parthenon.

MILLS, A.M., WILKINSON, C.L., BROMHAM, D.R. *et al.* (1996) Guidelines for prescribing combined oral contraceptives (letter). *British Medical Journal*, **312:** 121.

MONTGOMERY, J.C. and STUDD, J.W.W. (1991) Psychological and sexual aspects of the menopause. *British Journal of Hospital Medicine* **45:** 300.

NILAS, L. and CHRISTIANSEN, C. (1988) Rates of bone loss in normal women: evidence of accelerated trabecular bone loss after the menopause. *European Journal of Clinical Investigation* **18:** 529.

NOP (1992) *National Opinion Poll Survey – The Menopause Revolution, How Far Have We Come?* London: NOP.

OPCS (Office of Population Censuses and Surveys) (1987) *Mortality Statistics: Cause of Death England and Wales*. London: HMSO.

OLIVER, M.F. and BOYD, G.S. (1959) Effect of bilateral ovariectomy on coronary artery disease and serum lipid levels. *Lancet* **ii:** 690.

PAGANINI-HILL, A. (1996) Oestrogen replacement therapy and Alzheimer's disease. *British Journal of Obstetrics and Gynaecology* **103**, supplement 13, 80–86.

PATERSON, M.E.L., WADE-EVANS, T., STURDEE, D. *et al.* (1980) Endometrial disease after treatment with oestrogens and progestogens in the climacteric. *British Medical Journal* **280:** 822.

QUIGLEY, M.E.T., MARTIN, P.L., BURNIR, A.M. *et al.* (1987) Estrogen therapy arrests bone loss in elderly women. *American Journal of Obstetrics and Gynecology* **156:** 1516.

ROSENBERG, L., HENNEKENS, C.H., ROSNER, B. *et al.* (1981) Early menopause and the risk of myocardial infarction. *American Journal of Obstetrics and Gynecology* **139:** 47.

RCGP (Royal College of General Practitioners) (1991) Oral contraceptive study. *Lancet* **i:** 541.

SHERWIN, B.B. and GELFLAND, M.M. (1985) Differential symptom response to parenteral oestrogen and/or androgen administration in the surgical menopause. *American Journal of Obstetrics and Gynecology* **151:** 153.

SIDDLE, N., SARRELL, P. and WHITEHEAD, M.L. (1987) The effect of hysterectomy on the age of ovarian failure: identification of a subgroup of women with premature loss of ovarian function. *Fertility and Sterility* **47:** 94.

SMITH, R. and STUDD, J. (1993) *The Menopause and Hormone Replacement Therapy*. London: Martin Dunitz.

STEINBERG, K.K., THACKER, S.B, SMITH, S.J. *et al.* (1991) A meta-analysis of the effect of estrogen replacement therapy on the risk of breast cancer. *Journal of the American Medical Association* **265:** 1985.

STEVENSON, J.C., LEES, B., DEVENPORT, M. *et al.* (1989) Determinants of bone density in normal women; risk factors for future osteoporosis? *British Medical Journal* **298:** 924.

STEVENSON, J.C., LEES, B., FIELDING, C. *et al.* (1990) Exercise and the skeleton. In Smith, R. (ed.) *Osteoporosis*. London: RCP.

STUDD, J.W.W., WATSON, N.R. and HENDERSON, A. (1990) Symptoms and metabolic sequelae of the menopause. In Drife, J.O. and Studd, J.W.W. (eds) *Hormone Replacement Therapy and Osteoporosis*. London: Springer-Verlag, pp. 23–24.

STURDEE, D. (ed.) (1993) *Managing The Menopause II*. London: Fusion Communications.

SUHONEN, S.P., ALLONEN, H.O. and LAHTEEMAKI, P. (1995) Sustained-release estradiol implants and a levonorgestrel-releasing intrauterine device in hormone replacement therapy. *American Journal of Obstetric Gynecology*, **2:** 562–567.

WHITEHEAD, M.I. and GODFREE, V. (1992) *HRT Your Questions Answered*. Edinburgh: Churchill Livingstone.

WILKES, H.C. and MEADE, T.W. (1991) HRT in general practice: a survey of doctors in the MRC's general practice research framework. *British Medical Journal* **302:** 131.

15: Continence issues

Mary Dolman ♦

OBJECTIVES

After reading this chapter you will understand:

♦ urinary incontinence and its relationship to female sexuality

♦ the devastating effects that stress incontinence can have on the lives of otherwise healthy women

♦ the role of hormones in urinary incontinence

♦ how to inform women about how self-help can ameliorate the symptoms of incontinence

♦ how to encourage women to seek early treatment by informing them of available treatments.

Introduction

'Being incontinent makes me feel I am no longer a woman. I feel as though I have lost my femininity.'

These words were said by a young woman during an assessment at the continence clinic. This is not an isolated case and similar expressions are heard all too frequently.

Little is written on the subject of incontinence and its effect on sexuality, and nurses often fail to recognize that this symptom can be a real problem to women at any age. As Norton (1986) points out 'some women experience urinary incontinence during sexual activity, leakage most usually occurs during intercourse or at orgasm'. It is not known how common this is so it is not surprising that it is difficult to investigate. In a survey by Dolman (1994), 13.5% of the sample ($n = 155$) indicated leakage during sexual intercourse.

While assessing women at a continence clinic, nurses have an opportunity to ask if they experience dyspareunia. This is an excellent way to introduce the subject of incontinence during intercourse without asking a direct question. It may be difficult for a woman to talk about this problem and you should provide the opportunity and give appropriate prompts to make such a discussion possible. One woman admitted that she leaked during orgasm, but related that she had solved the problem by never allowing herself to have an orgasm.

The mechanism for urinary incontinence during sexual activity is unknown, but it is thought that mechanical pressure or a detrusor contraction underlie the problem. Sometimes treatment for a diagnosed bladder dysfunction will cure the problem, but reassurance that the symptom has no pathological significance is needed along with advice on how to possibly avoid the problem in future, e.g. by emptying the bladder before sexual intercourse.

When women are too embarrassed to talk to their partner about urinary incontinence during intercourse and make endless excuses for avoiding sex, it can sometimes lead to a breakdown of the relationship. Wet bedclothes and the fear of odour lead to such anxieties that intimate moments are avoided.

Incidence of urinary incontinence in women

Prevalence studies have been well-documented (Feneley *et al.*, 1979; Thomas *et al.*, 1980; Norton, 1990) but the results vary according to the type and age of the sample. However, it has been estimated that 1 in 4 women experience urinary incontinence varying from mild to severe leakage sometime in their life. One of the difficulties for accurate reporting of the symptom is the fact that many women are too embarrassed or ashamed to mention it. Recently the subject has gained more publicity in womens' magazines and other media, and incontinence has even been mentioned in the 'soaps'! This has helped women to realize that they are not alone with such a symptom, that treatment should be sought early and that surgery is not the only answer to the problem.

The so-called 'taboo' subject of urinary incontinence is now out in the open and you must feel confident to help and give advice to all women in your care. This chapter will provide you with the information and knowledge required to help women who may have urinary incontinence. It must be stressed that sexual counselling is a speciality in itself (see Chapter 2) and you must recognize your own limitations on counselling women with urinary incontinence and sexual dysfunction. After all, the incontinence may be the best excuse the woman has thought to use!

Before the 1970s the aetiology of urinary incontinence was poorly understood and women tended to put up with it as an inevitable event following childbirth. It is only in the last 20 years that bladder dysfunction has been better understood, and with the advent of urodynamic investigations for the diagnosis of bladder problems the outlook for women with urinary incontinence has greatly improved.

Development and anatomy of the lower urinary tract

Without going into details of the embryological development of the lower urinary tract, it is important to know that by the 12th week of intra-uterine life the upper bladder and lower part of the urethra have a common embryological origin with the vagina (Cardozo *et al.*, 1993). This will help you to understand the effects of oestrogen and progesterone which will be discussed later in the chapter.

The lower urinary tract is composed of the bladder and the urethra (Figure 15.1) and has a complex nerve supply from both the sympathetic and parasympathetic branches of the central nervous system (Figure 15.2). Urine is conveyed from the kidneys via the ureters which enter the bladder obliquely. The triangular area of the bladder bounded by the two ureteric orifices and the proximal part of the urethra (bladder neck) is known as the trigone. The bladder consists of the detrusor and trigone muscles which are composed of smooth muscle fibres. The capacity for urine storage is assured by elasticity of the detrusor muscle which allows the bladder to stretch to accommodate urine with minimal increase in pressure (Mundy, 1984).

The female urethra is about 4–5 cm long and conveys urine from the bladder to the external surface of the body at the meatus. The urethra is lined by transitional cell epithelium but distally the lining becomes stratified squamous epithelium. The submucosal folds along the urethra help to provide a watertight seal for maintaining

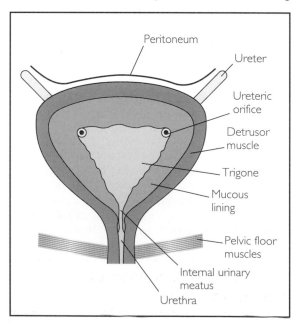

Figure 15.1 *Cross section of the female bladder.*

Figure 15.2 *Diagram of nerve pathways to the bladder.*

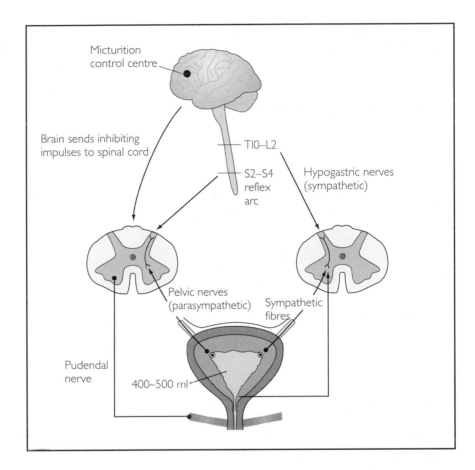

Micturition control centre

Brain sends inhibiting impulses to spinal cord

TlO–L2

S2–S4 reflex arc

Hypogastric nerves (sympathetic)

Pelvic nerves (parasympathetic)

Sympathetic fibres

Pudendal nerve

400–500 ml

continence. The mucosal folds are sensitive to oestrogen and, when fully oestrogenized, provide the watertight seal. When there is an oestrogen deficiency at the menopause, the mucosal folds become less effective and this may contribute towards stress incontinence.

The main support for the bladder is the pelvic floor striated muscle which forms a hammock-like sling from the pubic bone to the coccyx known as the levator ani. This subdivides into the pubococcygeus and iliococcygeus and the ischiococcygeus muscles through which the urethra, vagina and the rectum pass (Figure 15.3) (Sampselle *et al.*, 1989).

Physiology of micturition and continence control

According to Mundy (1984), the bladder should fill to a capacity of about 500 ml and empty at a rate 20–25 ml/second to completion. Emptying should be under voluntary control and occur in such a way that upper urinary tract function is not impaired.

The bladder can fill to this capacity because the detrusor muscle does not contract until voluntary voiding begins. As a result, the pressure within the bladder stays low (less than 15 cm H_2O). This is partly due to the inherent physical properties of the bladder wall, which allow it to be stretched without causing a rise in intravesical pressure, and partly due to a neurological mechanism which prevents nervous impulses being transmitted to the bladder, thereby preventing detrusor contraction until a capacity of approximately 400–500 ml is reached.

Continence is maintained as long as (a) the bladder neck stays closed and (b) the pressure within the urethra (the intraurethral pressure) is greater than the pressure within the bladder (the intravesical pressure). These two functions are achieved by two sphincter mechanisms:

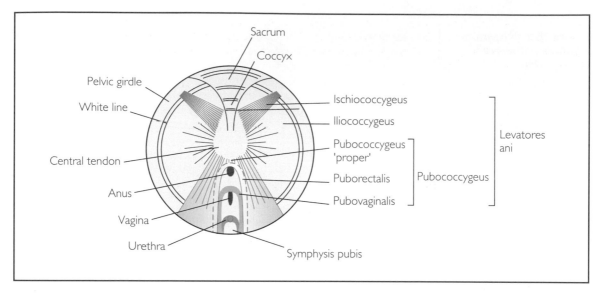

Figure 15.3 *The female pelvic floor muscles viewed from above.*

♦ The *internal sphincter* ensures that the bladder neck only opens when the detrusor muscle contracts, regardless of any rise in pressure around the bladder, e.g. coughing, sneezing or physical activity.

♦ The high urethral closure pressure below the bladder neck is maintained by the *external sphincter*, a group of muscles comprising the urethral smooth muscle, the striated muscle sphincter within the urethral wall and the rhabdosphincter striated muscle.

The bladder fills with urine at the rate of about 1 ml/min by a series of ureteric, peristaltic contractions. As the bladder fills, sensory fibres send impulses from the stretch receptors in the detrusor to the sacral roots of S2, S3 and S4 (Figure 15.2). These are suppressed by unconscious inhibitions mediated from the level of the basal ganglia. As the urine volume increases, impulses are relayed up the lateral spinothalamic tracts to the cerebral cortex, bringing the desire to micturate to a conscious level. This is suppressed by the cortex until a suitable time and place has been selected for micturition.

When the correct time and place has been selected, an appropriate position is adopted and, through the organization of the frontal lobes and hypothalamus, the bladder becomes converted to an active, dynamic, well co-ordinated expulsive unit. At the same time, active relaxation of the striated and smooth muscle components of the urethra causes a marked fall in intraurethral pressure. The inhibitory activity of the higher centres on the sacral reflex arc is lifted, allowing a rapid flow of efferent, parasympathetic impulses to cause the detrusor to contract and pull open the bladder neck. As a result, the intravesical pressure rises smoothly, sometimes augmented by the voluntary contraction of the abdominal muscles. As soon as the intravesical pressure exceeds the intraurethral pressure, urine flow commences.

At the end of micturition, the intravesical pressure falls and the urine flow diminishes. Eventually, the pelvic floor and external urethral sphincter are voluntarily contracted, causing the terminal flow to stop in the region of the mid-urethra, with 'milking back' of urine in the proximal urethra into the bladder. At the same time the abdominal muscles relax and inhibition of the higher centres on the sacral reflex is reapplied, so that the bladder becomes passive once again to allow the recommencement of the next micturition cycle.

Continence control

Under normal conditions, urine is retained in the bladder because the intravesical pressure is very much less than the intraurethral pressure. This is achieved by suppression of the sacral reflex arc by the higher centres which prevents detrusor contractions occurring during the filling phase.

The urethral lumen is kept closed at a higher pressure than the bladder by a combination of the smooth and striated muscle components around the bladder neck. The urethra is also held forward and upwards by the pubourethral ligaments so that increases in intra-abdominal pressure are equally transmitted to the bladder and upper third of the urethra which lie above the pelvic floor, thus maintaining the pressure gradient between the two. In addition, a reflex contraction of the levator ani compresses the mid-urethra; this is innervated by the pudendal nerve.

Urinary tract infection, cystitis and sexuality

Although a urinary tract infection alone does not cause incontinence, it can certainly affect sexual function and can cause considerable discomfort. At least 20% of women will have a urinary tract infection (UTI) during their lifetime and 3% experience recurrent infection (Nicolle and Ronald, 1987). It is probable that the majority of infections in adult women are asymptomatic and clear spontaneously; however, many women will be troubled by recurrent symptomatic infections. For women who do experience recurrent UTIs, the frequency of episodes is highly variable. After any one infection, approximately two-thirds will experience another infection within six months (Kraft and Stamey, 1977).

Factors which precipitate infection are poorly identified, but sexual intercourse and method of birth control, particularly diaphragm use, are two well-documented associations (Nicolle *et al.*, 1982). According to Cardozo *et al.* (1993), there is a double peak in the prevalence of UTI in women: one occurs in the 30–40 age group and the other between 55 and 65 years. In the younger of these two age groups, with a higher level of sexual activity, it is thought that intercourse predisposes women to UTI by microorganisms readily entering the bladder from the vagina and perineum. Newly sexually active women on honeymoon frequently experience cystitis and this is often called 'honeymoon cystitis'.

In the post-menopausal age group, the incidence of recurrent UTIs may be related to the reduced oestrogen status.

Urinary pathogens

The indigenous intestinal bacterial flora are the primary source for urinary pathogens. These organisms contaminate the vagina and perineum and ascend into the bladder. The most common organism is *Escherichia coli*, which accounts for up to 85% of acute infections. Less common pathogens are *Proteus mirabilis, Klebsiella pneumoniae, Aerobacter aerogenes* and, rarely, Gram-positive cocci.

A UTI can affect any part of the urinary tract, but it is the 'adherence' of the bacteria that is an important factor in the pathogenesis of infections. The urinary tract has a natural ability to resist bacterial colonization and the intruding bacteria are efficiently eliminated by the interaction of multiple mechanisms. Urine acidity, osmolality, organic acids and urea have a role in inhibiting bacterial adherence and growth. Bladder mucosa has intrinsic antibacterial properties and destroys those bacteria remaining on its surface after micturition. However, if a woman does not empty her bladder completely and leaves a residual urine, it reduces the host defence and makes her susceptible to UTI (Iravani, 1988).

Symptomology

A patient with a UTI will present with frequency of micturition, but may or may not complain of pain or difficulty in passing urine. With cystitis, however, frequency of micturition, urgency, dysuria and suprapubic discomfort are characteristic symptoms. Twenty to thirty per cent of women presenting with classical symptoms of cystitis will not have a urinary tract infection.

Many women with frequent episodes of cystitis live in dread of the next episode, and sexual dysfunction may occur due to the apprehension of acute cystitis following intercourse.

Investigation

In the investigation of UTI or cystitis, a midstream urine specimen is essential and antibiotic treatment should only be commenced according to the results of the culture and sensitivity. It is unsound practice to treat a patient with a presumptive diagnosis as many cultures are negative and antibiotics will not be required.

Upper-tract pathology may be adequately investigated by renal ultrasound along with a plain X-ray of kidneys, ureters and bladder. Cystourethroscopy may be performed and a bladder biopsy may show evidence of chronic inflammation. Cystourethroscopy is more relevant in the elderly, as recurrent UTIs may be the presenting symptoms of a transitional cell carcinoma.

Women under 40 years old should have a urodynamic investigation looking for detrusor instability, as this will give rise to urgency symptoms. Urodynamic studies will also reveal mechanical outflow obstruction which may have resulted from previous bladder neck surgery. These women may not be emptying the bladder completely and thus suffering from symptoms of cystitis, but will have negative urine cultures.

Treatment

Most urinary tract infections can be treated with an appropriate antibiotic, depending on the urine culture. However, before going ahead with treatment, you should check for underlying conditions or practices that may predispose to recurrent UTI (Box 15.1).

Box 15.1   UTI: predisposing factors

◆ *An incorrectly fitted diaphragm*   This may be causing pressure during intercourse, followed by dysuria and sometimes the onset of infection.

◆ *Spermicidal preparations*   These may cause dysuria secondary to a vaginitis due to an allergy.

◆ *Sexual partners*   Establish whether there has been any recent change in sexual partner or sexual practice. This may be a contributory factor.

◆ *Incomplete bladder emptying.*

◆ *Bladder instability* (see page 380).

◆ *Atrophic vaginitis*   This can be treated with oestrogen supplements (see page 380).

Various non-prescription treatments and hints can be recommended to your clients:

◆ Increase fluid intake by at least 500 ml per day. The diuresis will help to 'wash out' low-grade infections.

◆ Take a mixture of potassium citrate, 3 g in water, three times daily. This will relieve mild UTIs by restoring the urine pH.

◆ Take sodium bicarbonate, 3 g in water, every two hours. This also helps by reducing the acidity of the urine.

◆ Drink three glasses of cranberry juice daily (Box 15.2).

Box 15.2   Effects of cranberry juice
As early as the last century, American Indians used crushed cranberries as a herbal remedy for the treatment of urinary infections (Bodel *et al.*, 1959). Many studies have focused on the anti-adherence activity of cranberry juice and its alteration of the urinary pH (Blatherwick and Long, 1923, Schmidt and Sobata, 1988).

Although there is no conclusive evidence that cranberry juice is a cure for urinary infection and cystitis it can be effective for some people. It has been found with some women who complain of recurrent cystitis that drinking three glasses of cranberry juice a day during the acute phase can often help to alleviate the symptoms. As cranberry juice is quite harmless, it may be worth trying! Cranberry juice is available in most supermarkets, some chemists and independent health food stores.

You can also recommend that she consults her chemist. Many preparations can be bought over the counter without a prescription that can relieve symptoms.

Women should be advised that if their symptoms are not considerably improved after 48 hours then they should consult their doctor.

Types of incontinence

As can be seen from Table 15.1, there are several different types of incontinence and these may be found in isolation or in combination. The International Continence Society has defined incontinence as 'a condition in which there is involuntary

Table 15.1 *Overview of the types of incontinence*

Types of incontinence	Patient complains of	Usual cause
STRESS INCONTINENCE	Leaks with cough, sneeze, exercise, lifting	Incompetent urethral sphincter
URGE INCONTINENCE	Leakage with urgent desire to void Frequency, nocturia	Detrusor instability (unstable bladder) 1°; or 2° to neuropathy Sensory urgency
MIXED STRESS AND URGE	Pure stress, pure urge or mixture of both	Incompetent sphincter and detrusor instability
NOCTURNAL ENURESIS	Wet bed when asleep	Unknown Detrusor instability Delayed maturation
OVERFLOW INCONTINENCE	Frequency, nocturia, passive dribbling, incomplete emptying Symptoms of UTI	Outflow obstruction Hypotonic bladder Detrusor-sphincter dyssynergia
FUNCTIONAL	Inability to reach toilet or remove clothes in time	Impaired mobility Poor environment
INAPPROPRIATE MICTURITION (OR DEFECATION)	Carers complain patient makes no attempt to use toilet appropriately	Confusion, dementia

Source: Reproduced by kind permission of the Continence Foundation.

leakage of urine, which is objectively demonstrable and is a social or hygienic problem' (Abrams *et al.*, 1990).

Incontinence will occur whenever the intravesical pressure exceeds the urethral closure pressure. Thus, where detrusor contractions are uninhibited, where there is spontaneous relaxation of the urethral sphincter and when there is dysfunction of the urethral closure mechanism, urinary leakage will occur.

Stress incontinence

Stress incontinence is the most common type of incontinence found in females of all ages, and will be discussed in more detail than the other types of incontinence. It is defined as 'the involuntary loss of urine when the intravesical pressure exceeds the maximum urethral closure pressure in the absence of detrusor activity' (International Continence Society; Abrams *et al.*, 1990).

Stress incontinence occurs due to the deficiency in the urethral closure mechanisms during episodes of stress such as coughing, sneezing, running, etc. (Figure 15.4).

Weak pelvic floor muscles are rarely due to a single event (although there may be congenital weakness of the urethral closure mechanism which may go undetected) and usually it is a combination of factors which contribute to the weakening of the pelvic floor muscles. It is associated with pregnancy, vaginal delivery, previous incontinence surgery, the menopause, constipation and obesity (Box 15.3).

'Don't make me laugh or I will wet myself.'

Women frequently complain of small amounts of urine loss during activities such as playing with the children, running, jumping, laughing, dancing, etc. The degree of urine loss will be variable: for some it is only mild (damp pants) and for others it is quite severe (wet underclothes and wet outerclothes which require changing). One woman said 'I can no longer wear trousers as the wetness cannot be hidden'.

Careful history taking and a physical examination will give a nursing diagnosis of stress incontinence. However, assessment with urodynamic

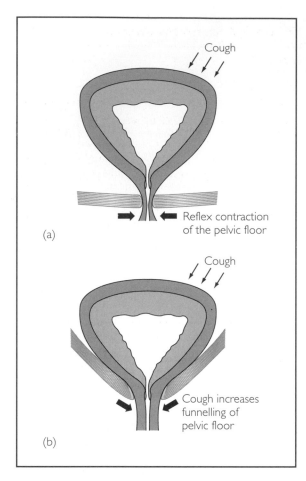

Figure 15.4 *(a) Normal contraction of the pelvic floor with raised abdominal pressure. (b) Contraction of the pelvic floor with stress incontinence.*

Box 15.3 Causes of stress incontinence

♦ Pregnancy and childbirth

♦ Obstetric trauma to pelvic floor muscles (episiotomy, tears, forceps)

♦ Laxity of pelvic floor muscles

♦ Prolapse of uterus

♦ Atrophy of pelvic supports

♦ Oestrogen depletion

♦ Collagen disorder in some women

♦ Obesity

♦ Chronic constipation.

---

studies will be necessary to make a clinical diagnosis and is essential prior to any surgery. Typically women try to keep the bladder empty prior to engaging in physical activity, and as such, may then develop voluntary frequency and perhaps urgency, thus presenting with 'mixed' symptoms.

Incontinence related to pregnancy and childbirth

Pregnancy

About 46% of women complain of incontinence during pregnancy (Chiarelli, 1991), but Cardozo and Cutner (1993) state that up to 55% of pregnant women have stress incontinence, depending on the gestation. When it occurs antenatally it is normally transient and will resolve postpartum. When it occurs for the first time postnatally it is likely to be more severe and permanent due to a weakened urethral sphincter closure.

There is an additional problem due to the hormone relaxin, which begins to circulate even before the ovum is fertilized in the Fallopian tube. Relaxin is responsible for softening all the ligaments and muscles of the pelvic outlet so that the baby's head can be pushed out during childbirth. When the ovum is fertilized, the levels of relaxin continue to rise and reach a peak at about the 12th week of pregnancy. Relaxin needs to start softening tissues early in the pregnancy so that the baby's increasing weight acts as a stretching force.

Allen and Warrell (1987) found stress incontinence in pregnancy to be significantly increased due to partial denervation of the striated muscle of the pelvic floor, which is supplied by the pudendal nerve and pelvic branches of the sacral plexus. This partial denervation caused by the expanding uterus results in reduced postural tone of the sphincter mechanism. It is usually resolved postpartum.

A combination of all these factors makes it more difficult to exercise the pelvic floor muscles ante-natally and it is debatable if this is an appropriate time to teach such exercises. Further research is required in this particular area.

Labour and delivery

Intra-partum events which may have a profound effect on postpartum lower urinary tract function include the method of delivery, the length of labour and the weight of the baby (Cardozo *et al.*, 1993). A long first stage and a long active second stage (pushing) have both been shown to result in urethral sphincter damage. Changes in the position of the bladder neck during labour may result in the stretching of supporting muscles and ligaments which can also cause damage to the urethral sphincter closure.

Poor bladder management during labour can result in voiding difficulties such as overflow incontinence, particularly if a spinal epidural has been administered (Dolman, 1992). Labour causes a decrease in bladder sensation and this, combined with epidural analgesia, may result in an over-distention of the bladder unless urine output is not monitored carefully. It has been shown that a single episode of overdistention of the detrusor can result in long-term voiding difficulties (Weil *et al.*, 1983), and may necessitate long-term intermittent self-catheterization.

Women who have a Caesarean section rarely have urethral sphincter damage, which is the main cause of postpartum stress incontinence, but the effects of hormones and the pregnancy itself will still apply.

Perineal damage: episiotomy and forceps-assisted delivery

Trauma to the perineal body, perineum and layers of the pelvic floor muscles which results from overstretching, forceps, tearing or episiotomy will cause damage to the pudendal nerve. Denervation causes loss of sensation and the ability to exercise the muscles. If suturing has to take place, this will leave scar tissue, which will not be innervated. The muscle around the scar tissue needs to be kept healthy and strong by pelvic floor exercises.

Other factors precipitating stress incontinence (Figure 15.5)

Other factors which put pressure on the pelvic floor muscles causing weakness are obesity, chronic chest problems with coughing, constipation and occupations which require heavy lifting. An eminent male urogynaecologist advises that women should never lift anything heavy as the strain damages the pelvic floor, so they should always ask a male to do the lifting for them!

Treatment for stress incontinence

The various routes for treatment of stress incontinence are summarized in Box 15.4.

> **Box 15.4** Summary of treatment for stress incontinence
> ♦ Pelvic floor exercises
> ♦ Weighted vaginal cones
> ♦ Neuromuscular stimulation
> ♦ Surgery
> ♦ Oestrogen replacement

Pelvic floor exercises

An American gynaecologist, Arnold Kegel (1948) was the first to describe pelvic floor exercises in the treatment of urinary incontinence in women and the exercises are often referred to as 'Kegel exercises'. He reported a 'cure' rate of 84%, although 'cure' was not defined. Little activity in this field followed Kegel's presentation, but in the last two decades there has been renewed interest in the pelvic floor exercises.

Early published data on these exercises showing a 'cure' or improvement were based on the patients' own reports. The variation in success rates may be partly explained by the different duration of exercise periods, which varied from

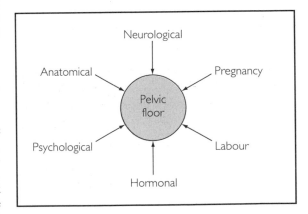

Figure 15.5 *Factors affecting the pelvic floor.*

four weeks to four months. It may also be explained by the lack of reliable and valid measurements of the degree of urinary leakage and pelvic floor muscle strength. On an uncontrolled study of 500 women, Kegel recommended 300 contractions a day with the added use of a perineometer for resisted exercises twice a day. He reported that 84% became continent, including obese and elderly women. He described the weak muscles as a 'syndrome of lack of awareness of function and co-ordination of the pubococcygeus muscle', he also noted that 30% of women could not elicit a contraction on command.

In 1963, Gomer-Jones adopted Kegel's methods of exercises and he emphasized the importance of teaching awareness of the pubococcygeus muscle and its ability to draw in, draw up and retract the perineum. He also emphasized the need to hold the muscles in this contracted state and then relax the muscles completely during half-hourly exercise sessions. Gomer-Jones maintained that more than ten contractions at each session would cause fatigue and would therefore be counter-productive. Recent studies by Laycock *et al.* (1992), however, suggest that individual exercise programmes are needed to ensure maximum effort without fatigue and such exercise programmes will depend on the initial pelvic floor assessment.

Purpose of pelvic floor exercises

Simply explained, the purpose of pelvic floor exercises is to increase the muscle volume. Hypertrophy of the muscle will result in an increase of maximum urethral closure pressure and stronger reflex contractions following a quick rise in intra-abdominal pressure (Bo *et al.*, 1991). The striated muscle comprises fast and slow twitch fibres which are innervated by the pudendal nerve. When re-educating the pelvic floor muscle, attention must be paid to the needs of these fast and slow twitch muscle fibres (Gosling, 1979). These two fibre types have differing roles to play in maintaining continence and will respond to different types of exercises.

Fast twitch fibres tire easily, but are responsible for the fast reflex response associated with coughing, sneezing etc., and also for providing a maximum voluntary contraction. This is important to enable a woman to quickly and strongly elevate and occlude the urethra prior to a stress-provoking act such as coughing, lifting or sneezing. When providing a strong maximum contraction, the fast twitch fibres also suppress urgency and relax detrusor contractions, thus activating the perineodetrusor inhibitory reflex. This reflex, which travels from the pelvic floor back to the bladder, 'informs' the detrusor muscle to stop contracting and pushing urine out.

The *slow twitch fibres*, on the other hand, do not tire so readily. They provide a postural tone which generally supports the bladder and the sphincteric action for long periods of time. Pelvic floor weakness will reduce the ability of both of these types of fibres to function in their important role of sustaining continence.

Sexual responses and the pelvic floor muscles

The pubococcygeus has also been referred to as the 'love muscle'. Women with strong pelvic floor muscles seem to enjoy the bonus of good sexual responses. In a study of orgasm, Graber and Kline-Graber (1979) found that orgasm was significantly related to maximum pubococcygeal squeeze pressure.

The pelvic floor muscles are directly responsible for the amount of sensation that a woman feels during intercourse. The lining of the vagina is not well endowed with sensation (you can test this by drawing your finger down the inside surface) and most vaginal sensations come from the pelvic floor muscles that loop around behind the vagina. The pubococcygeus also directly affects the amount of sexual sensation male partners feel (Chiarelly, 1991).

The nerve endings in the muscles respond to being stretched, so the firmer and stronger the muscle is, the more it responds to the erect penis. As the glans of the penis moves back and forth during intercourse, the firm muscles will rhythmically stretch and relax, thus heightening vaginal sensations. The ability to achieve orgasm will be enhanced as pelvic floor muscle strength increases. The pubococcygeus is also responsible for helping to lubricate the vaginal walls during foreplay and intercourse, so, sexually speaking, these muscles play a vital role (Box 15.5).

Box 15.5 The effects of strong pelvic floor muscles on sexual response will:

♦ increase vaginal lubrication during foreplay/intercourse

♦ increase sexual sensation felt vaginally

♦ increase orgasmic response

♦ give you a better grip on your partner.

Making an assessment of the pelvic floor muscles

The role of the nurse is increasing in many spheres of practice and they are nowadays expected to undertake new skills. One such skill could be that of making a pelvic floor muscle assessment thereby avoiding the need for a woman to see her doctor. This type of assessment requires training and you will not understand the principles without adequate instruction. It will be necessary for you to make enquiries about courses in pelvic floor assessment in your area. However, even without extended training it is hoped that by reading this section you will have a better understanding of pelvic floor exercises and be able to advise and help your patients.

Awareness of the pelvic floor muscle and its contraction is best assessed by a digital vaginal examination (Laycock, 1987). The woman can then be shown what is expected from an exercise programme.

Having obtained permission to do a vaginal examination, the women lays supine on the couch, hips flexed and abducted. A gloved, lubricated index finger is inserted 5 cm into the vagina and the rim of the pubococcygeus palpated. This will determine muscle bulk and any asymmetry, and will detect a change in tone as the woman contracts and relaxes the muscle (Laycock, 1992). Next, the index and middle fingers are inserted into the vagina in the antero-posterior (A-P) position with fingers spread apart. When the woman is squeezing and lifting the fingers, you should be able to detect the lift movement of the coccyx towards the pubis and evaluate the squeeze potential of the pubococcygeus (Brink *et al.*, 1989).

The Oxford grading system is widely used by nurses and physiotherapists for assessing pelvic floor muscle strength:

0 = nil, no squeeze
1 = flicker only
2 = weak contraction
3 = moderate contraction
4 = good contraction
5 = strong contraction.

Fatigue assessment

When assessing for muscle fatigue the length of time the muscle is contracted is recorded in seconds. The woman must be in charge of the muscles' relaxation and note if the contraction has already faded away. If the contraction has faded before you finish counting the seconds, repeat with fewer seconds until the woman consciously relaxes the muscle herself. That will be her starting point for her individual exercise programme.

Example: Moderate contraction (3) held for 4 seconds.

It is then necessary to determine the number of repetitions which can be tolerated to further evaluate endurance.

Example: Moderate contraction (3) held for 4 seconds, repeated 4 times.

This individual's starting point would therefore be: four contractions each to the count of 4, relaxing to the count of 4, repeated a minimum of ten times a day.

So far you have been concentrating on the slow twitch fibres of the muscle which are responsible for the endurance qualities. As the woman progresses and has had time to practice what you have taught her, the next visit will be the time to introduce the 'quick flick' contractions. This re-educates the fast twitch fibres, which are used whenever a maximum voluntary contraction, or speed, is required.

Example: Five 'Quick flick' contractions lasting 1 second.

Total exercise programme from above example:
1 Moderate contraction (grade 3)
2 4 second contraction, 4 second relaxation
3 Repeat this group four times each session
4 Do ten daily sessions
5 Start each session with five quick flick contractions.

Each woman will have a different starting point according to her own muscle capabilities and this can only be determined from a proper pelvic floor assessment.

Once the pelvic floor assessment is complete and an individual home exercise programme has been discussed, the woman needs to be encouraged to adhere to this programme. Compliance will depend on individual motivation, remembering to do the exercises and trying to fit them in during a busy lifestyle (Dolman, 1994).

Women do not have an innate ability to perform pelvic floor exercises in the Western world, and as such, the quality of the teaching of the exercises is of vital importance. According to Bump *et al.* (1991), some women are unable to locate and contract the proper muscles when given either verbal or written instructions, and this is obviously inadequate preparation for a woman about to pursue a pelvic floor exercise programme. Some women bear down instead of squeezing and lifting. It is also important to eliminate the use of other muscle groups such as the abdominal, glutei and thigh abductors which are often used instead of the pelvic floor muscles.

Dolman (1994) found from a postal survey that a significantly higher proportion of women were doing pelvic floor exercises who had been examined vaginally (71%) compared to those who were not examined vaginally (59%). However, it is not always possible, or desirable by the woman, to do a vaginal examination, and verbal or written instruction in these cases will have to suffice. A guideline for written instruction that you can give and discuss with your clients is given in Box 15.6.

Alternatives to pelvic floor exercises

What happens when a woman cannot contract the pelvic floor muscles? How can she be helped?

Vaginal cones

In 1985, Plevnik devised the weighted vaginal cone as a means to test and strengthen the pelvic floor muscle. The tampon-shaped cone, with a nylon 'tail' for easy removal, is available in two sets of three (Femina 3) (Figure 15.6). The lightest weight cone is approximately 20 g and there is a 12.5 g increase for each cone from weight one to weight

Box 15.6 Guidelines for pelvic floor exercise
1 Sit comfortably with knees slightly apart. Without moving your tummy muscle or bottom, try to squeeze the muscle around the back passage. Pretend you are trying to stop wind from escaping and squeeze and lift the muscle, this tightening should give you a feeling of being lifted away from the chair.
2 Now try the same with the front part of the muscle. Again, without moving the tummy and bottom, squeeze and lift the muscle into the vagina. Alternatively, pretend you are on the toilet and want to stop the flow of urine. Moving this front part of the muscle is harder than exercise one above and takes some time to practice.
3 Once you can tighten the muscles, pull up as hard as you can and hold for at least 5 seconds, then relax for 5 seconds. Repeat this 5–10 times at least five times a day.
4 Also try to pull up the muscles quickly, a one second flick and then relax. Repeat this five times in conjunction with the exercises in No. 3.
5 These two exercises combined will strengthen your pelvic floor muscle and as you progress you will be able to hold the contraction longer and do more repetitions without an aching muscle!
6 If you are in any doubt about exercising the muscles correctly, please seek advice. You do not want to think you are doing the exercises correctly only to find out years later you have wasted your time.
7 Looking after a healthy and strong pelvic floor muscle is a life-long exercise.

six cone. The cone is inserted into the vagina and the feeling of 'losing' the cone causes a sensory feedback to make the pelvic floor contract to retain the cone in the vagina. Cones can be used to assess muscle capabilities and to help a woman become aware of the action required to contract the pelvic floor muscle (Dolman, 1994).

Once the function of the cone has been explained to the woman, she is instructed to insert the lightest weight cone into the vagina, not quite as high as a tampon, and walk around for about two minutes, trying to keep it *in situ*. If the cone is retained it is then removed by pulling on the nylon 'tail' and the next heaviest cone inserted. The weighted cone which slips out of the vagina while the woman is walking around is the cone with

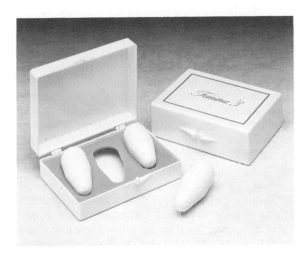

Figure 15.6 *Weighted vaginal cones. (Photo courtesy of Colgate Medical Ltd.)*

which to start exercising. The suggested regime is to retain the cone of the appropriate weight for 15 minutes twice a day. Several studies have shown an improvement in the resting tone of the pelvic floor muscle after using the cone therapy (Peattie *et al.*, 1988).

Wise *et al.* (1993) suggested that a combination of cone therapy and supervised pelvic floor exercises was more effective than either treatment used alone. It has been suggested by Laycock (1992) that to increase the exercise value of the cones, women should try retaining the appropriate one during coughing, jumping or any physical activity which raises the intra-abdominal pressure to provoke incontinence. This will reinforce the reflex pelvic floor contraction and the muscle power necessary to retain the cone.

Dolman (1994) reported that non-compliance to cone usage was sometimes caused by the following:

♦ Women found it difficult to find the time to use them with a busy daily lifestyle

♦ Women found the cone difficult to keep *in situ*

♦ Women did not know if they were using them correctly.

Weighted cones have been part of physiotherapy for many years but unfortunately this treatment was restricted to physiotherapy depart-

ments. Since 1988, the cones have become available to the general public through mail order only (Colgate Medical Ltd., Windsor). They are not available on prescription or at a chemist. You may recommend cones as a treatment, but many women buy the cones without any professional advice. Dolman (1991) found women's urinary symptoms greatly improved after cone treatment where conventional exercises had failed, but also found motivation and compliance to use the cones was maintained because of the professional input through the clinical trial.

Cones should not be recommended when:

♦ the woman is pregnant;

♦ she suffers from any type of vaginitis;

♦ she objects to inserting it in herself;

♦ there is a noticeable prolapse (cystocele, rectocele or uterine); or

♦ there is menstruation.

The cones are designed for single-person use only and need careful washing and drying after use. They can be stored in the container provided. Women should be reminded not to 'share' the cones with a friend. Autoclavable cones are available for professionals and can be autoclaved up to 10 times.

Some women buy the cones not because they have incontinent symptoms, but for simply 'toning up the pelvic floor muscles'. A growing area of interest in the use of the cones is where vaginal laxity is associated with sexual dysfunction.

Scenario (Olah, 1992)

Emma, 21-year-old woman and her 22-year-old husband, Steven were seen in the outpatient clinic. *They had been married for one year, throughout which time they had experienced problems with intercourse. Vaginal penetration resulted in insufficient stimulation to cause male ejaculation, which could only be achieved by masturbation. Prior to ejaculation the penis was inserted into the vagina to allow for insemination. Though the problem had not been a major concern to them, they were anxious to have children and were worried that conception might be impeded. Emma had been a virgin prior to marriage, and Steven had experienced no problems with other sexual partners. Examination of both Steven and Emma was completely normal.*

The problem appeared to be due to a lack of vaginal stimulation of the penis; there were no obvious psychosexual problems, and the couple appeared to have a stable relationship. It was considered that their present practice would probably not delay conception, as long as insemination was occurring. However, the possibility of pelvic floor physiotherapy to improve the pelvic floor tone was suggested, and they were keen to try this.

The physiotherapist felt that Emma had very poor pelvic floor tone. As she could not contract the appropriate muscles, weighted vaginal cones were used to 're-train' the muscle groups. By performing pelvic floor exercises on a daily basis, the strength of the muscles improved rapidly and after four weeks' treatment Emma could retain a 60 g weight in her vagina.

When reviewed in outpatients there had been a vast improvement, with male ejaculation resulting in over half the couple's attempts at intercourse. Emma was advised to continue the exercises to maintain this improvement.

As mentioned earlier in this chapter, psychosexual counselling with incontinence and vaginal laxity is a specialized subject in itself and you must be aware of this fact and know to whom you can refer your patient when necessary.

Electrical stimulation of the pelvic floor muscles

Women with no ability to contract the pelvic floor muscles at will, or who find it difficult to identify the muscles, can receive help from neuromuscular stimulation. This method of treatment has traditionally been one that physiotherapists administer. However, with the advent of home devices for women to purchase for self-administration, it is necessary for nurses to be made aware of the principles of treatment and to know how to answer enquiries from women in their care.

Principles of neuromuscular stimulation

In order for a muscle to contract, impulses pass from the anterior horn cell to the neuromuscular junction where a chemical reaction causes the muscle fibres to shorten. The frequency of these impulses depends on the type of muscle fibre to be supplied, i.e. slow or fast twitch fibres. The slow twitch fibres receive 10–20 pulses per second and the fast twitch fibres receive 30–60 pulses per second (Eccles *et al.*, 1958).

Neuromuscular stimulation 'mimics' a muscle contraction by passing an electrical impulse along the efferent nerves using low frequencies of 10–60 Hz. It is used as a treatment for women who are unable to contract their pelvic floor muscles on command and it aims to teach them the correct action. They will learn to voluntarily contract the muscles with the electrical stimulus.

As well as being a treatment for stress incontinence, neuromuscular stimulation can also be used for treating an unstable bladder which may lead to urge incontinence. By stimulating the pelvic floor and external urethral sphincter via branches of the pudendal nerves (S2, 3, 4), the perineodetrusor inhibitory reflex is also activated, thus reducing bladder instability (see page 380).

There are no side-effects to electrical stimulation, although there may be some discomfort as the sensory nerves are activated, so the intensity of the current must be kept below the patient's tolerance level. This treatment should only be used on women who can understand the procedure and who can verbalize any discomfort. Contraindications for use would be pregnancy, vaginitis, someone with a pacemaker and those with a diagnosis of pelvic malignancy.

It must be emphasized that any woman who cannot voluntarily contract the pelvic floor muscles and is in need of electrical stimulation treatment should be referred to a physiotherapist (preferably specialized in obstetrics and gynaecology). Electrode pads may be placed on the skin suprapubically, inner thigh, perineum or sacrum depending on the type of treatment the physiotherapist is using, or a vaginal probe may be placed in the vagina.

Once a woman can contract her pelvic floor muscles, electrical stimulation will no longer be necessary and this may be a 'once only' treatment.

Most treatments consists of 20 minute sessions twice a week for a minimum of six weeks at the physiotherapy department. This is clearly time-consuming and inconvenient for many women. Some departments can now offer a session which teaches the woman the mode of electrical stimulation, and then rents or provides a compact machine for home use. The treatment is self-administered in the comfort and convenience of her own home daily for anything from 4 to 12 weeks. The individual assessment will dictate the length of time required for use.

The 'home treatment' is becoming a popular alternative to visiting a hospital, but, as yet, only a few centres offer this facility. There are several devices on the market for purchase (see Resources, page 388) but it is confusing to know which is the most suitable and you should first ask advice from the professionals who specialize in this treatment before making any recommendations to your patients.

Surgery for stress incontinence

No one would choose surgery as a first option for treatment of incontinence but obviously it may be the only choice in some cases. Rigorous assessment, investigations and urodynamic studies should be done prior to any urogynaecological surgery. Conservative treatments, already discussed, should have been attempted before surgery. No woman should be persuaded to have surgery if she does not want or need it.

Details of the surgery for incontinence are discussed in Chapter 17, but there are over 100 different operative procedures. The most commonly used operations are listed in Box 15.7.

Many of the operations are adaptions or modifications of previous procedures which is evidence of the desperation many surgeons face in operating on this difficult condition. There is a definite role for surgery for urinary stress incontinence, but it is most important that the first operation that is performed is the correct procedure, as subsequent operations are more difficult and less likely to be successful. The aims of surgery are

> to elevate the bladder neck and proximal urethra into an intra-abdominal position where intra-

---

Box 15.7 Operations for stress incontinence

Vaginal

♦ Anterior colporrhaphy + urethral buttress (pelvic floor repair)

♦ Urethrocliesis

Abdominal

♦ Marshall–Marchetti–Krantz

♦ Burch colposuspension

Combined

♦ Endoscopic bladder–neck suspension, e.g. Stamey, Raz

♦ Slings

Complex

♦ Neourethra

♦ Artificial sphincter

♦ Urinary diversion

---

abdominal pressure will act as an additional closing force. Surgery should also support the bladder neck and align it to the postero-superior aspect of the pubic symphysis which will, in some cases, increase outflow resistance.

> (Cardozo *et al.*, 1993, p.82)

Post-operative complications which may result from surgery for stress incontinence are:

♦ Detrusor instability (frequency and urgency of micturition)

♦ Voiding difficulties (incomplete emptying of the bladder, poor stream, residual urine which may lead to UTI)

♦ Bladder pain

♦ Dyspareunia

♦ Surgical failure (stress incontinence symptoms might recur either immediately or at a later date).

The success or failure of surgery for urinary stress incontinence lies mainly in the competence and skill of the surgeon. A full explanation of the procedure must be given pre-operatively and the chances of success should be honestly discussed so that the woman can make an informed choice before deciding on surgery.

Hormonal influences and the menopause

The embryological development of the vagina, trigone and urethra was explained earlier in the chapter so you should understand why oestrogen affects the urethra. In pre-menopausal women when oestrogen levels drop just prior to menstruation, the resting urethral pressure falls, and some women say that their stress incontinence tends to be worse in the week before the period. The urethral wall is soft and convoluted, forming many folds, and when fully oestrogenized creates a watertight seal. When hormone levels fall, the urethral walls become less soft, the folds less pronounced and the closure is less efficient.

In post-menopausal women, the oestrogen levels may take some years to fall, but some women remain well oestrogenized into old age. The lower oestrogen levels after the menopause combined with pelvic floor trauma from pregnancy and childbirth leads to stress incontinence. Lack of oestrogen may cause urethritis and trigonitis, often associated with atrophic vaginitis. This can easily be recognized by looking at the vulva which will appear red, inflamed and often dry. Vaginal dryness means there is a loss of sexual lubrication and intercourse can be uncomfortable and painful.

Some women experience discomfort while passing urine due to the urine being in contact with the inflamed vulva. They may be treated for a urinary infection when in reality they have atrophic vaginitis.

Treatment for atrophic vaginitis is with low-dose oestrogen replacement therapy. Local application of creams, pessaries, tablets or a ring into the vagina at night is often recommended although some older women dislike doing this and find it difficult to use the applicator. Oral hormone replacement therapy may produce side-effects such as a monthly bleed which the older women may not want to tolerate. Oestrogen supplementation improves the vaginal, urethral and trigonal epithelium and leads to a restoration of the pre-menopausal vaginal flora.

Hysterectomy

In effect, a hysterectomy can be considered as surgical menopause, particularly if accompanied by bilateral oophorectomy. If hormone replacement therapy is not commenced the woman will have the symptoms described above, and you may frequently hear women say 'I was alright until I had my hysterectomy'. In addition to the oestrogen depletion following a hysterectomy, post-operative scarring and infection were suggested by Smith *et al.* (1970) as aetiological factors for urinary symptoms. Occasionally urethra obstruction is due to peri-urethral fibrosis and damage to the bladder base and proximal urethral during a total abdominal hysterectomy resulting in scar formation. When the bladder is not emptied completely the women may have symptoms of needing to void again soon after the initial void: 'I have to go to the toilet again about 2 minutes after I've just been'. The symptom may be frequency of micturition or repeated urinary tract infections. Often a simple dilatation of the urethra will resolve the problem. A women can be taught to self-dilate the urethra using a nelaton intermittent catheter.

Detrusor instability

The second most common type of urinary dysfunction in menopausal women is detrusor instability (also referred to as the unstable bladder or uninhibited bladder). It is a condition characterized by involuntary detrusor contractions occurring during bladder filling. The normal inhibiting impulses are not sent from the cortical centre to prevent completion of the sacral reflex arc, and so the bladder begins to contract before micturition is voluntarily initiated (Figure 15.7). The symptoms are usually frequency and urgency, sometimes resulting in urge incontinence, nocturia or even nocturnal enuresis. In the majority of cases there is no known cause and it is called idiopathic detrusor instability. It is sometimes thought that poor bladder control learnt in infancy may be a cause for example, if the woman was always told as a child to go to the toilet when it was not really necessary. Later in adulthood a woman adopts bad toileting habits by going to the toilet 'in case' rather than waiting for the bladder signals that it needs emptying. When a woman has a dreaded fear of wetting herself and does not know when or where this may happen, it is easy to understand how she may begin to withdraw from social activities. These women

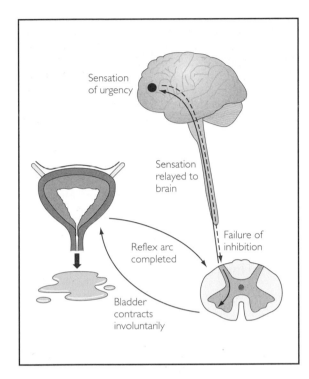

Figure 15.7 *Detrusor instability (the unstable bladder).*

learn where all the public toilets are so that they can go shopping without being 'caught out'.

> 'I don't go to my friends anymore because I am so embarrassed about always going to the toilet, nobody else seems to need the toilet as much as I do.'

Women with urge incontinence suffer greater disruption to daily activities than those with stress incontinence. However, in 20% of women the two symptoms coexist. Leaking urine during sexual intercourse and at orgasm is associated with detrusor instability, as mentioned earlier.

In some women detrusor instability may be secondary to an upper motor neurone lesion such as multiple sclerosis and there is increased evidence that detrusor instability may occur after surgery for stress incontinence (Cardozo, 1991).

Treatment

First, objective assessment for detrusor instability must be confirmed by a urodynamic investigation (briefly described at the end of this chapter), but some women with mild or intermittent symptoms may be helped with reassurance and simple measures such as:

♦ Explanation of how the bladder should function

♦ Reducing fluid intake if in excess of 2 litres

♦ Avoiding tea, coffee or alcohol which are bladder stimulants

♦ Retraining the bladder to hold more urine, i.e. increase the interval time between toileting.

Bladder retraining

This technique can be very successful when used properly and it is important that you understand the principles of bladder retraining before advising your clients.

The most important element for success is to use the correct regime for each individual person and their situation. A prior assessment is essential to identify those who will benefit from bladder retraining. Other contributing factors such as UTI and constipation must be treated first. A frequency/volume chart needs to be recorded by the individual for a week as this will show the extent of the problem. Every time she goes to the toilet she will use a jug to measure the amount of urine passed. No special 'chart' is needed, simply a plain piece of paper recording day-to-day frequency and volume (Box 15.8).

After explaining the function of the bladder and its ability to hold urine the client is encouraged to increase the interval time between voiding by not answering the first signal from the bladder as it is filling and by contracting the pelvic floor muscles to suppress detrusor contractions. The 'urgency' feeling should diminish and the client can 'hold on' for longer periods.

After four weeks another chart can be recorded and compared to the base-line chart to check the reduction in frequency episodes and to note the increased volumes of urine being voided. Bladder retraining can take as little as two weeks or as long as six months to show some improvement.

When there is little improvement after three months a referral for urodynamic investigation (centres are available in most areas throughout the country) is required to diagnose detrusor instability, and once confirmed bladder retraining should

| **Box 15.8** Example of a frequency/volume chart | | | |
Day 1	Day 2	Day 3	Day 4 etc.
7am/200 ml	*6.15/220 ml*	*7.15/150 ml*	*7am/220 ml*
7.30/50 ml	*7am/20 ml*	*7.30/30 ml*	*7.45/40 ml*
8am/125 ml	*7.45/50 ml*	*8am/100 ml*	*8am/50 ml*
9am/-	*9am/125 ml*	*9.30/-*	*9am/30 ml*
10.30/-	*11am/-*	*11am/120 ml*	*10am/-*

be used in conjunction with a low dose of an anticholinergic drug (oxybutynin). You will need to warn your client about the side-effects of these drugs, the most common of which is a dry mouth. Some women will not tolerate this. Sometimes constipation and blurred vision can affect the elderly. The side-effects of oxybutynin are dose related and 3 mg twice a day causes fewer problems than 5 mg twice a day.

Once the bladder has been retrained using the combined drug therapy and bladder retraining schedule a reduction in drug dosage can commence until drugs are no longer required. Much support and encouragement is required from you to help your client succeed with bladder retraining, particularly if you have to retrain someone who has lived with years of bad toileting habits.

In severe cases of detrusor instability (e.g. every 20 minutes 24 hours a day) surgery may be indicated. The bladder can be overdistended with water while the patient is under anaesthetic, thus producing ischaemic nerve damage which reduces the nerve stimulation to the bladder. A bladder retraining programme should follow this procedure.

More drastic surgery is a clam augmentation cystoplasty, in which the bladder is divided and augmented with a section from the large bowel or ileum. All cystoplasties produce mucus which can be kept less viscous by a high fluid intake, but the reduction in bladder contraction may mean the patients have difficulty in voiding. Straining to void or the use of self-intermittent catheterization will probably be required to empty the bladder.

Voiding difficulties

Voiding difficulties may be due to a weak bladder contraction (hypotonic detrusor contraction) or an outflow obstruction, or the two causes may coexist. Some of the causes have already been mentioned in this chapter and are listed in Table 15.1.

General measures

♦ If drugs with anticholinergic side-effects are being taken, try to withdraw them if possible, e.g. anticholinergics, tricyclic antidepressants.

♦ Encourage the woman to double void, i.e. when she thinks she has emptied the bladder, wait 50 seconds and bear down using the abdominal muscles to try to cause another bladder contraction. This may prevent residual urine and a UTI.

♦ A change in voiding position may help the bladder to empty completely if there is a problem after incontinence surgery or a hysterectomy.

♦ The woman may need to learn intermittent self-catheterization after each void until the residual is less than 100 ml, then the procedure can stop. Detrusor hypotonia may be the result of acute retention, i.e. following epidural anaesthesia or general anaesthetic.

♦ Cholinergic drug therapy, e.g. distigmine bromide, may help chronic voiding difficulties. These drugs stimulate bladder contractions. Response to treatment must be monitored by measuring the post-micturition urinary residual.

♦ Where there is long standing detrusor hypotonia the only treatment may be intermittent self-catheterization. This is preferable to an indwelling catheter as the incidence of UTI is much lower and a more normal lifestyle can be resumed.

Intermittent catheterization

As the name suggests, this involves introducing a catheter into the bladder intermittently to remove any residual urine then removing the catheter so the woman is catheter-free between catheterizations. The catheter used for single use is a Jacques or Nelaton plastic catheter Charrier 10/12. In a hospital the procedure must be strictly aseptic but in the home environment the woman learns a clean technique.

This technique is only used when the woman has a persistent residual urine volume greater than 100 ml and is experiencing problems of overflow incontinence and/or recurrent bladder infections. A competent urethral sphincter mechanism is required to maintain continence.

The techniques must be discussed fully with the woman and the final choice whether to proceed lies with her. Booklets are available for teaching this procedure (EMS and Simcare produce helpful literature) but dexterity and good eyesight are important factors towards the success of the technique. Good teaching by a competent nurse will enhance the chances of success with this technique.

Most women are not aware of the position of the urethral meatus and many find that touching themselves in that area is not acceptable. The psychological aspect of this technique must be fully discussed with them.

Assessing female bladder dysfunction

Before you can advise women complaining of any bladder dysfunction you must take an accurate and detailed history of the problem. You must also have a basic knowledge of the subject and understand the significance of her answers. The history is a tool to aid diagnosis and to help in planning treatment and care and it provides a baseline from which to monitor progress. It will also highlight when referral to another discipline is necessary. The assessment form in Box 15.9 (pages 384–385) can be used as a guide or a memory prompt to assist you with your patients.

Various investigations can be performed by nurses in assessing the woman with bladder problems (Box 15.10). Most of these will be familiar to you and others are described in detail in this chapter.

Box 15.10   Investigations nurses can perform

♦ Urinalysis

♦ Mid-stream specimen of urine if required

♦ History of condition and assessment (see Box 15.9)

♦ Vaginal examination for prolapse or vaginitis

♦ Vaginal examination for pelvic floor muscle action

♦ Rectal or abdominal examination for constipation

♦ Post-micturition residual urine (in/out catheter)

♦ Dry/wet pad test

♦ Bladder charting for frequency/volume (see Box 15.8).

Pad test

This test can be used to quantify the degree of urinary incontinence and to verify that there is incontinence. A dry pad is pre-weighed, in grams, and then weighed wet. Any increase in weight will indicate the degree of incontinence. As a guide, 1 g is equivalent to 1 ml of urine. Therefore, if a pad weighs 95 g when dry and then 125 g when wet, the urine loss is 30 ml. In the standard test the patient drinks 500 ml of fluid and then wears the pre-weighed dry pad while certain activities are carried out, e.g. walking, jumping, coughing, etc. The pad is then re-weighed and the urine loss estimated. More recently it has been suggested that a 24-hour home pad test is more representative as the woman can carry out her normal activities while wearing the pre-weighed pad.

Specialist investigations

Investigations must be tailored to the individual's needs and referral to specialist centres may be required to complete the assessment and final diagnosis (Box 15.11).

When women are told they need a special test, they are often so worried that they fail to hear the explanation of what to expect. The term 'urodynamics' often confuses the client and you will usually need to explain what the test entails (a

Box 15.9 Assessment for female bladder dysfunction

NAME: . . . . DoB . . . .

ADDRESS: . . . .

TEL. NO . . . . GP . . . .

DURATION OF PRESENT URINARY PROBLEM:

Less than a year [ ] No. years [ ] Lifelong [ ]

HISTORY:

MEDICAL . . . .

. . . .

SURGICAL . . . .

. . . .

CONSULTANT/HOSPITAL . . . .

OBSTETRIC:

Number of pregnancies . . . . Live births . . . .

Difficult deliveries: Forceps [ ] Breech [ ]

Caesarian [ ] Tear [ ] Episiotomy [ ] Epidural [ ]

No. weight over 8.5 lbs . . . . Dyspareunia [ ]

Leakage during intercourse? Penetration [ ] Orgasm [ ] No [ ]

MEDICATION: Diuretic   [ ]
                Anticholinergic [ ]
                Antidepressant [ ]
                HRT   [ ]
                Other . . . .

                . . . .

URINARY SYMPTOMS: Urge incontinence   [ ]

                       Frequency   [ ]

                       Urgency   [ ]

                       Nocturia   [ ] No. times   [ ]

                       Stress incontinence   [ ]

                       Reflex incontinence   [ ]

                       Dribbling   [ ] Before void   [ ]

                                                      After void   [ ]

                       Hesitancy   [ ]

                       Slow stream   [ ]

                       Dysuria   [ ]

                       Wet bed   [ ] No. nights   [ ]

BOWEL SYMPTOMS:

                       Constipated   [ ]

                       Diarrhoea   [ ]

                       Other   [ ] State . . . .

                       Normal habit . . . .

                       Medication/Diet . . . .

MOBILITY: Good [ ] Impaired [ ] Walks with aid [ ] Cannot stand [ ] Chairbound [ ]

DEXTERITY: Good [ ] Limited [ ] Poor [ ]

MENTAL STATE: Alert [ ] Forgetful [ ] Confused [ ] Dementia [ ]

Box 15.9 *(continued)*
FLUID BALANCE:

Per 24hrs . . . . cups/litres
Restricted intake . . . .

PHYSICAL ASSESSMENT
Vaginal examination consent . . . .
Done [　] 　　　　　Not done [　]
Vagina: Healthy [　]　Vaginal Discharge [　]　Atrophic vaginitis [　]
Prolapse: Cystocele [　]　Rectocele [　]　Urethrocele [　]　Uterine [　]
Constipation [　]

PELVIC FLOOR MUSCLE ASSESSMENT:
Vaginal Squeeze:　　0 = nil [　]　1 = flicker [　]　2 = weak [　]
　　　　　　　　　　3 = moderate [　]　4 = good [　]　5 = strong [　]
Endurance:　. . . . .　　seconds
Repetitions:　. . . . . . .　　number of times

Pad Test:
Weight of pad dry　. . . . . . .　grams　Weight wet　. . . . . . .　grams

URINALYSIS:　　SG Multistix . . . .
　　　　　　　　N.A.D. [　]
　　　　　　　　MSU required [　]　Sent [　]
　　　　　　　　Result . . . .
Frequency/Volume Chart Commenced　. . . . .　(date)
Results/Comments . . . .
. . . .

RESIDUAL URINE:　P.U　. . . . .　mls RU =　. . . . .　mls
Repeat 1 . . . .　2　. . . . .
　　　　3 . . . .

ACTION PLAN:
Pelvic Floor Exercise Programme:
Muscle strength　=　Contraction hold . . . .　secs
　　　　　　　　　　Repeat . . . .　times　Group of . . . .
　　　　　　　　　　5 quick flicks　yes [　]　no [　]
Straining to void　　　　　　　　[　] Yes　[　] No
Bladder Retraining　　　　　　　[　] Yes　[　] No
For intermittent catheterization　[　] Yes　[　] No
For drug therapy　　　　　　　　[　] Yes　[·] No
For urodynamic investigation　　[　] Yes　[　] No　Referral date . . . .
Rectal examination　　　　　　　[　] Yes　[　] No
Pads required:　How many per day? . . . .　Type . . . .
For Leakage:　Slight [　]　Moderate [　]　Severe [　]

PLAN OF TREATMENT/REFERRAL TO:
. . . .
. . . .
. . . .

DISCHARGE RESULTS:

Signature　. . . . .

diagrammatic representation is shown in Figure 15.8). For this reason, a brief outline of urodynamic investigations is given in Box 15.12 that will help you to answer questions. Some of the books mentioned in the reading list have excellent sections on urodynamics.

Many women find such investigations uncomfortable, embarrassing and very stressful and will need support and encouragement from you in order to go ahead with the investigations, rather than continue to put up with an existing problem.

> **Box 15.11** Diagnostic investigations
> ♦ Urodynamic investigations
> ♦ Ultrasound
> ♦ Micturating cystography
> ♦ X-ray: kidneys, ureters, bladder
> ♦ Intravenous urography
> ♦ Cystourethroscopy.

Prevention is better than cure

There are many opportunities for nurses in the community and in hospital environments to approach the subject of bladder problems with women. The conversation can take place casually while assessing or advising them on other issues. You can give women a chance to talk about and maybe admit to bladder problems in a friendly atmosphere, but you must be able to understand the meaning of their symptoms. Asking the right questions at the right time will often be a relief to the woman that the subject has been mentioned and taken seriously rather than glossed over. During cytology, family planning and well-woman clinics you could ask 'have you noticed an increase in the number of times you go to the toilet each day?' A typical question to ask at a chest clinic could be 'do you leak urine during a coughing attack?' Pelvic floor muscle exercise can be mentioned at any clinic and should be part of your routine vocabulary. Key points to bear in mind are listed in Box 15.13.

Figure 15.8 *A diagrammatic representation of urodynamics. (Redrawn by kind permission of Coloplast Ltd.)*

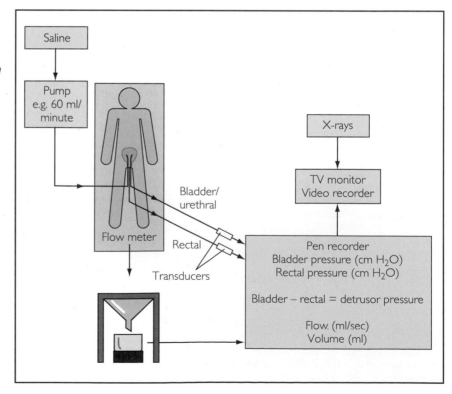

Box 15.12 Urodynamic investigations: a patient's guide

1. Urodynamics investigates the function of the bladder.
2. The test takes about 40–60 minutes.
3. Try to drink 500 ml (one pint) prior to the test so that you arrive with a fairly full bladder. You will not have to wait long for the test to begin.
4. You will undress and put on a gown which is provided.
5. You will be asked to empty your bladder into a commode-like toilet which is electronically connected to a recording machine, this measures the rate of the flow of urine.
6. You will then lie on a couch (or X-ray table, if pictures are to be taken) so that two small catheters can be put into the bladder. One fine catheter measures the pressure inside the bladder, the larger one is for filling the bladder with water.
7. A small rubber balloon is placed just inside the rectum, this measures the pressure in the abdomen.
8. Water enters the bladder slowly and any bladder activity is recorded on the machine.
9. When you feel full the water flow is switched off and the larger catheter removed. You will be asked to cough while still lying down and any leakage noted.
10. When you stand up you will be asked to give a series of coughs and/or gentle movements to see if leakage occurs.
11. Finally you empty the bladder again on the commode-like toilet before the pressure catheters are removed.
12. The way your bladder is functioning will have been recorded and a diagnosis of any problem can be made.

Box 15.13 Key points to help you help your client

♦ Teach pelvic floor exercises at all stages of a woman's life from puberty onwards.

♦ Where possible, assess pelvic floor muscle function by doing a vaginal examination.

♦ Use every opportunity to explain *why* pelvic floor muscle exercises are important. Discuss the advantages of a strong, healthy pelvic floor.

♦ Remember, most urinary incontinence can be avoided if a woman understands bladder function and exercises her pelvic floor muscles throughout her life.

per cent of women can be cured if their symptoms are treated in the early stages.

There are many instances in a woman's life when she is in contact with a nurse and every opportunity should be used by you to open the lines of communication about pelvic floor function. Nurses working in pre-conceptual care, family planning, ante- and postnatal clinics, well-woman clinics, cytology, gynaecology in/out patients – the list is endless – have daily occasions when they can broach the subject.

It is hoped that this chapter will help you to take on the role of trying to prevent incontinence, thus ensuring that your clients are fully informed of the advantages of strong pelvic floor muscles. Try to remember that a woman with urinary incontinence frequently feels that she has lost her femininity and sexuality.

Conclusion

The disruption of normal daily and social activities due to the symptoms of urinary incontinence has a devastating effect on women. The psychological aspect has not been fully discussed within this chapter, but I am sure you can perceive for yourself the range of feelings, including anger, experienced by most women who suffer from incontinence.

The sad part about incontinence is that this distressing situation can be prevented. Eighty-five

Resources

Association for Continence Advice
Winchester House, Kennington Park, Cranmer Road, The Oval, London SW9 6EJ
Tel. 0171 820 8113

The Continence Foundation
The Basement, 2 Doughty Street, London WC1N 2PH, Tel 0171 404 6875
Provides information and education for professionals and the public.

InconTact
2 Doughty Street, London WC1N 2PH

An organization for people with continence problems and their carers. Tel. National helpline: 0191 213 0050. Mon–Fri, 9am–5pm.

Suppliers

Acupad Therapy: Donald Wardle & Son
Ratton Street, Hanley, Stoke-on-Trent ST1 2HH
Tel. 01782 202142

Colgate Medical Ltd
Burney Court, Cord-Wallis Park, Maidenhead, Berks SL6 7BZ
Tel. 01628 594500
Maker of vaginal cones.

Coloplast Ltd
Peterborough Business Park, Peterborough, Cambs PE2 6FX
Tel. 01733 233348

N.H. Eastwood & Son Ltd
118 East Barnet Road, Barnet, Herts EN4 8RE
Tel. 0181 441 9641

EMS Medical Group Ltd
Unit 3, Stroud Industrial Estate, Stonedale Road, Oldends Lane, Stonehouse, Gloucester GL10 2DG
Tel. 01453 791791

Genesis Medical Ltd
Freepost WD 1242, London NW3 4YR
Tel. 0171 284 2824

Simcare Ltd
Peter Road, Lancing, West Sussex BN15 8TJ
Tel. 01903 761122

Further reading

CARDOZO, L., CUTNER, A. and WISE, B. (1993) *Basic Urogynaecology*. Oxford: Oxford Medical Publications.

MANDELSTAM, D. (ed.) (1980) *Incontinence and its Management*. Beaconsfield, Bucks: Croom Helm.

MUNDAY, A.R., STEPHENSON, T.P. and WEIN, A.J. (eds) (1994) *Urodynamics: Principles, Practice and Application*, 2nd edn. Edinburgh: Churchill Livingstone.

NORTON, C. (1986) *Nursing for Continence*. Beaconsfield, Bucks: Beaconsfield Publishers.

ROE, B. (ed.) (1992) *Clinical Nursing Practice: The Promotion and Management of Continence*. New York: Prentice Hall.

For patients

CASTLEDEN, C.M. and DUFFIN, H. (1991) *Staying Dry: Advice for Sufferers of Incontinence*. Quay Publishing.

FADER, M. and NORTON, C. (1994) *Caring for Continence: A Care Assistant's Guide*. Better Care Guides, Hawker Publications.

FENELEY, R.C.L. and BLANNIN, J.P. (1984) *Incontinence: Patient Handbook*. Edinburgh: Churchill Livingstone.

MARS, P. (19) *In Control – Help with Incontinence*. London: Age Concern.

The Continence Guide '94. The Continence Foundation, 2 Doughty Street, London WC1N 2PH.

References

ABRAMS, P., BLAIVAS, J.G., STANTON, S.L. and ANDERSON, J.T. (1990) The Standardisation of terminology of lower urinary tract function. *British Journal of Obstetrics and Gynaecology* (Suppl). **6**: 1–16.

ALLEN, R.E. and WARRELL, D.W. (1987) The role of pregnancy and childbirth in partial denervation of the pelvic floor. *Neurology and Urodynamics* **6**(3):183–84.

BLATHERWICK, N.R. and LONG, M.L. (1923) Studies of urinary acidity: the increased acidity produced by eating prunes and cranberries. *Journal of Biological Chemistry* **57**: 815–18.

BO, K., HAGEN, R.H., KVARSTEIN, B. *et al.* (1991) Effects of two different degrees of pelvic floor muscle exercises. *Journal of the Association of Chartered Physiotherapists in Obstetrics and Gynaecology* **69**: 12–17.

BODEL, P.T., COTRAN, R. and KASS, E. (1959) Cranberry juice and the antibacterial action of hippuric acid. *Journal of Clinical Medicine* **56**(4): 881–87.

BRINK, C.A., SAMPSELLE, C.M., WELLS, T.J. *et al.* (1989) A digital test for pelvic muscle strength in older women with urinary incontinence. *Nursing Research* **38**(4): 196–99

BUMP, R.C., HURT, W.G., FANTL, J.A. and WYMAN, J.F. (1991) Assessment of Kegel pelvic muscle exercise performance after brief verbal instruction. *American Journal of Obstetrics and Gynecology* **165**(2): 322–29.

CARDOZO, L. (1991) Urinary incontinence in women: have we anything new to offer? *British Medical Journal* **303**: 1453–56.

CARDOZO, L.D. and CUTNER, A. (1993) Is disturbed bladder function after pregnancy normal? *Maternal and Child Health* 180–83.

CARDOZO, L., CUTNER, A. and WISE, B. (1993) *Basic Urogynaecology*. Oxford: Oxford Medical Publications.

CHIARELLI, P.E. (1991) *Women's Waterworks: Curing Incontinence.* Gore & Osment.

DOLMAN, M.E. (1991) Stress incontinence: Weights prove an advance in treatment. *Professional Care of Mother and Child* 1(3): 110–11.

DOLMAN, M.E. (1992) Midwives' recording of urinary output. *Nursing Standard* 6(27):25 27.

DOLMAN, M.E. (1994) Female Incontinence: Awareness, Expectations, and Compliance to Treatment. Unpublished Survey. University of Surrey, Guildford.

ECCLES, J.C., ECCLES, R.M., and LUNDBERG, A. (1958) The action potentials of the alpha motoneurones supplying fast and slow muscles. *Journal of Physiology* **142:** 275–91.

FENELEY, R.C.L., SHEPHERD, A.M., POWELL, P.H. and BLANNIN, J. (1979) Urinary incontinence prevalence and needs. *British Journal of Urology* **51:** 493–96.

GOMER-JONES, E. (1963) Non-operative treatment for stress incontinence. *Clinics in Obstetrics and Gynaecology* **6:** 220–35.

GOSLING, J. (1979) The structure of the bladder and urethra in relation to function. *Urologic Clinics of North America* 6(1):31–38.

GRABER, B. and KLINE-GRABER, G. (1979) Female orgasm: Role of pubococcygeus muscle. *Journal of Clinical Psychiatry* **40:** 348–51.

IRAVANI, A. (1988) Causes, diagnosis and treatment of bacterial infections of the urinary tract. *Comprehensive Therapy* 14(11): 49–53.

KEGEL, A. (1948) Progressive resistive exercise in the functional restoration of the perineal muscles. *American Journal of Obstetrics and Gynaecology.* **56:** 238–48.

KRAFT, J.K. and STAMEY, T.A. (1977) The natural history of symptomatic recurrent bacteriuria in women. *Medicine* **56:** 55–60.

LAYCOCK, J. (1987) Graded exercises for the pelvic floor muscles in the treatment of urinary incontinence. *Physiotherapy* 73(7): 371–73.

LAYCOCK, J. (1992) Pelvic floor re-education for the promotion of continence. Chapter 5 in Roe, B (ed.) *Clinical Nursing Practice: The Promotion and Management of Continence.* New York: Prentice Hall.

LAYCOCK, J., FARRAGHER, D., GARDNER, J. *et al.* (1992) Standardisation of physiotherapy: clinical practice in the management of female urinary incontinence. in Roe, B. (ed.) *Clinical Nursing Practice: The Promotion and Management of Continence.* New York: Prentice Hall.

MUNDY, A.R. (1984) Clinical physiology of the bladder, urethra and pelvic floor. in Mundy, A.R. Stephenson, T.P. and Wein, A.J. (eds) *Urodynamics: Principles, Practice and Application.* Edinburgh: Churchill Livingstone, pp. 14–25.

NICOLLE, L.E. and RONALD, A.R. (1987) Recurrent urinary tract infection in adult women: diagnosis and treatment. *Infectious Disease Clinics of North America* 1(4): 793–806.

NICOLLE, L.E. *et al.* (1982) The association of urinary tract infection with sexual intercourse. *Journal of Infectious Diseases* **146:** 579 83.

NORTON, C. (1986) *Nursing for Continence.* Beaconsfield: Beaconsfield Publications.

NORTON, P.A. (1990) Prevalence and social impact of urinary incontinence in women. *Clinical Obstetrics and Gynaecology* 33(2): 295–97.

OLÁH, K.S. (1992) Sexual dysfunction associated with vaginal laxity. *Journal of Sexual Health* March: 23.

PEATTIE, A.B., PLEVNIK, S. and STANTON, S.L. (1988) Vaginal cones: A conservative method of treating genuine stress incontinence. *British Journal of Obstetrics and Gynaecology* **95:** 1049–53.

PLEVNIK, S. (1985) New method for testing and strengthening of pelvic floor muscles. *Proceedings International Continence Society.* London, pp. 267–68.

SAMPSELLE, C.M., BRINK, C.A. and WELLS, T. (1989) Digital measurement of pelvic muscle strength in childbearing women. *Nursing Research* **38:** 134–38.

SCHMIDT, R.D. and SOBATA, A.E. (1988) An examination of the anti-adherence activity of cranberry juice on urinary and non-urinary bacterial isolates. *Microbias* **55:** 173–81.

SMITH, P., ROBERTS, M. and SLADE, N. (1970) Urinary symptoms following hysterectomy *British Journal of Urology* **42:** 3–9.

THOMAS, T.M., PLYMAT, K.R., BLANNIN, J. and MEADE, T.W. (1980) Prevalence of urinary incontinence. *British Medical Journal* **281:** 1243–46.

WEIL, A., REYES, H., ROTTENBERG, R.D. *et al.* (1983) Effect of lumbar epidural anaesthesia on lower urinary tract function in the immediate postpartum period. *British Journal of Obstetrics and Gynaecology* **90:** 428–32.

WISE, B.G., HAKEN, J., CARDOZO, L.D. and PLEVNIK, S. (1993) A comparative study of vaginal cone therapy, cones + Kegel exercises, and maximal electrical stimulation in the treatment of female genuine stress incontinence. *Neurology and Urodynamics* 12(4): 436–37.

16: Common gynaecological problems

Jill Steele

OBJECTIVES

After reading this chapter you will understand:

♦ how to recognize some of the disorders which women encounter during their reproductive lives

♦ how to respond supportively

♦ the alternative methods available for women for whom orthodox treatment is not working or is not acceptable

♦ that things are not always what they seem and that it is important to be aware of hidden problems and unspoken anxieties.

Introduction

An attempt has been made in this chapter to remind you of the basic anatomy and physiology of the female reproductive system and the physiology of menstruation. The topics covered are various, but they have been grouped so that you will think of the problem as it affects your client rather than as a problem on its own, although many gynaecological problems are interrelated.

Women's disorders are often complicated by events which have nothing at all to do with gynaecology. Some disorders are 'everyday' matters and common occurrences, others are less common and some you may never meet but should be aware of, simply because they are complex and sensitive.

Anatomy and physiology of the reproductive system

The female reproductive system consists of the pelvic organs: the uterus and cervix, the vagina, two ovaries, two Fallopian tubes; and the external genitalia. The pelvis is the name given to the basin-shaped structure formed by the ilium, the sacrum and the coccyx at the back and the symphysis pubis (the joint between the pubic bones) at the front (Figure 16.1).

Uterus

During the reproductive years, the uterus is normally the size and shape of a small pear. It is made up of the fundus, body and cervix (Figure 16.2). The uterus has three distinct layers:

♦ *Endometrium* This is the uterine lining which varies in thickness both between individual women and also at different stages in the menstrual cycle. It grows in each cycle and is largely shed during menstruation.

♦ *Myometrium* This middle layer contains the muscle fibres which run both transversely and longitudinally to allow the uterus to accommodate a growing baby and to produce the strong

Figure 16.1 *Median sagittal section of the female pelvis.*

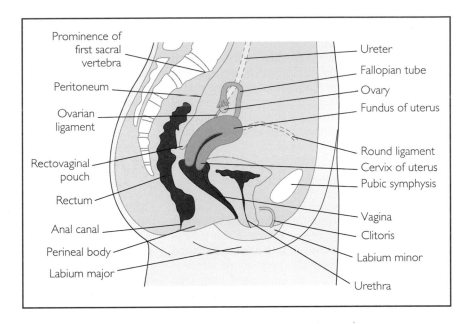

contractions necessary for the baby to be born. The uterus may enlarge when fibroids are present, depending on their size.

♦ *Peritoneum* This is the serous layer which forms the outer covering of the uterus, apart from the lower anterior segment where the uterus lies in close proximity to the bladder and the peritoneum is reflected over the bladder.

The uterus usually lies in an anteverted position but in 20% of women it is retroverted without causing any problems. The broad ligament, round ligament and utero-sacral ligament help to maintain the uterus in its anteverted, anteflexed position. Having said this, the uterus is by no means 'fixed' and will alter position slightly when the bladder is full and rises to an almost upright position in the pelvis during sexual arousal and orgasm.

Cervix

The cervix of the uterus is situated partly above the vagina and partly within it. The cervix is 2–3 cm long and opens into the uterus via the cervical isthmus or internal os. The isthmus dilates and becomes part of the uterus during labour. The external os at the lower end is normally closed and plugged with mucus which protects the uterus from

infection. It dilates and opens up completely during labour.

The endocervical canal is lined with columnar epithelium and connects the internal and external os. The outer cervix in the vagina is covered with squamous epithelium up to the external os. The junction of these two types of cells forms the transformation zone where the abnormal cell changes,

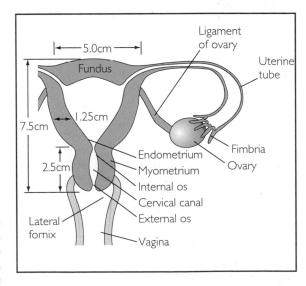

Figure 16.2 *The uterus and left uterine tube and ovary.*

known as cervical intraepithelial neoplasia (CIN), take place (see Chapter 11).

The cervix undergoes the same cyclical changes as the uterus but the endocervical mucosa is relatively thin compared with the endometrium and so does not bleed. The cervical glands secrete mucus that is thin after menstruation, profuse at the time of ovulation and thick after ovulation.

Fallopian tubes

Two Fallopian tubes join the uterus just below the fundus, or upper part of the uterus. Each tube is 10–14 cm long and opens out into a funnel-shaped structure of small, finger-like projections which is called the infundibulum or fimbriated end. One fimbria of each tube is slightly longer than the rest and is attached by its tip to one of the two ovaries which lie close to the ends of the tubes. The tubes are mobile to enable them to pick up ova. At ovulation the fimbriae wrap around the adjacent ovary.

The function of a tube is to carry the fertilized ovum along its three parts:

♦ the ampulla (where fertilization usually takes place);

♦ the isthmus; and

♦ the interstitial section where the tube joins the cornu of the uterus.

The epithelial lining is coated with fine, hair-like, mobile processes called cilia which waft the ovum along the tube.

Ovaries

Ovaries are normally similar in size and shape to an almond. The surface is usually irregular. At birth the ovaries contain some 2–3 million follicles. Most of these develop incompletely and regress before puberty, although the number left is well in excess of those needed for childbearing. During the years of fertility with regular menstruation a woman will ovulate about 400 times. Each follicle contains an oocyte which if matured will be released as an ovum ready for fertilization by a sperm. Ovulation occurs 14 days before the onset of menstruation and therefore mid-cycle in the usual 28-day cycle. The ovaries form part of the endocrine system and secrete the hormones oestrogen and progesterone and small amounts of testosterone in response to stimulation by the gonadotrophins secreted by the anterior pituitary gland.

The vagina

The vagina is a tubular structure connecting the uterus to the external genitalia. It is about 8 cm long. Normally the anterior and posterior walls lie in contact. They are lined with mucous membrane and lie in folds (rugae) which makes the vagina capable of distending to accommodate a baby in childbirth.

The pockets caused by the insertion of the cervix into the vagina are called the anterior, posterior and lateral fornices (singular, fornix). Cervical swabs and smears are taken from the external os and high vaginal swabs from the fornices.

During the reproductive years the vagina is kept moist by mucus from the cervix and from glands. Transudation of fluid into the vagina during sexual arousal also has a lubricating effect on the tissues.

Under the influence of oestrogen, glycogen is produced which, when fermented by the Doderlein's bacilli (a form of lactobacillus which normally inhabits the vagina), produces lactic acid. This helps to keep the vagina free from infection by maintaining an acid balance in the vagina with a pH of 3.4–4.5. The growth of other bacteria is inhibited.

In the absence of oestrogen, or when there is trauma or haemorrhage, the vagina becomes more susceptible to infection. This can happen after childbirth, before puberty, after the menopause and when antibiotics are taken and the acid balance is disturbed, or the hormonal status changed, eg. whilst taking the contraceptive pill. The vaginal orifice is the midline opening of the vagina. In the young child it is incompletely closed by the hymen, a thin fold of tissue covered with squamous epithelium. There is a variable opening for blood to escape during menstruation. It is stretched during sexual intercourse and the first coitus usually causes slight bleeding. The hymen is virtually destroyed during childbirth.

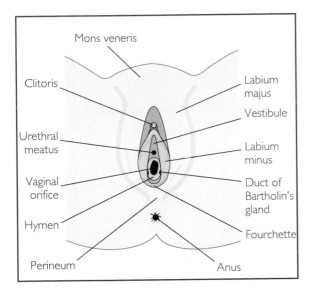

Figure 16.3 *The external genitalia.*

The external genitalia (Figure 16.3)

The pelvic floor is the name given to the group of muscles which support the organs in the pelvis. They run from front to back and side to side so the effect is of a sling or hammock with openings in the middle for the urethra, vagina and the rectum. The perineal body is a fibromuscular node between the vagina and the anus with attachments to eight muscles. If the perineum is damaged in childbirth it can lead to later problems of weakness in the pelvic floor. Teaching your clients, especially after childbirth and also those approaching their middle years, how to do regular pelvic floor exercise before their muscles lose tone may help prevent such problems as prolapse and stress incontinence (see Chapter 15).

The normal menstrual cycle

Menstruation is the cyclical activity involving the partial shedding of the endometrium. It usually occurs every 21–35 days with a 28-day cycle being regarded as normal. While many women do have a 5/28-day cycle, variations of a few days are common. This is how a period is usually described in the patient's notes, with 5 representing the days of bleeding and 28 the length of the cycle (i.e. from the first day of one bleed to the first day of the next). If the cycle is irregular you may see it written as, for example, 5–7/26–32. Longer variations can be worrying and shorter cycles troublesome.

Variations in cycle length are most common at either end of the reproductive years but can occur at any time when ovulation may be delayed, e.g. by a change in body weight, stress or disease. A vegetarian diet has been known to disrupt cycle length when adopted for the first time but this settles as the body adjusts to the change (Balen, 1993).

The menstrual cycle (Figure 16.4) is controlled by the hypothalamus and the anterior pituitary gland with feedback pathways between the brain and the ovaries involving circulating levels of oestrogen. When gonadotrophin-releasing hormone (GnRH) is released from the hypothalamus the anterior pituitary is stimulated to release first follicle stimulating hormone (FSH) then luteinizing hormone (LH). FSH starts activity within one or other ovary and stimulates a few sensitized follicles to mature. Oestrogen is released from these follicles and one dominant follicle progresses to maturity while the others are subject to atresia. (This is the degenerative procedure which affects most ovarian follicles.) The mechanism is complex but as the oestrogen level reaches a peak there is a surge of LH from the anterior pituitary gland which causes the ripened follicle to rupture and release the ovum (Figure 16.5).

Ovulation occurs about 30 hours after the LH surge. Some women experience pain which may be sharp or of a cramp-like nature. It may last for a day or two and is sometimes replaced by a dull ache. Known as *mittelschmerz*, the cause of this pain is unknown, but is thought to be due to irritation of the peritoneum by the fluid and blood which come from the ruptured follicle.

When ovulation occurs the follicle collapses, becoming the corpus luteum which secretes progesterone. Oestrogen and progesterone are responsible for the changes which take place within the uterus during the menstrual cycle:

♦ Proliferative or follicular phase

♦ Ovulation

♦ Secretory or luteal phase

♦ Menstruation.

During the proliferative phase, the stroma and glands in the endometrium are regenerated in a process of thickening from the basal layer which

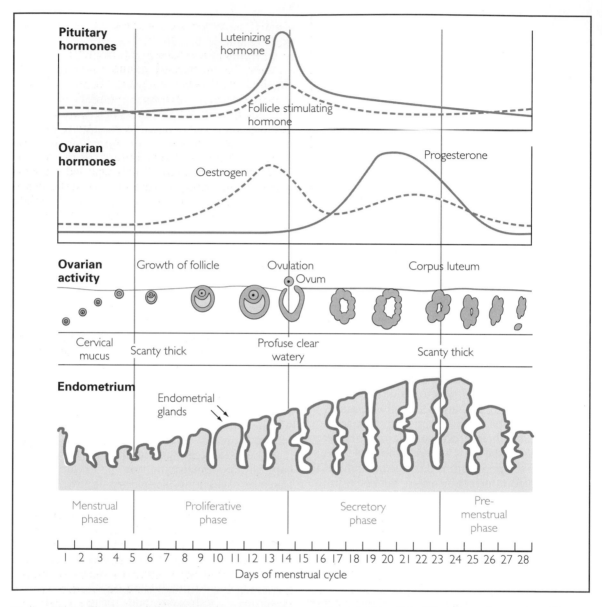

Figure 16.4 *Schematic description of menstruation and ovulation. (Modified from Scambler and Scambler, 1993, with permission.)*

remains after the previous menstruation (now about 0.5 mm thick). Usually 10–14 days long, the proliferative phase will vary in length where the cycle is irregular.

Ovulation and the start of the secretory phase usually occur 14 days before the onset of menstruation. Progesterone continues the thickening process and produces secretions to fill the endometrial glands ready for the fertilized ovum. The endo-

metrium will be 5–6 mm thick before menstruation, but again this varies between women and it can be several millimetres thicker than this. The thickness of the endometrium can be measured by pelvic ultrasound.

If fertilization does not take place, the corpus luteum normally degenerates into a corpus albicans. As the corpus luteum function decreases, a fall in progesterone occurs which causes changes

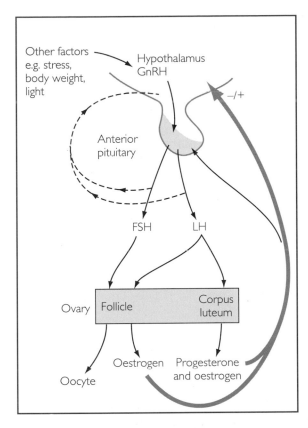

Figure 16.5 *Possible pathways controlling the release of female reproductive hormones (GnRH, gonadotrophin releasing hormone; FSH, follicle stimulating hormone; LH, luteinizing*

in the endometrium. Spasm of the arterioles occurs in the basal layer of the endometrium. The resulting ischaemia leads to shedding of the endometrium down to the basal layer which receives its blood supply from the artery below and is not involved in the vasoconstriction. The mechanism is similar to that which is involved in cardiac ischaemia.

Menstruation has begun on day one of the menstrual cycle. Bleeding usually lasts 4–5 days with a normal range of 1–7 days. Normal blood loss is estimated to be 30–40 ml with bleeding in excess of 80 ml being described as menorrhagia. Eighty per cent of menstrual loss is blood, with less than 25% consisting of endometrial tissue, tissue fluid and mucus. The blood contains minimal fibrinogen and does not clot, although rapid bleeding can result in clot formation within the

uterine cavity before the blood is seen in the vagina.

Nurses need to be aware of the different cultural attitudes to menstruation and the importance attached by many women to the cleansing effect of a regular show of menstrual blood. At the same time many nationalities use a colloquial word which supports the view that menstrual blood is polluting and unclean – 'the curse' in the UK, 'avadi' (polluted) in India, 'kotoran' (dirt) in Java.

Despite this, menstruation is regarded as a symbol of youth, fertility and usefulness and the menopause is an event which many women contemplate with dismay (Snowden and Christian, 1983).

Menarche

Menarche, the onset of periods, is being reached at an increasingly early age. The normal range in the UK is now 10–16, with some girls starting as early as 9 years old. The onset of periods can be delayed by intensive sport and physical activity and it seems that a critical weight needs to be reached for menarche to occur. A normal body mass index (BMI) is 20–25; amenorrhoea is common when the BMI is 19 or below (see also pages 19 and 84).

Occasionally precocious puberty may happen before 8 years with the first period before 10. For children, identification with a peer group is important and having periods before the rest of your friends can be frightening and confusing and may well lead to teasing or bullying. During the first year or two the cycles may be anovular. Because of this, periods though free from pain may be heavy or irregular. This can be distressing and possibly frightening both to a young girl and her parents. Preparation for the event at such a young age needs careful, sympathetic handling and many mothers find this a difficult task. You may be able to help both the child and her parents by offering support and reassurance.

We can only hope that with increasing openness about sexual matters the situation described by Deutsch (1944), where mothers were so inhibited that they found it easier to talk to their daughters about conception, pregnancy and birth than menstruation, has improved so that young girls are no longer quite so unprepared as they were then.

Scenario

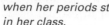

Jean, now aged 37, described her introduction to menstruation. She was 10 years old when her periods started – the first in her class.

'I was reading in my bedroom when I felt my pants were wet and sticky. I found that I was bleeding. I can remember feeling terrified and I started screaming. My parents came rushing up stairs. My father was sympathetic but taken aback. My mother told me to stop being stupid and making such a noise – it was only my periods and every one has them. I did not know what she was talking about and was convinced that I was going to die. She showed me some sanitary towels and told me to go to the chemist to buy some for myself. He was a man and I felt embarrassed although I didn't know why. It was the chemist who explained what was happening to me and told me about menstruation. I have always had trouble with periods – I don't know if that is why.'

The menopause

The menopause (the last period) marks the end of the female reproductive life and normally occurs between 45 and 55 years of age, with an average age of 51 (Chapter 14).

Once a woman in this age group has had six months without a period she is usually defined as post-menopausal, although she may have a further period. If this happens, it must be differentiated from post-menopausal bleeding, which may be a symptom of serious disease such as carcinoma of the endometrium.

Women experience the menopause in different ways. Periods may stop suddenly, gradually, or there may be problems with irregular and/or heavy bleeding. It may be welcomed if the woman has experienced problems with menstruation, but more often it raises feelings of regret and misgiving. The menopause may come at a time when there are other problems in her life, such as children leaving home, ageing parents to worry about, possible redundancy for herself or her partner. It will certainly mean that she can no longer have a child unaided. On the other hand she will be free to enjoy her sexuality with no fear of pregnancy.

With correct information this stage of life can be very positive and active but unfortunately many women do not know where to find such information. You, as a nurse, can offer advice and support and may be the person she feels able to ask for help at this potentially difficult time of her life.

Menstrual problems

Menstrual disorders are among the ten conditions most frequently seen by the GP (Scambler and Scambler, 1993). Common menstrual problems include:

♦ Menorrhagia

♦ Amenorrhoea

♦ Oligomenorrhoea

♦ Dymenorrhoea

♦ Dysfunctional uterine bleeding

♦ Inter-menstrual bleed (IMB)

♦ Irregular periods/irregular bleeding.

Because menstruation is not a subject which is generally talked about, it can be difficult for a woman to realize she has a problem. She may seek help and advice from a doctor or nurse for a number of reasons. The pattern of her periods may have changed and be causing her concern. She may be experiencing pain or she may be subject to stresses in her life which are affecting her tolerance towards menstruation which she has hitherto regarded as normal.

Menorrhagia

Menorrhagia occurs in about 10% of women and is usually regarded as bleeding in excess of 80 ml. The bleeding may be heavy or prolonged, or both. In young women occasional heavy periods do not require investigation, but any marked change in menstrual pattern in an older woman should be investigated thoroughly.

Causes

Common causes of menorrhagia are listed in Box 16.1.

Box 16.1 Causes of menorrhagia

♦ Fibroids

♦ Polyps

♦ Endometrial hyperplasia

♦ Intrauterine contraceptive device (IUCD)

♦ Underactive thyroid gland

♦ Psychosomatic causes

♦ Endometriosis and adenomyosis (are associated with menorrhagia)

♦ Polycystic ovaries

♦ Pelvic inflammatory disease

♦ Blood coagulation disorders

♦ Endometrial carcinoma and cervical carcinoma.

Uterine fibroids (Figure 16.6). Uterine fibroids occur in 25% of women over 40. They are benign, oestrogen-dependent growths of fibrous and muscular tissue. They can occur singly but are usually multiple. Much of the time they do not cause any problem but if they are in the submucous layer, distorting the endometrium then menstruation may be heavier. If the fibroid protrudes into

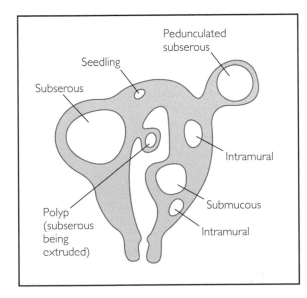

Figure 16.6 *Uterine fibroids. (Reproduced from Steele 1985, with permission.)*

the endometrium enough to stretch and thin it, inter-menstrual bleeding may occur and there may be a vaginal discharge. Occasionally, submucous fibroids develop into polyps which may reach the cervix and will cause dysmenorrhoea and severe menorrhagia. Fibroids do not usually cause pain but may cause symptoms of pressure on the bladder or the bowel.

Malignant change within a fibroid is rare.

Endometrial polyps. These are benign growths which protrude into the cavity of the uterus. They are common, vary in size and there may be several. Inter-menstrual bleeding, a vaginal discharge, or increased bleeding during a period are all possible symptoms. Some polyps are asymptomatic. They are removed during a hysteroscopy and curettage, which is a minor procedure (see page 423).

Endocervical polyps are also common, usually benign, and may cause discharge or inter-menstrual bleeding.

Endometrial hyperplasia. Disruption of the balanced levels of oestrogen and progesterone can occur as a woman approaches the menopause, when she may find her periods become irregular both in length and in the amount of bleeding that she experiences. Some cycles will be anovular and the period may be very heavy, due to excessive thickening of the endometrium. Urgent medical intervention may be indicated. It is important to exclude serious disease and establish a diagnosis. This will usually be done with the help of a pelvic ultrasound and endometrial sampling before treatment is started, as once hormones have been given, the histology of the sample will be affected.

Intrauterine contraceptive device. Periods may become heavier after the insertion of an intrauterine contraceptive device (IUCD). This usually settles in 2 or 3 months and the bleeding and any associated pain may be helped by one of the non-steroidal anti-inflammatory group of drugs such as mefenamic acid (Guillebaud *et al.*, 1978). If menorrhagia continues, the device may have to be removed. IUCDs are generally not recommended for women with heavy periods although it is expected that the recent introduction of a new levonorgestrel containing device, known as 'Mirena', will change this situations as it becomes more widely available. It has been shown to reduce menstrual loss considerably.

Underactive thyroid. This condition is easy to miss as the symptoms may be masked by the menorrhagia. As well as having no energy and feeling more tired than usual (both common symptoms of menorrhagia), the woman may be overweight and complain of being unable to lose this weight. Diagnosis is confirmed by a blood test and the treatment will be replacement thyroxine.

Hyperthroidism may also cause menstrual disorders and amenorrhoea.

Psychosomatic causes. Life events, such as a recent bereavement, break-up of a relationship or redundancy, can be traumatic enough to disturb normal endocrine function and contribute to menorrhagia. Long-term stressful situations at home or at work can have the same effect. It is quite possible for the woman herself not to be aware of the connection, therefore such events may well not be mentioned while she is with the doctor. Most patients hesitate to 'waste the doctor's time'.

Time spent with you following the consultation with an opportunity to discuss different treatment options, may provide the helpful environment needed for your client to discover the underlying cause of her problem and consider ways of dealing with it.

In some cases the present difficulty seems relatively small and the stress belongs to an event or situation from the past, maybe even from childhood, which was repressed at the time. Such problems will probably need specialist help from a clinical psychologist, skilled psychotherapist or counsellor and must certainly be resolved before major surgery such as hysterectomy is considered.

Endometriosis, see page 415.

Polycystic ovaries, see page 403.

Pelvic inflammatory disease, see page 407.

Blood coagulation disorders, e.g. thrombocytopaemia will cause menorrhagia.

Endometrial carcinoma. This occurs most commonly after the menopause with about three-quarters of sufferers being over the age of 50. At present there is no screening test for this disease so it is especially important to advise all women to seek medical advice without delay if they have any post-menopausal bleeding, or irregular bleeding around the time of the menopause.

Carcinoma of the cervix. This is usually preceded by dysplasia of the cervix and cervical intraepithelial neoplasia (CIN grade I–III), which can be detected by cervical cytology and colposcopy (see Chapter 11).

The woman may be asymptomatic or may complain of:

♦ abnormal bleeding; post-coital, inter-menstrual or post-menopausal bleeding, or menorrhagia;

♦ discharge which may be offensive or blood-stained; and

♦ with advanced disease, a fistula or pain.

Other causes. Women who have been sterilized may complain of heavier periods. If the woman has been taking the Pill, normal menstruation afterwards will almost always be heavier. While there is no evidence that modern methods of sterilization cause menorrhagia, it could be that sometimes the perception of heavier periods may be due to the psychological disturbance caused by menstruation when fertility has been removed (Pearce, 1991).

Other conditions and diseases can contribute to menorrhagia, sometimes because of the medication needed, e.g. anti-clotting drugs (e.g. warfarin) for the patient who has had heart-valve replacement surgery. Menorrhagia may make a pre-existing condition such as rheumatoid arthritis or lupus erythematosus more difficult to cope with. Because it is not always possible to find compatible drugs, patients in this situation may be recommended to consider hysterectomy and referred to a gynaecologist for an opinion. You may be able to offer extra support while a decision is reached.

Other causes of menorrhagia include endometriosis, polycystic ovaries and pelvic inflammatory disease which will be discussed later in the chapter.

Dysfunctional uterine bleeding. Frequently no explanation for menorrhagia will be found and it will be described as dysfunctional uterine bleeding which probably means that, despite all the research into the subject, scientists have still not fully identified the cause of the disturbance. Clearly the woman's perception of her situation is important and it is not helpful for her to be dismissed by medical staff because she is not anaemic or because no abnormality in the pelvis has been found. This effectively discounts what for her is a major problem.

Assessment of menorrhagia

Assessment of menorrhagia is for the most part subjective although researchers have long recommended scientific measurement (Haynes *et al.*, 1977) because of the variability of a woman's idea of her own blood loss (Chimbira *et al.*, 1980). The equipment for this is not available to most practices or hospital departments and by careful listening a nurse or doctor can form a good idea of the situation by finding out, for example:

♦ if her nights are disturbed and if the sheets need changing;

♦ if she has to wear towels as well as tampons and how frequently she has to change them;

♦ if she passes clots and/or experiences flooding; or

♦ if her activities are restricted during menstruation.

However, there are clinicians who argue that this is not a satisfactory way of assessing the problem (Fraser *et al.*, 1984).

Some women overestimate the amount they are losing during menstruation, but the nature of a woman's job or employment can make loss of a small amount seem intolerable and she may need help in understanding and managing the situation. A two-hour spell of duty at a supermarket checkout where unscheduled breaks to change a towel or tampon are frowned on can cause great anxiety. 'Flooding', the rapid loss of blood, can be particularly embarrassing and is not always related to a total heavy loss. A board meeting in a City office where all the other directors are men may be difficult for the woman trying to cope with menorrhagia while striving to resist being made to feel inadequate.

Investigations

Women with known or suspected pathology will be referred to a gynaecologist for an opinion. Investigations may be necessary to confirm the diagnosis and exclude serious disease (Box 16.2).

Treatment

This may be medical or surgical and will depend on the diagnosis and the preference of the patient (Box 16.3).

Box 16.2 Investigations for menorrhagia

♦ *Blood tests* These will determine hormonal and endocrine status, also anaemia.

♦ *Pelvic ultrasound* The ovaries can be seen and the thickness of the endometrium estimated. Fibroids or other tumours may be noted and measured.

♦ *Endometrial biopsy* This can be done as an outpatient procedure using a pipelle or vabra (see also page 422).

♦ *Hysteroscopy and curettage* Hysteroscopy alone can be done as an outpatient procedure, without anaesthetic, allowing examination of the endometrium.

♦ *Laparoscopy* This allows inspection of the pelvic organs.

Box 16.3 Treatment for menorrhagia

Medical options

♦ Reassurance

♦ Hormonal treatment

♦ Non-hormonal drugs
  - prostaglandin inhibitors
  - anti-fibrinolytic agents

♦ Iron

♦ Removal of IUCD.

Surgical options

♦ Endometrial resection

♦ Endometrial ablation

♦ Hysterectomy

♦ Myomectomy.

Hormonal treatment. This may include progestogens and, in appropriate women, oral contraception. These will control ovarian activity.

In an emergency the bleeding may be controlled by giving moderately high doses of progestogen or oestrogen. Oral medroxyprogesterone acetate (MPA) (Provera), norethisterone (Primolut N) or dydrogesterone (Duphaston) should be effective but are disappointing in the majority of cases.

It takes 48 hours or more for progestogens to become effective. If the bleeding does not respond to treatment by then it may be necessary for the patient to have a hysteroscopy and curettage to remove some of the thickened endometrium. The curettage will not have a lasting effect and the patient will normally be prescribed further hormonal treatment. Usually this will be a progestogen taken from mid-cycle or from day 5 of the cycle. If there are no contraindications she may prefer to take a form of oral contraception instead. Treatment will usually only be needed for 3 or 4 cycles until the hormonal balance is restored.

Women who become anaemic will need maintenance courses of iron until the situation has improved.

Hormones in the LHRH analogues group will control the cycle by preventing ovulation through intervention at the pituitary level, e.g. leuprorelin acetate (Prostap). Women using these drugs may experience a surge of oestrogen initially which can cause extra or heavier bleeding, but once suppression is achieved, menstruation will be minimal or non-existent. A temporary menopausal state will be induced by taking the drug. It is worth warning your client that she will experience menopausal symptoms such as hot flushes, night sweats and dryness in the vagina. This situation is reversible and as soon as treatment stops the hormone levels will return to normal.

Some women find this treatment unpleasant and may decide to discontinue, while others welcome the break from heavy periods and would like to be able to continue for longer. The treatment is expensive and for short-term use only because of the effect of oestrogen withdrawal on bone density, leading to osteoporosis. It is particularly useful for reducing the size of fibroids before surgery and the thickness of the endometrium before an endometrial resection. Some forms are taken nasally by sniffing, others are given by injection. One injection lasts a month.

Danol (Danazol) inhibits ovarian activity in a similar way with different side-effects which are dose-dependent. Low-dose treatment is worth trying as it may improve menorrhagia. It can be given for longer than the LHRH analogues (usually nine months). Side-effects are a problem and they can be unpleasant – including weight gain, depression, hirsutism, acne and voice changes. Danol is not the treatment of choice for singers as changes to the voice may be permanent. Other side-effects are temporary.

Although periods may be suppressed some form of contraception (not hormonal) must be used during treatment. This is especially important when danol is used because of the possibility of masculinization of a female fetus should pregnancy occur.

Non-hormonal treatment. Anti-prostaglandin synthetase inhibitors (also called non-steroidal anti-inflammatory drugs) can be useful in controlling menorrhagia and are effective analgesics. They are a large group which includes mefenamic acid, naproxen and ibuprofen. A form of ibuprofen called Nurofen is available without prescription. To avoid gastrointestinal upset always advise patients using drugs from this group to take the tablets with food.

The anti-fibrinolytic agents aminocaproic acid and tranexamic acid can be effective in reducing menorrhagia, particularly when an IUCD is thought to be the problem. Ethamsylate, a haemostatic agent, has a similar effect.

Surgical options. Surgical options are discussed in Chapter 17. Fibroids are particularly common in African women and if hysterectomy is being considered as a possible method of treatment, it is vital that the woman and her partner if she wishes, should be included in the discussion. In many cases the ability to have children is most important and without sufficient counselling and time to reflect, the woman could accept a cure for her distressing symptoms which might leave her relationship in pieces.

Amenorrhoea

Amenorrhoea is classified as primary or secondary and is defined in the Oxford Concise Medical Dictionary as 'the absence or stopping of the menstrual periods'.

Primary amenorrhoea

This refers to the delayed onset of periods or menarche. Puberty, which is the onset of sexual maturity, may or may not be delayed. Some causes are listed in Box 16.4.

Whether the cause of the delay is endocrinological or congenital, it will be a source of concern and distress for the parents, and as time

> **Box 16.4** Causes of primary amenorrhoea
>
> ♦ Constitutional or physiological
>
> ♦ Absent uterus, with or without a vagina
>
> ♦ Androgen insensitivity syndrome
>
> ♦ Cryptomenorrhoea due to transverse vaginal septum or imperforate hymen
>
> ♦ Eating disorders
>
> ♦ Ovarian dysgenesis, e.g. due to Turner's syndrome
>
> ♦ Hyperprolactinaemia
>
> ♦ Hypothalamic and pituitary dysfunction and tumours
>
> ♦ Polycystic ovary syndrome
>
> ♦ Systemic disease, e.g. diabetes, thyroid disease.

progresses for the young woman as well. A mother may appreciate the opportunity to talk to a nurse about amenorrhoea before involving her daughter in the process of investigations. Figures vary, but the incidence of endocrine disorders being the cause of primary amenorrhoea is in the order of 40% (Ross and Vandewiele, 1985). Ninety-five per cent of girls menstruate before they are 16. In the absence of the development of any secondary sexual characteristics (breast development indicates that the gonads are active and producing oestrogen) investigation may be justified at 14 but this will depend on the family history and the level of anxiety shown by the parents. Delayed puberty is often familial or constitutional and will need no treatment other than time. Primary ovarian failure or dysfunction of the hypothalamus or anterior pituitary need to be excluded (Brook, 1985).

Management of primary amenorrhoea is specialized and the young woman will usually be referred to the care of an endocrinologist or a gynaecologist with a particular interest in paediatric gynaecology and/or endocrinology.

The commonest cause of ovarian dysgenesis (the ovaries develop and then fail) is Turner's syndrome. This is a chromosomal abnormality in which spontaneous menstruation and development of secondary sex characteristics are rare.

Turner's syndrome is treated with the administration of oestrogen to establish breast develop-ment. Oestrogen is essential for growth and bone development and for maintaining health in the female. If it is not produced or its production is inhibited then hormone replacement at an early age is indicated. If the patient has a uterus, HRT including a progestogen, will achieve a monthly bleed and maintain the health of the endometrium. The chances of a normal pregnancy are small.

In cases of *androgen insensitivity syndrome* (AIS) (or testicular feminization syndrome) the girl will look female and will have normal breast development but no pubic or axillary hair. She will have no uterus and only a short vagina. Fortunately this is a rare condition but, when it does occur, skilled ongoing support for the young woman and her family are essential in order to achieve a successful psychological and sexual adjustment to a complex situation (Goodall, 1991; Balen, 1993).

Occasionally, investigations for primary amenorrhoea will reveal functioning ovaries but an absent uterus, with or without a vagina. Sometimes an adequate vagina can be obtained by indentation and stretching of the skin. If this is not possible, a vaginoplasty may be performed. This is a major operation and the constructed vagina will stenose if not dilated artificially or by coitus. Again, careful counselling and support will be needed for the young woman and her parents. The mother particularly may feel guilty in these circumstances and the relationship with her daughter may be put under great strain.

Local support groups for these conditions are starting to be formed. Up to date information can be obtained from the organization Contact-A-Family and the AIS support group (see Resources, page 418).

Scenario

Lucy, a 19-year-old in her first year at university, was referred to the gynaecologist because she was unable to have sexual intercourse and attempts at penetration were distressingly painful for her. She was accompanied by her anxious, distressed mother. Examination was not possible and so Lucy was admitted for an examination under anaesthetic and a laparoscopy. She had

been having periods and had developed as a normal female.

At this stage Lucy asserted her independence as a young adult and requested that she should be told the results of the investigations. She would tell her parents and any further conversations with them were to be in her presence. This caused considerable consternation within the family but Lucy's wishes were respected. Laparoscopy confirmed the findings of the ultrasound scan which had shown two ovaries and a uterus. The examination under anaesthetic (EUA) revealed that there was no practical vagina present, just a small track through which menstrual blood could escape. Initially Lucy was angry and refused to see the psychologist she was referred to for an assessment. After some weeks of silence, however, she phoned to say that she would like to return for treatment and that she would see the psychologist first.

The vaginal opening was enlarged surgically and when the tissues had healed Lucy was taught how to gently stretch her new vagina with dilators. The instructing nurse and Lucy got on well together and Lucy was able to talk about some of the issues that were bothering her. Her partner was supportive and understanding and together they went for psychosexual counselling. Her relationship with her parents changed to one where Lucy was treated as an adult, capable of making her own decisions.

Fortunately cases such as that described in the Scenario are rare, but they are highly specialized, difficult areas of female health, requiring a multidisciplinary approach. This is best provided by a hospital where all the resources needed are available on one site, and there is good communication between all carers, particularly the general practitioner.

Cryptomenorrhoea is a physical cause of primary amenorrhoea where menstrual blood is unable to escape from the uterus either because of a transverse vaginal septum or an imperforate hymen. Both are rare conditions but will require surgical intervention.

The symptoms are cyclical pain with lower abdominal swelling. Surgery is usually straightforward although the Fallopian tubes may have been damaged by retrograde menstruation (the menstrual blood flows backwards up the tube).

Secondary amenorrhoea

This refers to absence of menstruation for six months in a woman who has previously menstruated. The fact that she has a menstrual history means that she is known to have produced gonadotrophins and must therefore have ovaries, a uterus and a vagina. Investigations are therefore less extensive. Some causes of secondary amenorrhoea and oligomenorrhoea (i.e. infrequent menstruation with gaps of six weeks or longer) are listed in Box 16.5.

Box 16.5 Causes of secondary amenorrhoea and oligomenorrhoea

◆ Pregnancy

◆ Eating disorders

◆ Stress, emotional upset

◆ Strenuous exercise

◆ Pituitary tumour or hyperprolactinaemia

◆ Uterine adhesions (Asherman's syndrome)

◆ Polycystic ovary syndrome

◆ Premature ovarian failure

◆ Radiotherapy and chemotherapy.

The most common cause of secondary amenorrhoea is pregnancy, sometimes overlooked by the woman herself.

Scenario

Dina, a 41-year-old woman with a history of infertility and no children went on holiday to Baghdad to visit her family for three months. While there she developed severe abdominal pain and was admitted to hospital. She gave birth to a healthy 3.75 kg baby girl.

Lactation may prolong amenorrhoea when breastfeeding is frequent and demand-led.

Eating disorders. Being underweight can delay menarche or at a later age can cause secondary amenorrhoea (Adams *et al.*, 1986). Fat should comprise at least 17% of body weight for the onset and maintenance of regular menstruation to be achieved (Frisch *et al.*, 1973). Anorexia nervosa and bulimia are both psychosomatic illnesses where the individual has a disturbed pattern of eating which is linked to a disturbed body image (see Chapter 7). If psychological treatment is successful and a satisfactory body mass index can be attained, regular menstruation will return.

It has been suggested that dieting is an aetiological factor in the onset of bulimia (Treasure, 1990).

There are many women for whom weight and body image becomes an obsession. Dieting is big business and for over a decade the fashionable figure has been slim not fat. It is perhaps not surprising that eating disorders are so common and that some women who present in the infertility clinic are unable to conceive because their low weight is suppressing regular menstruation. (Obesity can have a similar effect.)

A brief period of amenorrhoea may result from psychological stress and emotional upset (Franks, 1987). Unless associated with a marked loss in weight it is unlikely to last longer than two or three cycles. Hypothalamic GnRH secretion is temporarily disturbed.

Strenuous exercise. Athletes, particularly runners, are more prone to oligomenorrhoea and amenorrhoea than the general population. The combination of stress, intensive exercise and weight loss appears to be the factor which affects GnRH secretion. Menstruation usually resumes when training is less strenuous, even if there is no accompanying change in weight.

Ballerinas and other dancers where height, weight and shape can influence their career prospects, are also more likely to experience amenorrhoea. Puberty and menarche may be later than average because of a low body mass index. Ballerinas are also susceptible to eating disorders. Low levels of circulating oestrogen over an extended period can result in osteoporosis and scoliosis (Warren, 1983). Stress fractures and soft tissue injuries are the result of the osteoporotic changes and lower than normal levels of collagen. Intensive exercise in these circumstances can only slightly compensate for the oestrogen deficiency. Appropriate counselling is

needed and in some cases dietary advice. When the body weight is increased menstruation will start again.

Hyperprolactinaemia. This is a disruption of the normal secretion of prolactin from the pituitary. It is most commonly due to a tumour but may occasionally be a symptom of polycystic ovary syndrome (PCOS). If due to PCOS the woman will not be short of oestrogen but if a tumour is present she will show symptoms of low oestrogen.

Hypothyroidism must be excluded and treatment will be according to the diagnosis.

Asherman's syndrome. This is a condition where intrauterine adhesions are formed following vigorous curettage or a severe intrauterine infection (including tuberculosis). While the full syndrome is rare, it is not unusual to see cases where adhesions restrict the growth of the endometrium causing scanty periods and occasionally amenorrhoea.

Treatment where possible is by hysteroscopic division of adhesions followed by a course of oestrogen or a cyclical oestrogen/progestogen preparation. Sometimes steroids are given for three weeks and an IUCD may be inserted temporarily to prevent further adhesions forming.

Polycystic ovary syndrome (PCOS). Surveys have found that about one in five women have polycystic ovaries (Polson *et al.*, 1988), which will be observed on a pelvic ultrasound scan (Figure 16.7). Ninety per cent of women investigated for oligomenorrhoea have PCOS, while only 25% of women with amenorrhoea will be found to have the same condition (Adams *et al.*, 1986).

Polycystic ovaries contain at least ten small cysts. Normally these cysts do not cause any problem.

A woman has polycystic ovary syndrome when she has other symptoms in addition to the cysts on the ovaries, such as:

♦ Irregular periods

♦ Acne

♦ Hirsutism

♦ Tendency to be overweight

♦ Pelvic pain

Figure 16.7 *Polycystic ovaries. (Photo courtesy Organon.)*

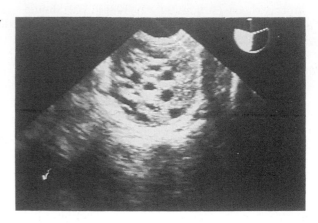

♦ Possible infertility

♦ Recurrent miscarriage.

Diagnosis is confirmed by pelvic ultrasound scan, blood test to confirm raised LH, and/or raised testosterone level.

The cause of polycystic ovary syndrome is not known although it may be that the ovary does not secrete the right balance of hormones which causes an abnormal feedback to the pituitary gland. The pituitary then releases high amounts of LH in an attempt to correct the problem. There is also an hereditary element in some families.

The hormonal imbalance results in either irregular ovulation or anovulation, resulting in oligomenorrhoea and occasionally amenorrhoea. With irregular ovulation the chances of conception are reduced. If she does become pregnant, a woman with PCOS has an increased risk of miscarriage, probably because the high level of LH affects development of the ovum and the implantation of the embryo in the wall of the uterus.

Raised testosterone levels from the ovary and metabolism of oestrogen in fat may cause both acne and hirsutism. These are embarrassing symptoms and women with unwanted hair have to cope with additional expenditure on depilatory creams or electrolysis.

Weight control is often a problem for women with PCOS and they will be asked to diet in order to achieve a satisfactory weight-to-height ratio. In fact some women only have symptoms as their weight increases. Just as being underweight can affect ovulation so obesity can have a similar effect and has to be considered when fertility treatment is being contemplated. Any encouragement that you can give to a woman to enable her to reduce weight before she is seen and investigated in hospital will help to make treatment more likely to succeed.

Polycystic ovary syndrome is treated by establishing control of and regularizing ovarian activity.

For women who have no wish to become pregnant, the oral contraceptive pill is the easiest solution. Ovarian activity is suppressed and a regular withdrawal bleed achieved. A short course of an LHRH analogue will control symptoms in the short term, but, as mentioned earlier, cannot be used for longer than six months. In the hyperandrogenic woman an anti-androgen such as cyproterone acetate can be given. Acne often responds quickly but any effect on hirsutism will take some months.

Drugs to induce ovulation, e.g. clomiphene citrate, will be used when infertility is a problem, although spontaneous ovulation may occur when excess weight is lost.

Sometimes surgical intervention is indicated. A new minimally invasive technique known as laparoscopic ovarian diathermy or laser laparoscopy offers an alternative to wedge resection which used to be the standard surgical treatment for PCOS, although it was associated with a high incidence of adhesion formation. With this new technique the hormonal abnormalities are corrected and a high success rate has been reported with subsequent ovulation and conception (Armar *et al.*, 1990). Follow-up of treated patients will be needed to assess the long-term effects on the ovary of this procedure.

Premature ovarian failure. The most commonly accepted definition of premature ovarian failure is the cessation of periods before the age of 40 years (Abdalla, 1993) (see also page 338). This can happen as early as the mid- to late twenties and can be a totally devastating event which requires gentle understanding from all involved and careful counselling.

Although the diagnosis and outcome usually come as a dreadful psychological shock, it is estimated that between 1 and 3% of young women in the UK are affected. The news triggers the emotions and feelings of bereavement and need to be dealt with as such. Hopes of fertility without medical intervention are very unlikely. Occasionally a pregnancy will occur with or without treatment, but the outlook is poor.

In many cases the reason for the early ovarian failure will not be known. The woman will have been referred to the clinic with amenorrhoea. She may have had occasional periods with longer spells without bleeding. Some possible causes are listed in Box 16.6.

Box 16.6 Causes of premature ovarian failure

♦ Resistant ovary syndrome

♦ Chromosomal abnormalities, e.g. Turner's syndrome

♦ Previous radiotherapy or chemotherapy

♦ Bilateral oophorectomy

Resistant ovary syndrome is a relatively rare condition which may be an autoimmune disorder. The patient has amenorrhoea, high FSH and LH levels indicating a post-menopausal state but the ovary still contains follicles.

Premature ovarian failure is investigated using blood tests for FSH/LH, oestrodial and ovarian antibodies, and pelvic ultrasound scan. An ovarian biopsy will confirm the absence of follicles but is rarely done because of the likelihood of causing antibodies and adhesion formation. If there are no follicles there will be no further activity from the ovaries.

The only way that a young woman with premature ovarian failure can contemplate a family, apart from adoption, is by oocyte donation and *in vitro* fertilization (IVF) or gamete intra-fallopian transfer (GIFT) (see Chapter 9). These options need to be approached with caution and should not even be considered until the woman and her partner are both strong enough to be able to cope with the investigations, medications and interventions involved. But most of all they have to be strong enough to accept the disruption of their sexual privacy and the disappointment of no baby should the procedure fail. Assisted conception is not acceptable to every couple.

Women with premature ovarian failure will be advised to take a form of hormone replacement therapy (HRT) or the Pill to prevent adverse effects of lack of oestrogen. This may not be an easy decision and you may be able to help by talking it through with her and explaining the reasons and benefits. She will also need to be given time to understand and come to terms with her feelings of acute loss and disbelief.

Scenario

Beverley, a 32-year-old woman who had been married for eight years, came to the clinic asking for advice about her periods which had been infrequent since she stopped taking the oral contraceptive pill 7 months previously. She and her husband wanted to start a family. Taking her history the nurse learnt that she had been treated for Hodgkin's disease with chemotherapy ten years ago and again for a recurrence five years later.

At no time had it been suggested to Beverley that her fertility might be affected. Blood tests and a pelvic ultrasound scan confirmed the diagnosis of premature ovarian failure.

Beverley had several sessions with the counsellor in which she expressed her sadness, anger, feelings of guilt and resentment that she had had no counselling before chemotherapy nor been given any hint of the possibility of ovarian failure. On the contrary, she had been prescribed the Pill so that she would avoid the risk of pregnancy until her body had time to recover from the effects of the second course of treatment. The irony of the situation made it more difficult to accept. Investigation showed that it was possibly the first treatment which had caused the damage. Beverley was encouraged to tell her doctor at the *next check-up how she was feeling, and eventually agreed to start HRT.*

Her husband joined her for counselling and they discussed their future hopes and plans, including the possibility of life without children. She obtained information about infertility treatment which she shared with her counsellor. There followed a period of no contact and then a phone call came to say that she was on a waiting list for IVF (with ovum donation).

Hormone replacement therapy will quickly relieve the immediate symptoms of oestrogen deficiency so that the woman will regain some of her former sense of well-being. In the long-term the protection against osteoporosis and cardiovascular disease afforded by HRT is essential.

There is still concern about the effect of long-term HRT on the breasts and a small increase in the risk of developing breast cancer (Hunt and Vessey, 1991). Regular examination of the breasts is wise but it is generally agreed that in these cases the benefits of HRT outweigh the risks, except perhaps in those with a strong family history of carcinoma of the breast.

Dysmenorrhoea

Dysmenorrhoea is painful menstruation. Many women experience some discomfort with the onset of a period, but dysmenorrhoea is more severe, with pain often felt in the lower back and radiating down the tops of the legs.

Primary dysmenorrhoea

Primary dysmenorrhoea occurs within one or two years of the onset of menstruation (the first cycles are usually anovular and not painful). Many young women experience troublesome pain with periods and it is estimated that 50% of women between the ages of 15 and 24 are affected.

It is thought that prostaglandins, present in the uterus in large numbers during menstruation, cause the pain. Other possible causes that may need to be considered include pelvic inflammatory disease, congenital abnormalities and endometriosis.

Symptoms associated with severe dysmenorrhoea include:

♦ Nausea/vomiting

♦ Pallor/fainting

♦ Headache/migraine

♦ Bowel disturbance

♦ Bladder irritability.

Treatment. Primary dysmenorrhoea can be treated with an anti-prostaglandin synthetase inhibitor such as mefenamic acid, flufenamic acid, or naproxen to lessen the pain. Treatment must be started as soon as the period starts. An alternative in cases of severe pain is the combined oral contraceptive pill which will suppress ovulation, and reduce the amount of blood lost. Occasionally the symptoms are so severe that a hysteroscopy is performed to exclude pathology within the uterus. A laparoscopy may also be needed as endometriosis has been found to occur as early as 3–4 years after the onset of menstruation (Hoshiai *et al.*, 1993).

If symptoms persist and you have a good relationship with your client she may indicate that she would like to talk to you about the pain and the difficulty it causes her. If still at school she may be under undue pressure, perhaps related to her own wish to succeed. There may be problems at home or difficulty with a relationship. Tension affects perception of pain and she may find some relief when given the opportunity to talk freely with someone who is outside her circle of friends and family. You can offer practical advice on managing pain, too. Sometimes pain is soothed by cuddling a hot-water bottle whilst others find that exercise encourages the release of endogenous endorphins which have natural analgesic properties.

Secondary dysmenorrhoea

Secondary dysmenorrhoea occurs later in life and is related to acquired disorders such as pelvic inflammatory disease, endometriosis and adenomyosis (endometriosis occurring in the myometrium). Less commonly, it is caused by uterine fibroids, cervical stenosis, psychological factors or an IUD.

The treatment will depend on finding the underlying cause of the pain.

Pelvic inflammatory disease (PID).   This is infection or inflammation in the pelvis and is usually an ascending infection via the cervix (Box 16.7). The infection tends to centre on the Fallopian tubes or the endometrium with varying involvement of the peritoneum and surrounding structures, e.g. the ovary. It may be acute, subacute or chronic.

Box 16.7 Causes of pelvic inflammatory disease

♦ Ascending infection, usually sexually transmitted (often *Gonorrhoea* or *Chlamydia*).

♦ After surgery: curettage, termination of pregnancy, hysteroscopy, hysterosalpingography.

♦ Transperitoneal: appendicitis or abdominal surgery.

♦ Blood-borne infection, e.g. tuberculosis. This is rarely seen in the UK but the incidence may be increasing.

A woman with acute pelvic inflammatory disease may present with

♦ Pyrexia, headache, malaise

♦ Lower abdominal pain, usually bilateral

♦ Vaginal discharge

♦ Dyspareunia

♦ Abnormal bleeding (e.g. heavier than normal).

Occasionally, she may have late onset of nausea and vomiting (in appendicitis the vomiting is usually an early symptom).

The onset of symptoms often coincide with the start of a period, and the lower abdominal pain is at its worst during or sometimes immediately after a period. Examination of the patient will reveal a tender abdomen and occasionally a mass may be felt. In severe, acute PID there may be signs of peritonitis. Pelvic examination will be very painful. A mass felt in one of the fornices will usually indicate that an abscess has formed.

Investigations for PID include vaginal, urethral and cervical swabs for culture, blood tests (white cell count and ESR) and pelvic ultrasound scan. Laparoscopy is the only reliable way to confirm the diagnosis. The pelvis can be inspected and swabs taken from any site of infection.

Inflammation with no infection is usually due to pelvic surgery, haemorrhage or endometriosis.

Once diagnosed, the patient with PID may be admitted to hospital or she may stay in the care of her GP or be treated by the department of genito-urinary medicine. Rest is essential. Antibiotic coverage will be given for at least two weeks, probably using two different antibiotics. The aim is to cure the condition in the acute stage and to prevent it from recurring and becoming chronic.

After one attack of PID the patient is vulnerable to further episodes. She should have been warned about this and you will be able to reinforce the advice to take life quietly until she has had time to recover fully. This will include avoiding energetic sexual activity. Barrier methods of contraception are protective. Explanation is needed that the risk of the disease becoming chronic is quite high and brings with it the scenario of future problems with fertility, considerable pain, menstrual problems, periods of ill-health and dyspareunia.

You can also provide the understanding and sympathy which she will need. As well as the condition being painful and unpleasant there are additional feelings of guilt and self-reproach, particularly if the disease has been sexually transmitted, fear of future attacks and also implications for her fertility. She may feel resentment if the disease has been transmitted by her regular partner and she herself has not been promiscuous and will need help in managing the situation she finds herself in. It may be helpful to suggest seeing a counsellor or therapist. You will find it useful if you know what resources are available in your area and the method of referral, e.g. self-referral, or by the nurse or doctor.

Salpingitis.   This is an infection or inflammation in the Fallopian tubes and is commonly caused by *Chlamydia*. Seen through the laparoscope the tubes appear red, swollen and oedematous. At this stage the openings into the uterus are still patent and if successfully treated with antibiotics there will probably be no long-term damage. Tubal patency will be maintained.

If the disease progresses to subacute salpingitis a tubo-ovarian abscess or a pyosalpinx will have developed.

With chronic salpingitis the lumen of the tube becomes blocked at the fimbrial end with fluid in the tube. This is a hydrosalpinx. Hydrosalpinges cause infertility and pain and are usually associated with dyspareunia. The patient may also complain of dysuria.

If, after treatment with antibiotics, a pyosalpinx or tubo-ovarian abscess does not resolve it may have to be drained or the tube removed.

In some cases, where the pain misery and disruption of PID is affecting quality of life to such an extent that it has become disabling, hysterectomy with removal of both tubes may be considered an appropriate option. The ovaries could remain if unaffected but if they are removed oestrogen replacement should be given. Clearly this is a big decision for any woman to make, especially in the light of the emotional agenda that often accompanies the onset of PID. To have reached the stage of considering major surgery, much suffering will have already been endured. The chance to talk the issues through with an informed and sympathetic nurse before coming to a decision may help her to feel she is more in control of the situation.

One of the major considerations will be future fertility. If the infection has been controlled but she has been left infertile, the option of IVF remains. After a hysterectomy she will have no hope of having children unless by surrogacy.

Even if a hysterectomy is what she wants as her family may be complete or she may not want children, it is still important that she has an opportunity to explore her feelings with a nurse or counsellor before surgery. Feelings of loss after the operation are better coped with when they are recognized beforehand. Many women find that it is one thing to decide that they do not want a family but quite another to know that the option no longer exists.

Toxic shock syndrome (TSS). This is an infection caused by the bacteria *Staphylococcus aureus* which can enter the body via the vagina wall from a tampon which has been left in too long, or was contaminated before insertion. Tampons should be changed about every four hours and one with reduced absorbency used if changing is not necessary. Damage to the membrane lining can be caused by a fingernail, a tampon applicator, or a tampon inserted with difficulty into a dry vagina. TSS is rare (an average of eighteen cases are notified annually) but can be fatal. The symptoms are severe and include a sore throat, pyrexia, rash, diarrhoea, aching muscles and inflamed, sore eyes. Early diagnosis and removal of the tampon are essential. An appropriate antibiotic will be prescribed.

Pelvic pain

Some of the causes of pelvic pain have already been discussed and will be mentioned again. There are many gynaecological reasons for such pain but sometimes it may be related to other systems of the body, such as the urinary tract, intestinal tract or musculoskeletal system, or to a systemic disorder (porphyria) or psychosomatic causes.

Pelvic pain is a complex subject and can be acute or chronic (Box 16.8).

Box 16.8   Causes of pelvic pain

Acute pelvic pain

♦ Associated with pregnancy

  – Ectopic
  – Miscarriage
  – Degenerating fibroid

♦ Gynaecological causes

  – Onset of PID
  – Ruptured corpus luteum
  – Rupture or torsion of ovarian cyst
  – Ovulation pain.

Chronic pelvic pain

♦ Endometriosis

♦ Pelvic inflammatory disease

♦ Adhesions

♦ Prolapsed ovary in the pouch of Douglas

♦ Ovarian cyst

♦ Uterine prolapse

♦ Psychological causes.

Acute pelvic pain associated with pregnancy

This is pain that starts suddenly with little if any prior warning. It is usually caused by ectopic pregnancy, miscarriage or degenerating fibroids.

Ectopic pregnancy

An ectopic pregnancy is a pregnancy occurring outside the uterus. Ninety-five per cent occur in one or other tube. The most common sites are the ampulla and the isthmus of the Fallopian tube and the cornual angle of the uterus. A pregnancy may less commonly be implanted on the interstitial section and the fimbriated end of the tube and rarely on the ovary and cervix or in the abdominal cavity. The condition occurs in about 1 in 200 pregnancies (Winston, 1993) and is often the result of fibrosis or damage to the cilia in the tube following salpingitis.

Other contributing factors include:

♦ IUD or progestogen-only pill

♦ Tubal surgery, including sterilization

♦ Postpartum or post-abortion infection

♦ Tuberculosis

♦ Low-grade pelvic inflammatory disease

♦ Congenital abnormality of the upper Mullerian duct (this forms the Fallopian tube)

♦ Endometriosis

♦ Uterine fibroids in or near the cornu

♦ Previous ectopic pregnancy (there is a 10% risk of a second ectopic occurring).

Depending on the site of the implantation the patient's symptoms will vary. If the event occurs within 4–6 weeks of her last period she may not realize she is pregnant.

As most ectopic pregnancies are tubal, the space available for the developing ovum will affect the time before the woman has symptoms. She may or may not have had amenorrhoea or a minimal bleed coinciding with an expected period.

Diagnosis of an intact ectopic pregnancy can be difficult. Symptoms usually include lower abdominal tenderness or discomfort on one side and vaginal bleeding. If it is not recognized and treated, a tubal pregnancy has three possible outcomes:

1 *Tubal mole* The ovum separates. It is surrounded by blood which forms a clot. It may be reabsorbed or be expelled from the fimbriated end as a tubal abortion.

2 *Tubal abortion* Haemorrhage is followed by separation of the ovum from the wall which is then passed from the fimbriated end into the peritoneal cavity. Very rarely the pregnancy may continue in the abdominal cavity. The ovum implants or re-implants on a site such as the external surface of the uterus which has an adequate blood supply to sustain the developing fetus.

3 *Tubal rupture* The trophoblast erodes the wall of the tube. This is followed by severe haemorrhage.

A woman with tubal rupture may not realize that she is pregnant but often will have missed one or two periods and may be feeling tenderness and tingling in her breasts. Presentation is sudden and the condition serious (Box 16.9 and page 430).

Box 16.9 Symptoms of tubal rupture

♦ Sudden severe pain

♦ Vaginal bleeding

♦ Shoulder tip pain when lying down caused by irritation of the diaphragm by blood in the peritoneal cavity

♦ Pallor and signs of shock and blood loss

♦ Distended abdomen due to bleeding.

Treatment for an ectopic pregnancy is usually salpingectomy. There will not be time for investigation when the patient has collapsed and is in a state of shock. Her condition will be assessed and treatment given as indicated while arrangements are made to take her to theatre as quickly as possible.

There were 19 reported ectopic pregnancy deaths in the three years 1988–90 (Hibbard *et al.*, 1994).

A diagnosis of ectopic pregnancy can be confirmed using a serum βhCG pregnancy test, which is accurate two weeks after conception, and a pelvic ultrasound scan or a transvaginal scan.

Bimanual examination may reveal the site of the pain and any tender mass, but this has to be done with great care as it is possible to rupture an ectopic pregnancy and is also likely to be extremely painful.

If the diagnosis remains doubtful, laparoscopy will provide the answer. If an ectopic pregnancy is confirmed a laparotomy may be performed to remove the pregnancy or tube, although new less invasive techniques have been developed which allow conservation of the tube (Laatikainen *et al.*, 1993).

In some cases of tubal abortion the ovum and debris will be reabsorbed without intervention. The patient will be admitted to hospital for observation while the BhCG levels fall.

An ectopic pregnancy is a distressing event, calling for supportive skills and understanding. As well as having lost the pregnancy, the woman will have to come to terms with the fact that there is an increased risk of subsequent pregnancies being ectopic as well. She will be understandably apprehensive when she next realizes she is pregnant until (hopefully) implantation can be confirmed by pelvic ultrasound scan. If she has had previous pelvic inflammatory disease she may experience feelings of guilt or anger which will complicate her adjustment to the situation.

IVF, an already stressful procedure, carries an increased risk of ectopic pregnancy. Grieving is an important part of healing and your awareness of this can help you encourage the process and relieve the guilt.

Early miscarriage

Miscarriage or spontaneous abortion is the loss of a pregnancy before the fetus is legally viable at the 24th week of pregnancy. It is estimated that about 25% of pregnancies end in miscarriage during the first trimester (Pearce, 1991), due to a variety of causes (Box 16.10).

Box 16.10   Causes of early miscarriage

♦ Blighted ovum – an empty sac, no foetus

♦ Fetal abnormality of chromosomal origin

♦ Uterine abnormality – fibroids, divided septum

♦ Maternal disease – renal problems, diabetes, *Listeria*, tuberculosis, syphilis, rubella if infection between 4 and 8 weeks

♦ Endocrine problems – high LH levels, raised androgen levels may affect fetus and implantation

♦ Chorionic villus sampling – about 2% around 8–12 weeks.

Pregnancy is divided into three trimesters – the first trimester refers to the first 12 weeks and it is during this period that early miscarriage or spontaneous abortion occurs. Miscarriage risk decreases as the pregnancy continues. Many women think that the word abortion refers to a pregnancy which has been terminated deliberately. It has been suggested that the term 'miscarriage' should be used when referring to a spontaneous abortion and it is important for nurses to appreciate that, for most women in these circumstances, the word 'abortion' adds to their distress.

Bleeding will occur after a period of amenorrhoea where pregnancy is either suspected or has been confirmed. If, on gentle digital examination, the cervical os is found to be closed, a pelvic ultrasound scan should be arranged as soon as possible to confirm whether the fetal heartbeat is present and whether the pregnancy is still viable.

The only symptom of threatened miscarriage is bleeding. The likelihood of this pregnancy continuing is good and it is usually advisable for the woman to rest in bed until 24 hours after any bleeding has stopped. Opinions vary as to whether intercourse should be avoided until the second trimester.

With an inevitable or incomplete abortion the os will be found to be open on vaginal examination. The bleeding will be heavier with clots. Some women experience uterine contractions which are so painful that they are comparable with labour pains (Weideger, 1975). Miscarriages of this kind before six weeks are often complete with the fetus and placenta being expelled together and the woman may not realize that she was pregnant.

Later than this, although many abortions are complete, it is more likely that the placenta will be left behind. The bleeding and the pain can be severe. The woman will be taken to theatre and evacuation of the retained products of conception will be performed (ERPC) (see also page 429). This will be done without delay to avoid causing further distress to the patient who knows her pregnancy is lost, and also to avoid the possibility of a subsequent infection or haemorrhage.

In the same three-year period 1988–1990 11 women died following a spontaneous abortion. Six died from post-abortion sepsis (Hibbard *et al.*, 1994).

The differential diagnosis between a ruptured ectopic pregnancy and an incomplete abortion can be difficult to make. If the pain is one-sided it is more likely to be due to an ectopic pregnancy, while the pain felt during an incomplete abortion is central lower abdominal.

Many women are unaware that miscarriage is not a rare event and feel isolated and distressed in their misery at losing the pregnancy. Even in the early weeks miscarriage is felt as a great loss, a bereavement, and the support needed will be of the same quality as that offered after an ectopic pregnancy. Because for many women miscarriage is not something they have anticipated, these feelings can be bewildering. A woman struggling to come to terms with the event will welcome the chance to talk to you and the use of open-ended questions may help her to find a way of expressing her feelings. You may enable her to organize her emotions into a form she is able to cope with. It can help to put her in touch with a support group. Too often follow-up in the community is haphazard and she has to cope alone in the best way she can.

Degenerating fibroids (red degeneration)

This is the most important complication of fibroids during pregnancy. Usually the woman will be known to have fibroids which will provide a clue to the diagnosis. The onset of symptoms are often sudden and include severe pain localized over the fibroid, possible vomiting with a raised temperature and pulse rate. If there is no improvement after 24 hours of treatment with analgesics, bedrest and a local application of heat, then the diagnosis will be reconsidered.

Acute gynaecological pain

Onset of pain will be sudden. There will probably be no previous similar history. Possible causes include the onset of PID, ruptured corpus luteum, torsion of an ovarian cyst (associated with vomiting and bleeding), rupture of an ovarian cyst, and *mittelschmertz* (ovulation pain).

PID, ruptured corpus luteum and torsion of an ovarian cyst all feature in the differential diagnosis of an ectopic pregnancy which must be considered if there is any possibility of the woman being pregnant, even though there is no history of amenorrhoea or unusual vaginal bleeding.

Investigations to establish a diagnosis include:

♦ Pelvic examination
♦ Pregnancy test
♦ Pelvic ultrasound scan
♦ Laparoscopy.

Treatment will be conservative except where bleeding into the peritoneum occurs when the bleeding point will have to be ligated. The twisted ovary or cyst may have to be removed. If the ovary is still viable an ovarian cystectomy will be performed.

Chronic pelvic pain

Chronic pelvic pain is one of those conditions that causes a 'heartsink' reaction in the GP and the nurse as the patient comes through the surgery door. This is because it is a condition that can persist over many years, causing considerable disability despite extensive investigation and treatment. Sometimes the onset and cause of the pain cannot be identified.

Various disorders cause chronic pelvic pain (see Box 16.8). Whilst some of the clinical causes have already been discussed, endometriosis, ovarian cysts and uterine prolapse will be discussed in greater length at the end of this chapter. It is worth remembering that patients presenting with chronic pelvic pain run the risk of being overinvestigated or inappropriately treated. Sometimes the problem turns out to have a psychological origin.

Some points to consider when a client presents with chronic pelvic pain are as follows:

♦ Are there any previous life events or unresolved problems that may be relevant?
♦ Why is the woman seeking help now?
♦ What is the effect on her relationships or family life?
♦ What is the effect on her ability to work?

Psychological causes

Sometimes, chronic pelvic pain turns out to be functional – i.e. no physical cause can be found for the symptoms. This may be difficult for a woman to accept and then all your listening and counselling skills will be needed.

Considerable research has been done into the

psychological aspects of women who have pelvic pain but the incidence of unexplained pain varies. One of the most comprehensive studies found that about two-thirds of the women presenting with pelvic pain had no obvious pathology to explain it (Gillibrand, 1981).

A history taken carefully and with time for the woman to talk may reveal unsuspected problems which at first sight seem quite unrelated. With experience you will begin to recognize the external factors which can make the perception of pain more intense. For instance, she may have been the subject of sexual abuse as a child and be showing signs of the unresolved consequences.

Scenario

Carol was referred to the gynaecologist for advice *about PMS. The nurse taking her history soon realized that the symptoms she was describing did not fit the definition of PMS. She was encouraged to talk about the issues in her life which put pressure on her, about her relationships and her job. There were no obvious contributing factors although she was clearly not happy but did not appear to understand why. Carol was then asked to think back to her childhood. Had she been happy at school? Had she had any lengthy period of separation, e.g. in hospital? She described a stable family background and there was no apparent answer as to why she was having the symptoms she described.*

There was a spell of silence, broken only when Carol began to talk about a single episode of sexual abuse which had happened to her when she was eleven. She had felt guilty at the time, not really understanding what had happened but knowing that it was wrong and that she hated it. She had never talked about it before. It seemed that her first sexual relationship had triggered the onset of her 'PMS' symptoms.

Carol agreed to see the clinical psychologist. There was a three-week delay before her first appointment. The nurse, concerned about her in the meantime, phoned to see how she was coping. She said that she had cried a lot and that having started to talk about it she couldn't stop. She was looking forward to seeing the psychologist and

wished she had had the opportunity to reveal the event before.

The psychologist reassured the nurse that Carol would be able to cope with her distress while waiting, knowing that an appointment had been made.

What you do when you have identified these stressful situations is another matter. To some extent this will depend on what confidence you have in your own counselling skills, what other resources are available and the complexity of the problem.

It is important for health care professionals listening in depth to the worries and problems of clients to have access to another member of staff to talk to if needed, rather in the way a counsellor will have a recognized support system. Such a system of clinical supervision not only benefits you by sharing a problem that could become overwhelming, but enables you to look at aspects of the problem in a different light in order to help your client. This does not involve breaking a confidence but gives you a useful sounding-board. Other people's problems when off-loaded on to you can feel quite stressful and to be of further use to your client, you have to avoid taking those problems home with you. It is important to remember that no-one should attempt to undertake a therapeutic counselling role until trained to do so.

If you are genuinely interested in your clients and show that you have time to listen, then you may well find yourself hearing some distressing information (Tschudin, 1991). Your response can trigger further confidences, but you should be aware of your own clinical boundaries and limits in dealing with such patients and not 'hang on' to a problem when you are out of your depth. This will certainly not help you or your client. Awareness that this may happen will enable you to plan your strategy of referral in advance of it being needed. Ideally it is helpful if you have a regularly updated list of local agencies, support groups and counsellors which can be shared by all members of the health care team. Comments from previous clients who have used the resources are also very helpful.

Other things can affect the perception of pain and previously unresolved life events can intensify the effect of pain without the sufferer being aware of what is happening to her (Holmes and Rahe,

1967). Some examples of such 'events' are:

♦ Bereavement – either recent or unresolved from the past

♦ Disturbed family relationships

♦ Marital problems

♦ Employment problems

♦ Stressful lifestyle

♦ Abuse
  – a violent relationship
  – child abuse
  – sexual abuse
  – rape.

The suggestion that there may be a psychological element to pain is something which many of us find difficult to understand or accept. Your client may resist the idea that her pain is anything other than completely physical. Before you can help her to find a way acceptable to her of coping with the pain and making the perception of it less intense, you will have to convince her that you believe her, that you care about her problem and that you are on her side. Let her know that you do not think the pain is in her mind, and if she is referred, for example to a psychologist, reassure her that you and her doctor are not trying to get rid of her and you will always be happy to see her again. Anything less than this does not justify the trust she has already put in you by confiding in you. The fact that she has been able to talk about and identify areas of her life which are hurting her may leave her feeling vulnerable and sensitive.

The help you will be able to suggest for your client will depend on what is available locally and the impression you have from her as to what is acceptable and what she will feel comfortable with. Supportive therapies such as relaxation techniques, hypnotherapy, acupuncture, massage with aromatherapy, reflexology or shiatsu may be available and may appeal to your client (Wells and Tschudin, 1994).

You will probably want to discuss the problem with the doctor involved who may have ideas on this. It is sometimes useful to ask yourself why has your client come for help *now*. For example, feelings attached to a previous termination of pregnancy may have been repressed or denied at the time. Still unresolved, these feelings will continue to cause unhappiness which can be disregarded by

the patient until a totally unrelated event proves to be the last straw which makes her seek help. The termination will not be the cause of the pain but will affect her perception of it.

Feelings attached to a bereavement can intensify pain and referral to a bereavement counsellor or CRUSE may be the place to start (see Resources, page 419).

In some cases of PID or endometriosis the pain can become incapacitating. Major surgery such as hysterectomy and removal of both ovaries and tubes may be suggested as the only solution. Allowing your client to ventilate her feelings of anger or guilt may help her in the process of recognition that relief may be available to her.

Your ability to appear receptive to clients and then hear what they are saying, will depend on your professional communication skills. Books are available which, although often targeted at doctors and medical students, contain suggestions on how these skills may be improved which apply equally well to nurses (Davis and Fallowfield, 1991).

Referral to a psychologist or counsellor with an interest in gynaecological pain may be acceptable to your client and help her to come to terms with the situation and to decide how to cope in the future.

Much has been written during the last 30 years on helping relieve pelvic pain where investigations have failed to reveal any identifiable gynaecological disorder or pathology (Pearce and Beard, 1984). A 'model of pain' may be agreed upon with the patient before the psychologist takes a history (Erskine and Pearce, 1991). Such a history will include past episodes of pain and any psychosexual experiences. A pain diary can be kept and brought to the next appointment.

Clients are often resistant to accepting a referral of this kind and may need time to think about it. Some will be referred to a hospital pain clinic.

Dyspareunia

Many conditions can give rise to painful intercourse or dyspareunia, which is clearly a distressing symptom not only for the woman but also for her partner.

Dyspareunia can be defined as either *deep* – referring to problems within the pelvis – or *superficial* – relating to pain or discomfort at or near the introitus. The causes are listed in Box 16.11.

Box 16.11   Causes of dyspareunia

Deep dyspareunia

♦ Endometriosis

♦ Pelvic inflammatory disease

♦ Adhesions

♦ Prolapsed ovary in the pouch of Douglas (usually associated with a retroverted uterus)

♦ Ovarian cyst.

Fibroids rarely cause pain but may make intercourse uncomfortable.

Superficial dyspareunia
This occurs with most vaginal and vulval infections and irritations.

♦ Vaginal atrophy

♦ Vaginitis

♦ Vaginismus – muscle tension or spasm in the lower third of the vagina that prevents penetration

♦ Painful perineal scar

♦ Bartholin's cyst

♦ Vulvodynia – pain in the vulva which is triggered by intercourse and which often remains unexplained.

Whatever the cause of dyspareunia it will be made worse by dryness in the vagina. This may be due to a physiological lack of oestrogen, as happens after the menopause, or in response to fear of pain which can inhibit lubrication. Whatever the cause it is helpful to suggest a topical lubricant to apply until treatment takes effect. 'Senselle' and 'KY jelly' can both be bought from a chemist. 'Replens' and 'Astroglide' are examples of non-hormonal vaginal moisturizers which you can safely recommend to the post-menopausal woman complaining of a lack of vaginal lubrication.

Dyspareunia needs to be taken seriously as it is the cause of much unhappiness. It can be a precursor to vaginismus, which will prevent the woman having intercourse or using tampons. The cause may be physical or psychological, or a combination and may need expert help from a psychosexual counsellor or a psychologist. A sensitive nurse may become aware of the woman's difficulty in this area when carrying out a speculum examination. Careful counselling and steps taken to alleviate the cause will help to avoid the onset of vaginismus.

Bartholin's cyst

Bartholin's glands lie on each side of the vulva with a duct which opens at the vaginal introitus. They are susceptible to infection by the sexually transmitted diseases and also the general organisms such as staphylococci and *Escherichia coli.* If the duct becomes blocked the mucus secretions which lubricate the vaginal opening during intercourse are unable to drain and a cyst forms. Sometimes the cyst may resolve, or resolve and recur with sexual arousal. The usual treatment is excision of part of the wall of the gland (marsupialization) (see page 427).

If the gland is infected, an abscess will occur which is extremely painful (Bartholin's abscess). The treatment is admission to hospital and marsupialization.

Endometriosis

Endometriosis is a strange condition which is not completely understood but it occurs in women of reproductive age and continues to be the subject of current research (Ramey and Archer, 1993). There is a familial tendency.

There are three accepted theories as to why endometriosis occurs. It is generally agreed that none of these hold the complete answer (Olive and Schwartz, 1993).

1   *The transplantation theory*   This was first proposed in the 1920s. During menstruation some blood mixed with cells flows backwards up the tubes and escapes into the peritoneal cavity. This is called 'retrograde menstruation'. Since then it has been widely established by laparoscopy that this is a common event in normal menstruating women. The unknown factor is why some women and not others develop endometriosis.

2   *Involvement of the autoimmune system* has been suggested.

3   The role of *peritoneal fluid* is also being researched.

Endometrial tissue is found in deposits outside the uterus, where it is subject to the same hormonal changes and during menstruation, continues to function in the same way as the endometrium lining the uterus. The blood released has no way of escape and is reabsorbed into the bloodstream. The inflammation caused gives rise to scarring which, if extensive, forms adhesions that distort the normal anatomy in the pelvis.

Endometriosis is most commonly found on the ovary. It also occurs on the outside of the uterus, on the utero-sacral and broad ligaments and the peritoneum. Other less common sites include the bowel wall, the bladder, cervix, vagina, vulva, and umbilicus and in scar tissue. It occasionally, but rarely, occurs in the lung.

Another puzzling thing about endometriosis is that the symptoms experienced by the woman do not necessarily reflect the degree of the disease.

Patients with minimal disease can have considerable pain and dyspareunia with no signs on examination, while some women with severe endometriosis do not have symptoms which upset them unduly.

Endometriosis has been classified by the American Fertility Society into four stages according to severity:

Stage I = minimal
Stage II = mild
Stage III = moderate
Stage IV = severe.

In severe endometriosis the ovaries, Fallopian tubes, uterus and bowel are stuck together and may be fixed by dense adhesions. An ovary may be out of position on the back of the uterus or in the pouch of Douglas. This gives rise to deep dyspareunia with pain persisting for several hours. The partners of these women are frequently affected by the fact that they initiate the pain and this frequently has a harmful effect on the sexual side of the relationship. Release of an ovum and subsequent passage through the tube in such circumstances may be difficult and the woman may have problems with conception.

Some symptoms of endometriosis are listed in Box 16.12. Some women experience tiredness and depression. A survey carried out amongst members of the Endometriosis Society showed a range of about 20 symptoms, most of which do not generally appear in medical textbooks. The findings were presented in a paper at an international symposium (Hawkridge, 1989).

Box 16.12 Symptoms of endometriosis

♦ *Dysmenorrhoea* The pain tends to last throughout the period and may get worse towards the end rather than tailing off.

♦ *Menorrhagia* Patients with endometriosis often find their periods start with 2 or 3 days spotting of dark blood and that their periods are heavy.

♦ *Dyspareunia*

♦ *Infertility* About a third of known cases are affected. This may be the only symptom.

Diagnosis

Initial diagnosis of endometriosis is by pelvic examination and pelvic ultrasound scan. Pelvic examination may reveal tenderness and nodularity. Pelvic ultrasound scan is not very helpful although it can pick up an ovarian cyst which may be an endometrioma or 'chocolate cyst'. Diagnosis is confirmed by laparoscopy.

The deposits may be seen as tiny black spots or larger cysts known as 'chocolate cysts' from the appearance of altered blood. Depending on the stage of development of the disease the colour of the deposits range from almost colourless, through pink, to red, to purple and then black when endometriosis is longstanding.

Treatment of endometriosis

Medical treatment

Endometriosis rarely occurs after the menopause and then only in women taking HRT. Pregnancy has a limiting, often curative effect on the disease but even if a baby is wanted, infertility may be one of the symptoms of the disease. Medical treatment therefore is based on suppressing ovarian function, as was described earlier in treatment of menorrhagia (page 399).

Danol (Danazol). This may be used for up to nine months and where the side-effects (discussed earlier) are tolerated, can dampen down the endometriosis. It may well recur when the normal menstrual cycle is re-established although some women find their symptoms are improved.

The combined contraceptive pill. The Pill can be successful in the treatment of mild cases, particularly when contraception is also needed. It is particularly effective when the tricycling method is used (page 191). Breakthrough bleeding and spotting may occur but be less of a problem than the endometriosis.

Progestogens. Norethisterone, dydrogesterone or medroxyprogesterone acetate given in high doses will have the same hormonal effect as a pregnancy. The side-effects are symptoms similar to those of PMS, and breakthrough bleeding may be a problem.

LHRH analogues. These are effective in suppressing the disease but can only be taken in the short-term because of the risk of osteoporosis.

Alternative and complementary therapies. Many women report an improvement in their symptoms when they take vitamins, mineral trace elements or herbal remedies. It is an area of therapy which has not attracted research but the interest in these sort of cures for PMS has encouraged endometriosis sufferers to try them. Mood swings, pain, dryness in the vagina and cramp-like pain, are all reported to have been relieved by oil of evening primrose. The B vitamins (particularly B_6) and trace elements such as zinc and magnesium are also found to be effective. Without the support of reputable scientific studies, the part played by the placebo effect in these treatments is unknown. It will be helpful if you have knowledge of some of the alternatives available and can advise your client where she can go for more information if she expresses an interest. The National Endometriosis Society produces literature and there are recent books written for sufferers which you may wish to read and recommend.

Endometriosis is similar to chronic pelvic pain in that some women suffering from the disease may have taken a long time to find a doctor to make the diagnosis. Your client may wish to discuss her progress with you. It can be therapeutic and reassuring for her to find a professional who understands and is willing to listen. She may have had to curtail her social activities and her quality of life may have suffered. Dyspareunia can have a disastrous effect on a relationship. Unfortu-nately, symptoms may persist in some patients even after the disease has been successfully treated and laparoscopy reveals no evidence of active disease.

Surgical treatment

Techniques using local ablative treatment, with diathermy or laser laparoscopes, have been developed in some centres with mixed reports of success. Ovarian cystectomy or oophorectomy may be advised. There is less recovery time needed when micro-surgical techniques are used but the equipment is expensive and availability is limited. Consequently many women have to undergo major surgery. The problem of recurrence may remain although treatment with suppressive therapy prior to surgery may be helpful in this respect.

Hysterectomy and bilateral salpingo-oophorectomy may be considered as the final option available to the woman who has suffered pain and its consequences over a number of years. The implications are similar to those discussed for women with chronic pelvic pain. The decision to have surgery may come as a relief but again it is wise if you help the patient to examine her feelings about fertility beforehand.

Ovarian cysts

There are many types of ovarian cysts. The most common types are described in Box 16.13.

Ovarian cysts are often asymptomatic and the woman may not consult the doctor until the cyst has grown quite large and is causing pressure symptoms such as abdominal distension, interference with normal micturition, altered bowel habit, dyspareunia and pelvic or epigastric discomfort.

Pain will be a symptom of rupture or torsion of a cyst.

All cysts larger than 5 cm in diameter will usually be removed as soon as possible because of the risk of malignancy. Benign cysts are usually resected in younger women leaving as much ovarian tissue intact as possible. Cysts occurring in the peri-menopausal and post-menopausal woman must always be investigated, and a hysterectomy with bilateral salpingo-oophorectomy will be advised if malignancy cannot be excluded. If you are involved in helping a woman make this difficult

Box 16.13   Ovarian cysts

Distension or non-neoplastic cysts

♦ *Follicular cysts* These are common and usually single. They seldom grow to be larger than 5 cm in diameter and most are discovered incidentally during a pelvic ultrasound scan or laparoscopy. Most regress spontaneously and require no treatment.

♦ *Corpus luteum cysts* These may be associated with amenorrhoea and can occur in the pregnant or non-pregnant woman. They usually regress, but occasionally rupture, when the symptoms may be similar to those of an ectopic pregnancy. The pain, which can be severe, is usually short-lived. A pelvic ultrasound scan may help in making the diagnosis, if this is in doubt.

♦ *Theca lutein cysts*   These are multilocular and associated with hydatidiform mole.

Cystic neoplasms   These occur between the menarche and the menopause.

♦ *Serous cystadenoma* This is an epithelial cyst which may be simple or multilocular. Usually not larger than 15 cm in diameter, it may be bilateral.

♦ *Mucinous cystadenoma* These are common and can grow to an enormous size. They are multilocular in structure and contain mucus which may be thick or thin. If a mucinous cyst ruptures, the rare condition myxoma peritonei may occur. Large collections of mucinous material accumulate in the peritoneal cavity and progressively spread, even after removal.

♦ *Benign cystic teratomas, or dermoid cysts* These occur most commonly in young women, and again may grow to a large size. They are derived from germ cells. The cysts are covered in a firm, fibrous capsule and may contain sebaceous material, hair, teeth, bone, cartilage, thyroid and neural tissue and gastrointestinal mucosa. Dermoid cysts are heavy and are susceptible to torsion.

decision, if she is already taking or considering HRT it is worth remembering she will be able to take oestrogen replacement without progesterone. This will be a positive aspect of surgery to discuss with her.

Carcinoma of the ovary

There is as yet no safe and reliable screening method to detect this cancer, which remains a silent and deadly disease. There is often no pain or discomfort until the tumour is quite advanced when the woman may present with loss of weight and ascites. Some cases may be detected earlier when the woman is found to have an adnexal mass on abdominal examination. Carcinoma of the ovary is responsible for about 4000 deaths in England and Wales each year. This is about the same number as the combined deaths from cervical and endometrial cancer. Every year nearly 2% of women develop cancer of the ovary.

The incidence is higher in women in their fifties and sixties and among single and nulliparous women. Pregnancy and the oral contraceptive pill both have a protective effect and it is thought that repeated ovulation without any gaps may be responsible for the development of this cancer.

A pelvic ultrasound scan, with a laparoscopy if the findings are doubtful, will aid diagnosis. The exact nature and spread of the disease will be assessed during a laparotomy and the amount of surgery will depend on the staging of the disease. Generally the prognosis is poor and surgery will usually be followed by radiotherapy or chemotherapy. Unfortunately many women with this disease present late and the survival rate is only about 30%, irrespective of the grading of the tumour.

Uterine prolapse

Uterine prolapse can cause symptoms of pelvic pain or ache, backache, urinary symptoms and dyspareunia. It occurs because of inadequacy of the muscles or ligaments of the pelvic floor. It may be due to pregnancy and delivery, atrophy due to oestrogen deficiency or intra-abdominal pressure. Occasionally it is seen in women with no children and so presumably there may be a congenital factor, such as an unusually large vagina, involved as well. Pelvic floor exercises in the puerperium and later in life when muscle tone decreases, are aimed at preventing this from happening. In all types of prolapse the woman will have a bulge into the vagina. Further than this she may be asymptomatic or have minimal problems.

There are three degrees of uterine prolapse:

♦ *1st degree*   The cervix does not reach the introitus

♦ *2nd degree*   The cervix descends to the introitus

♦ *3rd degree*   The cervix is below the introitus.

In extreme cases the uterus prolapses right outside the vagina. This is called a *procidentia*.

Other types of prolapse can still occur after hysterectomy. These include the following:

♦ *Vault prolapse*   The vaginal vault prolapses.

♦ *Cystocele*   The bladder bulges through a weakness in the anterior vaginal wall.

♦ *Cysto-urethrocele*   The urethra is involved as well. The symptoms reflect problems with the bladder and include: difficulty emptying the bladder, recurrent cystitis, stress incontinence and dyspareunia.

♦ *Enterocele*   The upper third of the posterior vaginal wall is covered by peritoneum and lies adjacent to the pouch of Douglas. A weakness may result in a hernia, usually containing bowel or omentum.

♦ *Rectocele*   This is a prolapse in the middle third of the posterior wall which lies adjacent to the rectum. The woman may have backache and a dragging feeling in the pelvic floor. A rectocele can cause dyspareunia and a heavy 'bearing down' sensation. If the perineal body is damaged, the rectocele will extend lower down the vaginal wall. (A rectal prolapse may be associated with vaginal prolapse and cystocele but is a separate condition in which the rectum prolapses through the anal sphincter.)

Treatment

Treatment for a prolapse will depend on the nature of the symptoms and how the woman herself views them and their effect on her life. Any decision to operate should be made only when the nature of the surgery and the likely outcome of the procedure has been fully explained and discussed with the patient. Full recovery time varies considerably with repair operations. She will need time to consider the implications of surgery in the light of her present symptoms and to discuss these with her partner or family. You may be involved in helping her come to a decision.

If she is elderly and unfit for an operation, she may be fitted with a ring pessary. These are changed every 4–6 months and work quite well in this situation by supporting the pelvic organs, although vaginal tissues may become irritated and sore. Intermittent courses of vaginal oestrogen help to prevent atrophic changes, infection, inflammation and discharge.

Conclusion

This chapter can only be an introduction to some of the common gynaecological problems you will meet. Often women seeking help may be confused by the changes that they are aware of in their bodies. You may be the first person your patient can talk to about her problems and difficulties. Once a diagnosis has been made, a knowledge of the implications of a condition may enable you to support and reassure her, if this is what she needs from you.

Often people do not ask for help because they do not realize that they have a problem. This is especially true where pain is involved and it is not easy helping in such cases. Sometimes it can be distressing, which is why you need to consider the support available to you in your working environment. Finding an empathetic listener can be the first step your patient takes in coming to terms with a difficult situation.

Resources

Androgen Insensitivity Syndrome (AIS) Support Group
c/o Mrs Jackie Burrows, 2 Sherburn Avenue, Mansfield, Notts NG18 2BY
Tel. 01623 661749

British Association for Counselling
1 Regents Place, Rugby CV21 2PJ
Tel. 01788 578328

Contact-A-Family
Tel. 0171 383 3555
For advice and information on handicapping diseases and less familiar conditions. Very helpful concerning available support groups etc. where parents and families feel isolated.

Coloplast Advice Service
Tel. 0800 220622
For advice on how to obtain free copies of a useful leaflet about pelvic floor exercises and a healthy diet. Called *Regaining Bladder Control*, the leaflet is issued free to nurses.

Cruse Bereavement Line
Tel. 0181 332 7227
Will provide number and a local address to contact for bereavement counselling (self-referral accepted).

Cruse Bereavement Care (Head office)
126 Sheen Road, Richmond TW9 1UR

National Endometriosis Society
Suite 50, Westminster Palace Gardens, 1–7 Artillery Row, London SW1P 1RL
Tel. 0171 222 2781
Helpline: 0171 222 2776
Offers support and advice to endometriosis sufferers.

Relaxation for Living
12 New Street, Chipping Norton, Oxon OX7 5LJ
Tel. 01608 646100
Large SAE for information pack.

Westminster Pastoral Foundation
23 Kensington Square, London
Tel. 0171 937 6956
Self-referral for counselling. There is usually a waiting list for those over 25.

Further reading

BROOME, A. and WALLACE, L. (eds) (1984) *Psychology and Gynaecological Problems*. London: Tavistock Publications.

DAVIS, H. and FALLOWFIELD, L. (eds) (1991) *Counselling and Communication in Health Care* Chichester: John Wiley.

HAWKRIDGE, C. (1989) *Endometriosis*. London: Macdonald Optima.

HAYMAN, S. (1991) *Endometriosis*. London: Penguin.

MACKAY, E.V., BEISCHER, N.A., COX, L.W., and WOOD, C. (1992) *Illustrated Textbook of Gynaecology* 2nd edn. Sydney: W.B. Saunders/Baillière Tindall.

SCAMBLER, A., and SCAMBLER G. (1993) *Menstrual Disorders*. London: Routledge.

TSCHUDIN, V. (1991) *Counselling Skills for Nurses*, 3rd edn. London: Baillière Tindall.

WELLS, R. and TSCHUDIN, V. (eds) (1994) *Wells Supportive Therapies in Health Care*. London: Baillière Tindall.

References

ABDALLA, H.I. (1993) Oocyte donation. In Asch, R.H. and Studd, J.W.W. (eds) *Annual Progress in Reproductive Medicine*. Carnforth, Lancs: Parthenon Publishing.

ADAMS, J., POLSON, D.W. and FRANKS, S. (1986) Prevalence of polycystic ovaries in women with anovulation and idiopathic hirsutism. *British Medical Journal* **293:** 355.

ARMAR, N.A., McGARRIGLE, H.H.G., HONOUR, J., HOWLONIA, P., JACOBS, H.S. and LACHELIN, G.C.L. (1990) Laparoscopic ovarian diathermy in the management of anovulatory infertility in women with polycystic ovaries: endocrine changes and clinical outcome. *Fertility and Sterility* **53:** 45.

BALEN, A. (1993) Amenorrhoea – causes and consequences. In Asch, R.H. and Studd, J.W.W. (eds) *Annual Progress in Reproductive Medicine*. Carnforth, Lancs: Parthenon Publishing.

BROOK, C.D.G. (1985) Management of delayed puberty. *British Medical Journal* **290:** 657.

CHIMBIRA, T.H., ANDERSON, A.B.M., NAISH, C. *et al.* (1980) Reduction of menstrual blood loss by danazol in unexplained menorrhagia: lack of effect of placebo. *British Journal of Obstetrics and Gynaecology* **87:** 1152.

DAVIS, H. and FALLOWFIELD, L. (1991) Evaluating counselling communication. In Davis, H. and Fallowfield, L. (eds) *Counselling and Communication in Health Care*. Chichester: John Wiley.

DEUTSCH, H. (1944) *The Psychology of Women*. New York: Grune & Stratton.

ERSKINE, A. and PEARCE, S. (1991) Pain in gynaecology. In Davis, H. and Fallowfield, L. (eds) *Counselling and Communication in Health Care*. Chichester: John Wiley.

FRANKS, S. (1987) Primary and secondary amenorrhoea. *British Medical Journal* **294:** 815.

FRASER, I.S., McCARRON, G., MARKHAM, R. *et al.* (1984) A preliminary study of factors influencing perception of menstrual blood loss volume. *American Journal of Obstetrics and Gynecology* **149:** 788.

FRISCH, R.E., REVELLE, R. and COOK, S. (1973) Components of weight at menarche and the initiation of the adolescent growth spurt in girls: estimated total water, lean body weight and fat. *Human Biology* **45:** 469.

GILLIBRAND, P.N. (1981) The investigation of pelvic pain. Communication at the Scientific Meeting on 'Chronic Pelvic Pain – a gynaecological headache'. Royal College of Obstetrics and Gynaecology, London.

GOODALL, J. (1991) Helping a child to understand her own testicular feminisation/Y chromosome. *Lancet* **337:** 33.

GUILLEBAUD, J., ANDERSON, A.B.M. and TURNBULL, A.C. (1978) Reduction by mefenamic acid of increased menstrual blood loss associated with intrauterine contraception. *British Journal of Obstetrics and Gynaecology* **85:** 53.

HAYNES, P.J., HODGSON, H., ANDERSON, A.M. *et al.* (1977) Measurement of menstrual blood loss in patients complaining of menorrhagia. *British Journal of Obstetrics and Gynaecology* **84:** 763.

HAWKRIDGE, C. (1989) *Endometriosis.* London: Macdonald Optima.

HIBBARD, B.M., ANDERSON, M.M., O'DRIFE, J. *et al.* (1994) *Maternal Mortality Report: Report on the Confidential Enquiries into Maternal Deaths in the United Kingdom* 1988–1990. London: HMSO.

HOLMES, T.H. and RAHE, R.H. (1967) Social events readjustment rating scale. *Journal of Psychosomatic Research* **11:** 213.

HOSHIAI, H., ISHIKAWA, M., SAWATARI, Y. *et al.* (1993) Laparoscopic evaluation of the onset and progression of endometriosis. *American Journal of Obstetrics and Gynecology* **169:** 714.

HUNT, K. and VESSEY, M. (1991) The risks and benefits of hormone replacement therapy; an updated review. *Current Obstetrics and Gynaecology* **1:** 21.

LAATAIKINEN, T., TUOMIVAARA, L. and KALEVI, K. (1993) Comparison of a local injection of hyperosmolar glucose solution with salpingostomy for the conservative treatment of tubal pregnancy. *Fertility and Sterility* **60:** 80.

OLIVE, D.L., and SCHWARTZ, L.B. (1993) Endometriosis. *New England Journal of Medicine* **328:** 1759.

PEARCE, J.M. (1991) Spontaneous abortion. In Varma, T.R. (ed.) *Clinical Gynaecology.* London: Edward Arnold.

PEARCE, S. and BEARD, R.W. (1984) Chronic pelvic pain. In Broome, A. and Wallace, L. (eds) *Psychology and Gynaecological Problems.* London: Tavistock Publications.

POLSON, D.W., ADAMS, J., WADSWORTH, J. *et al.* (1988) Polycystic ovaries – a common finding in normal women. *Lancet* **1:** 870.

RAMEY, J.W. and ARCHER, D.F. (1993) Peritoneal fluid: its relevance to the development of endometriosis. *Fertility and Sterility* **60:** 1.

ROSS, G.T. and VANDEWIELE, R. (1985) The ovary. In Wilson, J.D. and Foster, D. (eds) *Textbook of Endocrinology.* Philadelphia: W.B. Saunders.

SCAMBLER, A. and SCAMBLER, G. (1993) Menstrual disorders. In Fitzpatrick, R. and Newman, S. (eds) *The Experience of Illness Series.* London: Tavistock/ Routledge.

SNOWDEN, R. and CHRISTIAN, B. (eds) (1983) *Patterns and Perceptions of Menstruation.* A World Health Organization International Study. Beckenham: Croom Helm.

STEELE, S.J. (1985) *Gynaecology, Obstetrics and the Neonate,* London: Edward Arnold.

TREASURE, J.L. (1990) Anorexia nervosa. In Studd, J.W.W. (ed.) *Progress in Obstetrics and Gynaecology* Vol. 8. Edinburgh: Churchill Livingstone.

TSCHUDIN, V. (1991) *Counselling Skills for Nurses,* 3rd edn. London: Baillière Tindall.

WARREN, M.P. (1983) Effects of under nutrition on reproductive function in the human. *Endocrinology Reviews* **4:** 363.

WEIDEGER, P. (1975) *Female Cycles.* London: Women's Press.

WELLS, R. and TSCHUDIN, V. (eds) (1994) *Wells' Supportive Therapies in Health Care.* London: Baillière Tindall.

WINSTON, R.M.L. (1993) *Infertility.* London: Martin Dunitz (for Organon).

17: Gynaecological investigations and surgery

Imogen Rider ◆

OBJECTIVES

After reading this chapter you will understand:

◆ the most common gynaecological operations and investigations currently performed

◆ what women will experience whilst in hospital and during recovery at home and how to explain this

◆ how to investigate the sexual aspects of surgery and discuss both practical and emotional issues

◆ the importance of being aware of recent surgical developments and research within the field of women's health.

Introduction

Surgery on any part of the body can cause pre-operative anxiety, and gynaecological surgery (however minor and routine a procedure may be) is no exception. A woman's anxieties relating to gynaecological problems are unique. Not only does she worry about vaginal examinations, but impending surgery also poses a threat to her concept of body image, her role as a woman and mother, her sexuality and her relationship with her partner (Broome and Wallace, 1984).

Aspects of sexuality within the sensitive field of gynaecological surgery are a major area of concern for women but unfortunately this is often forgotten by health care professionals. The potential role of nurses in relation to sexual issues is vast, both in hospital and community work, and yet this role is not really being fulfilled. Webb (1985) stresses that the more knowledge people have about human sexuality, the more open and flexible they are likely to be in their attitudes towards their own and others' behaviour. Nurses who have this knowledge will be better able to help their patients.

Gynaecological outpatient procedures

Pelvic ultrasound scan

Ultrasound is used as a means of examining various organs of the body by means of high-frequency sound waves. These form pictures on a screen and enable any abnormalities to be detected.

The patient must fill the bladder by drinking one and a half litres of fluid (not fizzy drinks) during the two hours before the appointment. The very full bladder feels uncomfortable but is important since it helps to push the uterus and ovaries into a better position for examination.

A cold gel is applied to the woman's abdomen which helps the sound waves to pass into the abdomen by forming a good contact with the skin. A small scanning device is then pressed firmly against the abdominal wall and is moved backwards and forwards across the abdomen to produce a picture on the nearby screen. The picture is built up from the differing times echoes take to bounce back from structures of varying density. The scanning room is darkened so that images on the screen are more clearly visible.

The procedure takes between 5 and 10 minutes, is not painful but may be uncomfortable. This is because the radiographer has to press firmly against the abdomen and full bladder in order to produce a clear picture. Once the scan has been performed, the bladder can be immediately emptied. The results of the scan are then explained to the woman.

Transvaginal ultrasound scan

This type of scan facilitates a much clearer view of the pelvic organs than a pelvic ultrasound scan. The tip of a round-edged probe is inserted into the vagina. The probe is covered by a condom which is changed for each patient. A full bladder is not required for this procedure, making it easier for the doctor or radiographer and certainly more comfortable for the patient. The scan cannot harm a pregnancy.

Vabra curettage

It is possible to obtain a biopsy of the endometrium, without general anaesthesia, using a Vabra aspirator. This is a sharp instrument – a curette – with suction attached, that passes through the cervix and collects a small sample.

This procedure is performed in the outpatients clinic and may be uncomfortable for a brief moment. It is not suitable for women who have not had children. A slightly easier and less painful option is to use a pipelle (no additional suction) to obtain an endometrial biopsy.

The advice to women following a Vabra procedure is similar to that following a D and C.

Hysterosalpingogram (HSG)

A hysterosalpingogram is an X-ray examination of the female genital tract and takes about 15–20 minutes. It is a diagnostic aid and demonstrates internal uterine abnormalities, such as fibroids, bicornuate uterus and occasionally cervical incompetence. The test also illustrates the site of tubal occlusion in cases of infertility. If the Fallopian tubes are patent, radio-opaque dye will spill into the pelvic cavity. However, in many cases of infertility, the usefulness of this procedure has now been superseded by the 'laparoscopy and dye' test, which gives more detail about the nature of the tubal occlusion.

The test must take place during the first ten days of the cycle, after menstruation has ceased but before ovulation. It must not take place during the follicular phase as it could disturb a pregnancy if conception has occurred. An HSG should not take place if there is evidence of active infection since infected material could enter the tubes.

A speculum is inserted and radio-opaque dye is injected into the cervical canal via a cannula. The dye may cause a warm flush in the abdomen combined with some abdominal cramping pains.

Progress of the dye through the uterus and Fallopian tubes can be followed on a television screen. The dye is harmlessly absorbed into the bloodstream and excreted via the urine.

Women should be advised that period-type pains may be felt afterwards for which paracetamol may be taken. Slight vaginal bleeding is common which may be mixed with a small amount of clear sticky fluid – the liquid used in the test. The woman should be escorted home and should rest in bed for 12 hours.

Gynaecological surgery

Cystoscopy

A cystoscopy is a minor operative procedure that takes about 15 minutes and allows a thorough examination of the bladder. It is usually performed under a general anaesthetic.

This operation is carried out to investigate the cause of recurrent urinary tract infections or to find out why blood is present in the urine. A small polyp may also be removed from the bladder during the procedure, or a caruncle at the urethral entrance.

A fine telescope-like instrument – a cystoscope – with a light source is inserted into the urethra and passed along into the bladder. This enables the urogynaecologist to view inside the bladder, and a biopsy may be taken if necessary. Occasionally, a woman may have a urethral catheter inserted at the end of the procedure.

Cystoscopy is usually performed as a day-case. It is important that the woman has passed urine before she goes home. Initially there may be blood in the urine due to bleeding from the biopsy site. If the woman has a catheter she will usually stay in overnight. The catheter will be removed in the morning and once she has passed urine she may go home. A bath or shower may be taken but bubble baths or perfumed bath oils are not recommended.

Most women will feel well enough to return to work and their usual activities within 2–3 days.

It is probably advisable to refrain from sexual intercourse following cystoscopy for up to a week to avoid infection or trauma to the urethra. A vaginal lubricant may reduce friction. Women should also be advised to empty their bladder before and after intercourse.

Dilatation and curettage (D and C)

A dilatation of the cervix and curettage of the uterus is the most common minor gynaecological procedure. It is an investigative operation which gives information about the size and shape of the uterine cavity and the endometrium.

The procedure may be diagnostic where there has been occurrence of post-menopausal bleeding, post-coital bleeding or any instance of increased bleeding, both during menstruation and inter-menstrually. It is also used as a therapeutic intervention to treat menorrhagia where the cause is an endometrial polyp, and to remove the retained products of conception following a miscarriage. A similar procedure is also used to perform an early suction termination of pregnancy.

The cervix is gently dilated and a curette (a spoon-like instrument) is used to scrape away the lining of the uterine cavity. The curettings are sent for histology. The procedure only takes a few minutes and the cervix closes naturally afterwards.

The woman either has a gynaecology out-patient appointment or returns to her GP for the results.

A D and C is usually performed as a day-case but occasionally an overnight stay in hospital may be recommended. It is common to have some bleeding after the procedure which may be bright red at first and should gradually decrease to a brown stain that can last for up to a week. If the bleeding becomes heavy, offensive smelling or there is a raised temperature then medical advice should be sought as these are indications of an infection.

A D and C is not normally painful but some women do experience period-like pains which can be relieved by mild analgesia, such as paracetamol. If the pain becomes prolonged or severe medical advice should again be sought.

You should advise the woman to use sanitary towels rather than tampons to reduce the risk of infection, although the latter may be used at the next period. Sexual intercourse should be avoided for two weeks to allow healing and to reduce the risk of infection. Most women ovulate and menstruate as usual following a dilatation and curettage and their next period should be at the expected time.

Hysteroscopy

A hysteroscopy is a minor operation, performed under light general anaesthesia or local anaesthetic, to enable the gynaecologist to view directly inside the uterus and examine the endometrium.

It may be used to diagnose the cause of post-menopausal bleeding. In this instance a D and C is often carried out simultaneously. It may also be combined with a therapeutic intervention, such as an endometrial ablation or resection to treat menorrhagia.

A small fibre-optic telescope is passed through the cervix into the uterus. The walls of the uterus are separated with gas or fluid to enable the telescope to view inside the uterus. This procedure is not carried out when the woman is menstruating or experiencing any bleeding, since this can impair the view.

The operation takes about 10 minutes and is usually performed as a day-case. Afterwards there may be some slight abdominal cramps which can be relieved by paracetamol. If a general anaesthetic is used it is advisable for a woman to take 2–3 days off work but, if a local anaesthetic has been chosen, she can return the following day.

Transcervical resection of the endometrium (TCRE)

Also known as hystero-resection or an endometrial ablation, this procedure involves the use of the hysteroscope in conjunction with other instruments to remove the endometrial lining of the uterus, and is monitored on a video screen. It is a relatively new type of minimally invasive surgery which was initially pioneered in Oxford in 1987.

Women usually have a D and C at some stage prior to the operation to ensure their suitability for such surgery. A drug, such as Danazol, may well be given for 4–6 weeks beforehand to reduce endometrial thickening.

A TCRE is performed as a therapeutic intervention to treat menorrhagia. Prior to the development of this procedure, the traditional treatments for heavy menstrual bleeding were drug therapy, a D and C (no longer considered curative) or the option of major surgery in the form of a hysterectomy. Obviously the length of stay in hospital and the risks of undergoing a major surgical procedure, with its associated psychological implications, mean that to some women a TCRE is considered preferable to a hysterectomy. In addition, a recuperation of several weeks' following a hysterectomy must be compared to the early return to work following a TCRE.

After a TCRE a woman can expect her periods to become lighter and, in some cases they may cease altogether. However, period pains and premenstrual symptoms will not necessarily stop and the woman cannot be assured that she will not need a hysterectomy eventually. On rare occasions, a hysterectomy may need to be performed at the time of the TCRE if bleeding does not stop during the operation. All women should be aware of this possibility when signing their consent form.

The advantages and disadvantages of having a TCRE compared with a hysterectomy are outlined in Table 17.1.

It was originally felt that TCRE would challenge the hysterectomy as a routine treatment for menorrhagia. However, results of long-term studies looking at women post-TCRE are not encouraging and 50% will need either another endometrial ablation or else go on to hysterectomy. TCRE for menorrhagia is not appropriate for all women. Contraindications are listed in Box 17.1.

Box 17.1 Contraindications to TCRE

♦ Any woman with a vaginal prolapse would be advised to have a hysterectomy.

♦ Conditions of the uterus, such as endometriosis or fibroids, will not necessarily be cured by a TCRE. It is not possible to remove fibroids transcervically if they are larger than the size of a 12-week pregnancy.

♦ If there is a suspected or known malignancy, a total abdominal hysterectomy, where biopsies may be taken from other sites in the pelvis, is required. It will also be more difficult to perform endometrial biopsies at a later date due to possible stenosis of the cervix and reduced endometrial thickness.

How it is performed

The cervix is dilated to allow the passage of the resectoscope into the uterine cavity. Endometrial tissue is then removed, drawing away from the fundus in strips towards the cervix. The endometrium is excised using an electrical diathermy current passed through a variety of wire-cutting attachments. These attachments also coagulate bleeding vessels and minimize blood loss.

Several different instruments may be used via the resectoscope. Diathermy-powered cutting loops may be used and also laser ablation. This involves the passage of a small Nd:YAG laser (Nd:YAG = neodymium: yttrium-aluminium-garnet) into the uterus and heating the endometrium with laser energy. This can be time-consuming and the laser is very expensive.

In America a roller-ball is frequently used since it is cheaper and reduces the risk of perforating the uterus. It involves a small 25-mm oval-shaped roller-ball electrode that is passed, via the resectoscope, quickly over the surface of the uterus. A diathermy blade may be used to cut away the base of the polyp or fibroids.

Table 17.1 *Comparison between TCRE and hysterectomy*

TCRE	HYSTERECTOMY
Disadvantages	
Potential risk of fluid overload	High risk of haemorrhage
Potential risk of uterine perforation	Potential wound infection
Potential haemorrhage	Increased anaesthetic time

Cannot guarantee total cessation of periods or sterility	Post-operative complications:
	  Chest infection
	  Deep vein thrombosis
	  Constipation
	  Need for strong analgesics

Long-term effects unknown	
May still require hysterectomy for fibroids and ovarian problems	Altered body image with change in sexual function
	Large abdominal scar
	Long convalescence required
Advantages	
Can be carried out under sedation and local anaesthetic	No further periods
Greatly reduced need for analgesia	Sterility guaranteed
Rapid recovery and convalescence	No need for further surgery for fibroids etc.
No visible scar	
Short hospital stay, therefore cheaper	
Retains womb, symbol of feminity and fertility	
Quickly resume sexual function	

These electrical techniques are all performed while fluid is circulated through the uterus. The resectoscope is attached to a hysteromat pump which irrigates and expands the uterine cavity with glycine 1.5% irrigation fluid. This fluid is a non-conductive, transparent medium through which the gynaecologist maintains visibility whilst operating. The fluid, blood and debris are drawn out by suction into a separate container (see Figures 17.1 and 17.2). Due to the intrauterine pressure the fluid can be absorbed, causing dilational hyponatraemia (low sodium) and fluid overload. During the procedure a precise fluid balance is maintained. If an excess of 200 ml is absorbed the procedure is quickly finished and the patient is given a diuretic.

An even more recent method of performing transcervical endometrial resection is radio-frequency endometrial ablation (RaFEA). An intrauterine probe is inserted via the cervix into the uterine cavity. The probe tip emits radiofrequency energy at a reorganized medical frequency (27.12 mHz).

The probe, in conjunction with an abdominal diathermy plate, creates an electric field around the active probe tip sufficient to cause rapid movement of water molecules in surrounding cells. This creates sufficient localized heating to destroy the surrounding endometrium. A temperature of between 63 and 65°C is required to destroy the endometrium and the basal layer on which it regenerates.

The advantage of RaFEA is that it does not require the gynaecologist to visualize the uterine cavity, thereby removing the need for large volumes of flushing medium which can cause fluid overload and pulmonary oedema.

Women with pacemakers or implanted spinal

Figure 17.1 *The hysteromat pump and associated tubing.*

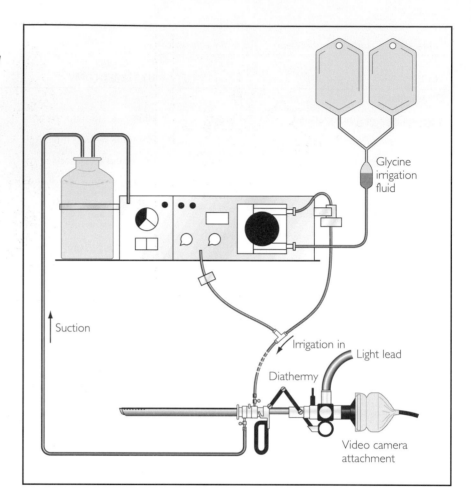

Glycine irrigation fluid

Suction

Irrigation in

Light lead

Diathermy

Video camera attachment

anaesthetic coils should be excluded from RaFEA ablation since these devices may be altered by the radiofrequency equipment. Women should not be menstruating during this procedure since this reduces the effectiveness of the treatment. Those patients who have experienced other methods of TCRE are also not suitable since the myometrium will be too superficial for the treatment to be effective.

Pinion *et al.* (1994) found that women treated by hysteroscopic surgery had less morbidity and a significantly shorter recovery period (2–4 weeks) than those treated by hysterectomy (2–3 months.)

Advice to women

Light bleeding is usually experienced for several days, followed by a watery discharge, which may continue for 2–3 weeks. Sanitary towels rather than tampons should be used to reduce the risk of infection. Menstrual bleeding usually decreases progressively during the next two to three periods. Slight cramping pelvic pain may be experienced for several hours but should be relieved by paracetamol or voltarol. Any temperature or offensive-smelling discharge is suggestive of infection and medical advice should be sought.

Sexual intercourse may be resumed when the vaginal bleeding has ceased. Pregnancy is unlikely in those women whose periods become lighter or disappear, but sterility cannot be guaranteed so contraception remains necessary: some hospitals offer women a simultaneous laparoscopic sterilization. Women usually return to work within 1–2 weeks.

Menopausal women using hormone replacement therapy still need to take cyclical progestogen with their oestrogen as small patches of

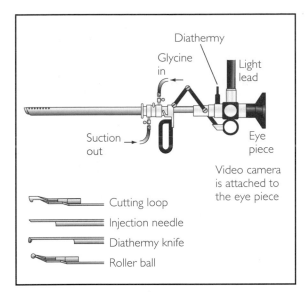

Figure 17.2 *The assembled resectoscope and attachments.*

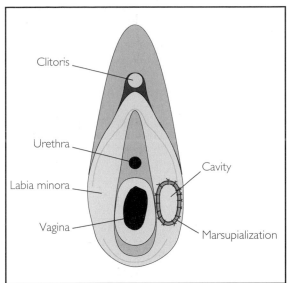

Figure 17.3 *Marsupialization of a Bartholin's abscess.*

endometrium may remain in the uterus and these may be subject to excessive growth (hyperplasia) if the oestrogen is not opposed.

In conclusion, many women prefer the idea of endometrial ablation since it is a far less invasive procedure than a hysterectomy and, in terms of effects on a woman's sexuality, is less likely to cause problems. However, it is advisable and relevant when considering this type of treatment to discuss with the woman any worries she or her partner may have about the effects of having a hysterectomy on their sexual feelings and correct any misinformation if present. It is important that the woman feels she has made the decision about which procedure to have for herself.

Marsupialization of a Bartholin's abscess

The Bartholin's glands, which lubricate the vulva, lie behind the vestibule. The duct can become blocked, giving rise to a painless swelling, which becomes palpable, called a Bartholin's cyst. The cyst may become infected resulting in a painful Bartholin's abscess which is often initially noticed during sexual intercourse. The abscess can be extremely painful and appear hot, red and swollen. The woman may have difficulty in walking, be unable to sit down and is reluctant to pass urine.

It is preferable not to excise the gland because

it provides lubrication for sexual intercourse. Instead, marsupialization is performed (from the Greek *marsipos* = bag). The abscess is opened to facilitate drainage and the walls of the abscess are sutured to the surrounding skin to leave a large orifice to facilitate drainage of the pus (see Figure 17.3). A new duct forms as healing occurs. During the operation a swab will be taken for microscopy, culture and sensitivity, and antibiotics may be prescribed. The cavity is loosely packed with ribbon gauze impregnated with an antiseptic solution such as proflavin.

This operation is often performed as an emergency and women usually go home 24 hours later, once they have passed urine. The vaginal pack will be removed either by the nurse or by the woman herself. This can be helped by sitting in a soothing bath of warm water. Regular use of a bath, shower or bidet is important to keep the area clean. A hair dryer can be used instead of a towel for drying. Antibiotics are not given routinely unless infection is proven. It is probably advisable not to have sexual intercourse for two weeks following the operation to avoid re-infection and to allow the area to heal.

Laparoscopy

Laparoscopy may be described as the direct visualization of the pelvic organs with a fibre-optic light and a telescope-like instrument, known as a laparoscope.

The procedure may be diagnostic when there is unexplained abdominal and pelvic pain, dyspareunia or infertility. In these instances, adhesions, infection, endometriosis or polycystic ovarian disease may be diagnosed. It is also possible to perform therapeutic interventions through the laparoscope. These include laparoscopic sterilization, division of pelvic adhesions, aspiration of small benign ovarian cysts and vaporization of endometriosis using a carbon dioxide laser and video screen. Infertility investigations and procedures are also carried out laparoscopically. A laparoscopy may also be required for the surgical diagnosis and treatment of an ectopic pregnancy.

Under general anaesthesia the woman is catheterized and placed in the Trendelenburg's position. The table is tilted downwards to allow the upper abdominal contents to fall away from the pelvic organs. A small incision is made below the umbilicus and 2–3 litres of carbon dioxide is introduced into the abdominal cavity. This produces a pneumoperitoneum which helps to displace the intestines and allows the pelvic and abdominal organs to be viewed easily via the laparoscope. A second instrument is inserted through a small cut near the upper pubic hairline.

At the end of the operation the carbon dioxide is expelled by abdominal pressure and the small incisions may be sutured or steristrips applied. Any remaining gas is absorbed over the next few days.

This operation is mostly performed as a daycase. Some gynaecologists prefer women to have the top 2 cm of pubic hair shaved for the lower incision in the suprapubic region. You should warn the woman that she may feel bloated and have an aching pain around the shoulders following a laparoscopy. This is quite usual and is caused by the carbon dioxide in the abdomen irritating the phrenic nerve. Paracetamol and hot peppermint water can give relief. Occasionally, opiate analgesia is necessary. Sometimes the incisions may bleed or ooze a little but an ordinary plaster should be sufficient covering. If they become painful or produce an offensive smelling discharge, medical advice should be sought.

It normally takes a woman a few days to recover fully from a laparoscopy and she should resume normal activities and work when she feels ready. Sexual intercourse may be resumed when she feels comfortable.

Laparoscopy and dye test

This test involves a laparoscopy as outlined above. In addition, a blue dye, methylene blue, is injected through the cervix and observed as it passes from the uterus through the Fallopian tubes and out via the fimbrial ends into the pelvic cavity. The dye illustrates any blockages in the tubes which might prevent the eggs from the ovaries reaching the uterus. If the dye flows through (referred to as 'fill and spill') the tubes are assumed to be patent. The test is performed during the follicular phase of the cycle so that any developing follicles may be viewed.

After the operation, you should warn the woman that there may be a blue stain on the sanitary towel and urine may appear green or blue as it mixes with dye from the vagina. The gynaecologists should explain their findings to the woman and her partner and any further appointments for tests or referral to a specialist infertility clinic will be made (see Chapter 8)

Adhesiolysis or salpingolysis

This is the most successful operation for tubal blockage causing infertility. It consists of dividing the peri-tubal adhesions around the upper ends of the Fallopian tubes. If the fimbriae are not damaged and the adhesions are not too extensive, the lining epithelium of the Fallopian tubes is likely to be intact and its function may be restored. Thirty per cent of patients are likely to become pregnant (Lewis and Chamberlain, 1991) but there is an increased risk of ectopic pregnancy and reformation of adhesions. A peritoneal lavage of 5% dextran solution may be required for 24–48 hours following surgery to prevent the tissues adhering together.

Laser laparoscopy

The word 'laser' refers to light amplification by stimulated emission of radiation. The carbon dioxide (CO_2) laser vaporizes tissue so that malignant or unwanted tissue, such as adhesions and endometriosis, may be removed painlessly and completely under the enhanced vision of the laparoscope.

The laser has a sealing effect on the blood vessels and the risk of bleeding is greatly reduced. The Nd:YAG laser is an exceptional coagulator which delivers an invisible beam near to the infra-red region of the spectrum.

Laser laparoscopy may be used to treat endometriosis and polycystic ovarian disease (see Chapter 16). In the latter case it replaces the old-fashioned wedge resection which was often followed by spontaneous ovulation. Cauterization and multiple ovarian biopsy have also been used to mimic a wedge resection, but can cause formation of adhesions and haematomas. Using a laser, multiple holes in the ovary are made causing drainage of the subcapsular cysts which contain high levels of androstenedione. This will lead to a rise in FSH secretion and ultimately spontaneous ovulation should occur. The laser drill technique results in about 60% of patients returning to spontaneous ovulation and the remaining 40% will usually respond to clomiphene, even though they were resistant to it before surgery. Although the effect is usually temporary, it allows 'a window of opportunity' for women to attempt conception without having to resort to expensive infertility options.

Laparoscopic sterilization (see also page 210)

In the past, it was necessary for women to have a laparotomy (large incision of the abdominal wall) if they wished to be sterilized. Nowadays it is usually possible to perform the operation via the laparoscope. Occasionally, a mini-laparotomy (8–10 cm scar) may be necessary if access and visualization of the Fallopian tubes is difficult. In this instance a stay of one or two days in hospital will be recommended and heavy lifting should be avoided for about three weeks.

Sexual aspects of sterilization. Alder (1984) stresses that when a couple request sterilization they should be given an opportunity to discuss any queries or worries, and be offered sexual counselling if necessary. If the operation is straightforward, this will be the last time the couple ask for contraceptive advice and may be the last opportunity they have to ask for professional help with the sexual relationship, without making it a particular issue. You should, therefore, facilitate

discussion about any sexual concerns a couple may have.

Miscarriage

An abdominal or transvaginal ultrasound is usually carried out to aid diagnosis. In the case of an inevitable miscarriage, the woman may be in pain and bleeding, whilst those with a missed miscarriage may not have either of these symptoms and can be even more distressed to discover their baby has stopped growing and died.

Women are particularly sensitive at this time and appreciate health professionals recognizing their loss as significant and as a real baby (not as a 'fetus'). Women not only need physical and emotional support at this time but they require information to be given clearly, honestly and in a sensitive manner.

Surgical intervention

An evacuation of the retained products of conception (ERPC) is carried out to remove any remaining tissue which might cause infection or excessive bleeding. This procedure is similar to a D and C. Again, the language you use is important and it is advisable that you do not refer to it as a D and C or a 'scrape', since this can understandably upset some women. An ERPC is usually performed under general anaesthesia, although some hospitals do offer a spinal block or local anaesthesia. Recent research in Sweden has shown that expectant management (i.e. no surgical intervention) in selected cases of spontaneous miscarriage has a similar outcome to ERPC (Nielsen and Hahlin, 1995).

These operations are often performed at the end of a booked theatre list and for this reason women may have to wait several hours for surgery. This can further add to their distress, particularly when they have not been allowed to eat or drink and the nursing staff have no idea when the operation will be performed. The woman will be allowed home after recovery so long as she has no heavy vaginal bleeding.

Discharge advice

The advice for women following an ERPC is similar to the advice given following a D and C. Women who have had a miscarriage are only in hospital for a short time so it is important that relevant dis-charge advice is given, and backed up by the hospital's own leaflet (if available) with a contact telephone number. Vaginal bleeding may continue for a few days but should not be heavier than a normal period. Breast tenderness may be a prob-lem, especially if the miscarriage occurred later in the pregnancy and women should be warned as this can be a distressing problem for them. A well-supporting bra will help reduce discomfort but it is not usually felt that medication is necessary.

Women should be advised that it is probably better to wait until at least two normal menstrual periods have occurred before trying to conceive again.

A follow-up appointment is not usually offered unless the woman has had three consecutive mis-carriages, or has a miscarriage in the second trimester of pregnancy. The Miscarriage Associa-tion and SANDS (Stillbirth and Neonatal Death Society) have a useful range of booklets that you can recommend to your patients (see Resources, page 448).

Ectopic pregnancy

The word 'ectopic' comes from the Greek *ektopos*, meaning 'misplaced', and an ectopic pregnancy occurs when the fertilized ovum implants and develops outside the uterus. Approximately 1 in 200 pregnancies are ectopic and the condition is discussed more fully in Chapter 16.

A woman with a suspected ectopic pregnancy should always be treated as a gynaecological emergency since this condition is potentially life-threatening. Despite medical advances in the past decade there has been no decrease in the number of women dying from an ectopic pregnancy. This is because the sudden rupture of the Fallopian tube can lead to a massive intra-peritoneal haemorrhage.

Some women arrive in a state of collapse in the accident and emergency department requiring resuscitation, blood transfusions, and immediate surgery by laparoscopy or laparotomy.

Laparoscopic treatment of an ectopic pregnancy

Since the development of minimally invasive sur-gical techniques, it has been possible to treat unruptured ectopic pregnancies laparoscopically. Forceps may be used to 'milk' the pregnancy from the tube, or the tube may be irrigated via a supra-pubic cannula and also by hydrotubation through the cervix to flush out any remaining products of gestation. Alternatively, linear salpingostomy (opening of the tube) may be carried out using a laser to carefully open the tube and remove the pregnancy. Aspiration under ultrasound control may be possible in some hospitals.

Another new development in this area has been the use of embryotoxic drugs, such as metho-trexate, which is injected directly into the fetal sac. Methotrexate is a folic acid antagonist that induces dissolution of trophoblastic tissue.

Tulandi (1994) suggests that administration of methotrexate systemically in the form of an intra-muscular injection is a promising treatment in a selected group of patients. Tulandi also mentions the use of laparoscopic intratubal prostaglandin and hyperosmolar glucose. Hyperosmolar glucose probably acts by dehydrating the cells and causes necrosis of the trophoblastic tissue.

Laparoscopic treatment of unruptured ectopic pregnancies is not widely available at present and a woman undergoing a laparoscopy for a sus-pected ectopic pregnancy should understand that there is always a risk of laparotomy, even in centres where laparoscopic salpingostomy is performed.

Laparoscopy proceeding to laparotomy

This will be carried out when an ectopic pregnancy is diagnosed or in hospitals where scanning and BHCG radioassay are not available at all times. If an ectopic pregnancy is visualized via the laparo-scope, the gynaecologist may proceed to a lapar-otomy and remove the damaged tube (salping-ectomy) and the remainder of the pregnancy. Any bleeding will be stopped and a Redivac drain and urinary catheter may be inserted.

Psychological aspects of an ectopic pregnancy

Women are often very distressed when an ectopic pregnancy is diagnosed, particularly if they were using contraception (commonly the IUD or pro-gestogen-only pill) and had not even realized they were pregnant. On the other hand, a couple may have been trying to conceive for many years, have had a previous ectopic, or are on an IVF programme. An ectopic pregnancy in these situations is even more distressing.

Women and their partners should receive sensitive care and an opportunity to discuss their concerns. Information about the Miscarriage Association may be helpful and staff should remember that ectopic pregnancy not only involves the feelings of loss and bereavement, but also involves major surgery.

Women usually remain in hospital for about five days following laparotomy and one or two nights following laparoscopy. The woman's rhesus status will be ascertained before she goes home.

Sexual intercourse may be resumed once any bleeding has stopped. It is probably advisable for the couple to wait until one or two normal periods have occurred before they try for another pregnancy. Contraception should therefore be discussed (preferably not the IUD or progestogen-only pill) and this conversation can provide a starting point for discussion of any sexual concerns.

Aftercare following loss of a pregnancy

Sexual healing

Loss of a pregnancy or baby, for whatever reason – miscarriage, intrauterine death, stillbirth, ectopic pregnancy or even termination of pregnancy – can all cause psychological problems for the woman and her partner for some time after the event. Guilt is a common feeling and it can take a very sympathetic partner to help a woman through this time.

Miscarriage may create problems with self-concept, inner feelings of failure, loss of faith in her physical body, and other conflicts in the marriage and family relationships. Some studies indicate a serious increase in marital conflict after the loss of a pregnancy. Peppers and Knapp (1980) attribute some of this difficulty to what they term 'incongruent bonding' where the mother has had the biological bonding experience of carrying her child, while the father's process has been on a mental, intellectual level. Couples often experience sexual difficulties after the loss of a pregnancy and may not understand the relationship between these difficulties and their loss (Schiff, 1977).

Some couples may shy away from love-making in order to avoid intercourse and the memory of

the dead child's conception. Others may be fearful of another pregnancy too soon, and be unwilling to trust contraception. Some women may feel able to receive love-making but feel so drained by their grief that there is no energy to give in return. For those parents who are fearful of intercourse and therefore tense and anxious, a very gentle and slow return to love-making can be recommended. Panuthos and Romeo (1984) advise:

> Releasing all thoughts of performance and all goals of orgasmic completion. Initially, your return to love-making might merely be an exchange of tender back-rubs. You might then desire intimate caresses and physical closeness, still with no goal of completing intercourse or reaching orgasm. Talking about sexual love-making is difficult to many couples, but agreeing ahead of time on what your needs are would free your love-making from hidden fears and constraints.

Some parents feel guilty about forgetting their dead child if they allow the pleasure of love-making. In fact, they may view any kind of pleasure or happiness as the deepest disloyalty to their lost child. Some may always have conscious thoughts of their child when they make love. In such cases Panuthos and Romeo (1984) recommend the following exercise:

> Before love-making, visualise your lost child. Call her before you in your mind's eye and then visualise creating a peaceful haven for her. Create it as being completely safe and protective as well as sensorialy beautiful and peaceful. Then ask her to stay in that sanctuary, perfectly safe, while you are with your spouse or partner. If you feel the need, visualise calling another dead loved one to be with your child – a grandparent perhaps, or a favourite aunt. Promise to return to your child later, and then 'leave' with her blessing in your heart.

Often at this time, a common emotional response is a feeling of vulnerability – a harkening back to the vulnerability of childhood. The terrified 'child' within the bereaved parent may need to be comforted and held, not as a lover, but as a child would be held by a parent. Sexual intimacy may be just too much for the 'child' within. Bereaved couples may need to explore other means of physical comfort rather than sexual intimacy.

In addition, pregnancy losses often involve physical invasions (an ERPC, laparotomy, traumatic delivery, different types of TOP) of the sexual parts of a woman's body. A couple who have had a miscarriage should be advised to wait until the woman has had one normal period before trying for another pregnancy. Obviously, this is often the last thing the couple want to do, and it is important that health professionals give correct advice rather than 'go home and get pregnant again'. Finally, it is always important to include the partner in any discussions and consider his feelings of loss as well.

Rhesus status

After a pregnancy loss, whether a miscarriage or an ectopic pregnancy, it is crucial that the woman's rhesus status is checked to prevent haemolytic disease of the newborn. The rhesus factor is found in the red blood cells of 85% of the population (rhesus positive), the other 15% are rhesus negative. If a woman with rhesus negative blood becomes pregnant by a man with rhesus positive blood, the fetus will have rhesus positive blood. A small amount of blood will pass into the woman's blood which will form antibodies. If the woman continues with the pregnancy, there will be no harm to the fetus, but if she becomes pregnant again by a rhesus positive man, the woman's body will 'attack' the fetus. This will either cause a miscarriage or the child will be born with haemolytic disease of the newborn and will require a full exchange of blood. Rhesus disease may be prevented by the injection of 'Anti-D' which destroys any rhesus positive cells that have entered a woman's bloodstream. It therefore prevents the woman's body from making the antibodies, but must be given within 72 hours of the pregnancy finishing.

Hysterectomy

Over 1000 hysterectomies are performed in the UK every week and one in five women can expect such surgery by the age of 60 years. A hysterectomy is a routine but major gynaecological operation which involves the removal of the uterus and its neck, the cervix. There are various types of hysterectomy (see Figure 17.4) and it is important that the woman knows which procedure she is having. The type used will depend on the reason for the hysterectomy (Box 17.2).

Box 17.2 Reasons for hysterectomy

♦ Painful or irregular periods or episodes of unexplained vaginal bleeding.

♦ Fibroids which can cause pain, heavy bleeding and occasionally pressure on other pelvic organs, e.g. the bladder.

♦ Uterine prolapse which may interfere with bladder and bowel function.

♦ Severe endometriosis – a condition where the endometrium grows in other parts of the body, such as the ligaments of the uterus or ovaries, causing inter-menstrual bleeding, dysmenorrhoea and dyspareunia.

♦ Chronic pelvic pain caused by pelvic infection.

♦ Gynaecological cancers of the vagina, cervix, endometrium, Fallopian tubes or ovaries.

♦ Occasionally a hysterectomy is performed in an emergency, e.g. in instances of postpartum haemorrhage or following a gynaecological procedure where haemostasis cannot be maintained.

Total abdominal hysterectomy

This involves the removal of the uterus and cervix through a horizontal cut in the abdomen just above the pubic bone: a Pfannenstiel or 'bikini-line' incision. Some women may require a vertical incision where there is a large abdominal swelling or a previous scar.

Bilateral salpingo-oophorectomy

This refers to the removal of both Fallopian tubes and ovaries and is often performed at the same time as a total abdominal hysterectomy – particularly where there is evidence of disease or if the woman is approaching the menopause or is already post-menopausal. Oophorectomy obviously prevents ovarian cancer in the future. For pre-menopausal women an attempt is made to conserve the ovaries if they are healthy, to avoid a sudden decrease in oestrogen which could cause severe menopausal symptoms. It has been shown, however, that if ovaries are conserved they may have a decreased hormonal function in pre-menopausal women, possibly because their blood supply may be compromised during surgery.

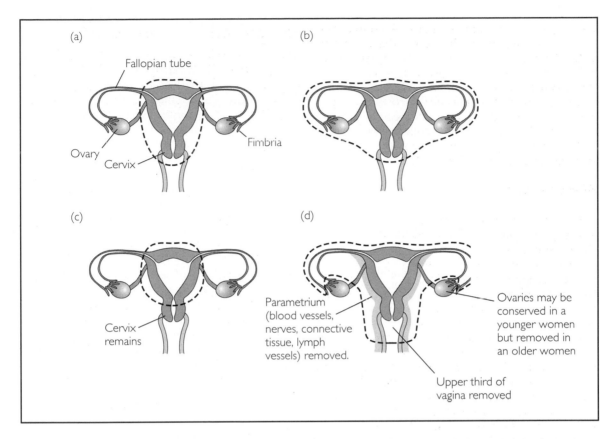

Figure 17.4 *Types of hysterectomy. (a) Total abdominal hysterectomy; (b) Total abdominal hysterectomy with bilateral salpingo-oophorectomy; (c) Subtotal hysterectomy; (d) Wertheim's hysterectomy.*

Subtotal hysterectomy

This procedure is rarely performed today but is growing in popularity, but it refers to the removal of the uterus while leaving the cervix behind. Regular cervical smears remain necessary.

Radical/Wertheim's hysterectomy

This operation is an extended hysterectomy where the uterus, ovaries, Fallopian tubes, adjacent pelvic tissue, lymph ducts and the upper third of the vagina are removed. This is necessary in cases of advanced cervical and endometrial cancer. The ovaries may be conserved in a younger woman.

Vaginal hysterectomy

This involves the removal of the uterus through the vagina, with conservation of the ovaries. A vaginal hysterectomy is usually performed on older women where there is a prolapse of the uterus. Contraindications to vaginal hysterectomy include a bulky uterus, (larger in size than a 14-week pregnancy), and suspected or known malignancy. This type of hysterectomy may be referred to as a 'suction hysterectomy' by women, although this is not an accurate description. There will be no abdominal scar.

One of the most recent developments in gynaecological surgery is that of laser-assisted laparoscopic vaginal hysterectomy including removal of the ovaries. This procedure is not designed to replace either abdominal or vaginal hysterectomy but it offers a less invasive option to women facing abdominal hysterectomy and oophorectomy. The operation takes no longer with a skilled surgeon and the hospital stay is reduced to two days. There is little post-operative pain, intra-operative blood loss is reduced significantly and four small incisions replace a large abdominal wound. This operation is not widely available.

Physical aspects of hysterectomy

What to expect in hospital. Normally, women are admitted to hospital the day before the operation and routine pre-operative procedures and investigations are performed including:

♦ Two glycerine suppositories or a small enema to ensure the bowel is empty before the operation.

♦ A pubic shave, performed by either the woman herself or her nurse.

♦ In some hospitals, women are measured for special support (anti-embolism) stockings which help prevent deep vein thrombosis.

New patients are usually introduced to each other and Wilson-Barnett (1975) found that patients derive considerable support from one another. Wise (1989) recommends the use of a few drops of lavender and geranium essential oils in a bath to reduce anxiety in the pre-operative patient.

The ward nurses will explain exactly what will happen and some gynaecology wards and clinics now sell an excellent booklet entitled *Hysterectomy and Vaginal Repair* by Sally Haslett and Molly Jennings (1992), which contains a useful section on pre- and post-operative exercises.

The woman may find during her stay in hospital that a ward round takes place which not only includes members of the medical team, but also several medical students. All women have the right to refuse to be part of the teaching round or to be examined vaginally by medical students. At some hospitals women may sign a consent form for medical students to perform vaginal examinations while they are in theatre under general anaesthesia. It is not always possible to ensure that a female doctor examines a woman but it is worth asking beforehand if this is what she would prefer. A nurse should always chaperone a male doctor.

After the operation. Surgery takes approximately 45 minutes and the woman should be warned that she will wake up in the recovery room rather than on the ward. She will often require oxygen for a while to help disperse the anaesthetic gases. She will usually have an intravenous infusion which will stay in for 24–48 hours and occasionally a blood transfusion in the case of severe blood loss during surgery. A urinary (Foley's) catheter might be present and a 'Redivac' drain will be protruding from a point near the incision site. This drain has a vacuum and removes excess blood from the wound to prevent a haematoma.

Women who have had a vaginal hysterectomy will have a 'vaginal pack' (a length of ribbon gauze soaked in proflavin antiseptic cream), which is inserted in the vagina rather like a large tampon instead of a Redivac drain. In some cases of vaginal hysterectomy a suprapubic catheter is used instead of a urethral catheter. This is inserted via the abdomen and is thought to reduce the risk of post-operative urinary tract infections.

Pain relief will be given by injection, e.g. pethidine, omnopon or morphine sulphate. Diclofenac sodium (Voltarol) suppositories are frequently used for their anti-inflammatory and excellent analgesic properties. In some hospitals, epidurals are available for hysterectomy patients or patient controlled analgesia (PCA) pumps which allow the patient to control their own pain relief.

Injections of prochlorperazine (Stemetil) or metoclopramide (Maxolon) may be given for nausea. Although not always successful, the aroma of peppermint oil can allay vomiting (Tisserand, 1988). A few drops may be placed on a tissue on the patient's pillow, or Wise (1989) recommends using one drop of peppermint oil in water to make a refreshing mouthwash. Wise (1989) also recommends placing bowls of hot water containing essential oils near the beds of patients who have just returned from theatre to promote deep breathing.

The next few days. The following day the woman will be encouraged to sit out of bed for a short while and a physiotherapist may visit to encourage leg exercises, pelvic rocking and deep breathing.

When bowel sounds are heard, the woman can start sipping water and gradually progress to light food. Her intravenous infusion will then be removed. A urinary catheter (if present) will be removed and fluid intake and urinary output measured. Sometimes women do contract urinary tract infections following hysterectomy and these will be treated with antibiotics. It is important that the woman empties her bladder fully and squeezes out the last few drops. Some women who are prone to urinary tract infections find drinking cranberry juice an effective prophylactic (see page 370).

The Redivac drain is removed when drainage is minimal and although not very painful, this will feel like a sharp tugging sensation which lasts for a few seconds.

By the second day following surgery the woman is usually able to walk to the bathroom without too much discomfort. Oral analgesics are now given as well as the Voltarol suppository. Women may worry about 'bursting their stitches' and need reassurance that this is not possible since there are several strong layers beneath the skin. The stitches are usually removed, without discomfort, on the fifth day for a horizontal wound, and on the seventh to tenth day for a vertical incision.

Many women experience griping 'wind' pain after the operation which can cause considerable discomfort. Hot peppermint water sipped slowly may help, and some doctors prescribe enteric-coated peppermint oil capsules (Colpermin) which are excellent. Walking around and sitting in a warm bath may also help. Constipation can be a problem and glycerine suppositories, lactulose syrup, Fybogel or Senokot are all remedies that can be offered.

It is very common for women to feel 'blue' on the third or fourth day following surgery and many women find themselves in tears for no apparent reason. They should be reassured that this is a normal reaction and will pass, although some women do experience similar feelings again on leaving hospital. Hormone replacement therapy will help many women, particularly those who are peri-menopausal and those who have had a bilateral salpingo-oophorectomy, but there may be many more subtle reasons for this feeling of depression.

Psychological aspects of hysterectomy

All major surgery has implications for an altered body image but the removal of a uterus can alter a woman's self-image and essentially her perceived femininity. The uterus is a symbol of reproduction and without it, and the associated menstruation, a woman may well feel she is not a sexual being.

To many women the suggestion of having a hysterectomy provokes fear and horror due to the misconceptions and old wives' tales surrounding this particular operation. In fact, the Ancient Greeks believed the uterus (hystero) to be the source of all emotions; hence the words 'hysteria' and 'hysterectomy'.

Studies have reported high levels of psychological problems both pre- and post-operatively. This higher than expected level of psychopathology is mirrored in gynaecology outpatient clinics (Worsley *et al.*, 1970) and therefore hysterectomy patients should be seen as a vulnerable group.

Women have often heard from relatives and friends prophesies of doom which make them wonder if a hysterectomy will cause them to grow hair on their face, gain weight, become unattractive to their sexual partners and, above all, lose all their own desires and feelings of pleasure. Some mistakenly believe that the vagina is sewn up at the vulva, and others think that a uterus is necessary for orgasm.

Naturally your role as a nurse is of utmost importance, to uncover anxieties and fears, to correct any myths and misconceptions and to give clear, accurate advice. Unfortunately, instead of the detailed information women require, they are often only given brief hints about 'not lifting' and important concerns such as when to resume sexual activity are neglected. Kreuger *et al.* (1979) reported that nurses volunteered little information to patients and were slow to initiate discussions which patients would have found helpful, particularly about sexual adjustment. Webb (1985) in her study of gynaecology nurses, found that although nurses did talk to their patients and were aware that hysterectomy patients feared 'losing their womanhood', they interpreted this as referring only to patients' sex lives and not to the wider aspects of sexuality, self-concept and self-esteem.

Some women do not realize they will no longer have periods following a hysterectomy, and in pre-menopausal women the cessation of menses and loss of fertility must be addressed and accurate information about hormone replacement therapy given (see Chapter 14). Those women who suffered from premenstrual syndrome and think that a hysterectomy will cure this problem may well find that cyclical symptoms persist following hysterectomy if the ovaries have been conserved, leading to the term 'ovarian cycle syndrome' (Backstrom *et al.*, 1981). The implications of oophorectomy can also be misunderstood and Williamson (1992) comments that some women believe that they will die at an earlier age if their ovaries are surgically removed.

Certain ethnic groups find hysterectomy particularly hard to accept and nurses should be aware of the impact this operation may have on different cultures and communities. West Indian women view menstruation as a cleansing act, ridding the body of impurities and are reluctant to have a hysterectomy. Some also fear they will be 'less of a woman' in the eyes of their men, who may be tempted to look for another 'whole woman'. For this reason they may not wish their partner or family to know exactly what operation they are having, and all staff should respect their right to confidentiality.

The cultural role of Muslim women is dependent on their fertility and, again, it may be difficult for both partners to come to terms with surgery. It can be of enormous value if you find time for discussion about impending surgery, not only with the patient but also with her partner and other members of the family.

The simple questions recommended by Shingleton and Orr (1987) (Box 17.3) provide an ideal framework for you to begin discussing any sexual concerns with your patients. Numerous authors have shown that proper information and counselling could alleviate many of the problems experienced by women following gynaecological surgery.

Box 17.3 Questions to open up discussion of sexual anxieties following hysterectomy

♦ What does your uterus mean to you?

♦ How will hysterectomy change your life?

♦ What is the most important function of your uterus?

♦ What are your thoughts about losing your uterus?

Williams (1986) revealed that women wanted specific advice to aid recovery and this was frequently lacking. Gould (1986) found that all the women in her study stated spontaneously that they were glad of the opportunity to talk to the researcher about their experiences and feelings, indicating an unmet need and a lack of support by hospital staff. In Gould's (1986) study, ward nurses

often expressed surprise that women's recovery from hysterectomy should be a topic worthy of investigation in view of its 'routine' nature and apparent lack of problems. Careful documentation of events after discharge from hospital suggested that many problems did, in fact, exist, and women would have worried less if they had been adequately prepared.

It is vital that all nurses, whether in hospital or primary care, realize how patients' home circumstances and need for information vary, and these must be assessed individually when care is planned. Some hospitals now organize pre-admission hysterectomy groups which can also meet following discharge. There is also a national network of Hysterectomy Support Groups (see Resources, page 448) and practice nurses could develop small support groups to meet the needs of their patients.

Discharge advice following hysterectomy and other major gynaecological surgery

Women normally stay in hospital for 5–10 days following major gynaecological surgery, and should be encouraged to go home when *they* feel ready to do so. Unfortunately, pressure on hospital beds means discharge is often too early. It is important that the whole family, particularly the woman's partner, understands what she can and cannot do whilst she is recovering at home. Women should be given discharge advice or a 'counselling' session with an opportunity to ask questions, and this should be backed up by written specific information, such as the 'Hysterectomy Hand-out' (*The Professional Nurse*, October 1989) with an assurance that she can ring the ward for advice at any time.

Bleeding. There may be a vaginal discharge for up to four weeks which will turn from red to a pale brown colour. If it becomes heavier, brighter in colour or offensive smelling, medical advice should be sought. Occasional red spotting may occur when stitches fall out. Sanitary towels rather than tampons should be used.

Resting. It is important that the woman should rest sufficiently during the first two weeks and go to bed when she feels tired. It is common to suddenly feel tired and exhausted, or occasionally have strange sensations in the abdomen (sometimes described as 'pinging elastic').

Exercise. Exercise is important and any exercises taught in hospital should be continued at home. It is advisable to go for short walks, increasing gradually to 45 minutes by six weeks after the operation. Swimming may be resumed after about four weeks if vaginal bleeding has stopped. Cycling and other light exercise may also be resumed at this stage.

Housework. No housework should be performed for the first two weeks but, after this, light chores can be safely done. It is very important to avoid lifting anything heavy for the first four weeks and very heavy items, such as shopping, wet laundry, full bin bags or toddlers, should not be lifted for at least three months. When anything is lifted it is important to remind the woman to bend her knees, keep her back straight and hold the object close to her. This avoids straining her abdomen.

Diet. Many women have heard that they will gain weight or develop a 'middle-age spread' after a hysterectomy. This is a myth and any weight gain is due to an increased calorie intake combined with a lack of exercise. It is advisable to eat a variety of foods, including fresh fruit and vegetables to avoid constipation. Some women find prune juice (available at some supermarkets and health food shops) effective. Other preventative measures, such as drinking at least eight glasses of water per day and taking high fibre foods are also recommended.

Work. Some women feel able to return to work 6–8 weeks following surgery, while others may feel the need to take another 6–8 weeks off. Obviously some jobs are more strenuous than others and women should judge for themselves when they feel ready. Some employees may allow women to return on a part-time basis initially which is an ideal way to readjust to the demands of a job. Rarely some women may take up to a year to feel completely fit.

Sexual intercourse. Generally speaking it takes about six weeks to feel both physically and emotionally ready to resume love-making after major gynaecological surgery, and most gynaecologists

recommend this time interval before attempting intercourse. In any event hysterectomy patients should certainly be advised to wait until any vaginal bleeding has stopped to prevent the risk of infection. The woman's partner should understand the importance of being gentle initially, to avoid undue trauma to the area. Tissue strength is adequate by this time, and the risk of infection is virtually non-existent in the presence of complete healing.

Even before the six weeks, however, you could advise the couple that other forms of sexual expression may be explored. Two weeks or so after surgery clitoral stimulation to orgasm without intercourse can be resumed, as can various methods for satisfying the partner, short of intercourse. Many women find that experiencing orgasm for the first time after surgery is best done alone through masturbation (Barback, 1975; Williamson, 1992). This allows them to take their time, tune in to any new sensations and experience an orgasm without the pressures of their partner. Barback (1975) recommends self-stimulation as a very reassuring strategy that can be recommended to women who do not object to the idea of masturbation, because it confirms their potential to reach orgasm.

It should be remembered that the latter two authors are American and their suggestions may be more liberal than what might be considered normal advice to perhaps more reserved British patients on a gynaecology ward!

The hormonal effects of oophorectomy, i.e. reduced oestrogen and testosterone, may cause loss of libido, vaginal atrophy and reduction of vaginal lubrication. This may be overcome by hormone replacement therapy or locally applied oestrogen cream. Vaginal dryness may also be helped by using an over-the-counter lubricant which will reduce chafing and discomfort, and increase sensitivity.

Sexual anxieties following hysterectomy. Blundell (1829), who performed the first hysterectomy in Britain in 1828, commented: 'the continuance of sexual desires . . . is very remarkable'. Many women fear that they will become 'frigid' following a hysterectomy and they can be assured that this is not correct. Some women feel more relaxed about love-making when there is no risk of pregnancy and those undergoing hysterectomy for fibroids or endometriosis may find sexual intercourse less painful and more enjoyable than before.

However, Shingleton and Orr (1987) stress that if surgery is perceived as 'mutilating' it is likely to become damaging rather than restorative. The woman who expects hysterectomy to decrease her sexual excitability and enjoyment often exhibits a self-fulfilling prophecy when she experiences decreased libido post-operatively. Women who depend on their gynaecological illness to secure relief from sexual commitments to their partners may develop anxiety if they believe the removal of the source of their symptoms will lead to the expectation that they will become more responsive sexually (Shingleton and Orr, 1987). Thus, surgery may constitute a threat to the relationship in opposing ways.

In general, however, the single most significant factor in post-operative sexual behaviour is pre-treatment sexual adjustment. The woman who has had a satisfying sexual relationship prior to surgery is likely to resume such a relationship post-operatively, while those with sexual problems pre-operatively, will find them likely to continue, not cease, following surgery.

Although post-operative tenderness may persist for as long as 12 weeks post-operatively, the couple need to resume their sexual relationship in some form as soon as possible. You could talk to them about different positions for intercourse in order to avoid abdominal or vaginal discomfort. Hysterectomy usually includes removal of the cervix which can slightly decrease the length of the vagina, but not to the extent of limiting intercourse. A change in position may be more comfortable initially such as female astride or 'legs together'.

Some women do report decreased sexual response after hysterectomy. This may be because the scar tissue at the surgical site within the vagina is not as tactile and will not engorge and stretch as well as other genital tissues during the excitement and plateau phases of sexual arousal. Sensory nerve pathways to the vagina and perineum may also have been interrupted. While the inner vagina does not contain tactile nerve endings, it has pressure-sensitive nerves that can prompt sexual engorgement. Pre-operatively, deep penile thrusting may have been very enjoyable because of the pressure it placed on the inner vagina and cervix.

Penile thrusting can also produce pleasurable feelings through the movement of internal abdominal organs caused by the motion of the cervix and uterus during intercourse. If this has been part of a woman's enjoyment and arousal pattern, she should be encouraged to focus on other sensations that will assist in building her sexual response (Williamson, 1992).

The character of orgasm for women who have had a hysterectomy may change. This is due to the lack of any uterine contractions, but does not usually affect overall satisfaction.

Finally, it should always be remembered that not all hysterectomy patients are in a heterosexual relationship. Lesbian women will also need reassurance that love-making will continue to be pleasurable. These women and their partners will need your support and care like any other couple.

Myomectomy

A myomectomy is a major operation to remove fibroids from the uterus. A fibroid (also known as a myoma or leiomyoma) begins as a single cell in the endometrium of the uterus, which multiplies to become a mass of muscle and fibrous connective tissue. Most fibroids are no larger than a pea but they can grow to the size of a grapefruit. Fibroids seem to occur more frequently in West Indian and West African women, although the reason for this is not clear. Fibroids have been discussed in more detail in Chapter 16.

It is not entirely clear why fibroids develop although it has been thought that they are hereditary. Their growth is dependent on oestrogen since they tend to grow faster during pregnancy and shrink after the menopause. Before a myomectomy, a woman is often prescribed Zoladex (goserelin) to suppress the release of oestrogen and cause the fibroids to shrink.

It is important that women are reassured that fibroids are benign tumours of connective tissue. In very rare cases a fibroid may turn into a fast-growing malignant tumour (leiomyosarcoma) and a hysterectomy will be performed.

Reasons for myomectomy

Small fibroids are asymptomatic and treatment is not required. However, where diagnosis of the pelvic mass is in doubt, where the mass is larger than the size of a 16-week pregnancy, or where there are unpleasant symptoms, surgery is advised.

Menorrhagia is a common problem caused by the larger area of endometrium that is shed at menstruation. Large fibroids may press on the bowel causing constipation, or on the bladder causing urinary frequency or retention.

How it is performed

A myomectomy involves the 'shelling out' of the fibroids and is preferable for women who still want children. If no further pregnancies are desired then a hysterectomy may be the operation of choice.

Lewis and Chamberlain (1991) consider the risks of a straightforward myomectomy or a hysterectomy are about equal but, if a large number of fibroids are present, myomectomy can be more difficult with a risk of considerable haemorrhage at surgery. Women should always be aware of the risk that if bleeding cannot be controlled a hysterectomy will be performed.

A vertical incision is usually necessary. Women will often return to the ward with a blood transfusion and therefore this operation is not always suitable for women who do not accept the transfusion of blood, e.g. Jehovah's witnesses.

After the operation

The woman will often stay in hospital for 7–10 days following the operation, depending on the healing of the wound. There is a risk of the formation of a haematoma and adhesions may develop between the intestines and the suture lines on the uterus. The suture line may weaken the wall of the uterus, requiring a Caesarean section at subsequent births.

There is a very real risk that new fibroids will grow after surgery and women cannot be assured that a pregnancy will occur. Although most women with fibroids have normal pregnancies, the risk of miscarrying and premature labour is higher. Since the development of new techniques in microsurgery, it has been possible to remove subserous and intramural fibroids via a laparoscope. Since this is minimally invasive surgery, women are able to return to an active life 7–10 days following surgery, and have no scar.

Discharge advice

This is similar to the advice given for women who have undergone hysterectomy. Some gynaecologists recommend that a woman tries to become pregnant during the first three to six months following surgery, before fibroids have had a chance to recur. There should be no problems sexually once the scar has healed and any bleeding has stopped. However, it is worth mentioning that a woman with multiple fibroids may have had a 'full feeling' during intercourse and she and her partner may now experience an 'empty sensation' once the fibroids are removed.

Continence surgery

The aims of continence surgery are discussed in Chapter 15 (page 379). There are several different operations that aim to improve incontinence and these may be done vaginally or by the abdominal approach (Box 17.4).

Box 17.4 Types of operations to relieve incontinence

Vaginal approach

◆ Anterior colporrhaphy

◆ Posterior colporrhaphy

◆ Manchester or Fothergill repair.

Suprapubic or abdominal approach

◆ Marchall–Marchetti–Krantz

◆ Burch colposuspension.

Vaginal approach

The most common vaginal repair operations include anterior colporrhaphy (anterior repair), posterior colporrhaphy (posterior repair) and the Manchester repair which is not so frequently performed these days.

Anterior colporrhaphy

An anterior repair is carried out to cure a cystocele or cystourethrocele with or without stress incontinence. However, recent evidence suggests that a suprapubic operation may be a more effective cure for genuine stress incontinence rather than a vaginal repair. Gould's (1986) study suggested that women who had undergone a repair operation in conjunction with vaginal hysterectomy were less satisfied with the result than those undergoing abdominal surgery, but this sample was small.

The anterior vaginal wall is incised and a triangular portion of vaginal skin from below the external urethral opening to the front of the cervix is excised. One or two sutures are placed deep around the bladder neck. The edges of the wound are sutured together to provide extra support for the bladder and urethra.

Posterior colporrhaphy

This procedure is used to repair a rectocele or a rectocele and enterocele.

A triangular portion of posterior vaginal wall, with its apex at the mid-vaginal level and its base at the introitus, is removed by an inverted T incision to expose the levator ani muscles. These muscles are brought together with one to two interrupted sutures, closed in a Y-shape to avoid narrowing the entrance to the vagina. The operation also involves the excision of any enterocele and repair of the perineal body (perinorrhaphy)

Manchester or Fothergill repair

This operation is not as common these days as a combined vaginal hysterectomy and pelvic floor repair which is now considered the operation of choice for a uterovaginal prolapse where there is descent of the cervix and vault as well as cystocele and rectocele. This operation involves amputation of the cervix and shortening of the cardinal ligaments, in addition to an anterior repair.

Physical aspects of vaginal repair surgery

The pre-operative care is very similar to that of women undergoing vaginal hysterectomy. Again, all women will require a full explanation of the proposed surgery, and discharge planning should commence at the time of admission, since these patients are often elderly.

Repair operations take about 45 minutes. On return to the ward a woman can expect:

- ♦ An intravenous infusion
- ♦ A vaginal pack
- ♦ A urethral catheter (occasionally suprapubic).

Drinking is often resumed later in the day provided any nausea has passed.

Following vaginal repair surgery:

- ♦ The vaginal pack will be removed the following day.
- ♦ The urinary catheter will be removed in the first couple of days.
- ♦ Pain can be a particular problem for those women who have had a posterior repair. Regular opiate injections will be given initially and Voltarol suppositories are very effective in reducing inflammation and pain.
- ♦ Ice packs can be useful, or advising the woman to change her position in bed, e.g. lie on her tummy, and the physiotherapist may have helpful advice.
- ♦ Women need reassurance as the pain and discomfort initially appears to be worsening due to the bruising 'coming out' and the fact that she is probably moving around more than on the day after the operation.

Discharge advice

This is similar to the advice given for women who have undergone hysterectomy. However, more care needs to be taken to avoid constipation or straining at stool. Wright (1974) stresses that hospital, with its strange environment and unfamiliar routines, is not the best place to learn new bowel habits. For this reason, health education and discharge advice is crucial. Some women may like to hold a sanitary towel supporting the perineum when they first have their bowels open.

Women undergoing repair procedures need to be told about their internal sutures since no external wound is visible and they may not understand why precautions about lifting etc. are necessary.

Suprapubic or abdominal approach

Again there is a wide variety of abdominal operations that can be performed to improve urinary incontinence.

*Marshall–Marchetti–Krantz
(vesico-urethropexy)*

This operation is performed through a suprapubic incision. The urogynaecologist inserts a urethral catheter to help identify the bladder neck and cuts into the retropubic space. The tissues at the side of the urethra are sutured to the periosteum behind the symphysis pubis so the bladder neck is re-elevated above the urethrovesicular junction.

Burch colposuspension

This is a similar but preferable operation to the above procedure. The sutures inserted on either side of the bladder neck and urethra are passed through the paravaginal fascia which becomes elevated and is sutured to the ileopectinal ligaments. As well as raising the urethra and bladder neck to restore the urethrovesicular junction, this procedure elevates the vaginal vault, so any co-existing anterior vaginal wall prolapse is simultaneously repaired.

The results of both these suprapubic operations are better than those for traditional anterior colporrhaphy with bladder neck buttress.

The first operation for stress incontinence is the one most likely to succeed so it is important that the best operation is performed first. Most suprapubic operations in current use produce a subjective cure rate in excess of 85% in patients undergoing their first operation for correctly diagnosed stress incontinence (Cardozo, 1993, unpublished). Subsequent surgery may have to be performed on a vagina which is less mobile and where there is fibrosis of the urethra. In such cases a Sling operation or an endoscopic bladder neck suspension, such as the Stamey or Raz procedure may be easier to perform and more effective.

Physical aspects of abdominal continence surgery

The pre-and post-operative care is very similar to that of any major gynaecological operation.

The operation takes approximately 45 minutes. On return to the ward a woman can expect:

◆ An intravenous infusion

◆ A Redivac drain

◆ A suprapubic catheter will be used, rather than a urethral (Foley) catheter, to avoid the risk of urinary tract infection. A suprapubic catheter is a fine plastic tube which is inserted through the abdomen just above the wound and has a plastic disc with four sutures attached to the abdominal skin to prevent it from falling out.

Depending on the urogynaecologist's preference, the suprapubic catheter will be left to drain freely for 3–5 days. After this time a 'suprapubic clamping regime' will commence to test whether normal bladder function has returned. On the first day the catheter is usually clamped for a period of around six hours to observe whether the woman can pass urine urethrally. After this time the clamp is released and the residual that drains into the bag is measured. Initially the residual may be larger than the amount of urine passed urethrally, but after a few days the residual usually decreases and when it is less than approximately 150 ml the catheter may be removed. This is a painless procedure and the small hole in the abdomen heals quickly without the leakage of urine that women might expect.

The regime used in different hospitals does vary and initially can appear complicated. Time and patience is required whilst explaining to the woman about clamping and measuring residuals. Women are usually taught how to clamp their own catheter, empty the drainage bag using their own individual jugs, and recording their own fluid balance measurements.

Women often need considerable encouragement, especially when they compare themselves with other patients who may be progressing with the regime more rapidly. Occasionally women are unable to pass urine urethrally due to excessive trauma during surgery, and these women may go home with their suprapubic catheter *in situ*. They can either give their bladder a rest at home, or they may continue with the suprapubic clamping regime where the familiar home environment often produces better results. They are taught to strap their catheter correctly, how to use a leg bag during the day and how to change to an overnight bag when necessary. Some district nurses will supervise a clamping regime.

In rare instances of women being unable to pass urine urethrally after at least a month following surgery, intermittent self-catheterization will be taught (see page 383).

Sexual anxieties following continence surgery

It is important that the sexuality of women over 60 is not ignored but addressed in the same manner as a young woman's. Older women may be even less likely to initiate discussions about sexual concerns and you should act as a sensitive facilitator and advocate for her. You should ascertain whether she is still sexually active and the doctors should be aware of this when they are suturing near the introitus, to prevent future dyspareunia.

Sexuality in the elderly is difficult to discuss and Griffiths (1988) states that there are two main reasons for this. First, nurses have historically not been trained to cope with sexuality. Their own sexuality is 'suppressed and repressed' with the aim of 'purity' and 'asexuality', and they suffer from sexism and stereotyping at work. Secondly, the elderly themselves are reluctant to verbalize their sexual feelings, for fear of being seen as depraved or lecherous. It is vital that each woman is treated as an individual and such assumptions are not made.

It is probably wise for women to wait six weeks before attempting full sexual intercourse to prevent bruising to the urethra. Extra lubrication can be used. If a suprapubic catheter is in place, it need not interfere with love-making, especially if a leg bag is used, or the tube is clamped and spigotted. A high standard of hygiene should be maintained to prevent infection and both partners should wash around the genital area before and after intercourse.

Gynaecological cancers

Invasive gynaecological cancer is the second most common malignancy in women after breast cancer. It accounts for approximately 15 000 cases per year, just over 20% of all cancers in women (Lambert and Blake, 1992). A diagnosis of gynaecological cancer threatens not only a woman's life but also her self-esteem, body image and sexuality, and therefore has wide-ranging implications for the patient, her partner and family.

Cairns (1983) found that women with gynaecological cancers were just as depressed as women with breast cancer at the time of surgery

but, for women with gynaecological cancers, depression increased significantly one month after surgery, and lingered for up to 20 months postoperatively. The researchers explained this as a reflection of the loss of function rather than of the fear and pain of cancer.

Vulvectomy

Carcinoma of the vulva accounts for 5% of all cases of genital cancer in women. It is most often seen in elderly women, aged over 60 years. The most common malignancy of the vulva is squamous cell carcinoma which accounts for 95% of all vulval cancers. There are two kinds of vulvectomy – simple and radical.

Simple vulvectomy

A simple vulvectomy is carried out for chronic vulval dystrophy, intractable pruritus vulvae (vulval itchiness) and vulval intra-epithelial neoplasia (VIN) (a pre-cancerous condition with similar histological features to CIN – see Chapter 11). The term leukoplakia meaning 'white patches' has been used in the past to refer to a pre-cancerous condition but is outdated since it has no clinical or pathological precision (Lewis and Chamberlain, 1991).

The incisions made are shown in Figure 17.5. The skin and subcutaneous tissues of the vulva are removed using a lateral elliptical incision starting at the mons pubis. The incision runs down the

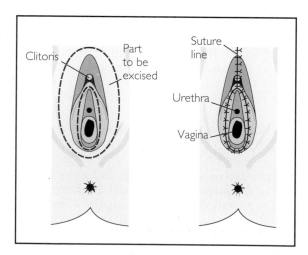

Figure 17.5 *Simple vulvectomy.*

lateral fold of the labia majora and meets the incision at the other side of the vulva at the posterior fourchette. The medial incision starts above the urethra and extends around the vaginal orifice. The muscles (levator ani) between the vagina and the anus are sutured together and the skin closed anteriorly at the mons pubis and posteriorly at the anus.

Radical vulvectomy

A radical vulvectomy is performed for invasive cancer of the vulva. It consists of extensive excision of the vulval tissue and bilateral lymph node groin dissection, including the superficial and deep inguinal nodes, Cloquet's gland in the femoral canal and nodes related to the external iliac vessels (Figure 17.6). Unfortunately, it is often necessary to remove the clitoris. A limited amount of skin is usually removed with the cancer and, since the vulval skin is stretchy, the remaining edges may be sutured together. However, if it is necessary to remove a large area of skin, a skin graft will be required from the thigh or abdomen. In cases of Stage I and II disease the inguinal nodes can be removed through separate groin incisions, but often a modified 'butterfly' incision is used. This technique reduces the area of skin removed which in the past led to frequent wound breakdown due to increased tension on the suture lines.

Physical aspects of vulvectomy

It is obviously vital that women have a full explanation of the operation and its implications. Patients may find it difficult to come to terms with the mutilating effects surgery will have and you will need to spend considerable time pre-operatively in discussion with women and, if necessary, their partners. There is an excellent BACUP booklet, *Cancer of the Vulva*, which you may find useful and recommend to your patients.

It is probably preferable that women undergoing vulvectomy are nursed in a side-room initially, due to the privacy and intensive nursing care required. However, if a woman would prefer to be with other patients, this should be arranged.

The pre-operative preparation for surgery is the same as that for any major gynaecological operation. In addition, a full shave will be given unless there are open or painful lesions, and anti-embolism stockings will be supplied since mobility will be impaired by pain and bulky bandages, and these patients tend to be elderly. Pre-operative deep breathing and leg exercises should also be taught.

The operation will take 2–4 hours. Regular injections of opiate analgesia will be given or an epidural may be in progress. A blood transfusion may be required due to excessive blood loss and intravenous fluid replacement is always necessary, since fluid loss is considerable during this complicated operation. After the initial drowsiness and nausea, drinking and eating may gradually be resumed. A low-fibre diet is necessary to avoid bulky stools and straining.

A urethral (Foley) catheter will be in place to ensure infection of the wound does not occur from spilling of urine, or urinary retention occur due to peri-urethral tissue being bruised during the operation. The catheter will remain *in situ* for 1–3 weeks while healing occurs. Although one-third to a half of the urethra may have been removed, spontaneous voiding is possible.

Some women find that urine no longer flows out in a steady stream, so they need to be taught how to squat and sit back slightly to avoid wetting their legs or the floor.

Two Redivac drains are inserted into the groins to prevent haematoma formation and will remain *in situ* for 7–10 days. There will be a non-adhesive dressing over the stitched areas, often held together by a T bandage between the legs. In some hospitals, the knees are gently tied together to prevent the legs being opened too wide and causing a pull on the sutures. Depending on the gynaecologist the bandages may be kept on for up to 4 or 5 days to

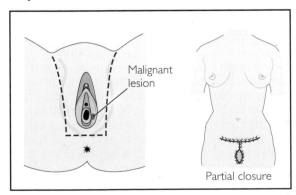

Figure 17.6 *Radical vulvectomy.*

allow undisturbed healing to occur. If the dressings do become very soiled they will be changed and the area will be irrigated with normal saline or a gentle antiseptic solution. It will then be dried thoroughly using a hair dryer. In some hospitals women return to theatre for a light anaesthetic before removal of sutures, or inhalational analgesia, such as Entonox is used.

Psychological effects of vulvectomy

All patients facing vulvectomy require psychologically sensitive nursing care. A full sexual history and assessment should be made, and at all times the woman's partner should be included, if possible. They both should be encouraged to discuss any sexual concerns pre-operatively and should be given clear explanations about the surgery and its implications.

Obviously, women may find it difficult to look at their new altered appearance and it is advisable they try to do so before going home. If possible, the woman should look with the help of a mirror, in her own time, but with her nurse present if she prefers. Many women in this age group are not used to looking 'down below' so you should act sensitively. This sensitive approach can really only occur if the nurse has already built up a relationship with the woman and her partner and discussed sexual concerns. It may be better to wait until the clips or stitches are removed since they can make the scarring look worse. Many women find it hard to visualize what the scar will look like. Due to the fatty, stretchy nature of vulval skin, the remaining skin can be stretched to leave a very neat scar. They need to be warned that because the labia have been removed, the opening of the vagina will be more visible. If the clitoris has been removed the area will now be flat skin, without the usual folds of the vulva. The groin may feel tight at first if lymph nodes have been removed and some women describe this feeling of tightness between their legs 'as though a sanitary towel is being pulled upwards'.

Women usually stay in hospital for 2–4 weeks and discharge planning from the time of admission is essential. Unfortunately, there is no special support group for vulvectomy patients, like the Hysterectomy Support Group or Mastectomy Association, but BACUP (see Resources, page 448) is a very helpful organization, and health care professionals can network between old and new patients.

Partner problems

At the same time as a woman is grieving for losses after learning she has cancer, her husband or partner also grieves. He, too, is threatened by her loss. Usually, men have difficulty in revealing and talking about their pain, and even more difficulty asking for help and, consequently they often face their fears alone.

Myths exist in society about cancer being transmittable, particularly by sexual activity when a genital site is involved (Lamont *et al.*, 1978), and this may lead to friends, colleagues or partners withdrawing from the woman. However, it is agreed that the quality of sexual relationships after a diagnosis of cancer has been made is more strongly related to the previous quality of the relationship than to any other factors. Partners may not want to have sex with cancer patients for fear of hurting them physically but, unfortunately, this can give patients feelings of self-disgust or undesirability (Derogatis and Kourlesis, 1981). Lamont *et al.* (1978) stress that the most important factor in total sexual rehabilitation for cancer patients is an educated and informed partner.

It has been shown that couples where one partner has cancer have a significantly increased need for affection and the need to show protectiveness towards their partners; an increased desire for physical closeness, including simply being together; holding hands, embracing and kissing, and an increased need for intercourse. Vachion (1977) explains that 'the attempt to continue intimacy is life-affirming'. Some couples, however, withdraw into their individual pain. Withdrawal is a frequent consequence of the many fears, depression and tensions caused by cancer and its treatment.

Johnson (1987) explains how, in her anguish, a woman can convince herself that it is not possible for her husband to still love her and still desire her. She can make it impossible for him to help her by sending conflicting signals. If he does want sex he is a 'selfish brute'. If he does not, he no longer desires her, he is 'heartless'. If he does grieve he is being weak and childish. If not, he is self-centred and uncaring. A man in this position cannot win.

Johnson (1987) reports several studies of sex after cancer and depending on the type of cancer, a woman's prognosis and what sex was like before cancer was diagnosed, from 30% to virtually all couples have sexual problems. Cairns (1983) found that about half the men suffer from secondary impotence after their partners have gynaecological cancer. Lamont (1978) found that sex stops temporarily or permanently for one in three couples after the woman has cervical cancer, and for four out of five couples coping with cancer of the ovaries or vulva. It is therefore very important that nurses involve partners at all times and be aware of their sexual concerns.

Sexual issues following vulvectomy

Rushton (1978) explains how cancer of the genital organs may be felt to be particularly shameful because it arises in an area of the body that we are conditioned from childhood into neither discussing nor revealing to any but those with whom we are most intimate. The psychosexual implications of vulvectomy are of utmost importance since genitals are intimately associated with a woman's sexuality, body image, gender identity and general quality of life.

Excision of the clitoris is likely to greatly reduce sensation and sexual arousability and orgasm is rare (Wabrek and Gunn, 1984). The scarred tissue at the remaining vaginal opening can be insensitive to penetration, or hypersensitive to friction. Removal of the pelvic lymph nodes can result in oedema of the legs which can cause embarrassment, and excision of fatty tissue can cause pain on sitting.

A woman who has undergone a vulvectomy should be advised that she may resume intercourse when she feels ready, probably 4–12 weeks following surgery. Couples should be advised to compensate for loss of perineal sensation by exploring other erotic areas – breasts, buttocks, thighs (Lamb, 1985). Massage, mutual masturbation and oral sex may be advised if penetration is not possible. Wallace (1987) recommends encouraging patients to use fantasy material, such as explicit accounts of female sexual experiences in books, such as *My Secret Garden* by Nancy Friday.

Limited hip abduction is advisable for the first 4–6 weeks to avoid putting undue stress on the groin and perineal sutures. Some women find it difficult to abduct their thighs and couples need to find the most comfortable position for love-making. A pillow under the woman's thighs may be helpful. The missionary position may be especially painful for the woman due to the deeper penetration. Other positions, such as the 'female superior' may allow the woman to control the depth of thrusting. It has to be remembered that couples may need explicit advice and information rather than vague generalizations about intercourse, since people's sexual experiences vary immensely.

Although such detailed discussion may or may not be accomplished by all nurses, depending on their personal expertise and degree of comfort, it is important not to neglect the issue of the patient's altered sexuality, since this will only reinforce the fallacy that her sexual role is over.

Total pelvic exenteration (TPE)

This extensive operation is used as a curative procedure in the treatment of certain types of pelvic malignancy, the most notable being recurrent cancer of the cervix. The surgery involves removal of the rectum and distal sigmoid colon, the urinary bladder, all reproductive organs and the entire pelvic floor, and necessitates the formation of both a urostomy and a sigmoid colostomy. These women, as with vulvectomy patients, require considerable nursing and a sensitive approach to their care in order to facilitate their recovery and rehabilitation.

Radiotherapy for gynaecological cancer

Radiotherapy is a well-established and effective method of treating malignant disease, either used alone, or with other interventions, such as chemotherapy and surgery. In cases of gynaecological malignancy it is used both as a curative treatment, particularly for cervical cancer, and palliatively for symptom relief.

Radiotherapy is the use of ionizing radiation to destroy cancer cells by inhibiting their ability to divide and proliferate. As radiation passes through a tissue, some of its energy is transferred to the cells of that tissue, causing ionization. This results in chemical changes which lead to cellular damage or death. The target of the radiation and, indeed, damage is DNA and therefore the greatest effects are seen during mitosis when the amount of DNA is doubled.

It is usually necessary to divide the calculated tumour lethal dose into smaller doses (fractionation) to prevent acute radiation exposure. The fractionated dose is normally delivered over a period ranging from two to eight weeks. This allows both normal and cancer cells to attempt repair between consecutive treatments.

External beam radiotherapy (teletherapy)

An external source is specifically focused on to the tumour which is about 100 cm from the source of ionizing radiation. Gamma rays or electrons are used – depending on which is felt to be the most appropriate.

Brachytherapy (pleoiotherapy)

The radioactive source is positioned either directly inside the tumour or inside an applicator which is as close to it as possible. The aim of radiotherapy in the case of cervical cancer is to deliver a lethal dose of radiation to the cervix, lower parts of the uterus, the upper vagina, the parametria and the proximal parts of the uterosacral ligaments.

The principle of radiotherapy for cervical cancer is that the local tumour and its immediate paracervical spread is attacked with intrauterine and intravaginal sources of radiation while the pelvic lymphatics and nodes are treated by mainly external radiation.

Afterloading

This is a type of intracavity therapy using a remote control radioactive microsource, such as 'microselectron'. Hollow applicators are inserted and positioned correctly in the uterus and ovoids are placed in the fornices under general anaesthesia. All the sources have tubes attached through which the radioactive material can be inserted. A remote afterloading system will deliver radioactive caesium pellets into the applicators in the patient by a pneumatic system using compressed air after the staff have left the radiation protected treatment area. If it is necessary to enter the room for nursing

care the sources are automatically withdrawn from the patient and stored in the machine. A scintillation counter measures the amount of radiation being received by the rectum and checks it is acceptable. If the bladder and rectum receive excessive irradiation, severe cystitis or proctitis will develop, possibly leading to necrosis and fistula formation.

Advice to women

Radiotherapy to this intimate area of the body can be a very anxiety-provoking experience for women, in addition to their already existing fears about the cancer. They need information about the procedures and side-effects they might experience and this advice should be backed-up by written information, such as Whale's patient handout 'Coping with Pelvic Irradiation' in *The Professional Nurse* (March 1991). Women who are commuting long distances to hospital to undergo treatment have additional problems and the local practice nurse is in an ideal position to provide close support to these women.

Effects on the bladder

Frequency and urgency of micturition may develop in addition to cystitis or urinary tract infection. Two litres of fluid should be taken every day. It has been noted that these symptoms only appear to develop in those patients who already have problems with their bladder.

Effects on the bowel

The bowel often becomes sensitive to the radiation and during the third or fourth week diarrhoea or loose stools may occur. Fresh fruit and vegetables, bran, wholemeal bread or highly spiced food should be avoided.

Effect on the skin

The skin may become more sensitive during radiotherapy. Warm (rather than hot) baths or showers are recommended and it is advisable not to soak for too long. Bubble baths, perfumed oils and talcum powder should not be used. However, Oilatum ointment in the bath and Johnson's Baby

Powder may be used. Any marks on the skin, usually gentian violet, to illustrate where the treatment area is, should not be washed off.

Sexual anxieties

Radiotherapy can result in temporary or permanent sexual dysfunction. It is important that women understand they are not a danger to their partner and that no radiation remains inside the body, and their cancer cannot be passed on during sexual intercourse.

Loss of pubic hair may occur but this will probably grow again. Cessation of ovarian function is common and will mean that a woman has a premature menopause. Radiotherapy may cause the fragile tissues in the genital area to become more fibrotic and lose their elasticity. This fibrosis will not disappear and scar tissue at the surgical site within the vagina will not engorge and stretch as well during intercourse as other genital tissue.

Vaginal fibrosis can also cause vaginal shortening and narrowing. Vaginal dilators, lubricants and new intercourse positions may relieve dyspareunia and preserve vaginal function. Sexual activity should be maintained during this time. This not only helps the couple to maintain a sense of sexual normality but also preserves the patency of the vagina which could be threatened by adhesion. Intercourse ideally should occur at least once per week. Fear of pain from friction, fibrosis, or even the sensation that semen can cause should not be reasons for abstaining. You should discuss these anxieties with your patients and if problems exist they can be ameliorated by using lubricants, vaginal dilators and condoms.

Even women who have no sexual partners can take steps to maintain vaginal function through masturbation, which increases blood circulation to the pelvis and vagina, or through use of a dildo or vaginal dilator. Without these precautions adhesions, fibrosis or loss of elasticity can result and corrective surgery may become necessary.

Use of vaginal dilators

The use of vaginal dilators should start two weeks after treatment has been completed and they should be used for ten minutes twice daily for four weeks, and then two or three times a week for two years. Their use will prevent stenosis and allow regular follow-up vaginal examinations to take place. Dilatation may be discontinued if regular intercourse is resumed.

Chemotherapy for gynaecological cancer

The correct definition of chemotherapy is the specific treatment of disease by the administration of chemical compounds, including sulphonamides and antibiotics. It is often misused to imply treatment only by the use of cytotoxic agents.

The treatment of cancer is by cytotoxic chemotherapy. The word cytotoxic literally means 'cell poisoning' and this is precisely what these drugs do. Cytotoxic drugs work by disrupting the process of cell division through a direct effect on DNA.

There are numerous side-effects from chemotherapy because cytotoxic chemotherapy cannot distinguish between cancerous cells and normal cells which are also dividing rapidly. Cytotoxic agents therefore produce unavoidable damage to normal proliferating tissues, such as bone marrow, lymphoid tissue and the epithelial lining of the intestinal tract. Side-effects of chemotherapy are discussed more fully in Chapter 10 (page 244).

Unlike radiotherapy, which is used to attack local and regional disease when the target has been identified, cytotoxic chemotherapy is chosen to attack systemic disease and is useful for metastatic disease, or after surgery when microscopic disease may be present. It has a major role in the palliative care of advanced and recurrent gynaecological malignancies, especially of the cervix and ovaries.

The drug may occasionally be given in tablet form, but is usually administered intravenously. A balance has to be achieved between killing malignant cells and allowing regeneration and recovery of normal healthy cells. For this reason, chemotherapy is often given on an outpatient basis every 3–4 weeks, or as an inpatient on a programme of 1–5 days' treatment every 3–4 weeks.

A single chemotherapeutic dose will not always achieve cure or a long-term remission, and there is a high risk of tumour resistance. Combination cytotoxic chemotherapy permits administration of smaller doses with fewer side-effects and achieves a larger cell kill than a large dose of a single agent.

Common cytotoxic drugs used in treating gynaecological cancer include platinum agents (cisplatin and carboplatin) and alkylating agents (cyclophosphamide and ifosfamide). Antimetabolites, such as methotrexate and 5-fluoracincil, are also used.

Advice to women before and after chemotherapy

The effects of chemotherapy on sexuality have been less well-documented than radiotherapy. However, loss of libido is commonly experienced due to the drugs themselves and to their side-effects, such as nausea and vomiting. The repeated hospital visits and admissions necessary for treatment are disruptive and limit the time and opportunity for sexual relationships.

Alopecia is a devastating blow to a woman's self-image. Loss of body hair from any site can have a profound effect on self-esteem, making people feel like babies. Unfortunately some women are not warned to expect alopecia and therefore have not had the opportunity to buy a wig, scarves or a hat. BACUP produce a helpful booklet on coping with hair loss.

Walbroehl (1985) states that younger women may be more severely disturbed by altered body image because they have not had as much time as older women to become sure of their self-image. They are also less likely to have a permanent partner to offer them support.

Women of reproductive age undergoing chemotherapy following unilateral oophorectomy, or with gestational trophoblastic disease will require advice about contraception and future childbearing. During chemotherapy ovulation may be suppressed and the patient may have amenorrhoea and menopausal symptoms. Return of fertility will be influenced by the drugs, the dose and the duration of treatment. Contraceptive precautions must be continued and a discussion of available methods may be required. A non-hormonal method of contraception is advisable and an intrauterine contraceptive device is contra-indicated during chemotherapy because of the increased risk of bleeding and infection due to bone marrow depression. It is also necessary to reinforce the importance of leaving a sufficient interval after completing treatment before planning a pregnancy (usually about two years) to permit assessment of disease-free status and absence of the risk of teratogenesis (drug-induced congenital abnormality).

Conclusion

This chapter has identified and described many of the commonly performed gynaecological operations. Most of the procedures are nowadays considered routine and are frequently performed. For the woman undergoing such surgery however no procedure should be considered 'routine' as each individual woman has her own fears and anxieties that are unique to her. Gynaecological surgery, by its very nature, can have an enormous impact on female sexuality and these issues should not be ignored but raised and discussed by all health care professionals when talking to women.

Looking into the future it is hoped that not only will there be further advances in minimally invasive gynaecological surgery, but also that the sexual anxieties of gynaecology patients will be considered and discussed by all staff whether in wards, clinics or in general practice.

Resources

BACUP
3 Bath Place, Rivington Street, London EC2A 3JR
Tel. 0800 181199 (Freephone); 0141 553 1553 (Glasgow)
Counselling service in London and Glasgow. Information service on all aspects of cancer. Booklets available on different types of cancer and practical and emotional issues.

Continence Foundation
2 Doughty Street, London WC1N 2PH

Hysterectomy Support Group
For nearest contact address send SAE to: The Venture, Green Lane, Upton, Huntingdon, Cambs PE17 5YE

Miscarriage Association
c/o Clayton Hospital, Northgate, Wakefield, West Yorks WF1 3JS
Tel. 01924 200799

National Endometriosis Society
Suite 50, Westminster Palace Gardens, 1–7 Artillery Row, London SW1P 1RL
Tel. 0171 222 2781; Helpline: 0171 222 2776

Sands (Stillbirth and Neonatal Death Society)
28 Portland Place, London W1N 4DE
Tel. 0171 436 7940 (Office); 0171 436 5881 (Helpline)
Will put in touch with other bereaved parents. Variety of booklets available.

SATFA (Support around Termination for Abnormality)
73–75 Charlotte Street, London W1N 4DE
Tel. 0171 631 0280 (Office); 0171 631 0285 (Helpline)
Provides support and befriending through similar experiences. Booklets available.

Further reading

CLARK, J. (1993) *Hysterectomy and the Alternatives*. London: Virago.

FRIDAY, N. (1976) *My Secret Garden*. London: Quartet.

GOULD, D. (1990) *Nursing Care of Women*. Herts: Prentice Hall.

HASLETT, S. and JENNINGS, M. (1992) *Hysterectomy and Vaginal Repair*. Beaconsfield, Hants: Beaconsfield Publishers.

HUNTER, M. (1994) *Counselling in Obstetrics and Gynaecology*. Leicester: BPS Books

JENKINS, J. (1985) *Caring for Women's Health*. London: Women's Health Concern.

JOHNSON, J.E. (1987) *Intimacy. Living as a Woman after Cancer*. Toronto: NC Press.

LAMBERT, H.E and BLAKE, P.E. (1992) *Gynaecological Oncology*. Oxford: Oxford University Press.

MOULDER, C. (1990) *Miscarriage*. London: Pandora.

OAKLEY, A., McPHERSON, A. and ROBERTS, H. (1984) *Miscarriage*. London: Fontana William Collins Sons.

THOMAS, J. *Supporting Parents when a Baby Dies: Before or Soon After Birth*, 2nd edn. Published privately. Available from: Mrs J Brown, 1 Millside, Riversdale, Bourne End, Bucks SL8 5EB.

WALTON, I. (1994) *Sexuality and Motherhood*. Cheshire: Books for Midwives.

References

ALDER, E. (1984) Sterilisation. In Broome, A.K. and WALLACE, L.M. (eds) *Psychology and Gynaecological Problems*. London: Tavistock.

BACKSTROM, T., BOYLE, H. and BAIRD, D.T. (1981) Persistence of symptoms of premenstrual tension in hysterectomised women. *British Journal of Obstetrics and Gynaecology* **88**: 530–36.

BARBACK, L.G. (1975) *For Yourself. The Fulfillment of Female Sexuality*. Signet/Doubleday: New York.

BLUNDELL, J. (1829) Extirpation of the uterus. *Lancet* 215.

BROOME, A.K. and WALLACE, L.M. (eds) (1984) *Psychology and Gynaecological Problems*. London: Tavistock.

CAIRNS, K.V. (1983) Sexual rehabilitation of gynaecological cancer patients. *SIECCAN Newsletter, Toronto* **18**(1).

CARDOZO, L. (1994) Objective and subjective assessment of 189 colposuspensions performed at King's College Hospital (1991–1992). Unpublished data 1993. From: Kelleher, C.J. and Cardozo, L.D. Treatment options in urinary incontinence. *Review of Contemporary Pharmocotherapeutics* **5**: 163–77.

DEROGATIS, L.R. and KOURLESIS, S.M. (1981) An approach to evaluation of sexual problems in the cancer patient. *Cancer Journal for Physicians* **31**(1): 46–50.

GOULD, D. (1986) Hidden problems after a hysterectomy. *Nursing Times* **82**(23): 43–46.

GRIFFITHS, E. (1988) No sex please, we're over sixty. *Nursing Times* **84**(1): 34–35.

HASLETT, S. and JENNINGS, M. (1992) *Hysterectomy and Vaginal Repair*, 3rd edn. Beaconsfield, Bucks: Beaconsfield Publishers

HASLETT, S. and JENNINGS, M. *Having Gynaecological Surgery*. Beaconsfield: Beaconsfield Publishers.

JOHNSON, J.E. (1987) *Intimacy. Living as a Woman. After Cancer*. Toronto: NC Press.

JOLLY, J. (1987) *Missed Beginnings: Death Before Life has been Established*. Reading: Austen Cornish Publishers.

KREUGER, J.C. HASSELL, J. GOGGINS, D.B. ISHIMATSU, T., PABLICO, M. and TATTLE, E. (1979) Relationship between nurse counselling and sexual adjustment after hysterectomy. *Nursing Research* **28**: 145–50.

LAMB, M. (1985) Sexual dysfunction in the gynaecological oncology patient. *Seminars in Oncology Nursing* **1**(1): 9–17.

LAMBERT, H.E. and BLAKE, P.R. (1992) *Gynaecological Oncology*. Oxford: Oxford University Press.

LAMONT, J.A. PETRILLO, A.D. and SARGEANT, E.J. (1978) Psychosexual rehabilitation and extenterative surgery. *Gynaecological Oncology* **6**: 238–42.

LEWIS, T.L.T. and CHAMBERLAIN, G.V.P. (1991) *Gynaecology by Ten Teachers*. London: Edward Arnold.

NIELSEN, S. and HAHLIN, M. (1995) Expectant management of first-trimester spontaneous abortion. *Lancet* **345**: 84–86.

PANUTHOS, C. and ROMEO, C. (1984) *Ending Beginnings. Healing Childbearing Losses*. Mass.: Bergin & Garvey.

PEPPERS, L.G. and KNAPP, R. (1980) *Motherhood and Mourning*. New York: Praegar.

PINION, S.B. PARKIN, D.E., ABRAMOVICH, D.R. *et al.* (1994) Randomised trial of hysterectomy, endometrial laser ablation and transcervical endometrial resection for dysfunctional uterine bleeding. *British Medical Journal* **309** (6960): 979–83.

RUSHTON, M. (1978) Nursing patients with gynaecological malignancies. In Tiffany, R. (ed.) *Oncology for Nursing and Health Care Professionals*. Beaconsfield: Harper & Row.

SCHIFF, H. (1977) *The Bereaved Patient*. New York: Crown.

SHINGLETON, H.M and ORR, J.W. (1987) *Cancer of the Cervix: Diagnosis and treatment*. Edinburgh: Churchill Livingstone.

TISSERAND, R. (1988) *The Art of Aromatherapy*. C.W. Daniel.

TULANDI, T. (1994) Medical and surgical treatment of ectopic pregnancy. *Current Opinion in Obstetrics and Gynaecology* **6**: 149–52.

VACHION, M.C.S. (1977) Breast cancer: a longitudinal study. Unpublished paper.

WABREK, A.J. and GUNN, J.L. (1984) Sexual and psychological implication of gynaecological malignancies. *Journal of Gynaecologic and Neonatal Nursing* **13**(6): 371–5.

WALBROEHL, G.S. (1985) Sexuality in cancer patients. *American Family Physician*. **1:** 153–58.

WALLACE, C. (1987) Sexual adjustment after radical genital surgery. *Nursing Times* **83**(51): 41–43.

WEBB, C. (1985) *Sex, Nursing and Health*. Chichester: Wiley & Sons.

WHALE, Z. (1991) A threat to femininity? Minimising side-effects in pelvic irradiation. *Professional Nurse* March: 309–12.

WILLIAMS, H.A. (1986) Nurses attitudes towards sexuality in cancer patients. *Oncology Nursing Forum* **13**(12): 39–43

WILLIAMSON, M.L. (1992) Sexual adjustment after hysterectomy. *Journal of Gynaecologic and Neonatal Nursing* **21**(1): 42–47.

WILSON-BARNETT, J. (1975) Factors affecting patients' response to hospitalization. *Journal of Advanced Nursing* (3): 221–28.

WISE, R. (1989) Flower power. *Nursing Times* **85**(22): 45–47.

WORSLEY, P. *et al.* (1970) *Introducing Sociology*. Harmondsworth: Penguin.

WRIGHT, L. (1974) *Bowel Function in Hospital*. London: RCN.

GLOSSARY

Adnexa: appendages (the ovaries and Fallopian tubes).

Amenorrhoea: absence of menstrual periods.

Amniocentesis: sampling and examination of the amniotic fluid in early pregnancy. A diagnostic test for chromosomal abnormality.

Androgens: hormones that produce male characteristics in either sex.

Anorexia nervosa: a condition in which the sufferer diets drastically to lose real or imagined weight: 'the slimmers' disease'.

Antiretrovirals: drugs that are active against the retrovirus family that HIV belongs to.

Atrophy: wasting away through lack of use or nutrition.

Atrophic vaginitis: depleted supply of oestrogen in vagina tissues causing dryness and inflammation.

Autonomic reaction: under the control of the sympathetic and parasympathetic nerves which control involuntary muscles and glandular secretion over which there is no conscious control.

Bartholin's glands: vestibular glands which lie on either side of the vaginal orifice.

Bone density: a measure of the amount of mineral (mainly calcium) in bone.

Bulimia: a condition in which the sufferer binges on large quantities of food, and then vomits, as a means of losing real or imaginary weight.

Caruncle: a small fleshy lump at the urethral opening.

Cautery: the application of searing heat by a hot instrument, an electric current or other means such as a laser. Cold cautery is cauterization by carbon dioxide, also called cryocautery.

Chorioamnionitis: inflammation of the membranes, the amnion (fetal surfaces) and the chorion.

CIN: cervical intraepithelial neoplasia.

Climacteric: the years around the menopause, before and after the final period, when menopausal symptoms are being experienced.

Coitus interruptus: a method of contraception in which the male withdraws his penis before ejaculation.

Collagen: part of the skin and bone in which calcium is deposited.

Colporrhaphy: repair of the vaginal wall due to lax pelvic floor muscles or following trauma, e.g. childbirth.

Colposcopy: examination of the cervix and vagina using an instrument called a colposcope.

Continuous combined HRT: a form of hormone replacement therapy in which oestrogens and progestogens are both taken continuously.

Corpus luteum: a yellow mass which develops in the ovarian follicle after ovulation and rupture of that follicle.

CVS: chorionic villus sampling by removal of a piece of early placental tissue to detect chromosomal abnormality.

Cystocele: prolapse of the bladder into the vagina caused by laxity of the anterior abdominal wall.

Detrusor: smooth muscle of the urinary bladder made up of longitudinal fibres that form the external layer of the muscular coat of the bladder.

Detrusor instability: a condition in which the detrusor contracts either spontaneously or on provocation during bladder filling while the patient tries to inhibit micturition.

Dysuria: difficulty or a burning sensation when passing urine.

Dyspareunia: painful sexual intercourse.

Dysplasia: abnormal development; often noted on

cervical smear reports referring to abnormal cells.

Ectopic pregnancy: implantation of the zygote outside the uterus, usually in the Fallopian tube.

Ectropion or ectopy: when the squamo-columnar junction of the cervix is on the ectocervix and looks red in appearance (used to be termed an 'erosion').

Endometrial hyperplasia: non-cancerous overgrowth of the endometrium.

Endometriosis: abnormal growth of endometrial tissue outside the uterine cavity.

Endometrium: the lining of the uterus.

Fibroid: non-cancerous muscle growth in the uterine wall.

Fornix: (plural = fornices). The recesses at the top of the vagina in relation to the cervix: anterior, posterior or lateral.

HCG: human chorionic gonadotrophin; a hormone secreted early in pregnancy. Pregnancy tests are based on the detection of HCG.

Hydatidiform mole: disordered development of the zygote resulting in a rapidly growing cystic mass.

Hydrosalpinx: distension of the Fallopian tubes with fluid.

Hypotonic detrusor contraction: a weak bladder contraction which may result in incomplete emptying of the bladder.

Koilocytes: cells invaded by wart virus; a term usually seen on cervical smear reports.

Libido: sex drive, interest in sex.

Leucoplakia: development of white or greyish patches on the vulva; these may become malignant.

Leucorrhoea: non-pathological, excessive white vaginal discharge.

Menarche: onset of menstruation.

Menorrhagia: heavy menstrual bleeding.

Micturition: the act of passing urine, also called urination.

Missed abortion: the embryo or fetus dies but it is not expelled by the uterus.

Mittelschmerz: pain caused by ovulation.

Neuromuscular stimulation: a process of passing an electrical current along the efferent nerves at low frequencies in order to elicit a muscular contraction.

Oligomenorrhoea: scanty menstruation.

Osteoporosis: a disease in which bone becomes so porous, brittle and fragile that it breaks very easily.

PID: pelvic inflammatory disease.

Procidentia: complete prolapse of the uterus into the vagina.

Pyosalpinx: the presence of pus in the Fallopian tube.

Rectocele: prolapse of the rectum into the vagina caused by laxity of the posterior vaginal wall.

Residual urine: a volume of urine remaining in the bladder after micturition.

Seroconversion: the development of certain antibodies that can be detected in the circulation. In an HIV infected person, seroconversion relates to the production of anti-HIV antibodies.

Skene's glands: a pair of glands which open into the posterior urethral orifice of the female.

Spinnbarkeit: clear thin 'elastic' cervical mucus at the time of ovulation.

Stress incontinence: involuntary leakage of urine when intra-abdominal pressure is raised, e.g. when coughing or laughing.

TOP: termination of pregnancy.

Trigone: a triangular area of smooth muscle of the bladder between the opening of the ureters and the orifice of the ureters.

Trimester: a third; usually referring to the first, second and third three months of pregnancy.

Tachyphylaxis: in the case of HRT this is a condition in which some women with implants experience a return of menopausal symptoms even though their blood oestrogen levels are normal or high.

Vaginismus: spasm of the vagina which is so severe as to prevent digital or penile penetration.

INDEX